ANNALS OF THE NEW YORK ACADEM... ... ...

VOLUME 166, ART. 2 PAGES 365–819

October 14, 1969

THE PHOSPHOHYDROLASES: THEIR BIOLOGY, BIOCHEMISTRY AND CLINICAL ENZYMOLOGY*

Consulting Editor
WILLIAM H. FISHMAN

Conference Cochairmen
OSCAR BODANSKY AND WILLIAM H. FISHMAN

CONTENTS

Introduction. *By* WILLIAM H. FISHMAN ... 367

Part I. Genetics

Formation and Localization of the Alkaline Phosphatase of *Escherichia coli*. *By* MILTON J. SCHLESINGER, JACQUELINE A. REYNOLDS AND SONDRA SCHLESINGER ... 368

Studies on the Purification and Properties of the Genetic Variants of Red Cell Acid Phosphohydrolase in Man. *By* R. A. FISHER AND HARRY HARRIS ... 380

Blood Groups and Their Relation to Serum Phosphohydrolases. *By* LARS BECKMAN AND D. C. ZOSCHKE ... 392

Activity and Regulation of Alkaline Phosphatase in Cells From Patients With Abnormal Chromosome Complements. *By* RODY P. COX ... 406

Regulation of Alkaline Phosphatase in HeLa Clones of Differing Modal Chromosome Number. *By* M. J. GRIFFIN AND R. H. BOTTOMLEY ... 417

Alkaline Phosphatase Constitutivity: A Marker for the Estimation of Somatic Cell "Mutation" in Man. *By* GEORGE M. MARTIN, MARY ANN DERR AND CURTIS A. SPRAGUE ... 433

Part II. Development and Physiology

The Differentiation of Alkaline Phosphatase in the Small Intestine. *By* FLORENCE MOOG, MARILYNN E. ETZLER AND ROBERT D. GREY ... 447

Physiology of Prostatic Phosphohydrolase Secretion. *By* HARRIS ROSENKRANTZ ... 466

Decidual Alkaline Phosphatase Activity in the Pregnant and Pseudopregnant Rat. *By* JOHN P. MANNING, BERNARD G. STEINETZ AND THOMAS GIANNINA ... 482

* This series of papers is the result of a conference entitled The Phosphohydrolases: Their Biology, Biochemistry and Clinical Enzymology, held by The New York Academy of Sciences on November 14, 15 and 16, 1968.

Mechanisms of Phosphohydrolase Transport and of Homeostasis. *By* R. KEIDING 510

Summation of the Session on Development and Physiology. *By* CLEMENT L. MARKERT 523

Part III. Intracellular Localization

Phosphohydrolases in Cell Organelles; Electron Microscopy. *By* R. E. Smith 525

5′-Nucleotidase of Plasma Membranes of the Rat Liver: Studies on Subcellular Distribution. *By* CHULL S. SONG, ATTALLAH KAPPAS, AND OSCAR BODANSKY 565

Soluble and Membrane-Associated Forms of Acid Phosphatase Associated With the Lysosomal Fraction of Rat Liver. *By* BARBARA FURIN SLOAT AND JOHN M. ALLEN ... 574

Summation of the Session on Intracellular Localization. *By* CHRISTIAN DE DUVE 602

Part IV. Biochemistry

Purification and Molecular Properties of Placental and Intestinal Alkaline Phosphatases. *By* NIMAI K. GHOSH 604

Biochemical Studies on Phosphohydrolase Isoenzymes. *By* D. W. MOSS 641

Influence of Structure of Substrate on the Hydrolysis of Alkyl and Aryl Phosphates by Phosphohydrolases: Mechanism of Acid and Alkaline Phosphatases. *By* R. L. NATH 653

Zinc and Cobalt Alkaline Phosphatases. *By* ROBERT T. SIMPSON AND BERT L. VALLEE 670

Discussion Paper: Some Considerations on Alkaline Phosphatase. *By* B. K. BACHHAWAT 695

Some Properties and Possible Physiological Functions of Phosphotransferase Activities of Microsomal Glucose-6-Phosphatase. *By* ROBERT C. NORDLIE 699

Oligo- and Polysaccharide Inhibition of Muscle Transferase *D* Phosphatase. *By* C. VILLAR-PALASI 719

Summation of the Session on Biochemistry. *By* BERNARD L. HORECKER 731

Part V. Clinical Enzymology

Placental Alkaline Phosphatase and Pregnancy. *By* SOLOMON POSEN, CORALIE J. CORNISH, MICHAEL HORNE AND PARMESH K. SAINI 733

Immunologic and Biochemical Approaches to Alkaline Phosphatase Isoenzyme Analysis: The Regan Isoenzyme. *By* WILLIAM H. FISHMAN 745

Clinical Application of Alkaline Phosphatase Isoenzyme Analysis. *By* LEO L. STOLBACH 760

Clinical Application of Phosphohydrolase Measurements in Cancer. *By* MORTON K. SCHWARTZ, MARTIN FLEISHER AND OSCAR BODANSKY 775

The Importance of Varying Molecular Size, Differential Heat and Urea Inactivation of Phosphatase in the Identification of Disease Patterns. *By* JAMES J. FENNELLY, JOSEPH DUNNE, KEVIN MCGEENEY, LEE CHONG AND M. FITZGERALD 794

Discussion Paper: Studies on Serum Alkaline Phosphatase Isoenzymes. *By* HIROSHI SUZUKI, MASAMI YAMANAKA AND TOSHITSUGU ODA 811

INTRODUCTION

William H. Fishman
Tufts University School of Medicine

This conference has made it possible for people from all over the world who have worked in the field of phosphohydrolases to get together for the first time and share their experiences and knowledge. The history of this gathering goes back to September, 1966, to the time when it first became apparent to the co-chairmen that developments in the field of phosphohydrolases had become so important that a conference seemed mandatory. Well, if this was the situation in September, 1966, those of you who are reading the literature in 1968 know that it is even more timely today.

We've witnessed in the interim some rather important events in world history—occasional war, earthquakes, gold crisis, balance of payments crisis. Somehow the event that has affected us most recently is the research-grant crisis, which has imposed travel difficulties on workers in the field. So it is with a feeling of great humility and thanks that I see we have managed to survive all these disasters, both of world politics and of grant politics, and can assemble here today in this room.

We should not forget the names of some of those individuals whose work in the phosphohydrolases has led the way for many of the discussions that we will have today. It should be recognized that the initial thrust was that of the clinical biochemists who had discovered that the alkaline and acid phosphatases of the serum were of some significance in disease. I mention the late Earl J. King of London and the two Bodansky brothers, Aaron and Meyer. In Australia, there was R. K. Morton, whose butanol extraction techniques many of us are using today. Intracellular localization owes a great deal to the late George Gomori who was the father of modern enzyme histochemistry.

It is the aim of this conference to bring together mainly those who have contributed over a period of years to the subject while also including, as much as it is possible, workers who have made more recent contributions. Our purpose here is to define the present status of knowledge concerning the phosphohydrolases in five different fields—the fields of genetics, development and physiology, intracellular localization, biochemistry and clinical enzymology.

To help us achieve the proper perspective in these sessions, each of five distinguished session chairmen is charged with the responsibility of presenting a summation following his session's discussions and papers. These summations will help us to orient ourselves in our individual fields with the information presented during the sessions. It has been impossible, of course, to include everyone on the program who has been working in this field; I am told that in the space of about a year, there have been approximately one thousand papers with titles carrying the words phosphohydrolase or phosphatase. However, other workers in the field will have the opportunity of participating in open discussions following presentation of each paper. We would like to encourage free discussion and honest appraisal.

I would like to express my personal thanks, and those of Dr. Bodansky, to all the participants for coming here and in particular to Admiral Schanze and the Administration, and to the members of The New York Academy of Sciences, who have sponsored this conference and have made it possible for all of our speakers to come here.

PART I. GENETICS

FORMATION AND LOCALIZATION OF THE ALKALINE PHOSPHATASE OF *ESCHERICHIA COLI**

Milton J. Schlesinger, Jacqueline A. Reynolds, and Sondra Schlesinger

Department of Microbiology,
Washington University School of Medicine,
St. Louis, Mo.

The alkaline phosphatase of *Escherichia coli* is a nonspecific phosphomonoesterase that enables the bacterial cell to utilize organic phosphates when these are the only source of phosphate present in the medium. The enzymatic properties, the structure, and the genetics of this protein have been studied in several laboratories. A partial summary of the results of these investigations follows:

1. The enzyme is a stable, globular, zinc metalloprotein (molecular weight = 86,000) composed of two identical subunits.[1-4]
2. The protein is localized exterior to the cell cytoplasm in the periplasmic space.[5,6]
3. The structural gene is a single cistron;[7] mutations in this gene can lead to inactive proteins (CRM) that cross-react with antienzyme and/or antisubunit antibodies.[1,8]
4. In exponentially growing cultures of *E. coli* K12, formation of alkaline phosphatase is repressed and enzyme appears only when the growth medium becomes depleted of inorganic phosphate.[9] Mutations in any one of three distinct gene loci lead to cells (constitutives) that form enzyme even when high levels of inorganic phosphate are present in the growth medium.[10]
5. The enzyme can act as a phosphotransferase,[11] and a phosphorylated enzyme has been isolated.[12,13]
6. Enzymatic activity varies with zinc content (3 to 4 Zn^{++} per dimer have been measured for the pure enzyme[14]). Removal of zinc abolishes enzymatic activity. Only one catalytically active site per dimer can be measured by equilibrium dialysis against inorganic phosphate, a competitive inhibitor.[14]

We have been studying the relation of structure to function of the *E. coli* alkaline phosphatase with particular interest in describing the conformational changes that occur in the protein when the unfolded polypeptide chains are assembled into an ordered, compact, enzymatically active dimer. One aim of this study has been to determine how this enzyme becomes localized to the exterior of the cell cytoplasm. In this paper, we review the results of several experimental approaches that have been carried out to investigate the formation and localization of alkaline phosphatase.

In Vitro FORMATION OF ENZYME FROM SUBUNITS

Although the alkaline phosphatase from *E. coli* is an unusually stable enzyme, purified preparations of this protein can be reversibly inactivated by (a) chelating agents,[2] (b) urea and mercaptoethanol,[15] (c) 6 M guanidine HCl,[16] and (d) low pH ($<$3.0).[16] The latter three reagents have been shown to dissociate the

* Supported by research grants from the Life Insurance Medical Research Fund (G–67–43), National Science Foundation (GB 5973) and National Institutes of Health (5–T1–AI–257; AI GM 08593–01; AM 09226–04).

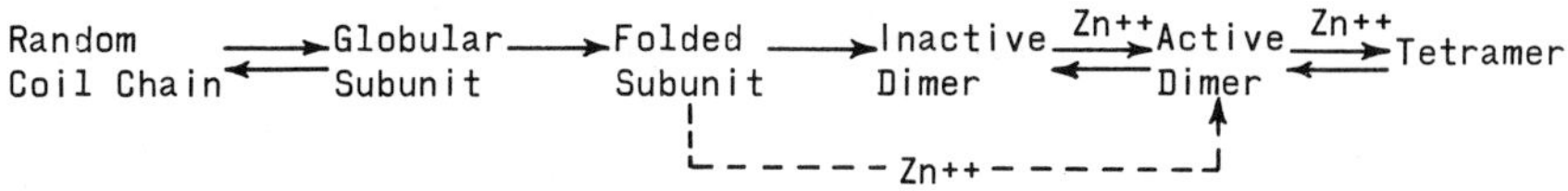

FIGURE 1. *In vitro* pathway to active enzyme from subunits prepared from acidified pure protein.

active dimer into inactive subunits. Recently, we have studied the conformational changes that occur in the polypeptide chain of this protein when the subunit, formed at low pH, is assembled into a catalytically active enzyme.[17]

In the pathway from subunit to enzyme, five states of the protein have been characterized (FIGURE 1). On the basis of hydrodynamic measurements, potentiometric titration of ionizable residues, and optical properties (optical rotatory dispersion, circular dichroism and ultra violet spectra), these different states were noted as follows:

1. Extended-coil unfolded monomer: The subunit at pH 2.0 appeared to be a random-coil chain containing no significant noncovalent interactions.[18]

2. Globular-unfolded monomer: At pH 4.0, the net positive charge on the extended coil was partially neutralized, resulting in a smaller hydrodynamic volume but no concomitant formation of secondary or tertiary structure.

3. Folded monomer: At pH 6.0, essentially all the "α-helical" content of the active dimer as measured by ORD was restored and four tyrosine residues per monomer were placed into hydrophobic regions.

4. Apodimer: At neutral pH, and in the presence of EDTA, high concentrations ($>$ 1 mg/ml) of the folded monomers associated to form an inactive zincless dimer. No differences have been observed in the optical properties between the folded monomer and the apodimer. This state appears to be identical to the inactive protein obtained when native active enzyme is denatured by chelating agent.[14]

5. Active enzyme: Addition of zinc ions to apoenzyme caused additional conformational changes in the protein, evidenced by changes in the difference spectrum between 2,500 and 3,200 Å, and led to active enzyme with properties essentially identical to pure native protein.

6. Active tetramer: At high protein concentrations and high zinc concentrations, the molecular weight doubled and the enzyme had a higher turnover number.[19]

The conformational changes that occurred in the polypeptide chain in the conversion of state 2 to 3 were detected as increasing dextrorotation at $\lambda =$ 2,100 Å and as a decrease in the U.V. difference spectrum at $\lambda =$ 2,700–2,900 Å, recorded between the unfolded subunit and native enzyme. A further decrease in the U.V. difference spectrum was observed in the conversion of the apodimer to enzyme. This activation step was also accompanied by a change in the CD spectra recorded for the two states (4 and 5).[14] The optical and hydrodynamic properties of the different states are summarized in TABLE 1.

Association of the folded subunits can occur in the presence of EDTA if high concentrations of the protein ($\geqslant$ 1 mg/ml) are used. At lower protein concentrations, formation of active enzyme from folded subunits required zinc ions and obeyed bimolecular kinetics.[16] The apodimer was indistinguishable from

TABLE 1

PROPERTIES OF *E. coli* ALKALINE PHOSPHATASE "PRECURSORS"*

State of Polypeptide Chain	Molecular Weight	$S_{20,w}$	[η] (cc/g)	[α] 2,100	[α] 2,330	No. of Tyrosines Exposed
Extended Coil	—	2.3	23.5	− 5,400	−5,400	20 ± 1
Globular-Unfolded	43,000	3.4	3.4	− 5,400	−5,400	20 ± 1
Globular-Folded	—	3.4	3.4	+10,000	−6,000	12 ± 1
Inactive Dimer	86,000	6.3†	3.4	+10,000	−6,000	12 ± 1
Active Dimer	86,000	6.3†	3.4	+10,000	−6,000	5 ± 1

* Data were obtained with enzyme purified from strain CW3747. Subunits were prepared by acidifying solutions of proteins to pH 2.0 with HCl. Experimental details are found in Reference 17.

† S°; pH 6.3; 22°.

folded subunits according to optical measurements, but these two states were distinct when tested for sensitivity to proteolysis (TABLE 2).

In Vivo FORMATION OF ENZYME FROM SUBUNITS

A. Characterization of Alkaline-Phosphatase Negative Mutants

As one approach to investigating the assembly process for alkaline phosphatase, we have been studying altered forms of this enzyme produced by alkaline phosphatase-negative strains (P^-) of *E. coli.* One of these mutants (U • 47 or C • 10 F • 18; the latter is a constitutive strain that carries the same structural gene as U • 47) formed an alkaline phosphatase that cross-reacted well with antienzyme antibody but was deficient in zinc.[20] The purified CRM from U • 47 was a stable dimer ($S_{20,w}$ = 6.0) that could be converted to an active enzyme

TABLE 2

EFFECT OF TRYPSIN ON FOLDED SUBUNIT AND APODIMER*

Sample Tested	Enzymatic Activity (U/mg) t = 0′; 0°	t = 30′ at 37°
1. Subunit dialyzed vs. EDTA at pH 6.5 for 24 hrs at 4°. (Apodimer).	50	50
2. Sample (1) incubated with trypsin.	50	50
3. Subunit (retained in) .01 N HCl.	0.08	30
4. Sample (3) incubated with trypsin.	0.11	0.14
5. Sample (3) incubated in absence of trypsin.	0.14	33

* Pure enzyme (2 mg/ml; 72.5 U/mg) was dialyzed against .01 N HCl, 0.1 M KCl, 1 mM EDTA at 4° for 16 hrs. One portion was then dialyzed against .01 M Tris-Cl, pH 6.5, 0.1 M KCl, 1 mM EDTA at 4° for 24 hrs. A second portion was kept at 4° in the .01 N-HCl solution. For measuring enzymatic activity (lines 1 and 3), a 10 μl sample of the treated enzyme was first diluted in 0.5 ml of .05 M Tris-Cl, pH 7.4, .5 mM $ZnCl_2$, 1 mM Mg Acetate at 0°; a 10 μl sample from this dilution was added immediately, and also after 30 min at 37°, to 1.0 ml of M Tris-Cl, pH 8.0 containing 0.2 mg/ml *p*-nitrophenyl phosphate at 37°. One unit equals 1 μmole nitrophenol ($\epsilon = 1.6 \times 10^4$ M^{-1} cm^{-1} at 410 mμ) formed per min in the assay tube. For measuring sensitivity to trypsin (lines 2, 4 and 5), .05 ml of the treated enzyme was added to 0.45 ml of .02 M Tris-Cl, pH 7.4, 0.1 M KCl, 1 mM EDTA and 50 μg of trypsin (Worthington). After an incubation period of 15 min at 25°, a 0.1 ml sample was added to 0.4 ml of .05 M Tris-Cl, pH 7.4, .5 mM $ZnCl_2$, 1 mM Mg Acetate and 200 μg of soybean antitrypsin inhibitor (Worthington). A 10 μl sample of this mixture was added directly to the assay tube, both immediately and again after 30-min incubation at 37°.

TABLE 3

ACTIVATION OF PURIFIED CRM FROM MUTANT*
C•10•F•18 WITH $^{65}Zn^{++}$

Treatment	Bound ^{65}Zn cpm/mg Protein	Molar Ratio, Bound ^{65}Zn:Protein	Enzymatic Activity U/mg
None†			0.12
Dialysis for 12 Hrs	1200	1.7	5.6
Sephadex Elution	130	0.2	0.12
Eluted Protein Incubated With Zinc at 37° for 2 Hrs			6.9

* Purified CRM (1.5 mg) was incubated with 0.1 μmole of $^{65}Zn^{++}$ (5.6×10^4 cpm/μmole) in 0.1 M Tris-Cl, pH 6.8 for 12 hrs at 23°. A sample was applied to a Sephadex G-25F column (0.2×25 cm) and fractions of the eluate assayed for $^{65}Zn^{++}$ and protein. Activity was determined in 0.1 M Tris-Cl, pH 8.0 with 0.2 mg/ml *p*-nitrophenyl phosphate as substrate.

† Direct Zn analysis showed 0.6 Zn: Protein when activity was 0.5 U/mg.

in the presence of zinc ions. Addition of $^{65}Zn^{++}$ led to a ^{65}Zn-labeled protein with enzymatic activity (TABLE 3). Subsequent loss of $^{65}Zn^{++}$ after Sephadex gel filtration led to inactive protein that was still activatable. Both the U.V. difference spectrum between active and inactive forms of this protein and differences in the fluorescence emission spectra of the active and inactive protein provided evidence that a conformational change occurred when zinc ions were bound to dimer.

The results with mutant U • 47 suggested that a zincless dimer was an intermediate in the pathway to active enzyme in the bacterial cell. However, the activated protein from U • 47 reverted to an inactive dimer in solutions of low zinc ion concentrations. This fact allowed for the possibility that, in the mutant, the inactive dimer that accumulated was formed by subunits associating *directly* to an active enzyme that subsequently lost metal rather than by subunits first forming a zincless dimer.

More recently, we have studied another P^- mutant that accumulates an inactive dimer. Like U • 47, this mutant was activated by zinc ions, but the activated protein was relatively stable in buffers of low zinc concentrations. Thus, the inactive dimer that accumulated in this mutant was derived directly from subunits in a pathway similar to that described for our *in vitro* results (FIGURE 1).

Studies with the P^- mutant S • 6 showed that the mutational defect led to a polypeptide chain that could not dimerize under normal conditions of cell growth.[21] The evidence that S • 6 (the constitutive strain is C • 10 F • 27) accumulated subunits was based on the following observations: (a) Cell-free extracts contained protein that cross-reacted well with antisubunit antibody but poorly with antienzyme antibody, (b) The immunologically reactive protein sedimented in a 5 to 20% sucrose gradient with an S value of 4 (similar to wild-type subunits), (c) Cell-free extracts containing the altered phosphatase protein were activated by zinc ions in a reaction that obeyed bimolecular kinetics, but that was inhibited by proteolytic enzymes and antisubunit antibody (TABLE 4). These properties were characteristic of the activation of wild-type subunits (at low concentrations) to active enzyme.

The enzymatically active form of alkaline phosphatase from C • 10 F • 27 was obtained in pure form, and it resembled the wild-type enzyme in many properties. However, unlike wild-type enzyme, treatment at low pH or with chelating agents produced an irreversibly denatured subunit. Based on immunological criteria, this form of the subunit was similar to the subunits that accumulated in the mutant cells (FIGURE 2). We have used antibodies directed against the denatured subunit to measure the amount of subunits synthesized by mutant S • 6 and to determine their location in the bacterial cell. Six percent of the total cell protein obtained from extracts of S • 6 cells that were grown for four hours in a P_i-free medium were precipitated as alkaline phosphatase sub-

TABLE 4

ACTIVATION OF ALKALINE PHOSPHATASE IN EXTRACTS OF MUTANT C•10•F•27*

Incubation Mixture	Enzymatic Activity at: 0 Min	30 Min
	(U/mg × 10^2)	
Complete (1.0 mg Extract)	0.75	2.0
Minus $ZnSO_4$	0.50	0.56
Complete + 100 μg of Pronase	0.56	0.62
Complete + Antisubunit Antibody	0.56	0.75
Complete (0.5 mg Extract)	0.25	0.56
Complete (2.0 mg Extract)	1.0	5.6

* Cell-free extracts (obtained by sonication of a culture of cells concentrated 150 times) were incubated in 1.0 ml containing 50 μmoles Tris-Cl, pH 6.0, 0.1 μmoles $ZnSO_4$, 10 μmoles Mg Acetate, 2 μmoles KH_2PO_4.

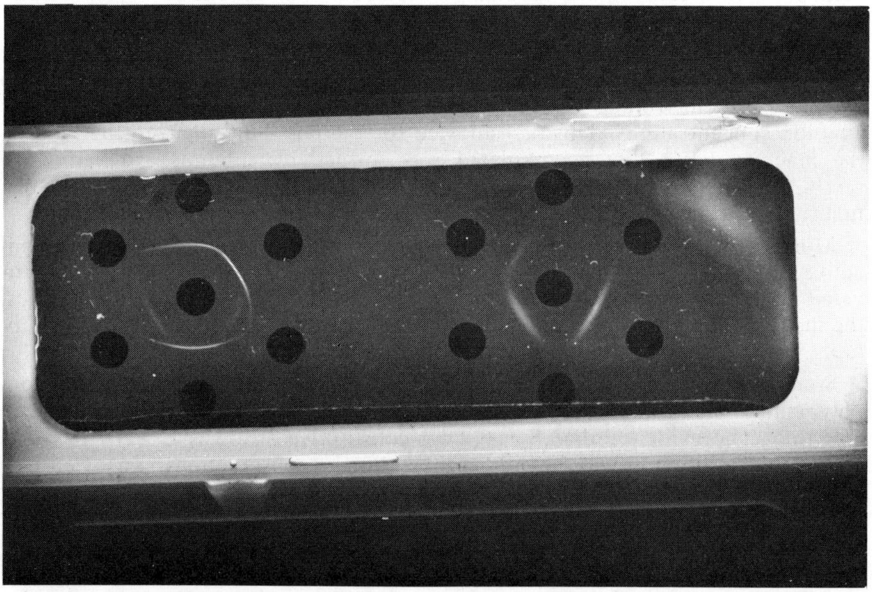

FIGURE 2. Precipitates in agar with P^- mutant S•6 and C•10 F•27 and antienzyme and antisubunit antibodies. The outer wells (from top reading clockwise) contained (1) wild-type enzyme (50 μg/ml), (2) purified active enzyme from C•10 F•27 (90 μg/ml), (3) enzyme from C•10 F•27 denatured by acidification to pH 2.0 (90 μg/ml), (4) wild-type enzyme (50 μg/ml), (5) concentrated extract from a culture of S•6 grown for four hours in phosphate-free medium (9.6 mg/ml), and (6) denatured wild-type subunits (50 μg/ml). The center well on the left contained antienzyme antibody; the center well on the right, antisubunit antibody. The preparation and properties of these antibodies have been described.[8]

TABLE 5

FORMATION OF ALKALINE PHOSPHATASE AND PROTEIN SYNTHESIS IN SPHEROPLASTS OF *E. coli**

Culture	Viable Cells/ml $\times 10^{-8}$		Alkaline Phosphatase Activity (U/ml)		^{14}C-Protein†
	Initial	Final	Initial	Final	cpm/ml
Intact Cells	3.9	7.0	4.7	6.9	55,000
Spheroplasts	0.20	0.37	4.5	4.5	35,000

* An exponentially growing culture of CW3747 was divided into two equal fractions. One sample was treated with EDTA and lysozyme to form spheroplasts, and incubated in a spheroplast medium. The second sample was incubated in the normal growth medium. Fractions (1.0 ml) were removed 1 min before and 30 min after addition of ^{14}C-amino acids (mixture from New England Nuclear Corp., Boston, Mass.), in order to measure viable colonies, enzymatic activity, and ^{14}C-protein formed. Experimental details are in Reference 22.

† Measured after 20-min incubation at 30°.

units. This value is the same as that reported for wild-type enzyme obtained from *E. coli* K12 grown under similar conditions. When spheroplasts were prepared with lysozyme, 64% of the subunits were released into the medium under conditions that released 90% of the active enzyme present in the cells. Thus, blocking of the pathway to active enzyme at the subunit stage, as occurs in S • 6, does not affect the continued synthesis of alkaline phosphatase polypeptide chains nor does it significantly alter the cellular localization of this protein to the periplasmic space.

B. Formation of Subunits in Spheroplasts of Wild-Type E. coli

To determine if the results obtained with S • 6 were applicable to wild-type cells, we measured alkaline phosphatase formation in cells whose outer walls had been altered by lysozyme. In these experiments, cultures of *E. coli* CW3747 (a strain that produces enzyme during the exponential growth phase) were converted to spheroplasts and resuspended in the growth medium supplemented with ^{14}C-amino acids and sucrose. After a 40-minute incubation at 30°, the spheroplasts and medium (concentrated 30-fold) were analyzed for (a) alkaline phosphatase activity, (b) ^{14}C-protein that was precipitated by antisubunit antibody, and (c) glucose-6-phosphate dehydrogenase activity. The latter measurement was used to ascertain the extent of cell lysis, since the dehydrogenase is considered a cytoplasmic enzyme. TABLE 5 shows that formation of active enzyme virtually stopped in spheroplasts, although ^{14}C-amino acids continued to be incorporated into protein. A fraction of this ^{14}C was found in alkaline phosphatase subunits that had been secreted into the medium (TABLE 6). A culture of cells (W3747) that did not form enzyme during exponential growth did not produce subunits when the cells were converted to spheroplasts. Conversely, the mutant C • 10 F • 27 which had been found to form altered subunits (see above) during exponential growth continued to form these subunits when the culture was converted to spheroplasts. These subunits were also detected in the medium of the spheroplast culture.

These results, together with those reported for the location of the subunits formed by mutant S • 6, clearly suggest that it is the alkaline phosphatase subunit that passes from the cytoplasmic site of biosynthesis to the extracellular periplasmic space. Subsequent dimerization and activation would then occur in the periplasm.

C. *Effect of Amino Acid Analogues on Formation of Alkaline Phosphatase*

Certain analogues of amino acids can be activated and attached to tRNA by the amino-acyl tRNA synthetases, and thus become incorporated into protein in place of the naturally occurring amino acid. If a particular analogue is added to a strain that requires the amino acid in a growth medium depleted of it, then only the analogue will be incorporated into protein. If the synthesis of a particular protein can be induced at same time as the addition of the analogue, then only the protein with analogue will be formed. We have used exactly these conditions to study the effects of several analogues on the formation and catalytic activity of alkaline phosphatase. Thus far, analogues of histidine (1,2,4-triazole-3-alanine and 2-methylhistidine), tryptophan (7-azatryptophan and tryptazan), and arginine (canavanine) have been tested.

In the case of the two tryptophan analogues, an active enzyme was formed that had enzymatic properties similar to those of native enzyme.[23] The analogue-containing proteins were slightly more heat labile and had ultraviolet spectra and fluorescence emission spectra characteristic of the analogue and distinct from the tryptophan-containing enzyme.

The alkaline phosphatase proteins formed in the presence of the histidine analogues were enzymatically inactive and gave strong precipitin lines in Ouchterlony double diffusion agar plates against antisubunit antibody.[24,25] Extracts of cells grown in ^{14}C-leucine and the analogues were sedimented in a 5 to 20% sucrose gradient, and fractions were tested for precipitation of ^{14}C-protein with antisubunit antibody. The fraction showing the largest amount of cross-reacting protein had an approximate S value of 4; this value is lower than active enzyme ($S_{20,w}=6$) and close to that of the subunits ($S_{20,w}=3.4$). The protein containing 2-methylhistidine was immunologically identical to the subunit prepared from mutant S • 6 when tested with antienzyme and antisubunit antibodies. The amount of subunits formed in the 60-minute period in the presence of 2-methylhistidine was equivalent to the amount of enzyme formed over the same time period when histidine was in the medium. Furthermore, like active enzyme, almost all of the subunits containing the analogue were released from spheroplasts prepared with lysozyme.

When canavanine was added to an arginine auxotroph of *E. coli* growing in

TABLE 6

DISTRIBUTION OF SUBUNITS AND ENZYME BETWEEN SPHEROPLASTS (S) AND MEDIUM (M)

Strain	Protein That Precipitates With Antisubunit Antibody (% ^{14}C in Precipitate)		Alkaline Phosphatase (Total Units)		G-6-P Dehydrogenase (Total Units)		^{14}C-Protein (% Total)	
	S	M	S	M	S	M	S	M
CW 3747	1.3	5.0	2.6	31	.14	<.01	75	25
W 3747	1.0	1.0	<.01	.01	.08	.01	80	20
C • 10 • F • 27	1.5	5.4	.06	1.0	.06	.02	71	29
CW 3747 (Not Spheroplasted)	2.6	<.1	9.1	.06	.06	<.01	99	1

Spheroplasts were separated from the medium by high-speed centrifugation, resuspended in a small volume of 10 mM Tris-Cl, pH 7.4, and 1 mM Mg acetate, and sonically disrupted. The medium was concentrated about 30-fold. See Reference 22 for experimental details.

TABLE 7

EFFECT OF ANALOGUES ON FORMATION AND LOCATION OF *E. coli* ALKALINE PHOSPHATASE

Analogue	Amino Acid Replaced	Type of Protein Formed	Location*
1,2,4-Triazole-3-alanine	Histidine	Subunit	Periplasmic Space
2-Methylhistidine	Histidine	Subunit	Periplasmic Space
Tryptazan	Tryptophan	Active Enzyme	Periplasmic Space
7-Azatryptophan	Tryptophan	Active Enzyme	Periplasmic Space
Canavanine	Arginine	Subunits and Active Enzyme (3:1 ratio)	Periplasmic Space

* Based on release by lysozyme spheroplasting.

the absence of arginine and inorganic phosphate (removal of inorganic phosphate induces enzyme formation), inactive subunits were detected in the periplasmic space.[26] Experiments with ^{14}C-leucine showed that the ^{14}C-protein that was precipitable by antisubunit antibodies had an S value of 4 (measured in sucrose gradients). Cells incubated in the presence of ^{14}C-canavanine formed ^{14}C-labeled subunits that accounted for 6% of the total soluble ^{14}C-protein released from spheroplasts. In addition to the formation of subunits by cells given canavanine, a small but significant amount of active enzyme was also made. This enzyme was purified, and contained about 16 residues of canavanine per active dimer (native enzyme has 20 to 22 arginine residues). Many of the properties (pH optimum, substrate specificity, K_m for *p*-nitrophenyl phosphate and K_i for inorganic phosphate) of the canavanine enzyme were similar to native alkaline phosphatase. However, the analogue enzyme was irreversibly inactivated by low pH or chelators, and was less stable to heating; these properties resembled those noted for the activated form of mutant S • 6 (see section *B*, above). In an experiment with cells prelabeled with ^{3}H-arginine, we found that the canavanine enzyme also contained some arginine residues (about two per dimer). This arginine was apparently derived from either the small pool present in the cells prior to addition of canavanine or from the small turnover of proteins that occurred.

A summary of the studies carried out thus far with analogues is presented in TABLE 7. They show that (a) histidine residues are essential to proper folding and assembly of the polypeptide chain, (b) that tryptophan, *per se* is not crucial to assembly or catalytic activity, and (c) that almost all the arginine residues can be substituted by canavanine without affecting the assembly process or enzymatic activity. The latter result may not be surprising in lieu of the fact that almost all the ionizable groups in alkaline phosphatase are at the surface of the protein,[18] suggesting that the contact points between subunits are not charge-charge interactions. The accumulation of abnormal subunits containing analogues in the periplasmic space, as found in mutant S • 6, again argues that dimerization is not required, either for continued synthesis of polypeptide chains or for transport of the protein out of the cytoplasm.

DISCUSSION AND SUMMARY

On the basis of our studies with structural gene mutants and with amino acid analogues, we have postulated that the assembly of alkaline phosphatase in the bacterial cell proceeds according to the pathway shown in FIGURE 3. Subunits, probably in the folded state, are transported from polyribosomes through the

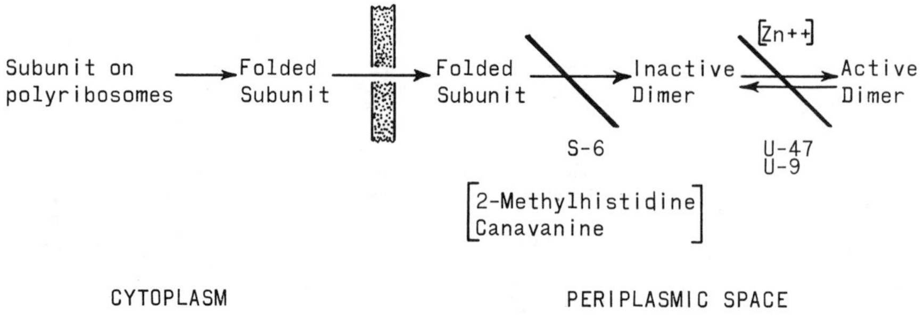

FIGURE 3. Postulated *in vivo* pathway to active enzyme from subunits formed in the bacterial cell.

cytoplasmic membrane to the periplasmic space, where dimerization and activation with Zn^{++} occurs. Further aggregation to a tetramer may follow, although no evidence has been obtained thus far for the presence of a tetramer in the bacterial cell. The postulated *in vivo* pathway closely follows that determined for the reformation of active enzyme from subunits prepared by acidification of the purified enzyme (FIGURE 1). Evidence has been presented for the accumulation of both inactive dimers[27] and inactive monomers[28] in wild-type cells where the bacteria were grown in media containing very low concentration of zinc ions. Thus, the role of zinc ions in the association of wild-type subunits *in vivo* can not yet be firmly stated.

The secretion of subunits by spheroplasts of *E. coli* is consistent with the scheme shown. A recent report by Torriani[28] showed that a small pool of subunits was detected in the cytoplasm of cells synthesizing alkaline phosphatase. The mechanism for transport of the polypeptide chain through the membrane is not known. We have found that the *E. coli* alkaline phosphatase was localized to the periplasmic space when the enzyme was synthesized in the cytoplasm of *Salmonella typhimurium,* an organism that does not have a structural gene for this enzyme.[29] This result had led us to postulate that no specific carriers are required for transport; rather it is the secondary and tertiary structure of the polypeptide chain (which follows from the amino acid sequence) that allows for the passage of the protein through the membrane and the subsequent localization to the periplasmic space.

ACKNOWLEDGMENTS

Dr. Joseph Attias carried out the studies with canavanine. Excellent technical assistance was provided by Mrs. Jo Ann Roberts and Mr. Robert Olsen.

REFERENCES

1. LEVINTHAL, C. 1959. Genetic and chemical studies with alkaline phosphatase of *E. coli.* Brookhaven Symposium in Biology **12:** 76.
2. GAREN, A. & C. LEVINTHAL. 1960. A fine structure genetic and chemical study of the enzyme alkaline phosphatase of *E. coli.* I. Purification and characterization of alkaline phosphatase. Biochim. Biophys. Acta **38:** 470.
3. ROTHMAN, F. & R. BYRNE. 1963. Fingerprint analysis of alkaline phosphatase of *Escherichia coli* K12. J. Molec. Biol. **6:** 330.
4. PLOCKE, D. J., C. LEVINTHAL & B. L. VALLEE. 1962. Alkaline phosphatase of *Escherichia coli*: A zinc metalloenzyme. Biochemistry (Wash.) **1:** 373.

5. Malamy, M. & B. L. Horecker. 1961. The localization of alkaline phosphatase in *E. coli* K12. Biochem. Biophys. Res. Comm. **5:** 104.
6. Neu, H. C. & L. A. Heppel. 1964. On the surface localization of enzymes in *E. coli*. Biochem. Biophys. Res. Comm. **17:** 215.
7. Garen, A. & S. Garen. 1963. Complementation *in vivo* between structural mutants of alkaline phosphatase from *E. coli*. J. Molec. Biol. **7:** 13.
8. Schlesinger, M. J. 1967. The reversible dissociation of the alkaline phosphatase of *Escherichia coli*. III. Properties of antibodies directed against the subunit. J. Biol. Chem. **242:** 1599.
9. Torriani, A. 1960. Influence of inorganic phosphate in the formation of phosphatases by *Escherichia coli*. Biochim. Biophys. Acta **38:** 460.
10. Echols, H., A. Garen, S. Garen & A. Torriani. 1961. Genetic control of repression of alkaline phosphatase in *E. coli*. J. Molec. Biol. **3:** 425.
11. Wilson, I. B., J. Dayan & K. Cyr. 1964. Some properties of alkaline phosphatase from *Escherichia coli*. Transphosphorylation. J. Biol. Chem. **239:** 4182.
12. Schwartz, J. H. 1963. The phosphorylation of alkaline phosphatase. Proc. Nat. Acad. Sci. U.S.A. **49:** 871.
13. Pigretti, M. M. & C. Milstein. 1965. Acid inactivation and incorporation of phosphate into alkaline phosphatase from *Escherichia coli*. Biochem. J. **94:** 106.
14. Reynolds, J. A. & M. J. Schlesinger. 1968. Alterations in the structure and function of *E. coli* alkaline phosphatase due to Zn^{++} binding. Biochemistry (Wash.) **8:** 588.
15. Levinthal, C., E. R. Signer & K. Fetherolf. 1962. Reactivation and hybridization of reduced alkaline phosphatase. Proc. Nat. Acad. Sci. U.S.A. **48:** 1230.
16. Schlesinger, M. J. & K. Barrett. 1965. The reversible dissociation of the alkaline phosphatase of *Escherichia coli*. I. Formation and reactivation of subunits. J. Biol. Chem. **240:** 4248.
17. Reynolds, J. A. & M. J. Schlesinger. 1967. Conformational states of the subunit of *Escherichia coli* alkaline phosphatase. Biochemistry (Wash.) **6:** 3552.
18. Reynolds, J. A. & M. J. Schlesinger. 1968. Hydrogen ion equilibria of conformational states of *Escherichia coli* alkaline phosphatase. Biochemistry (Wash.) **7:** 2080.
19. Reynolds, J. A. (Unpublished experiments.)
20. Schlesinger, M. J. 1966. Activation of a mutationally altered form of the *Escherichia coli* alkaline phosphatase by zinc. J. Biol. Chem. **241:** 3181.
21. Schlesinger, M. J. 1967. Formation of a defective alkaline phosphatase subunit by a mutant of *Escherichia coli*. J. Biol. Chem. **242:** 1604.
22. Schlesinger, M. J. 1968. Secretion of alkaline phosphatase subunits by spheroplasts of *Escherichia coli*. J. Bact. **96:** 727.
23. Schlesinger, S. 1968. The effect of amino acid analogues on alkaline phosphatase formation in *Escherichia coli* K12. II. Replacement of tryptophan by azatryptophan and by tryptazan. J. Biol. Chem. **243:** 3877.
24. Schlesinger, S. & M. J. Schlesinger. 1967. The effect of amino acid analogues on alkaline phosphatase formation in *Escherichia coli* K-12. J. Biol. Chem. **242:** 3369.
25. Schlesinger, S. & M. J. Schlesinger. J. Biol. Chem. In press.
26. Attias, J., S. Schlesinger & M. J. Schlesinger. J. Biol. Chem. In press.
27. Harris, M. I. & J. E. Coleman. 1968. The biosynthesis of apo- and metalloalkaline phosphatase of *Escherichia coli*. J. Biol. Chem. **243:** 5063.
28. Torriani, A. 1968. Alkaline phosphatase subunits and their dimerization *in vivo*. J. Bact. **96:** 1200.
29. Schlesinger, M. J. & R. Olsen. 1968. Expression and localization of *Escherichia coli* alkaline phosphatase synthesized in *Salmonella typhimurium*. J. Bact. **96:** 1601.

Discussion of the Paper

G. Martin: With respect to the histidine analogue experiments, I think there is some evidence from Hurwitz's laboratory at Albert Einstein that histidine is quite important in active sites for RNA polymerase. I don't remember for which of the several reactions they're studying–binding, initiation, elongation or termination. I was wondering if there is a possibility of interference with transcription when your organisms are grown with histidine analogues.

Dr. Schlesinger: After about 30 minutes, the analogues do affect general protein synthesis in the bacterial cell. Nevertheless, even if we carry out these experiments where we ask the cell to be induced for formation of alkaline phosphatase, we are able to show that the polypeptide chains are made in reasonably good yield. In fact, with 2-methylhistidine, taking into account this inhibition of general protein synthesis quantitatively, there's as much polypeptide chain containing 2-methylhistidine made under those conditions as made by cells given histidine.

DR. MARTIN: I was wondering if some protein important for the subsequent steps is interfered with by affecting transcription.

DR. SCHLESINGER: Our general feeling is that it's not necessary to have any other protein present to convert this polypeptide chain into active enzyme. I might point out, incidentally, that the work both of Dr. Reynolds and from Vallee's laboratory has implicated histidine as an important residue in the catalytic site of alkaline phosphatase. At least, it's known that a histidine residue is one of the ligands for the zinc.

DR. MARTIN: Dr. Gordon Dorn has a large number of loci mapped in *Aspergillus nidulans* for phosphatase. I think the current number is about 20. It would be very interesting to determine if some of these loci are related to the various *in vitro* and *in vivo* steps you so beautifully elucidated.

DR. SCHLESINGER: Are those regulatory genes or structural genes?

DR. MARTIN: I think there is no clear-cut information as to what proportion are regulatory or structural, but there seems to be clear correlation in the proportion of electrophoretic variations in the phosphatases of that group, which apparently involve both acid and alkaline phosphatases. I think his current notion is that there might be common polypeptide subunits that play a role both in acid and alkaline phosphohydrolases. It seems to be a very nice system to look at apropo of the different steps involved in producing functional protein. It seems the more we learn about the various human inborn errors of metabolism, and the more one particular entity is looked at in detail, the more heterogeneity one finds both biochemically and, we hope, someday, genetically, and this kind of work is the real basic science that will go into elucidating the nature of this heterogeneity.

C. DE DUVE: Is there any evidence for or against the possibility that these subunits are manufactured by body cells that are actually attached to the innerface of the cell membrane?

DR. SCHLESINGER: I don't know of any, but I think it's generally accepted that the site of protein synthesis in bacterial cells is probably on membranes in the bacterial cell cytoplasm. I don't particularly like to assign a specific membrane as a site for alkaline phosphatase formation because that means one has to say that the messenger RNA for alkaline phosphatase must have some information within it that says it must go to a specific site of synthesis. I prefer to think in terms of the secondary and tertiary structure of the polypeptide chain as having that information.

DR. DE DUVE: The reason I'm asking is that, of course, we have the same problem but multiplied by a factor of, I don't know, a hundred or a thousand, in the animal cell where the proteins that are actually secreted for export are, in fact, manufactured by body cells attached to membranes of the endoplasmic reticulum. There is a functional significance to this since, according to the work of Sabatini and Palade, a polypeptide chain is actually secreted at the same time as it is synthesized. Therefore, this bacterial system, if the polysomes were actually attached to the membrane, would be a bacterial model of secretion that would be comparable to that in animal.

DR. SCHLESINGER: Dr. David Schlessinger in the Microbiology Department at Washington University has clearly shown that polysomes are attached to bacterial cell membrane.

DR. DE DUVE: When you do your experiment using these histidine analogues, are all the histidines in the molecule replaced by the analogue?

DR. SCHLESINGER: We haven't actually shown this, but because of the way the experiments are done, the only histidine that could get in would be from a very small pool.

DR. DE DUVE: I wonder, going on from that, whether one or more are really critical and the rest really irrelevant in terms of the biological effect you're achieving by the replacement of the amino acid.

DR. SCHLESINGER: There are eight histidine residues per polypeptide chain, and one can't say at this stage if a specific residue is critical. The arginine case may be very different because of the fact that we do see active enzyme with probably one or two arginine residues. This is a situation where a specific residue may be critical.

DR. N. K. GHOSH: Did I understand correctly that when you induce the transition of active dimer to tetramer, you retain the enzyme activity completely?

DR. SCHLESINGER: Yes, these are Dr. Reynolds' results in which she has found that the tetrameric state of the protein actually appears to be more active in terms of the number of micromoles of nitrophenol produced per milligram of protein. It is actually higher by possibly twofold. Whether this means we're creating new catalytic sites we can not yet say, but the hint is there.

DR. GHOSH: Could you observe this tetramer in bacterial cells?

DR. SCHLESINGER: It's not yet been shown. Actually, the tetramer itself is very unstable to dilution. What one does with the bacterial cell is to open up the cells and, even if it were a tetramer in the confined periplasmic space, on release into the medium it probably dissociates.

DR. GHOSH: What are the experimental conditions you use to induce this transformation? Did you take the enzyme and treat it with zinc solution to get the tetramer?

DR. SCHLESINGER: The tetramer is obtained by working at relatively high protein concentrations (greater than 1 mg/ml) at about 10^{-3} M zinc at a pH close to 8.0.

M. ETZLER: I should like to know what the antiperiodate-treated subunit antibodies refers to.

DR. SCHLESINGER: That's a very detailed description. The point is that in order to get antibodies to the subunit, it's necessary to denature them because if you simply take subunits and inject them into a rabbit, what you find is that they apparently associate, and you only get antibodies to the active enzyme. So you have to freeze the subunit in a denatured state. We observed that one way of doing this, and it appeared to be a relatively mild way, was to treat the subunit at pH 2 with low concentrations of periodate. We don't know chemically what that does; the amino-acid analysis of the periodate-treated material suggests that a tyrosine or possibly a tryptophan residue has been destroyed. Nevertheless, the subunit product of that chemical reaction is completely denatured; it never dimerizes, and that molecule is a reasonably good antigen.

DR. ETZLER: Have you looked at the possibility that the periodate treatment might be degrading a carbohydrate on your subunits.

DR. SCHLESINGER: The *E. coli* alkaline phosphatase does not have any significant amount of carbohydrate present in the protein.

STUDIES ON THE PURIFICATION AND PROPERTIES OF THE GENETIC VARIANTS OF RED CELL ACID PHOSPHOHYDROLASE IN MAN

R. A. Fisher and Harry Harris

Medical Research Council, Human Biochemical Genetics Research Unit, The Galton Laboratory, University College, London, England

Red cell acid phosphatase is a phosphohydrolase and phosphotransferase with low pH optimum. It appears to be peculiar to the red cell (Davies 1934; Behrendt 1943; King, Wood & Delory 1945; Abul-Fadl & King 1949; Tsuboi & Hudson 1953, 1956). Its natural substrate and its normal function within the red cell are unknown. Nevertheless, it is of great interest because of its genetically determined polymorphism (Hopkinson, Spencer & Harris 1963). The different common variant forms are found in apparently normal individuals and as far as is known are not associated with any disease patterns (Valentine *et al.,* 1961; Modiano *et al.,* 1967). They must be regarded as different versions of biochemical normality.

Ten different phenotypes have been described (FIGURE 1), (Hopkinson *et al.,* 1964; Lai *et al.,* 1964; Giblett & Scott 1965; Karp & Sutton 1967), and these are evidently determined by a series of allelic genes at an autosomal locus. Three of these alleles, P^a, P^b and P^c, occur with frequencies of about 0.36, 0.60 and 0.04, respectively, in the English population (Hopkinson *et al.,* 1964), and give rise to six phenotypes, three of which (A, B and C) represent homozygous genotypes, while three others (BA, CA and CB) represent heterozygous genotypes. Each allele appears to be responsible for two isozymes, and there is no evidence of hybridization between types. Thus, the homozygous types show two isozymes, and the isozyme patterns in the heterozygous types appear to represent simple mixtures of those seen in the corresponding homozygotes.

There are marked differences in the relative activities of the two isozymes present in the different homozygous types. In type A, they are roughly equal in activity. In type B, the front (i.e., more anodal) band is more active than the back, and in type C, the back band is much more active than the front one. There are also striking differences in total activity between the types. (Hopkinson *et al.,* 1964). On the average, the acid phosphatase activity of type B red cells is about 50% greater than that of type A cells, and type C cells show an even greater total activity. (FIGURE 2).

The type A isozymes differ from types B and C in their electrophoretic mobilities, but some curious effects may be produced by certain additions to the buffer systems (Harris *et al.,* 1968). Thus, in a phosphate buffer system at around pH 6, they migrate more slowly toward the anode than the corresponding B or C isozymes. If, however, a tricarboxylic acid, such as citric acid, is added, the mobilities of both the A isozymes are increased relative to the corresponding B and C isozymes and migrate more rapidly toward the anode. (FIGURE 3).

No difference in Km or in pattern of substrate specificity have been found between the different acid phosphatase types (Scott, 1966; Luffman & Harris, 1967), but significant differences in thermostability have been noted (Luffman & Harris, 1967). The relative stabilities at raised temperatures and under standardized conditions were found to be in the order C>B>A. Such differences in stability may well be important *in vivo,* and could, at least in part, account for the differences in total activity observed between the several types.

These various findings pose two distinct problems: First, what is the nature of the differences between the genetically different types? Second, what are the differences between the two isozymes present within each of the homozygous types? The first question is concerned with the nature of the structural differences in the isozyme proteins produced by what we must presume to be single gene mutations. The second question is concerned with the differences between the two distinct isozyme proteins apparently specified by one gene.

In order to investigate these problems, it was clear that a fairly large quantity

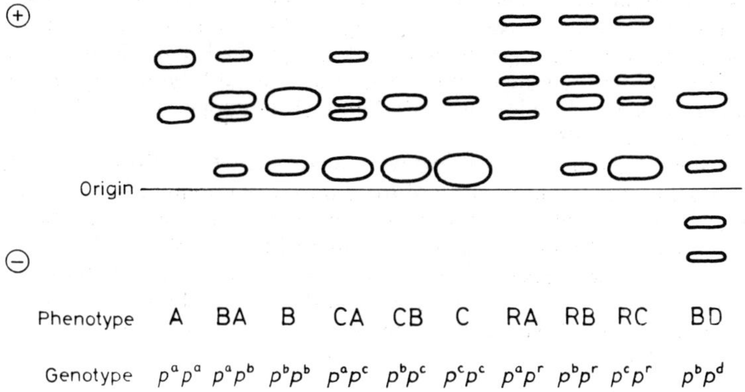

FIGURE 1. Patterns of red cell acid phosphatase types produced by starch gel electrophoresis using a citrate/phosphate buffer system at pH 5.9.

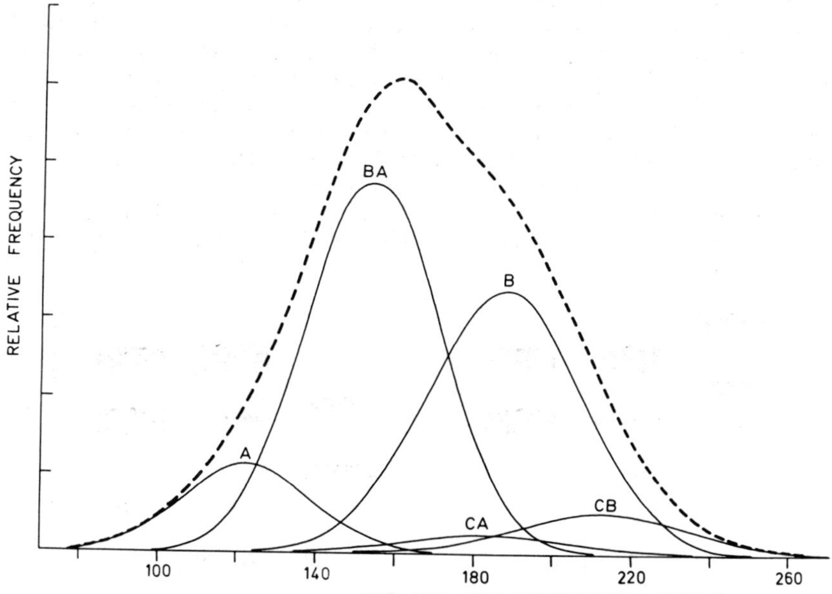

FIGURE 2. Distribution of red cell acid phosphatase activities in the English population (dotted line) and the common phenotypes (continuous lines). Diagram based on data of Hopkinson *et al.* (1964).

of purified material from each phenotype would be required. To begin with, it was decided to attempt the purification of the two homozygous types that occur most frequently in our population, i.e., B and A.

The laboratory scale preparation devised by Tsuboi and Hudson in 1954 was used first, and, although it gave good purification, the total yield was small and the percentage recovery poor. This is hardly surprising when it is considered that about 95 percent of the red cell is hemoglobin, and of the remainder, only a small fraction can be acid phosphatase. In the purer preparations, the dilution of protein was so great that the enzyme became extremely unstable. For this reason, we felt we would get better results by doing the first steps of the purification on a large scale, thus producing sufficient partially purified material to continue to the final stages without undue dilution. The Biochemical Engineering Department of University College, London, was kind enough to cooperate with us in a joint project (Fisher *et al.*, 1968).

In each step of the purification, we were anxious that conditions be such as to produce maximum possible stability of the enzyme. We required a good recovery not only in terms of activity, but also in terms of electrophoretic constancy; that is to say, the electrophoretic behaviour of the purified sample should be the same as that of the crude hemolysate. Thus, to find conditions under which the purification would be as efficient as possible, we investigated methods of stabilizing red cell acid phosphatase. Two of these methods were of particular interest, and will be discussed in detail.

Stabilization by Inorganic Phosphate

The first steps in the purification involved the selective adsorption of the enzyme onto a calcium phosphate gel, the removal of loosely bound hemoglobin by washing, and bulk elution of the enzyme with a buffer of low pH and high ionic strength (Tsuboi & Hudson, 1954). It became apparent that the enzyme was extremely stable both while it was adsorbed onto the gel, and while it was in the eluate. Whereas a crude hemolysate stored at 4° C lost all activity over a period of three to four weeks, the adsorbed or eluted enzyme, under the same conditions, had lost no activity after twelve weeks. However, the eluate was rendered unstable if dialyzed against distilled water.

Those factors that could be changed by dialysis included pH, ionic strength, and the concentration of various inorganic ions, including phosphate. Of these,

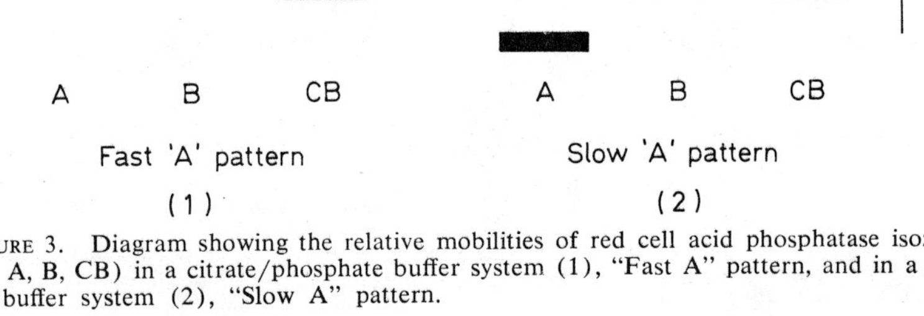

FIGURE 3. Diagram showing the relative mobilities of red cell acid phosphatase isozymes (types A, B, CB) in a citrate/phosphate buffer system (1), "Fast A" pattern, and in a phosphate buffer system (2), "Slow A" pattern.

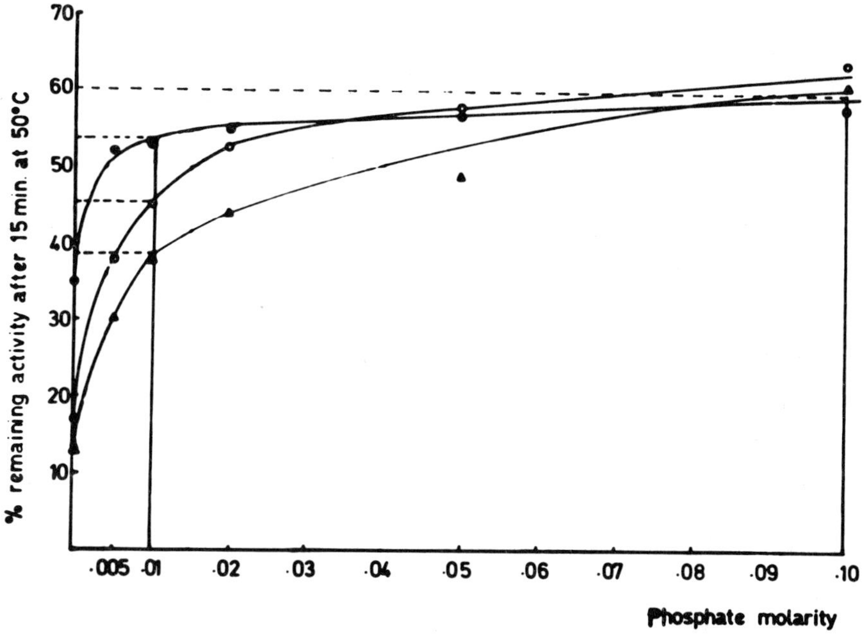

FIGURE 4. Plots of percentage remaining acid phosphatase activity in hemolysates of different phenotypes after incubation at 50° C for 15 minutes at various inorganic phosphate concentrations. Residual percentage activities in the presence of relatively high and low concentrations are indicated. (Type A: ▲——▲; Type B: ○——○; Type C: ●——●).

pH, ionic strength and phosphate ions were found to affect the stability. The enzyme was most stable between pH 5.0 and 6.5. Above pH 7.5, it became extremely unstable. As might be expected, it was also stabilized by a high ionic strength. The effect of phosphate ions on the stability was particularly marked, and differences were observed between types of enzyme.

Thermal stability tests had previously been carried out on crude hemolysates (Luffman & Harris, 1967), and, therefore, similar experiments were done to examine and compare the stabilizing effect of inorganic phosphate. One part washed cells were lysed with two parts of distilled water, and the hemolysate was then dialyzed for two hours against phosphate solutions of different molarities at pH 7.0. The hemolysate was then heated with mild agitation at 50° C. Samples were taken for assay at 0 and 15 minutes, and the percentage remaining activity was calculated. Types A, B and C were examined. (FIGURE 4).

The different stabilities of the types were still apparent at lower phosphate concentrations. Thus, after heating at 50° C for 15 minutes with a phosphate ion concentration of 0.01 M, type A had approximately 38% remaining activity, type B 45% and type C 54%, and the relative differences were repeatable and significant. However, when the phosphate ion concentration was increased to 0.1 M, the remaining activity was found to be around 60% for all three types. At lower temperatures, this concentration of phosphate gave a very good protection against denaturation and, acting on this evidence, we have found that by adding phosphate at certain stages during the purification, we have been able to increase the stability of the enzyme and considerably improve the yield.

Effect of Sulfhydryl Reagents and Oxidized Glutathione

Although acid phosphatase typing depends on the recognition of the main phenotype bands, the presence of several minor bands has frequently been noticed. Of these, the most obvious is seen in type B, running some way in front of the two main components. When purified and concentrated preparations were examined, a bewildering number of additional bands, with mobilities greater than either of the original bands, were produced. Bottini and Modiano reported in 1964 that oxidized glutathione affects the mobility of acid phosphatase, and for this reason, we decided to investigate the effects of oxidation further.

Washed red cells were lysed by sonication and three parts mixed with one part 0.1 M oxidized glutathione or 0.1 M mercaptoethanol, both at pH 7.0. Controls were incubated with distilled water. After incubation at +5° C for a number of days, activities were measured and the samples examined by starch gel electrophoresis.

The total activities were not found to differ significantly from those of controls of the same age, but the changes in electrophoretic mobility caused by oxidized glutathione were striking. In all cases, the mobilities of both bands were increased.

In a phosphate buffer system, all types showed a similar effect; the front band moving forwards, and the back band moving to a position just ahead of the normal front band (FIGURE 5). In a system incorporating citrate, types B and C showed the same kind of repositioning, but in type A, the back band appeared to reach a position just behind the original front band (FIGURE 6). In both systems, and for all phenotypes, the ratio of the distances moved by the front bands to the distances moved by the back bands was 1:1. The position taken up by the front B band corresponded to the extra, fast band seen in aged B hemolysates. The course of the reaction was followed over a period of 10 days, by which time all the original bands had been converted into the more mobile ones. It then became apparent that further increases of mobility with a similar 1:1 ratio were gradually occurring, but as the samples were by this time losing activity, the

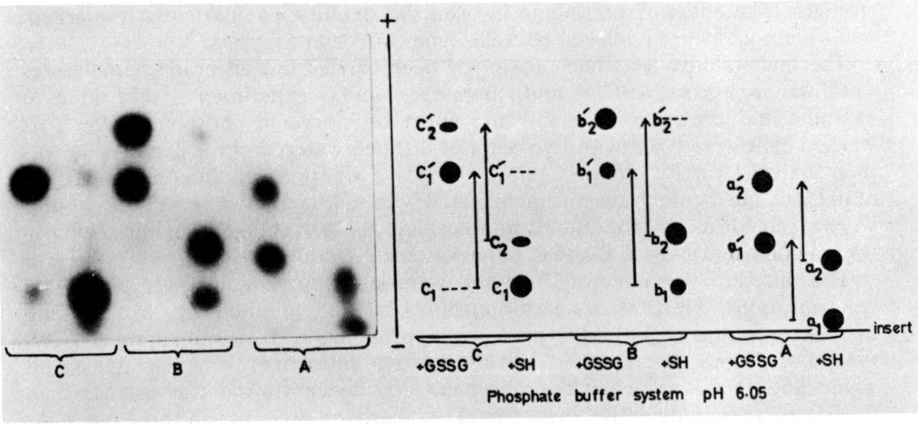

FIGURE 5. Photograph and diagram showing the increased anodal migration of acid phosphatase isozymes of different phenotypes produced by incubation of crude hemolysates with oxidized glutathione (GSSG), compared with the original pattern maintained in the presence of free sulfhydryl groups (SH) provided by excess mercaptoethanol. Electrophoresis was carried out with a phosphate buffer system (pH 6.0).

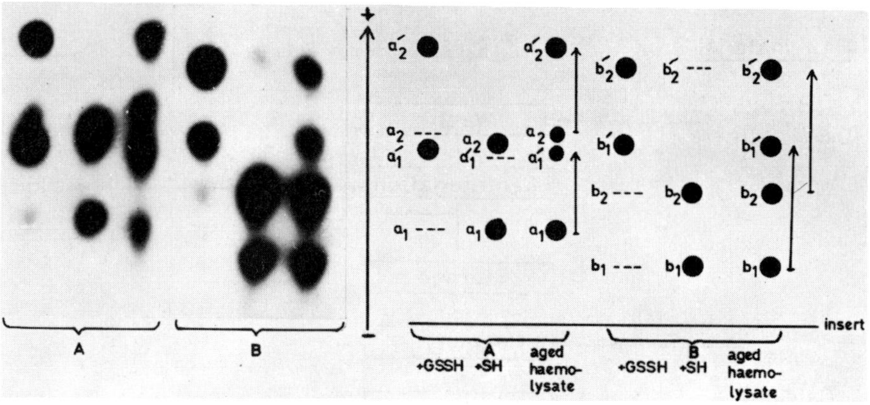

FIGURE 6. Photograph and diagram to show how the effect of ageing resembles the effect produced by incubation with oxidized glutathione (GSSG), and how incubation with free sulfhydryl groups prevents this effect. Electrophoresis was carried out in a citrate/phosphate buffer system (pH 5.9).

reaction could not be followed to its ultimate conclusion. The enzyme incubated in the presence of mercaptoethanol showed no changes in mobility. The control samples gradually produced extra bands similar in mobility to those appearing in the presence of oxidized glutathione, but complete conversion did not occur. It seems likely that the changes observed in ageing samples, and some of the changes produced by purification procedures, are due to oxidation of the isozymes. For all types of column work, therefore, fresh mercaptoethanol was added to the eluting buffer.

Large-Scale Preparation

We found that the initial steps of Tsuboi and Hudson's method (i.e., adsorption of the enzymes onto calcium phosphate gel and subsequent elution) could be scaled up 80 times without difficulty. This was about as much as could be handled conveniently by our pilot plant equipment, but there appeared to be no technical bar to further magnification (FIGURE 7).

Calcium phosphate gel was prepared to the same recipe as on a small scale and was harvested using a 6P "pressuretite" Sharples supercentrifuge (Sharples, Camberly, Surrey, England). Although the yields were variable, the consistency and absorptive qualities were as good as laboratory scale preparations. Bottles of out-dated red cells were kindly provided by the North London Blood Transfusion Centre in batches of 100 to 150, and were typed for acid phosphatase. The cells of similar types were pooled. Large-scale washing of red cells was, and still is, a problem. No general-purpose continuous centrifuge was found capable of separating cells from saline without damaging the cells, although several were suitable for separating cells from plasma. The cells were therefore washed in batches of 3 liters using a Mistral M.S.E. centrifuge (M.S.E., London, England) with a 6L head.

In the case of type B (36% of the English population), a sufficient volume of cells (10–20 l) could be collected over the course of one week, so that no storage problems arose. However, for type A, (13% of the English population), it was necessary to store the washed cells at −20° C until a sufficient volume

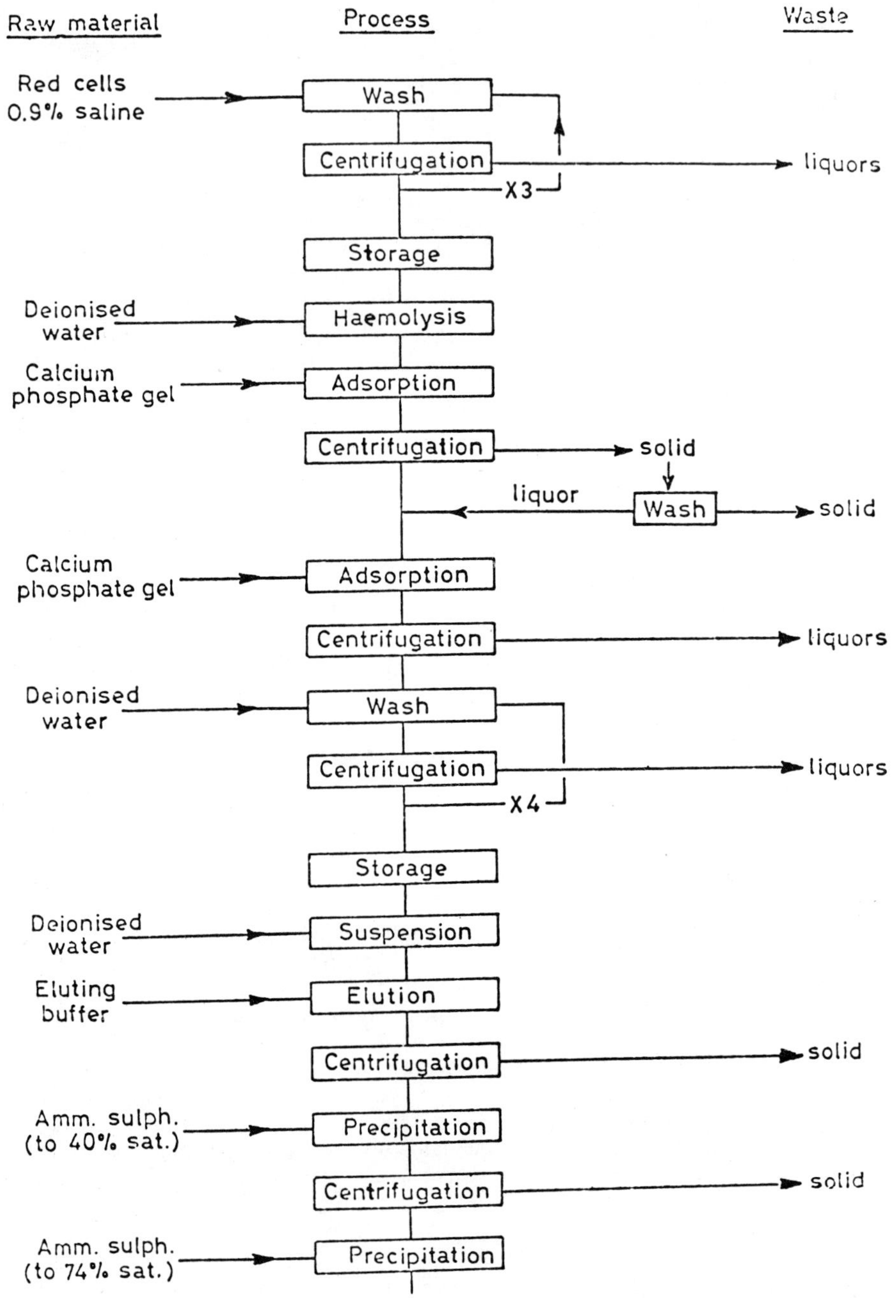

FIGURE 7. Flow diagram for the large-scale preparation of red cell acid phosphatase.

could be collected. The enzyme remained active under these conditions for several months, but it was found necessary to use up to twice as much calcium phosphate gel to adsorb the enzyme than if the cells had not been frozen.

After elution from the calcium phosphate gel, the enzyme was precipitated with ammonium sulfate between 40% and 74% saturation, and was harvested with a laboratory 1P Sharples supercentrifuge. The yield on a large scale was much greater than on a small scale, and the improvement was probably due to the better control of factors such as temperature, stirring speeds, etc. The precipitate remained active after storage for several months at −20° C.

The subsequent stages in the purification proved difficult at first because of the instability of the enzyme. These became less hazardous when we learned of the stabilizing effects of phosphate and mercaptoethanol. In all steps following the first ammonium sulfate precipitation, the enzyme was kept in as high a phosphate concentration as possible, and, where possible, in contact with fresh mercaptoethanol.

Gel filtration had previously been done on crude hemolysates to estimate the molecular size of the enzyme (Luffman & Harris, 1967). These experiments suggested a relatively low figure, (about 10,000), and incidentally produced a good separation from hemoglobin. Therefore, it was decided to include gel filtration as a purification step in the large-scale preparation. This was done using Bio-Gel P-60 (50–100 mesh) (Bio-Rad Laboratories, California) in two linked QVF glass columns, each 7.5 cm in diameter and 100 cm in length. The

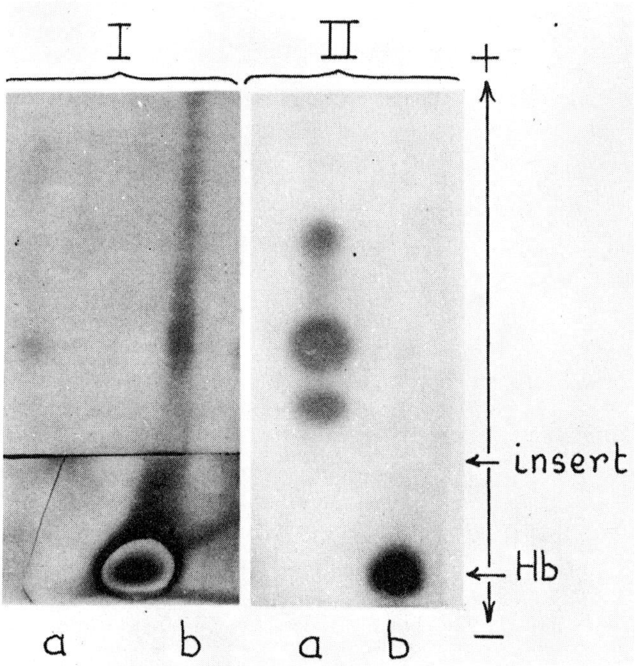

FIGURE 8. Starch gel electrophoresis (citrate/phosphate buffer system, pH 5.9) of a purified sample (a) following gel filtration, and of a crude hemolysate (b). Both samples are type B, (I) stained for protein, and (II) stained for acid phosphatase activity.

TABLE 1

EXPERIMENTAL RESULTS FOR THE LARGE-SCALE ISOLATION OF TYPE B ACID PHOSPHATASE FROM 16.4 LITERS OF WASHED RED CELLS

Stages	Total Volume (Liters)	Total Protein (g)	Total Units Activity	Mg Protein/ml	Units/mg Protein	Percent Recovery	Purification
Hemolysate	81.6	3990	224400	49.8	0.057		
Supernatant After 1st Gel Addition	89.0	4405	232290	49.5	0.053	100	
Eluate From 2nd Gel	33.0	29.4	120780	0.89	4.11	54	73
Supernatant From 1st Ammonium Sulfate	38.0		85500			38	
2nd Ammonium Precipitate in Solution & Dialyzed	0.355	19.5	82537	55.0	4.23	37	75
Pooled Fractions From Columns	2.057	0.82	60475	0.4	73.5	27	1305

ammonium sulfate precipitate from the previous stage was dissolved, dialyzed against the eluting buffer and centrifuged. The supernatant, whose final volume was about 300 ml, was then applied to the top of the first column. The eluting buffer was at pH 6.0, and contained 0.1 M phosphate as the sodium salt, 0.2% v/v mercaptoethanol; 0.01% sodium azide, which had previously been shown to have no detrimental effects on the enzyme, was also added to prevent bacterial contamination. The flow rate through the columns was between 3 and 4 ml/min and 15-ml fractions were collected. The whole procedure took about 30 hours, and was carried out at +5° C. The enzyme was eluted after the residual hemoglobin, and well separated from it. This was in good agreement with the previous experiments. Starch gel electrophoresis, carried out at this stage, showed bands of protein corresponding with the bands of acid phosphatase activity. (FIGURE 8).

The enzyme was then precipitated with ammonium sulfate at 74% saturation. A purification of about 1,300 times, with a yield of approximately 30%, was obtained at this stage (TABLE 1). This compared favorably with that obtained from the smaller scale by Tsuboi and Hudson in 1954, and by Scott in 1965. However, as we now had a relatively large quantity of material (about 5 g), further purification could be attempted.

The next stages of purification are still in the process of development. They involve ion exchange chromatography and are designed, first, to separate the enzyme as a whole from residual contaminating proteins, and then to separate the isozymes from one another.

It is known that the enzyme can be separated from most contaminants on DEAE cellulose using 0.02 M phosphate buffer at pH 6.0 with a sodium chloride gradient 0→ 0.4 M (FIGURE 9). Some separation of the isozymes is evident under these conditions, but not sufficient to be worth dividing the eluate at this stage. The active fractions are therefore pooled and precipitated with ammonium sulfate. An overall purification of about 4,000 times is achieved by this procedure. Further experiments indicate that good separation of the isozymes may be obtained by chromatography on CM cellulose.

Conclusions

Using these procedures, it is apparently possible to produce, from large volumes of typed red cells, reasonably stable acid phosphatase preparations with a high degree of purity, and to separate from each other the isozymes present in a given type. The procedures do not appear to result in any significant modification of the enzyme proteins, since the electrophoretic mobilities, as well as the catalytic properties, of the purified material seem to be the same as in the crude hemolysate. It should, therefore, become possible to characterize in structural terms the differences between these various phosphohydrolase isozymes.

Summary

Red cell acid phosphohydrolase shows genetically determined polymorphism. Each allelic gene appears to be responsible for at least two isozymes. To investigate the differences both between types and between isozymes within types, a relatively large quantity of each type material is required. We have presented a method for carrying out the first steps of the purification on a large scale. Ways of increasing the stability of the enzyme are discussed, and methods for further purification and separation of the isozymes are mentioned.

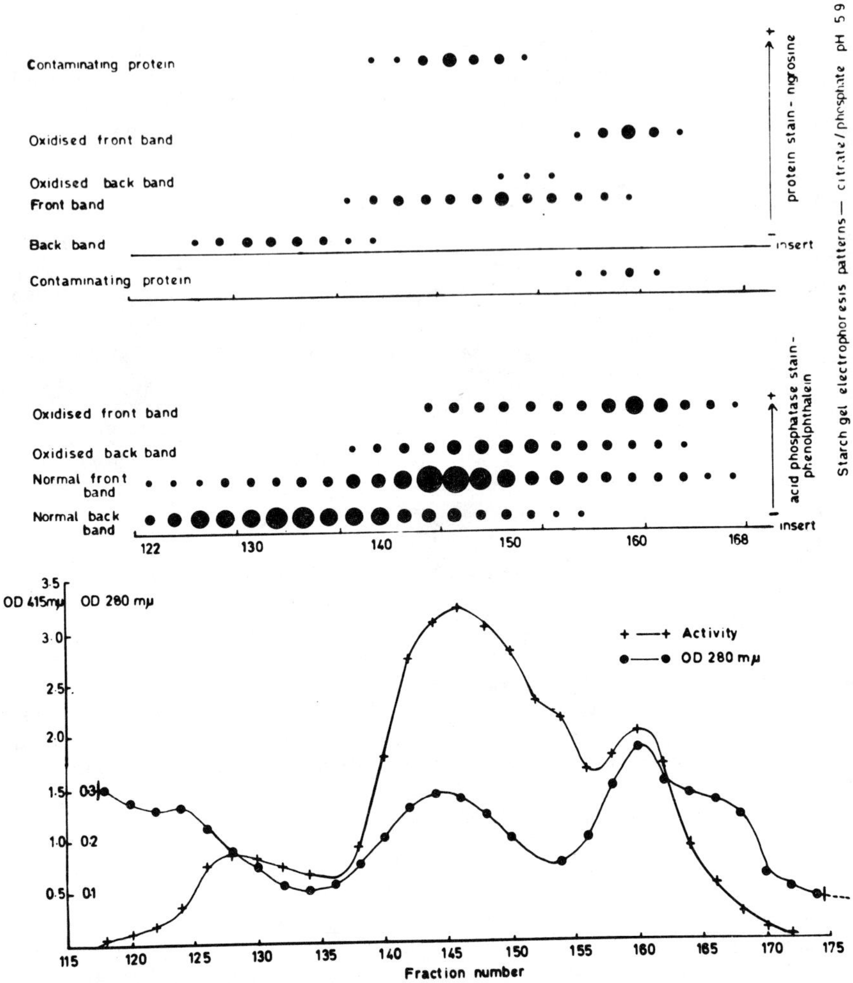

FIGURE 9. Diagram (bottom) shows part of the effluent (0.2 → 0.3 M NaCl) from a DEAE cellulose column. Buffer: 0.02 M phosphate, 0.2% v/v mercaptoethanol, 0.01% w/v sodium azide, pH 6.0. Overall gradient: 0 → 0.4 M NaCl. Diagram (top) shows starch gel electrophoresis of fractions stained for protein and for acid phosphatase activity.

References

ABUL-FADL, M. A. M. & E. J. KING. 1949. Properties of the acid phosphatases of erythrocytes and of the human prostate gland. Biochem. J. **45**: 51.

BEHRENDT, H. 1943. Phosphatase activity of human erythrocytes. Proc. Soc. Exp. Biol. Med. **54**: 268.

BOTTINI, E. & G. MODIANO. 1964. Effect of oxidised glutathione on human red cell acid phosphatase. Biochem. Biophys. Res. Commun. **17**: 260.

DAVIES, D. R. 1934. Phosphatases of the spleen. Biochem. J. **28**: 529.

FISHER, R. A., H. HARRIS, M. HOULDSWORTH, M. D. LILLY & P. DUNILL. 1968. Large-scale isolation of acid phosphatase from human erythrocytes. Biotechn. Bioengin. (In press.)

GIBLETT, E. R. & N. M. SCOTT. 1965. Red cell acid phosphatase: racial distribution and report of a new phenotype. Amer. J. Hum. Genet. **17**: 425.

HARRIS, H., D. A. HOPKINSON, J. E. LUFFMAN & S. RAPLEY. 1968. Electrophoretic variation in erythrocyte enzymes. *In* Hereditary Disorders of Erythrocyte Metabolism. (Chapt. 1) Grune and Stratton Inc.

HOPKINSON, D. A. & H. HARRIS. 1968. *In* Biochemical methods in red cell genetics. Chapt. 13. Academic Press, Inc., New York, N. Y. (In press.)

HOPKINSON, D. A., N. SPENCER & H. HARRIS. 1963. Red cell acid phosphatase variants: a new human polymorphism. Nature (London) **199:** 969.

HOPKINSON, D. A., N. SPENCER & H. HARRIS. 1964. Genetical studies on human red cell acid phosphatase. Amer. J. Hum. Genet. **16:** 141.

KARP, G. W. & H. E. SUTTON. 1967. Some new phenotypes of human red cell acid phosphatase. Amer. J. Hum. Genet. **19:** 34.

KING, E. J., E. J. WOOD & G. E. DELORY. 1945. Acid phosphatase of the red cells. Biochem. J. **39:** XXIV.

LAI, L., S. NEVO & A. G. STEINBERG. 1964. Acid phosphatase of human red cell. Predicted phenotype conforms to genetic hypothesis. Science **145:** 1187.

LUFFMAN, J. E. & H. HARRIS. 1967. A comparison of some properties of human red cell acid phosphatase in different phenotypes. Ann. Hum. Genet. **30:** 387.

MODIANO, G., G. FILIPPI, F. BRUNELLI, W. FRATTAROLI & M. SINISCALCO. 1967. Studies on red cell acid phosphatases in Sardinia and Rome: absence of correlation with past malarial morbidity. Acta Genet. (Basel) **17:** 17.

SCOTT, E. M. 1966. Kinetic comparison of genetically different acid phosphatases of human erythrocytes. J. Biol. Chem. **241:** 3049.

TSUBOI, K. K. & P. B. HUDSON. 1953. Acid phosphatase. I. Human red cell phosphomonoesterase: general properties. Arch. Biochem. **43:** 339.

TSUBOI, K. K. & P. B. HUDSON. 1954. Acid phosphatase. II. Purification of human red cell phosphomonoesterase. Arch. Biochem. **53:** 341.

TSUBOI, K. K. & P. B. HUDSON. 1956. Acid phosphatase. VI. Kinetic properties of purified yeast and erythrocyte phosphomonoesterase. Arch. Biochem. **61:** 197.

VALENTINE, W. N., K. R. TANAKA & M. D. FREDRICKS. 1961. Erythrocyte acid phosphatase in health and disease. Amer. J. Clin. Path. **36:** 328.

Discussion of the Paper

DAVID AMINOFF (*University of Michigan, Ann Arbor, Mich.*) It wasn't too clear to me what were the conditions for the adsorption of the calcium phosphate gel and the conditions for the elution.

DR. FISHER: Well, concerning conditions for the adsorption, we simply made a one-in-five hemolysate of the cells with distilled water, and then we added the calcium phosphate gel. A citrate-acetate buffer at pH 4.5 was used for elution. This was about .3 M with respect to citrate and about .03 M with acetate.

BLOOD GROUPS AND THEIR RELATION TO SERUM PHOSPHOHYDROLASES

Lars Beckman

Department of Clinical Bacteriology, University of Umea, Umea, Sweden

D. C. Zoschke

Department of Genetics, University of Wisconsin, Madison, Wis.

While the genetics and the chemical composition of many blood group substances are rather well known, the function of the red cell antigens and the surface mucoids in general has remained poorly understood. However, some of the discoveries in recent years concerning the relationships between blood groups and serum phosphohydrolases may provide some insight into problems having to do with the physiological role of the blood groups. A number of electrophoretically distinct forms of acid and alkaline phosphatase have been found in human serum. These isozyme variants originate from different tissues, and their concentrations may be influenced by a series of factors such as diet, age, sex, pregnancy, disease and blood groups. This paper is a review of present knowledge about the relations between blood groups and the quantitative variations of some serum phosphohydrolase isozymes.

Alkaline Phosphatase

Isozyme variants. By means of starch gel electrophoresis and subsequent enzyme staining (the zymogram technique), various molecular forms of alkaline phosphatase can be distinguished. At least four different organ-specific variants may be identified in human serum (FIGURE 1) by electrophoresis in a discontinuous buffer system at pH 8.6 (Poulik, 1957). Staining is performed in Tris/citrate buffer at pH 8.6 with α-naphthyl phosphate as substrate and Blue RR salt as a dye coupler.

The slow-moving alkaline phosphatase component seen in sample 3, FIGURE 1, is derived from the intestine (Hodson *et al.*, 1962). The intestinal alkaline phosphatase is more sensitive to inhibition by L-phenylalanine than the liver and bone enzymes (Fishman & Kreisher, 1963). This enzyme is also neuraminidase resistant and thus lacking sialic acid (Robinson & Pierce, 1964; Moss *et al.*, 1966). The fast-moving serum component may have contributions from liver, bone and intestinal alkaline phosphatase (Fishman & Ghosh, 1967). It shows higher activity and a somewhat reduced mobility in children (Boyer, 1961; Beckman, 1964), most likely depending on a contribution of bone alkaline phosphatase.

Normal, healthy individuals differ with respect to the concentration of the slow-moving intestinal enzyme. Somewhat variable electrophoretic techniques and scoring methods have been used to describe this variation (Beckman, 1968). Although the techniques vary with respect to their sensitivity, all studies so far have shown the same principal results concerning the correlation with blood groups. In the first studies in our laboratory (Arfors *et al.*, 1963a.; Beckman, 1964), we used a simple classification into two groups: those with (Pp 2) and those without (Pp 1) the slow-moving component. Bamford *et al.* (1965) used three classes: p° for sera with no detectable zone of intestinal alkaline phosphatase, p^{+} for sera with a weak zone and p^{++} for those showing a strong zone.

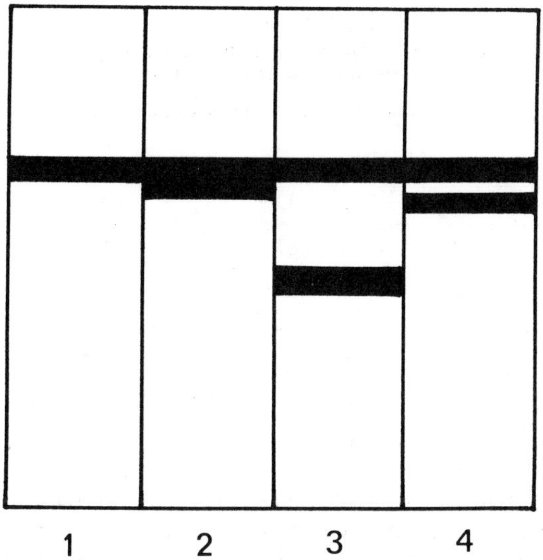

FIGURE 1. Electrophoretic variants of alkaline phosphatase observed in human serum at pH 8.6. The anode is at the top of the picture. 1 = adult type 1 (Pp 1), 2 = childhood, 3 = adult type 2 (Pp 2), 4 = pregnancy, variant S.

TABLE 1*

RELATION BETWEEN SERUM INTESTINAL ALKALINE PHOSPHATASE AND ABO BLOOD GROUPS IN BRAZILIAN FAMILY MATERIAL

Members	Pp†	7 Blood Groups						
		A_1	A_2	B	A_1B	A_2B	O	Total
		Number of Individuals						
Fathers	1	61	12	22	3	1	75	174
	2	0	0	14	0	0	42	56
Mothers	1	53	21	21	5	3	92	195
	2	0	0	6	0	1	36	43
Children	1	203	72	71	5	11	305	667
	2	7	3	30	2	2	128	172

* From Beckman, 1964.
† Pp 2 = presence of intestinal enzyme; Pp 1 = absence.

Effect of ABO blood type. In a study of a Swedish twin material (Arfors *et al.*, 1963a.), we were able to demonstrate a strong association between the serum alkaline phosphatases and the ABO blood groups. These results were confirmed in an investigation of Brazilian family material (Beckman, 1964). The frequency of individuals with the intestinal alkaline phosphatase was lower in the Brazilian material than in any other series tested by us (TABLE 1). This is most likely due to nutritional circumstances (cf. Langman *et al.*, 1966). In the Brazilian material, the association with the ABO blood groups is very clear. The intestinal alkaline phosphatase is found more frequently in the sera of individuals with blood groups B and O. These results have been confirmed by a number of investigators (Bamford *et al.*, 1965; Shreffler, 1965; Shinoda & Matsunaga, 1967; Walter *et al.*, 1967). TABLE 2 shows a series of blood donors from Hawaii

TABLE 2*

RELATION BETWEEN SERUM INTESTINAL ALKALINE PHOSPHATASE AND ABO BLOOD GROUPS IN HAWAII BLOOD DONOR SERIES 1

ABO Group	Serum Intestinal Alkaline Phosphatase Score			Total
	0†	1†	2†	
		Number of Donors		
A	150	13	1	164
AB	21	1	0	22
B	20	24	19	63
O	52	32	40	124
Total	243	70	60	373

* From Zoschke, 1968.
† 0 = absence; 1 = weak; 2 = strong.

where we have used the same classification as that used by Bamford *et al.* (1965). The table clearly shows that the frequency of individuals exhibiting the intestinal enzyme is blood group dependent and also that the concentration of the enzyme, when present, is higher in groups B and O. Bamford *et al.* (1965 have demonstrated that the average level of total serum alkaline phosphatase is higher in individuals of blood groups O and B than in people with blood groups A and AB. An interesting observation was made by Shinoda and Matsunaga (1967), who found also that the activity of the faster moving component of normal serum alkaline phosphatase was suppressed by the blood factor A.

Effect of secretor type. In 1963 we were able to demonstrate that the slow-moving serum alkaline phosphatase component was correlated with the Lewis blood groups and thus with the secretor trait (Arfors *et al.* 1963b). The intestinal enzyme was found less frequently in individuals of the Lewis blood group Le(a^+ b^-), which are all nonsecretors of ABH substances (Grubb, 1948). This result was confirmed in a study of the Brazilian family material mentioned before (TABLE 3). The correlation between intestinal alkaline phosphatase and ABH secretion appeared to be almost absolute in this material, while there was no association with Lewis secretion. Individuals with the slow-moving enzyme in their serum have been found among ABH nonsecretors (Bamford *et al.*, 1965;

TABLE 3*

RELATION BETWEEN SERUM INTESTINAL ALKALINE PHOSPHATASE AND THE SALIVARY SECRETION OF ABH AND LEWIS SUBSTANCES IN BRAZILIAN FAMILY MATERIAL

Members	Pp†	Individuals of ABH Secretion		Individuals of Lewis Secretion		Total
		SH	nh	Les	nl	
Fathers	1	130	44	148	26	174
	2	56	0	46	10	56
Mothers	1	145	50	151	44	195
	2	43	0	37	6	43
Children	1	493	174	522	145	667
	2	172	0	134	38	172

* From Beckman, 1964.
† Pp 2 = presence of intestinal enzyme; Pp 1 = absence.

Shreffler, 1965), but all investigations have clearly demonstrated that the intestinal alkaline phosphatase component is found in a much higher frequency among secretors.

Effect of other genetic factors. Arfors *et al.*, (1963a) studied the association with the Rh, MN and Hp systems, but with negative results. Shreffler (1965) also reported negative results for the MNSs, Rh, Kell, Duffy, Kidd and P blood groups and for the Gm, Gc and Hp serum groups. Beckman (1964) found no correlation with the Lutheran and P blood groups, but a significant association with the Duffy blood groups. The association with the Duffy system has not been possible to confirm, however, (Beckman *et al.*, 1966) and at present there is no evidence for an effect of the Duffy blood groups on the level of intestinal alkaline phosphatase in serum. Furthermore, there is no need to postulate the existence of genetic factors other than the ABO and the secretor genes to explain the residual variability observed by Beckman (1964) and Shreffler (1965) in their studies of twin and family data. This residual effect is in all probability caused by correlations between related individuals with respect to dietary factors (cf. Langman *et al.*, 1966).

Effect of diet. Langman *et al.* (1966) examined the effect of diet on the human serum alkaline phosphatases. The enzyme patterns of a series of individuals were studied in the fasting state and at different intervals after regular meals. In a group of individuals who were B or O and also secretors, a very marked effect of feeding on the amount of intestinal alkaline phosphatase was found. In contrast to this result, hardly any effect was observed in a group of non-secretor individuals. Another experiment demonstrated that the increase of intestinal alkaline phosphatase was found only after a fatty meal and not after a meal containing protein and carbohydrates only. These results illustrate an important principle, namely, the occurrence of an environmental metabolic influence restricted to individuals of a certain genotype.

Acid Phosphatase

Isozyme variants. The level of acid phosphatase is low in the serum of normal, healthy individuals. As a consequence, the demonstration of acid phosphatase isozymes by means of the zymogram technique meets with some difficulties, and there is considerable disagreement in the literature concerning the number of acid phosphatase isozyme components present in such serum. Thus Lundin and Allison (1966) were unable to find any acid phosphatase component by means of starch gel electrophoresis. Goldberg *et al.* (1966a), by using disc electrophoresis on polyacrylamide columns, found one acid phosphatase component of rather fast anodal mobility. Lawrence *et al.* (1960) described two distinct isozyme components by starch gel electrophoresis at pH 8.6. One of them was migrating between the albumin and transferrin zones, while the other zone was migrating close to the starting point. Similar results were obtained by Dubbs *et al.* (1960), who found one fast-moving zone and two slower moving zones. Variations in the fast- and slow-moving acid phosphatase components have been found in patients with various diseases (Czitober *et al.*, 1964; Goldberg *et al.*, 1966a; Ramot & Streifler, 1967). An increase in the fast-moving fraction was observed in patients with carcinoma of the prostate, lymphoma and monocytic leukemia, while patients with Gaucher's disease showed an increase in the activity and the number of zones in the slow-moving fraction.

Beckman & Zoschke (1968) were able to detect acid phosphatase activity in most individual sera by means of the following technique: Samples were applied in heavy filter paper inserts and examined by starch gel electrophoresis using a Tris-borate buffer at pH 7.5 (Allen *et al.*, 1963). The gels were pretreated at room temperature with 0.2 M acetate buffer at pH 4.0 for 30 minutes, and thereafter stained overnight at 37°C in acetate buffer at pH 5.0 using α-naphthyl phosphate as substrate and Black K salt as a dye coupler. It is important to examine the serum samples within a couple of days and to avoid heating during electrophoresis. Furthermore, in our experience, buffers containing citrate inhibit the slow-moving enzymes. Diazonium salts giving strong background staining (such as Fast Garnet GBC salt) should be avoided.

Four different electrophoretic variants of acid, phosphatase have been found rather frequently in human serum by means of the technique described above (FIGURE 2). The zone with the fastest anodal mobility (A) shows marked variations in its concentration. The second zone (A_1) is absent in many samples and usually weak when present. Close to the start of the electrophoresis there may be one or two zones. The major component (E_2) shows marked concentration variations. The minor component (E_1) is occurring less frequently and mostly in sera with a strong E_2 zone. These serum isozymes apparently do not correspond to the series of tissue acid phosphatases described by Beckman and Beckman (1967). All serum components are inhibited by L-tartrate and the electrophoretic mobility of the A zone decreased with about 15 percent after treatment with neuraminidase.

Sex and age differences have been found in relation to concentrations of serum acid phosphatase isozymes (Zoschke, 1968). The level of the A enzyme is higher among males. No sex difference was found concerning the E_2 component. No certain age difference was found in the level of the A component, whereas there was a very striking increase of the E_2 component among children.

Effect of ABO type. In a preliminary study of a hospital blood series from Sweden (TABLE 4), we found significantly higher levels of tartrate-inhibitable acid phosphatase among individuals of blood groups A and AB (Beckman &

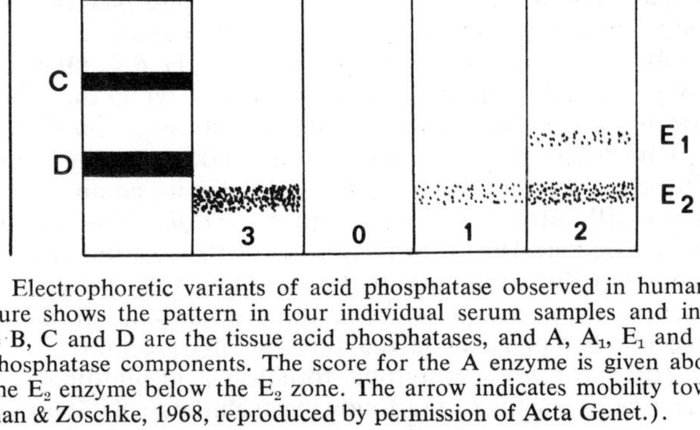

FIGURE 2. Electrophoretic variants of acid phosphatase observed in human serum at pH 7.5. The picture shows the pattern in four individual serum samples and in one placental extract where B, C and D are the tissue acid phosphatases, and A, A_1, E_1 and E_2 indicate the serum acid phosphatase components. The score for the A enzyme is given above the A zone and that of the E_2 enzyme below the E_2 zone. The arrow indicates mobility toward the anode (from Beckman & Zoschke, 1968, reproduced by permission of Acta Genet.).

TABLE 4*

RELATION BETWEEN TARTRATE-INHIBITABLE SERUM ACID PHOSPHATASE AND ABO BLOOD GROUPS. SWEDISH HOSPITAL SERIES.

ABO Group	Activity, B. L. Units Mean ± S. E.	Number of Donors
A	0.090 ± 0.0028	335
AB	0.092 ± 0.0083	39
B	0.077 ± 0.0066	62
O	0.079 ± 0.0032	254
Total	0.085 ± 0.0020	690

Difference A + AB/B + O. $0.005 > P > 0.001$.

* From Beckman & Zoschke, 1968.

Zoschke, 1968). There was no significant effect of the B factor, and the total phosphatase activity, measured at pH 5.0, showed no statistically significant relation to the ABO blood groups. The nontartrate-inhibitable phosphatase activity at this pH, however, was significantly higher in individuals of blood groups B and O, and may therefore represent background alkaline phosphatase activity.

Two series of blood donations from Hawaii collected over one month's interval were examined with respect to quantitative variations of the A and E_2 isozymes. A scoring method similar to the one used in studies of intestinal alkaline phosphatase was used. The relative strengths of the A and E_2 zones were classified as: 0 = no detectable zone and 1, 2 and 3 for increasing strength of the zone when present (FIGURE 2). In both blood donor series there was a highly significant association between the acid phosphatase component A and the ABO blood groups (TABLE 5). In agreement with the results from the Swedish hospital series, the highest levels were found in individuals of blood groups A and AB. There was no correlation between quantitative variations of the E_2 component and the ABO blood groups (TABLE 6).

DISCUSSION

The correlation between intestinal alkaline phosphatase and blood groups has been confirmed repeatedly, and a considerable number of blood and serum group systems have been tested regarding their relationship with serum alkaline phosphatase. Associations between blood groups and serum alkaline phosphatase have also been found in cattle (Rendel & Gahne, 1963) and in sheep (Rendel & Stormont, 1964).

Concerning serum acid phosphatase, our information is less complete; so far, only the effect of ABO type has been studied and in one laboratory only. Furthermore, the organ of origin of the blood-group-associated acid phosphatase isozyme is not known with certainty. The increased level of acid phosphatase in individuals of blood groups A and AB were found in three independent series with high levels of statistical significance; hence, there is strong evidence for the validity of this result. Studies of Japanese family material and a Swedish series have also been confirmatory.

There are similarities between the two phosphatase isozyme systems. In each system there are two main isozyme components, one of which shows quantitative variations associated with the ABO blood groups. The differences between these two systems are perhaps more important. The level of intestinal alkaline phosphatase is lower in individuals of blood groups A and AB, while the level of the fast-migrating acid phosphatase component is higher in the A and AB groups. There is also a difference in the carbohydrate content of the two enzymes involved. Intestinal alkaline phosphatase lacks sialic acid, while acid phosphatase A carries sialic acid on the molecule.

Langman *et al.*, in contrast to other investigators, claim that the mucosal concentrations of alkaline phosphatase show a correlation with the ABO and secretor types (cf. Langman *et al.*, 1968). They suggested that the ABO blood groups and secretor status affect the rate of production by the mucosal cell.

Beckman (1968) suggested an interpretation of the association between blood groups and alkaline phosphatase in terms of differential secretion. Further, he proposed that blood groups may influence the secretion to the extracellular environment of many glycoproteins (thus, the phenomenon may be rather general in nature) and that the mechanism of secretion was based on similarities between the carbohydrate composition of the cell membrane (blood groups) and the protein molecule. According to this hypothesis, one would expect that the secretion of some enzyme proteins would be favored by one blood group and other enzymes by another blood group factor. At present, there is no experimental evidence available for a secretion-controlling effect of blood groups on serum

TABLE 5*

RELATION BETWEEN SERUM ACID PHOSPHATASE COMPONENT A AND ABO BLOOD GROUPS IN TWO DIFFERENT SERIES OF BLOOD DONORS FROM HAWAII

Blood Donor Series 1

ABO Group	Acid Phosphatase A Score† 0	1	2	3	Total
	Number of Donors				
A	16	35	78	49	178
AB	2	4	14	6	26
B	13	19	20	11	63
O	27	45	43	13	128
Total	58	103	155	79	395

Difference A + AB/B + O with respect to high levels (score 2 + 3). $P < 0.001$.

Blood Donor Series 2

ABO Group	Acid Phosphatase A Score† 0	1	2	3	Total
	Number of Donors				
A	9	59	70	29	167
AB	1	8	9	3	21
B	2	30	17	5	54
O	24	77	57	13	171
Total	36	174	153	50	413

Difference A + AB/B + O with respect to high levels (score 2 + 3). $P < 0.001$.

* From Beckman & Zoschke, 1968.
† O = no detectable zone; 1, 2 and 3 represent increasing strength of zone when present.

TABLE 6*

RELATION BETWEEN SERUM ACID PHOSPHATASE COMPONENT E_2 AND ABO BLOOD GROUPS IN TWO DIFFERENT SERIES OF BLOOD DONORS FROM HAWAII

Blood Donor Series 1

ABO Group	Acid Phosphatase E_2 Score† 0	1	2	3	Total
	Number of Donors				
A	39	52	60	27	178
AB	4	8	11	3	26
B	17	18	18	10	63
O	28	40	45	15	128
Total	88	118	134	55	395

Difference A + AB/B + O with respect to high levels (score 2 + 3). $0.7 > P > 0.5$.

Blood Donor Series 2

ABO Group	Acid Phosphatase E_2 Score† 0	1	2	3	Total
	Number of Donors				
A	35	65	59	8	167
AB	7	7	5	2	21
B	8	19	22	5	54
O	39	54	67	11	171
Total	89	145	153	26	413

Difference A + AB/B + O with respect to high levels (score 2 + 3). $0.2 > P > 0.1$.

* From Beckman & Zoschke, 1968.
† O = no detectable zone; 1, 2 and 3 represent increasing strength of zone when present.

phosphohydrolases. It has been demonstrated, however, that an artificial alteration of the carbohydrate structure of the cell membrane by removal of sialic acid changes the secretion of alkaline phosphatase and ATPase from L 1210 leukemia cells in suspension (Goldberg *et al.*, 1966b). A secretion-controlling effect of cell membrane carbohydrates other than sialic acid (such as the immunodeterminant sugars of the ABO blood groups) is therefore a distinct possibility worth testing in future experiments. Another line of investigation is naturally to continue the search for further examples of blood group-serum protein associations. Finally, we should like to point out the interesting fact that levels of serum lipids also seem to be dependent on the ABO blood groups (Magis, 1960; Blankenhorn *et al.*, 1967). There is indication that some lipids may occur in higher levels in individuals of blood groups A and AB, while others show lower levels in these blood groups. The mechanism behind this correlation between ABO blood groups and serum lipids is not known. One possibility could be differential secretion of lipoproteins. A correlation between the formation of phospholipids and alkaline phosphatase activity has been reported (Przelecka *et al.*, 1962), and therefore, further investigations of the blood-group-associated variations of phosphatases and lipids as well as the phosphatase-lipid interrelations are needed.

REFERENCES

ALLEN, S. L., M. S. MISCH & B. M. MORRISSON. 1963. Genetic control of an acid phosphatase in Tetrahymena: Formation of a hybrid enzyme. Genetics **48:** 1635.

ARFORS, K.-E., L. BECKMAN & L. G. LUNDIN. 1963a. Genetic variations of human serum phosphatase. Acta Genet. (Basel) **13:** 89.

ARFORS, K.-E., L. BECKMAN & L. G. LUNDIN. 1963b. Further studies on the association between human serum phosphatases and blood groups. Acta Genet. (Basel) **13:** 366.

BAMFORD, K. F., H. HARRIS, J. E. LUFFMAN, E. B. ROBSON & T. E. CLEGHORN. 1965. Serum-alkaline-phosphatase and the ABO blood-groups. Lancet **1:** 530.

BECKMAN, L. 1964. Associations between human serum alkaline phosphatases and blood groups. Acta Genet. (Basel) **14:** 286.

BECKMAN, L. 1968. Blood groups and serum alkaline phosphatase. *In* Series Haematologica **1:** 137. Munksgaard. Copenhagen.

BECKMAN, L. & G. BECKMAN. 1967. Individual and organ-specific variations of human acid phosphatase. Biochem. Genetics **1:** 145.

BECKMAN, L., G. BJÖRLING & A. HEIKEN. 1966. Human alkaline phosphatases and the factors controlling their appearance in serum. Acta Genet. (Basel) **16:** 305.

BECKMAN, L. & D. C. ZOSCHKE. 1968. Serum acid phosphatase and ABO blood groups: A new blood group associated enzyme variation. Acta Genet. (Basel) **18:** 289.

BLANKENHORN, D. H., J. JENSEN, P. STURGEON, H. P. CHIN, N. W. ARMSTRONG & L. ENGELMAN. 1967. Effect of blood group on blood lipids in monozygotic twins. Nature **215:** 1499.

BOYER, S. H. 1961. Alkaline phosphatase in human sera and placentae. Science **134:** 1002.

CZITOBER, H., E. GRÜNDIG & B. SCHOBEL. 1964. Histochemische und biochemische Untersuchungen bei Morbus Gaucher. Klin. Wschr. **42:** 1179.

DUBBS, C. A., E. VIVONIA & J. M. HILBURN. 1960. Subfractionation of human serum enzymes. Science **131:** 1529.

FISHMAN, W. H. & N. K. GHOSH. 1967. Isoenzymes of human alkaline phosphatase. *In* Advances in Clinical Chemistry **10:** 225.

FISHMAN, W. H. & J. H. KREISHER. 1963. Stereospecific, organ-specific inhibition of intestinal alkaline phosphatase. Ann. N. Y .Acad. Sci. **103:** 951.

GOLDBERG, A. F., K. TAKAKURA & R. L. ROSENTHAL. 1966a. Electrophoretic separation serum acid phosphatase isozymes in Gaucher's disease, prostatic carcinoma and multiple myeloma. Nature **211:** 41.

GOLDBERG, A. R., J. L. GLICK & A. E. PARDEE. 1966b. Protein secretion from L 1210 leukemia cells regulated by sialic acid. Fed. Proc. **25:** no. 2, part 1.

GRUBB, R. 1948. Correlation between Lewis blood group and secretor character in man. Nature **162:** 933.

HODSON, A. W., A. L. LATNER & L. RAINE. 1962. Isoenzymes of alkaline phosphatase. Clin. Chim. Acta **7:** 255.

LANGMAN, M. J. S., E. LEUTHOLD, E. B. ROBSON, J. HARRIS, J. E. LUFFMAN & H. HARRIS. 1966. Influence of diet on the 'intestinal' component of serum alkaline phosphatase in people of different ABO groups and secretor status. Nature **212:** 41.

LANGMAN, M. J. S., A. CONSTANTINOPOLOUS & J. A. D. BUOCHIER. 1968. ABO blood groups, secretor status and intestinal mucosal concentrations of alkaline phosphatase. Nature (London) **217:** 863

LAWRENCE, S. H., P. J. MELNICK & H. E. WEIMER. 1960. A species comparison of serum proteins and enzymes by starch gel electrophoresis. Proc. Soc. Exp. Biol. Med. **105:** 572.

LUNDIN, L. G. & A. C. ALLISON. 1966. Acid phosphatases from different organs and animal forms compared by starch gel electrophoresis. Acta Chem. Scand. **20:** 2579.

MAGIS, C. 1960. Variation de l'extractibilité des lipides de sérum. Influence de facteurs physiques, chimiques et génétiques. Thesis, Lanord., Faculty of Science, University of Paris, Paris, France.

MOSS, D. W., R. H. EATON, J. K. SMITH & L. G. WHITBY. 1966. Alteration in the electrophoretic mobility of alkaline phosphatases after treatment with neuraminidase. Biochem. J. **98:** 32 C.

POULIK, M. D. 1957. Starch gel electrophoresis in a discontinuous system of buffers. Nature **180:** 1477.

PRZELECKA, A., G. EJSMONT, M. G. SARZALA & M. TARACHA. 1962. Alkaline phosphatase activity and synthesis of intestinal phospholipids. J. Histochem. Cytochem. **10:** 596.

RAMOT, B. & C. STREIFLER. 1967. Serum and tissue acid α-naphthyl-phosphatase isozymes in various diseases. Israel J. Med. Sci. **3:** 505.

RENDEL, J. & B. GAHNE. 1963. Interaction between phosphatases and the J blood groups in cattle. Immunogenetics Letter **3:** 38.

RENDEL, J. & C. STORMONT. 1964. Variants of ovine alkaline phosphatase and their association with the R-O blood group. Proc. Soc. Exp. Biol. Med. **115:** 853.

ROBINSON, J. C. & J. E. PIERCE. 1964. Differential action of neuraminidase on human serum alkaline phosphatase. Nature **204:** 4957.

SHREFFLER, D. C. 1965. Genetic studies of blood group-associated variations in a human serum alkaline phosphatase. Amer. J. Hum. Genet. **17:** 71.
SHINODA, T. & E. MATSUNAGA. 1967. Serum alkaline phosphatase variants and their association with ABO blood groups in a Japanese sample. Jap. J. Hum. Genet. **12:** 170.
WALTER, H., S. NEUMANN, C. YANNISSIS & H. STEEGMÜLLER. 1967. Untersuchungen über die alkalischen serumphosphatasegruppen. Humangenetik **4:** 174.
ZOSCHKE, D. C. 1968. Human serum acid phosphatase and the ABO blood groups. M.S. Thesis. University of Hawaii, Honolulu, Hawaii.

DISCUSSION OF THE PAPER

S. POSEN: Does intestinal alkaline phosphatase, which is located in the microvilli of the epithelial cells of the small intestine, enter the circulation, particularly in humans of a particular blood group? Were falsely elevated acid phosphatase readings found in his Swedish group?

DR. BECKMAN: First of all, I don't know anything very precise about the mechanism or transport, but do suggest that one could try to investigate the possibility that it is the secretion. Secondly, yes I said that in measurements of phosphatase level at pH 5.0, you may have a breakthrough possibly of alkaline phosphatase in hyperactive sera. It's a possibility since, if you make two measurements—with and without tartrate—and you compute the tartrate-inhibitible and noninhibitible fractions you will find that the tartrate-inhibitible one is dependent on blood types being higher in AB and A. Alkaline phosphatase has a higher level in sera from B and O subjects, and it's possible that you have some contribution from the alkaline phosphatase even at pH 5.0. I don't know what a clinical chemist would say about that.

W. H. FISHMAN: Actually Dr. Beckman's very first report with Arfors included reference to the possibility that the acid phosphohydrolases were blood-type associated, and the evidence today certainly bears that out. We have just one or two points to mention. Our placental alkaline phosphatase seems to travel between the bone and intestinal regions and therefore is slower than yours. We can probably straighten this difference out between us later. Two of my colleagues have found in their work some association of blood type with intestinal alkaline phosphatase, on the one hand, and placental alkaline phosphatase on the other, and, with the Chairman's permission, I wonder if Dr. Stolbach would present his finding.

L. L. STOLBACH: We've had the opportunity to study the blood-group factors and secretor status in relation to the chyle. We didn't have to cannulate thoracic ducts because we were able to study 11 patients who had accumulated chylous effusions (either chylous pleural fluid or chylous ascites). Significant levels of L-phenylalanine-sensitive alkaline phosphatase were present in the chylous fluid of patients with blood groups A and patients who are nonsecretors. In TABLE 1, the first patient, MM, is a nonsecretor, and yet she had 54.2% of the alkaline phosphatase in the pleural fluid, which was inhibited by L-phenylalanine and presumably of intestinal origin. Patient J.B. had lymphosarcoma, and developed both chylous ascites and chylous pleural fluid, and, again, high levels of intestinal alkaline phosphatase are seen in the pleural fluid, somewhat lower levels in the ascites. This opinion was confirmed both by finding an intestinal band on starch gel electrophoresis and by the L-phenylalanine sensitivity of the fluids. There are four patients here who are type A blood group, and, again, there doesn't seem to be any significant effect of the blood group on whether or not the intestinal alkaline phosphatase is present in the chyle. The genetic factor seems to act not at the intestinal level, or at the absorption level, but somehow after the material gets into the circulation from the thoracic duct. TABLE 2 shows data on some additional patients, and, essentially, the information is pretty much the same. We have one more nonsecretor who had a somewhat lower level of L-phenylalanine-sensitive alkaline phosphatase to only 28 percent, but again we have two A's and an AB, and the percentage inhibition of L-phenylalanine was 84.0, 61.7 and 67.4%, respectively. In each case, the amount of L-phenylalanine-sensitive alkaline phosphatase was higher in the chylous fluid than it was in the serum of each patient.

DR. BECKMAN: There's one thing I would like to ask you. You're postulating that the change you may see in intestinal alkaline phosphatase from the slower to the fast moving. Do you intend to say that there could be a transfer of these so that the faster moving component of serum, will have addition by time from the slower moving?

W. A. BARDAWIL (*St. Margaret's Hospital, Boston, Mass.*): At the recent meeting of the American College of Obstetricians and Gynecologists, in Halifax, Dr. Fishman and I reported the results of our studies in collaboration with Drs. Halim G. Habib and Robert V. Dandrow (St. Margaret's Hospital) on serum placental alkaline phosphatase levels in 123 pregnant women. 76 of whom were considered normal. In this study, efforts were directed at correlating the major blood groups of these patients with serum enzyme levels. It was found that patients with blood groups A, B or AB had generally higher serum phosphatase levels than those with group O. Thus, patients of groups A, B or AB are distributed

TABLE 1

TOTAL ALKALINE PHOSPHATASE AND L-PHENYLALANINE-SENSITIVE ALKALINE PHOSPHATASE IN SERUM AND EFFUSION FLUID

Patient	Diagnosis	Blood Type	Secretor Status	Alk. Phos. (K. A. Un.)			
				Sample	TAP	LPSAP	% LPSAP
M.M.	Lymphosarcoma	O	N.S.	S	9.3	1.5	16.1
				P.F.	8.3	4.5	54.2
J.R.	Cirrhosis	A	S	S	8.9	1.6	18.0
				A	3.7	2.5	67.7
M.G.	Lymphosarcoma	A	S	S	24.4	1.2	14.8
				P.F.	7.4	2.2	40.7
L.L	Carcinoma of Stomach	A	S	S	104.1	16.8	16.1
				A	24.2	7.5	31.0
J.B.	Lymphosarcoma	A	N.S.	S	8.1	1.1	13.6
				P.F.	17.1	11.1	64.9
				A	7.6	3.5	46.1

A = ascites.
TAP = total alkaline phosphatase.
LPSAP = L-phenylalanine-sensitive alkaline phosphatase.
P.F. = pleural fluids.
S = serum.

TABLE 2

TOTAL ALKALINE PHOSPHATASE AND L-PHENYLALANINE-SENSITIVE ALKALINE PHOSPHATASE IN SERUM AND PLEURAL FLUID

Patient	Diagnosis	Blood Type	Secretor Status	Alk. Phos. (K. A. Un.)			
				Sample	TAP	LPSAP	% LPSAP
M.B.	Lymphosarcoma	O		S	8.0	0.9	11.2
				P.F.	5.4	2.7	50.0
H.T.*	Lymphosarcoma	O	NS	S	12.2	0.8	6.6
				P.F.	8.1	2.3	28.4
E.C.	Lymphosarcoma	A	S	S	15.3	1.7	11.1
				P.F.	16.0	10.7	66.8
G.B.	Giant Follicular Lymphoma (? Lymphosarcoma)	O		S	20.9	1.47	7.0
				P.F.	9.2	7.7	84.0
A.T.	Reticulum Cell Sarcoma	AB		S	8.3	1.8	21.7
				P.F.	12.5	7.7	61.7
A.G.	Breast Carcinoma	A	S	S	10.4	2.1	20.2
				P.F.	10.1	6.8	67.4

* Pleural fluid obtained seven days after serum.
S = serum.
P.F. = pleural fluid.
TAP = total alkaline phosphatase.
LPSAP = L-phenylalanine-sensitive alkaline phosphatase.
NS = nonsecretor; S = secretor.

more or less equally above and below the level of 40 units, which represents the mean of the highest serum placental alkaline phosphatase value at or near term (FIGURE 1). Two-thirds of those patients with type O fell below the mean level. The Rh factor seemed to bear no important relationship to the serum enzyme levels. In FIGURE 2 blood groups of the patients were plotted against the product of the specific activity (S.A. defined as concentration of the enzyme/of mg of tissue protein), multiplied by the placental weight in kg. It may be observed that 9 of 16 patients (A) and 5 of 10 patients (B and AB) fall above the arbitrary line of 14 as compared with only 2 of 24 patients with type O. These findings clearly indicate a remarkable difference in the serum alkaline phosphatase levels from type A, B or AB as compared with O. This variance is statistically significant, although the next experiment (FIGURE 3) might lead one to consider it as being purely of a quantitative, rather than a qualitative, nature. FIGURE 3 represents starch gel electrophoresis of placental homogenates (P) and serum (S) from two pregnant patients, one with blood group A whose blood serum alkaline phosphatase was high, and another with blood group O whose serum level was low. The placental homogenates revealed two equal bands as represented in the P column. The above findings support the contention that: (1) the maternal blood group has influence on the serum level of placental alkaline phosphatase;

MATERNAL BLOOD TYPE

Highest Serum Placental Alkaline Phosphatase Value	A +	A -	O +	O -	B +	B -	AB +	AB -
0 - 19			2					1
20 - 29	6	1	6	1	3	1		
30 - 39	4	2	14	2	2			
40 - 59	7	1	10	2	3			
60 and over	3	1	1	1	1	1		

FIGURE 1.

MATERNAL BLOOD TYPE

A Measure of Placental Isoenzyme Production S.A. x Pl. wt (KG)	A +	A -	O +	O -	B +	B -	AB +	AB -
0 - 6		1	10	3	2			
7 - 13	7	1	6	3	1		1	1
14 - 19	3	1	1	1	2	1		
20 and over	3				2			
TOTAL	13	3	17	7	7	1	1	1

FIGURE 2.

and (2) difference in serum levels is of quantitative rather than qualitative nature. It remains to be determined whether the blood groups are directly or indirectly associated genetically with the mechanism of synthesis of the isoenzyme, although in this instance one suspects not. This work is still in an early stage of development. Additional studies in progress, such as correlation of blood groups of the babies with both synthesis and maternal levels of serum alkaline phosphatase, may resolve these questions.

B. LEVINE (*Mount Sinai Hospital, New York, N. Y.*): We've also been interested in the relationship, demonstrated this morning, between the intestinal band, secretor status, blood type and the ingestion of food. These relationships were precisely what our studies showed. It was not just a matter of the intestinal band being present, but rather the ability to induce intestinal band in people in whose blood it was not present to begin with. That is, many of these cases on a fasting blood specimen failed to show the presence of intestinal band, but with the ingestion of liquid diet, you were able to induce a band. This we thought was significant. Not only that, but we were able to demonstrate that there's a qualitative relationship between the lipids given and the ability to induce an intestinal band. We don't have the details worked out yet, but there definitely is a qualita-

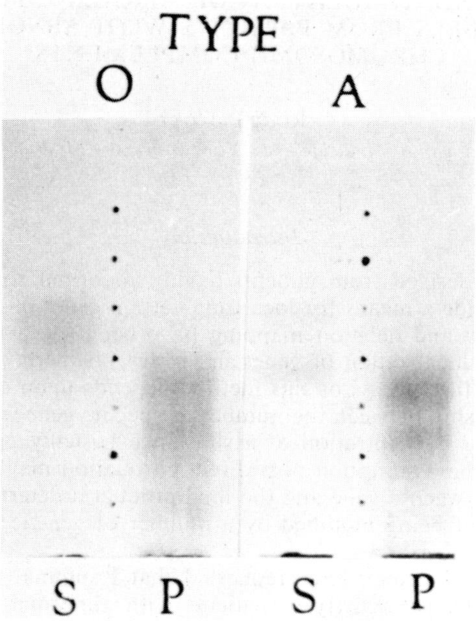

FIGURE 3.

tive difference. Some lipids cannot do this, while other lipids may. Also, there is a difference in the interval required for the intestinal band to appear. In addition, it is noteworthy that the intestinal band is much more prominent in the diabetic patient and that this, of course, may be related to abnormal metabolism. We, of course, understand now that any studies concerning the intestinal band should have baselines relating to the values in fasting blood specimens. Our particular interest is in the relationship between the secretor status and the ability to induce this intestinal band. The relationship of these factors to certain gynecologic malignancies and we hope that in the near future we'll have something to report.

DR. BECKMAN: Anyhow, I think this last comment is very fascinating because it brings in the relation between phosphohydrolases and lipids.

ACTIVITY AND REGULATION OF ALKALINE PHOSPHATASE IN CELLS FROM PATIENTS WITH ABNORMAL CHROMOSOME COMPLEMENTS*

Rody P. Cox†

Department of Medicine, New York University Medical Center
New York, N. Y.

Introduction

In theory, cells derived from patients having abnormal chromosome complements should provide a means for localizing certain genes on particular chromosomes. Duplication and deletion mapping have been successfully exploited for the definition and localization of genes in viruses,[1] bacteria[2] and certain higher forms.[3] However, the success of this method depends upon a reasonably simple and direct relationship between the number of specific gene replicas in a genome and the amount or concentration of a substance (usually protein) determined by the gene. But the assumption of a direct correlation may be incorrect, since the relationship between a gene and the final product it determines may be complex and capable of being modified by a number of genetic and environmental factors.

The conference chairmen have requested that I summarize the observations on alkaline phosphatase activity in patients with abnormal chromosome complements. I would like to do this with particular emphasis on the effect of gene dosage on enzyme activity and the problems that arise in getting clear-cut correlations.

One of the earliest attempts to associate a particular enzyme with a specific autosome in humans was in the suggestion that the gene determining alkaline phosphatase was located on chromosome number 21.[4-7] The basis for this hypothesis was the observation that the polymorphonuclear leukocyte alkaline phosphatase (LAP) *activity* seemed to vary with the number of chromosomes 21. For example, in chronic myelogenous leukemia, the alkaline phosphatase activity of leukocytes is reduced,[8] and in most cases, one chromosome 21—called the Philadelphia or Ph[1] chromosome—has a partial deletion of the long arm.[9,10] In contrast, polymorphonuclear leukocytes from patients with mongolism show an increased alkaline phosphatase activity.[4-7,11,12] This syndrome is characterized by the presence of an extra chromosome 21.[13]

Leukocyte Alkaline Phosphatase (LAP)

TABLE 1 summarizes data on LAP activity in normals and in patients with mongolism. It is apparent that in all of these studies LAP activity was greater in trisomic mongols than in controls. Although it is tempting to attribute the increased LAP activity in mongols to trisomy for chromosome 21, a simple gene-dose effect may not be the explanation. In two of the studies (TABLE 1), the enzyme activity ratio of mongol to control approached the expected 1.5, but in the other more extensive studies, the level of enzyme activity varied significantly from this predicted value. In one study,[11] 20 mongols out of a total of 200 had normal LAP. Chromosomal analysis on 18 of these 20 showed a typical trisomic

* Supported by grants GM 15508 of the U.S.P.H.S. and Research Contract U1296 of the Health Research Council of the City of New York.

† Career Scientist of the Health Research Council of the City of New York.

TABLE 1

COMPARISON OF LEUKOCYTE ALKALINE PHOSPHATASE ACTIVITY IN PATIENTS WITH MONGOLISM AND CONTROL SUBJECTS*

Study	Age of Patients	Mean Leucocyte Alkaline Phosphatase Activity† Trisomic Mongols	Trans-location Mongols	Chromosomal Analysis	References
Alter *et al.*	<10 $10>$	1.33 (41) 1.21 (17)	—	Not Done	4
Trubowitz *et al.*	12–50	1.50 (22 females)	—	Not Done	5
King *et al.*	6–46	1.22 (32 males) 1.22 (28 females)	—	Not Reported	6
Lennox *et al.*	—	1.44 (39)	—	Not Reported	7
O'Sullivan & Pryles	—	2.49 (124 males) 2.46 (76 females)	1.40 (3)	In Some Patients	11
Rosner *et al.*	—	2.37 (98)	0.95 (12)	In All Patients	12

* The units of measurement varied from one study to another. In most of these studies, the control population was matched for age, sex and race. In several studies, the control group comprised mentally defective patients from the same institution as the mongols. The numbers in parenthesis indicate the number of mongols studied.

† Leukocyte alkaline phosphatase activity is expressed as:

$$\frac{\text{mean alkaline phosphatase activity of mongols}}{\text{mean alkaline phosphatase activity of controls}}$$

mongol karyotype of 47 chromosomes including 5 small acrocentrics. Therefore, among trisomic mongols there appears to be heterogeneity with respect to elevated LAP. This heterogeneity might be expected since control of LAP activity per cell is known to be complex. Certain hormones, for example adrenal corticosteroids, are known to elevate LAP activity,[14] and increased enzyme activity is also associated with infection and other conditions in which leukocytosis occurs.[8] No correlation was found between the degree of leukocytosis, absolute neutrophil count, or the polymorphonuclear lobe count and the LAP activity in one of the studies reported in TABLE 1.[6] In translocation forms of mongolism, the LAP is either normal or only slightly elevated (TABLE 1). This finding does not exclude the possibility of a locus-determining alkaline phosphatase on chromosome 21, since it is well known that gene expression can be altered by translocation or by other position effects.[15]

Absence of a chromosome 21 would be expected to be accompanied by a decreased LAP, if this enzyme were determined by a locus on this autosome, and if a simple gene-dose relationship prevailed. Monosomy for an autosome is apparently incompatible with viability of the human fetus, since no instance of complete autosomal monosomy has yet been observed. However, two infants have been described with a mosaic chromosomal pattern showing most of the cells with only 45 chromosomes, and the missing chromosome was a member of the 21-22 group.[16,17] In one of these abnormal infants with absence of one of the G group chromosomes, the LAP was examined and found to be normal.[17]

As previously mentioned, LAP activity in chronic granulocytic leukemia is often very low, and this disease is accompanied by a small deletion in one of the chromosomes 21 (Ph^1 chromosome). However, several studies have clearly shown that, occasionally, chronic granulocytic leukemia with the Ph^1 chromosome may be associated with normal or increased activity of LAP.[18,19] Moreover, low LAP activity occurs at times in a variety of hematological and nonhematological diseases, as seen in TABLE 2.[20] In none of these diseases has a distinctive chromosomal abnormality been reported, nor has there been any morphological alteration reported in chromosome 21.

Aneuploidy involving chromosomes other than chromosome 21 have also been reported to alter LAP activity. Weber and his associates have described an elevated LAP in Klinefelter's syndrome.[21] Eight patients had an XXY chromosome complement, three were XXXY and one was XXYY. The LAP activities of these patients were compared to those of 24 mentally retarded controls (12 males and 12 females) closely matched in chronological and mental age. The results indicated that the mean LAP values of Klinefelter's were higher than those of controls. The increase over male controls was statistically significant, but that over female controls was not. These authors also found that the mean polymorphonuclear lobe count was low in Klinefelter's, and their results suggest a relationship between nuclear lobulation and the LAP activity in both Klinefelter patients and controls.

Alterations in Other Leukocyte Enzymes in Mongolism

If a locus on chromosome 21 determines either the structure or regulation of LAP, the elevation of this enzyme in mongolism would be expected to be relatively specific. However, as shown in TABLE 3, a number of other enzymes in whole blood, erythrocytes and leukocytes are also increased in mongolism. The elevation of leukocyte and erythrocyte glucose-6-phosphate dehydrogenase is of particular significance, since this enzyme is known to be determined by a gene located on the X chromosome. This multiplicity of increased enzyme activities in blood, leukocytes and erythrocytes, suggests that these alterations are not a direct consequence of the increase of structural genes resulting from trisomy for chromosome 21. Rather, some authors have attributed the increased enzyme activities to a general disorder of cellular metabolism. Leukocytes from patients with mongolism show certain morphological abnormalities,[25] a special liability to leukemic changes,[26] and a remarkable capacity for leukemoid reactions.[27]

Leukocyte life span or generation time in myelogenous leukemia is not shortened.[28] This suggests that the elevated white blood-cell count in myelogenous leukemia is not the result of increased cell proliferation, but is probably due to the accumulation of young leukocytes because of retarded cell maturation and

TABLE 2

LEUKOCYTE ALKALINE PHOSPHATASE ACTIVITY IN CHRONIC MYELOGENOUS LEUKEMIA AND OTHER HEMATOLOGICAL DISORDERS

Diseases	Number of Patients	Mean Leukocyte Alkaline Phosphatase Activity*	References
Chronic Myelocytic Leukemia	13	0.15	8
Paroxysmal Nocturnal Hemoglobinuria	7	0.22	20
Idiopathic Thrombocytopenic Purpura	7	0.38	20
Infectious Mononucleosis	24	0.67	20

* Leukocyte alkaline phosphatase activity is expressed as:

$$\frac{\text{mean alkaline phosphatase activity in disease}}{\text{mean alkaline phosphatase activity of normal controls}}.$$

Alkaline phosphatase activity was determined as milligrams of phosphorous liberated by 10^{10} neutrophils using as substrate beta-glycerophosphate at pH 9.9 for one hour incubation at 37° C.

TABLE 3

COMPARISON OF CELLULAR AND SERUM ENZYME ACTIVITIES* IN PATIENTS WITH MONGOLISM TO CONTROL SUBJECTS

Study	Number of Mongols Studied	Galactose-1-Phosphate Uridyl Transferase			Leukocyte Acid Phosphatase	Glucose-6-Phosphate Dehydrogenase		Leukocyte 5-Nucleotidase	Erythrocyte Phosphohexo-kinase	Refer-ences
		Leukocyte	Erythrocyte	Whole Blood		Leukocyte	Erythrocyte			
Mellman *et al.*	14	1.70			1.42	1.53				22
Rosner *et al.*										
Trisomic	98	2.42	1.59	1.73	1.85		2.44	3.08		12
Translocation	12	1.25	1.02	1.05	1.03		0.79	1.17		
Brandt *et al.*										
Trisomic	27			1.40						23
Translocation	2			1.21						
Baikie *et al.*	21								1.47	24

* Enzyme activity is expressed as: $\frac{\text{mean enzyme activity in mongols}}{\text{mean enzyme activity in controls}}$.

decreased cell destruction. It is known that the level and activity of certain intracellular enzymes in the red cell diminish with age,[29] and similar decreases might be expected in aging leukocytes. Therefore, the increased life span of leukemic leukocytes could explain the decrease in LAP and certain of the other metabolic abnormalities observed in leukocytes from patients with chronic myelogenous leukemia. On the other hand, cells with a shorter life span might have increased concentration of certain enzymes, particularly those enzymes with long half-lives. Thus, if the leukocytes of mongols were destroyed sooner than those of normals, the elevated LAP and other leukocyte enzymes found in mongols might be explained.[30,31] Measurement of the survival of granulocytes in patients with mongolism has produced conflicting results, one study showed a shortened survival[31] and in the other study the life span was found to be normal.[32]

Activity and Regulation of Alkaline Phosphatase in Skin Fibroblast Cultures From Patients With Aneuploidy

LAP activity is known to vary widely among normal subjects, and also to vary from one time to another in the same individual. Hormonal factors, "stress," infections and alterations in the age of cells can change the activity of LAP. Therefore, it seems desirable to study alkaline phosphatase activity and regulation *in vitro* where environmental factors can be carefully controlled and where feed back loops at the organismic level do not complicate interpretations. Tissue culture provides such a system where many of these factors can be controlled. Cultures of skin fibroblasts from mongols and from patients with other forms of aneuploidy can be studied and compared to euploid cells derived from normal subjects. TABLE 4 summarizes the results of two such studies.[33,34] The base-level alkaline phosphatase activity of skin fibroblasts from patients with trisomy 21, trisomy 18, trisomy D1, and XXY sex chromosome complement shows no significant differences from controls.

The findings in TABLE 1, and other evidence reviewed by King and her associates,[6] seem to indicate that there is no simple relationship between gene dose and LAP activity. King has postulated, therefore, that genes on chromosome 21, rather than determining the enzyme structure, may be involved in the regulation of alkaline phosphatase synthesis. To test this hypothesis, it seemed desirable to study alkaline phosphatase regulation in cell cultures derived from mongols and to compare them with normals. The alkaline phosphatase activity of most human-skin fibroblast strains can be increased manyfold by growth in medium containing a putative substrate of the enzyme,[36-39] while L-cysteine, an essential component of tissue culture medium, decreases the alkaline phosphatase activity of cells under either growth or maintenance conditions.[38,40] As seen in TABLE 4, the regulatory responses of skin strains derived from mongols and from patients with other types of aneuploidy are similar to those of diploid strains derived from normal donors. The findings in TABLE 4 indicate that neither an extra chromosome 21 nor other forms of aneuploidy affect either the level of alkaline phosphatase activity or its mode of regulation in skin cell cultures. The difference in regulatory response between alkaline phosphatase of skin fibroblast cultures and of leukocytes from trisomic mongols may be due to one or more of the following: (1) different isozymes of alkaline phosphatases occurring in different tissues with different control mechanisms; (2) tissue-specific variations in enzyme regulation; (3) cellular differences in genetic and environmental interactions that modify gene expression; (4) effect of tissue culture. With respect to the first possibility listed above, certain chemical and physical properties of

TABLE 4

COMPARISON OF ALKALINE PHOSPHATASE ACTIVITY IN SKIN FIBROBLAST CULTURES FROM EUPLOID AND ANEUPLOID SUBJECTS

Skin Cultures	Number of Patients	Alkaline Phosphatase Activity			References
		Base Level	With 2.0 mM cystine‡	With 2.0 mM phenyl-phosphate§	
Normal					
Nadler *et al.**	10	0.80 ± 0.10			33
Cox†	15	4.8 ± 2.8	2.1 ± 0.8	51.4 ± 8.1	34, 35
Trisomy 21					
Nadler *et al.**	5	0.81 ± 0.11			33
Cox†	4	4.6 ± 1.4	2.3 ± 0.6	53.0 ± 7.6	34, 35
Trisomy 18					
Nadler *et al.**	11	0.84 ± 0.12			33
Cox†	1	4.1 ± 0.8	2.6 ± 0.4	48.2 ± 9.1	35
Trisomy D_1					
Nadler *et al.**	4	0.83 ± 0.06			33
XXY					
Cox†	1	4.3 ± 1.2	1.8 ± 0.5	43.2 ± 8.8	35

* Nadler *et al*: Cultures were grown in medium F_{10} for seven days. Cells were harvested and then disrupted mechanically.[33] Enzyme activities are mean ± S.D. expressed as μmoles of *p*-nitrophenol formed per hr/mμg total protein.

† Cultures were grown in Waymouth's medium for seven to nine days. Cells were harvested and then lysed with 0.5% deoxycholate in 0.4% saline. Enzyme activities are means ± S.D. expressed as μmoles of *p*-nitrophenol formed per 30 min/μg cell protein. All experiments were done in duplicate. At least three different experiments were carried out on each fibroblast strain. Therefore, differences in specific enzyme activity between these studies probably are primarily due to differences in the efficiency of extracting the enzyme from cells. Deoxycholate lysis of cells is much more effective in liberating alkaline phosphatase than is mechanical disruption.[36]. Differences in medium and in methods of measuring alkaline phosphatase activity probably also contribute to the differences in specific activity observed in these two studies.[33,34]

‡ The cystine content of Waymouth's medium was increased from its usual concentration 0.5 mM to 2.0 mM. The cultures were harvested from seven to nine days later.

§ 2.0 mM phenylphosphate was added to Waymouth's medium, and the cultures were harvested from seven to nine days later.

alkaline phosphatases prepared from different tissues are known to be markedly different.[41]

Comparison of Chemical and Physical Properties and Mode of Regulation of Leukocyte and Skin Fibroblast Alkaline Phosphatase

TABLE 5 compares some of the chemical and physical properties of alkaline phosphatase preparations from leukocytes and skin fibroblast cell cultures. Both enzyme preparations were inhibited 50% by the same concentration of zinc and cysteine. Human-skin fibroblast alkaline phosphatase appears to require a higher concentration of histidine to produce an equal degree of inhibition than does the leukocyte enzyme. Unlike the inhibition observed with either the D or L form of cysteine and histidine, the L stereoisomers of phenylalanine and tryptophan are required to inhibit certain alkaline phosphatase prepartaions.[41] As seen in TABLE 5, LAP is more susceptible to inhibition by these L-amino acids than in the skin fibroblast enzyme. Fishman and his associates have pointed out the importance of these organ-specific differences in the response of various alkaline phosphatase preparations to L-phenylalanine as a means of characterizing the source of certain alkaline phosphatases.[42] The inhibition caused by L-tryptophan

TABLE 5

PHYSICAL AND CHEMICAL CHARACTERISTICS OF ALKALINE PHOSPHATASES PREPARED FROM HUMAN LEUKOCYTES AND HUMAN SKIN FIBROBLAST CULTURES

Source	Alkaline Phosphatase Specific Activity†	Inhibition Index*						
		Zinc pH 10.5	Cysteine pH 10.5	Histidine pH 10.5	L-Phenylalanine pH 10.5	L-Phenylalanine pH 9.0	L-Tryptophan pH 10.5	L-Tryptophan pH 9.0
Human Skin Fibroblasts	4.8	0.01	0.10	3.9	14.0	13.0	13.0	11.0
Human Leukocytes	182.6	0.01	0.12	2.0	8.5	7.0	6.0	5.5

* Inhibition index is the mean concentration of inhibitor in μmoles/ml required to produce a 50% inhibition of enzyme activity based on five separate experiments. Within an experiment, duplicate assays varied less than 10%. In different experiments in which enzyme preparations from the same source were used, the concentration of inhibitor required for 50% inhibition varied as much as 20%.

† Enzyme activities are expressed as μmoles of *p*-nitrophenol formed per 30 min/μg cell protein at 37° C.

appears to have a similar significance.[41] The electrophoretic mobilities and isozyme patterns of leukocyte and skin fibroblast alkaline phosphatases are also different, providing further evidence that these two proteins are different.[41] Because of these differences in the chemical and physical properties of alkaline phosphatases derived from human-skin fibroblast cultures and from human leukocytes, it seems probable that these two phosphatases are products of different genes. This speculation is also supported by their mode of induction. In skin fibroblasts, increased alkaline phosphatase activity is "induced" by putative substrates of the enzyme,* but not by glucocorticoid hormones.[36,37,39,43] On the other hand, human leukocyte alkaline phosphatase (LAP) activity is increased by glucocorticoid hormones.[14]

Studies on the Mechanism of Alterations in Alkaline Phosphatase Activity in HeLa Cell and in Human Leukocytes

Certain chemical and physical properties of LAP are similar to those of the HeLa cell enzyme, and their mode of induction is also the same.[41,44] Recent work on the mechanism of induction of increased alkaline phosphatase activity in HeLa cells by adrenal glucocorticoid hormones may, therefore, have relevance to changes in LAP activity. Studies of the kinetics of enzyme induction and the use of inhibitors of protein synthesis show that *de novo* protein synthesis is required for hydrocortisone induction of alkaline phosphatase in HeLa S_3 cell cultures.[45] However, there is neither an increased rate of alkaline phosphatase synthesis nor a hormone-mediated decrease in the catabolism of the enzyme, since both chemical and immunological methods show that, despite a 5 to 10-fold increase of enzyme activity in induced cells, the amount of alkaline phosphatase protein is about the same in induced, as in uninduced, cultures. Moreover, the physical and chemical properties of the induced enzyme differ from those of the base-level alkaline phosphatase with regard to speed and characteristics of elution from Sephadex G-200,[46,47] and in electrophoretic mobility when electrophoresis is carried out on starch gel using a high concentration of starch.[48] The previously reported[46] consistent differences in heat inactivation at 64.5° C between base-

* Current evidence indicates that substrate "induction" of alkaline phosphatase is probably, at least in part, substrate stabilization of the enzyme.[43]

level and induced alkaline phosphatase has not been reproduced in our recent experiments.[47] The base-level and induced enzyme, however, are similar with respect to certain other properties such as Michaelis constants and degree of inhibition by L-phenylalanine and L-tryptophan.[46] These findings suggest that prednisolone mediates a conformational change in alkaline phosphatase during its synthesis.[46,49] Such an alteration might lead to an increase in the number of catalytic sites or lowering of the energy level of the enzyme-substrate transition state. Maximal enzyme induction is not attained until the base-level enzyme has been replaced by enzyme synthesized in the presence of the hormone. The induction of glucocorticoid hormone of increased alkaline phosphatase activity in HeLa cell cultures, therefore, probably occurs at the level of protein synthesis (translation), and results in a steroid-mediated alteration in the conformational state of the enzyme.[46,49]

Somewhat analogous alterations in enzyme characteristics have been reported by Komma for glucose-6-phosphate dehydrogenase in *Drosophila,*[50] and by Endo and Schwartz for an esterase in maize.[51]

Bottomley and his associates have recently used similar methods to study LAP from normal subjects, patients with chronic granulocytic leukemia and reactive granuloycytosis.[52] Using an antiserum against a purified LAP prepared in rabbits, these authors showed that the enzyme from normal individuals, from patients with chronic myelogenous leukemia and from reactive granulocytosis is precipitated equally by antibody to normal LAP. Moreover, the antigen-antibody complexes of these three enzymes have *markedly different specific activities.* If one assumes that the ratio of antigen to antibody in the three types of enzyme-antibody complexes is approximately the same, then the finding of markedly different *specific* activities in the alkaline phosphatase from these three cell types suggests two possibilities: (1) that there are variable amounts of inactive alkaline phosphatase protein in these three types of leukoycytes that retain immunologic identity and dilute out the enzyme activity in the antigen-antibody complex, or (2) that in each condition, there is some alteration in the catalytic efficiency of the enzyme molecules, an alteration that does not change the immunologic reactivity but that does alter the specific enzymatic activity of the molecule. The decision between these possibilities rests upon the absence or presence of physical and chemical differences between these LAP's, and eventually upon purification of the enzyme to a point where primary, secondary and tertiary structure can be determined. The LAP's from these three groups of subjects were similar with respect to electrophoretic mobility, heat stability, kinetics of inhibition by L-phenylalanine, estimated molecular weight, immunological reactivity and apparent K_m for *p*-nitrophenyl phosphate.[52] Whether or not a relationship exists between hormonal induction of increased alkaline phosphatase activity in HeLa cells and alterations of LAP activity between cells from patients and from normal subjects is presently not clear. However, the striking similarities between the immunoprecipitation data obtained in these studies suggests that similar mechanisms could be involved in the control of alkaline phosphatase activity in these cell systems.

Conclusion

The level of LAP activity varies in a suggestively consistent manner in cells derived from patients with abnormal chromosome complements. In most mongols that are trisomic for chromosome 21, the LAP activity is increased; in many patients with chronic myelogenous leukemia, the LAP activity is reduced, and these subjects have a deletion of a portion of one chromosome 21 (Ph[1]). Although it is tempting to attribute these changes in LAP activity to a gene-dose effect for a locus-determining alkaline phosphatase on chromosome 21, the relationship is far from simple. A number of factors are known to alter LAP activity in normal subjects, and leukocytes of many patients with altered alkaline phosphatase activity also have striking changes in the activities of a number of other enzymes. When alkaline phosphatase levels and regulation are studied under carefully controlled conditions in a relatively simple system, such as skin fibroblast tissue cultures, the activity and regulation of the enzyme in aneuploid cells is similar to that observed in euploid strains. However, certain differences in the chemical and physical properties, and in the mode of regulation of alkaline phosphatases derived from leukocytes and from skin fibroblasts suggests that these two phosphatases may be products of different genes. Certain similarities between LAP and the HeLa cell enzyme in their chemical and physical properties, as well as in their mode of induction, suggest that studies on the control of the HeLa cell alkaline phosphatase may be important in understanding changes in LAP activity in a variety of aneuploid states. Evidence is discussed that supports this view.

As will be discussed in the following paper by M. J. Griffin and R. H. Bottomley, the base level activity of alkaline phosphatase in certain HeLa cell lines appears to correlate with the total number of group 21–22 chromosomes in these cells.[48,53] A clearer insight into the mechanism of the increased LAP observed in trisomic mongols probably could be obtained by immunologic studies on LAP from trisomic mongols similar to those reported by Bottomley and his associates using normal and leukemic leukocytes. On the basis of the evidence presented in this paper and in the one to follow, one can conclude that there may indeed be a complex gene-dose effect of chromosome 21 on human LAP activity that is modified by other genetic and environmental interactions. However, as yet the data are insufficient and too indirect to permit firm conclusions.

References

1. Benzer, S. 1955. Fine structure of a genetic region in bacteriophage. Proc. Nat. Acad. Sci. U.S.A. **41:** 344–354.
2. Ames, B. N. & P. E. Hartman. 1963. The histidine operon. Sympos. Quant. Biol. (Cold Spring Harbor) **28:** 349–356.
3. Muller, H. J. 1935. A viable two gene deficiency – phenotypically resembling the corresponding hypomorphic mutations. J. Hered. **26:** 469–478.
4. Alter, A. A., S. L. Lee, M. Pourfar & G. Dobkin. 1963. Studies of leukocyte alkaline phosphatase in mongolism: a possible chromosome marker. Blood **22:** 165–175.
5. Trubowitz, S., D. Kirman & B. Masek. 1962. The leukocyte alkaline phosphatase in mongolism. Lancet **2:** 486–487.
6. King, M. J., E. M. Gillis & A. G. Baikie. 1962. Alkaline-phosphatase activity of polymorphs in mongolism. Lancet **2:** 1302–1305.
7. Lennox, B., H. St C. White & J. Campbell. 1962. The polymorph alkaline phosphatase in mongolism. Lancet **2:** 991–992.
8. Valentine, W. N. & W. S. Beck. 1951. Biochemical studies on leukocytes. I. Phosphatase activity in health, leukocytosis and myelocytic leukemia. J. Lab. Clin. Med. **38:** 39–55.
9. Nowell, P. C. & D. A. Hungerford. 1960. Chromosome studies in normal and leukemic human leukocytes. J. Nat. Cancer Inst. **25:** 85–93.
10. Baikie, A. G., W. M. Court-Brown, K. E. Buckton, D. G. Harden, P. A. Jacobs & I. B. Tough. 1960. A possible specific chromosome abnormality in human chronic myeloid leukemia. Nature (London) **188:** 1165–1166.
11. O'Sullivan, M. A. & C. V. Pryles. 1963. A comparison of leukocyte alkaline phosphatase determination in 200 patients with mongolism and in 200 "familial" controls. New Eng. J. Med. **268:** 1168–1170.
12. Rosner, F., B. H. Ong, R. S. Paine & D. Mahanand. 1965. Biochemical differentiation of trisomic Down's syndrome (mongolism) from that due to translocation. New Eng. J. Med. **273:** 1356–1361.

13. LEJEUNE, J., M. GAUTIER & R. TURPIN. 1959. Étude des chromosomes somatique de neuf enfants mongoliens. C. R. Acad. Sci. (Paris) **248:** 1721–1722.
14. VALENTINE, W. N., J. H. FOLLETTE, D. H. SOLOMON & J. REYNOLDS. 1957. The relationship of leukocyte alkaline phosphatase to stress, to ACTH, and to adrenal 17-OH-corticosteroid. J. Lab. Clin. Med. **49:** 723–737.
15. DOBZHANSKY, T. 1936. Position effects on genes. Biol. Rev. **11:** 364–384.
16. LEJEUNE, J., R. BERGER & M. O. RÉTHORÉ. 1964. Monosomie partielle pour un petit acrocentrique. C. R. Acad. Sci. (Paris) **259:** 4187–4190.
17. REISMAN, L. E., S. KASAHARA, A. DARNELL, C. CHUNG & B. HALL. 1966. Antimongolism – Studies in an infant with a partial monosomy for the 21 chromosome. Lancet **1:** 394–397.
18. HEATH, C. W. JR. & W. C. MOLONEY. 1964. The Ph[1] chromosome in an unusual case of myeloproliferative disorder associated with high levels of leukocyte alkaline phosphatase activity. Hum. Chromosome Newsletter No. 12 : 14.
19. TEPLITZ, R. L., R. B. ROSEN & M. R. TEPLITZ. 1964. Granulocytic leukemia, Philadelphia chromosome, and leukocytic alkaline phosphatase. Lancet **2:** 418–419.
20. TANAKA, K. R., W. N. VALENTINE & R. E. FREDRICKS. 1960. Diseases or clinical conditions associated with low leukocyte alkaline phosphatase. New Eng. J. Med. **262:** 912–918.
21. WEBER, W. W., U. MITTWOCH & J. D. A. DELHANTY. 1965. Leukocyte alkaline phosphatase in Klinefelter's syndrome. J. Med. Genet. **2:** 112–115.
22. MELLMAN, W. J., F. A. OSKI, T. A. TEDESCO, A. MACIERA-COELHO & H. HARRIS. 1964. Leukocyte enzyme in Down's syndrome. Lancet **2:** 674–675.
23. BRANDT, N. J., A. FRØLAND, M. MIKKELSEN, A. NIELSEN & N. TOLSTRUP. 1963. Galactosaemia locus and the Down's syndrome chromosome. Lancet **2:** 700–703.
24. BAIKIE, A. G., P. B. LODER, G. C. GRUCHY & D. B. PITT. 1965. Phosphohexokinase activity of erythrocytes in mongolism – Another possible marker for chromosome 21. Lancet **1:** 412–414.
25. TURPIN, R. & G. BERNYER. 1947. De l' influence de l' hérédité sur la formule d' Arneth (Cas particulier du mongolisme). Rev. Hematol. **2:** 189–206.
26. HOLLAND, W. W., R. DOLL & C. CARTER. 1962. The mortality from leukemia and other cancers among patients with Down's syndrome (mongols) and among their parents. Brit. J. Cancer **16:** 177–186.
27. ENGEL, R. R., D. HAMMOND, D. V. EITZMAN, H. PEARSON & W. KRIVIT. 1964. Transient congenital leukemia in 7 infants with mongolism. J. Pediat. **65:** 303–305.
28. KILLMANN, S. A., E. P. CRONKITE, J. S. ROBERTSON, T. M. FLIEDNER & V. P. BOND. 1963. Estimation of phases of the life cycle of leukemic cells from labeling in human beings *in vivo* with tritiated thymidine. Lab Invest. **12:** 671–684.
29. HARRIS, J. W. 1963. *In* The Red Cell : 209. Cambridge, Mass.
30. HOOK, E. B. & R. R. ENGEL. 1964. Leukocyte life-span, leukocyte alkaline phosphatase and the 21st chromosome. Lancet **1:** 112.
31. MELLMAN, W. J., S. O. RAAB & F. A. OSKI. 1967. Abnormal granulocyte kinetics: an explanation for the atypical granulocyte enzyme activities observed in trisomy-21. *In* Mongolism. G. E. W. Wolstenholme & R. Porter, Eds. CIBA Foundation Study Group No. **25:** 77. Little, Brown and Co., Boston, Mass.
32. GALBRAITH, P. R. & L. S. VALBERG. 1966. Granulopoiesis in Down's syndrome. Pediatrics **37:** 108–110.
33. NADLER, H. L., T. INOUYE & D. Y. Y. HSIA. 1967. Enzymes in cultivated human fibroblasts derived from patients with autosomal trisomy syndromes. Amer. J. Hum. Genet. **19:** 94–99.
34. COX, R. P. 1965. Regulation of alkaline phosphatase in skin fibroblast cultures from patients with mongolism. Exp. Cell Res. **37:** 690–692.
35. COX, R. P. (Unpublished.)
36. COX, R. P. & C. M. MACLEOD. 1962. Alkaline phosphatase content and the effects of prednisolone on mammalian cells in culture. J. Gen. Physiol. **45:** 439–485.
37. COX, R. P. & G. PONTECORVO. 1961. Induction of alkaline phosphatase by substrates in established cultures of cells from individual human donors. Proc. Nat. Acad. Sci. U.S.A. **47:** 839–845.
38. COX, R. P. & C. M. MACLEOD. 1964. Regulation of alkaline phosphatase in human cell cultures. Sympos. Quant. Biol. (Cold Spring Harbor) **29:** 233–251.
39. MARTIN, G. M. 1964. Alkaline phosphatase of human skin fibroblast cultures II Kinetics of various "inductions." Exp. Molec. Path. **3:** 634–647.
40. COX, R. P. & C. M. MACLEOD. 1963. Repression of alkaline phosphatase in human cell cultures by cystine and cysteine. Proc. Nat. Acad. Sci. U.S.A. **49:** 504–510.

41. Cox, R. P. & M. J. Griffin. 1967. Alkaline phosphatase I Comparison of physical and chemical properties of enzyme preparations from mammalian cell cultures, various animal tissues and *Escherichia coli.* Arch. Biochem. **122:** 552–562.
42. Fishman, W. H., S. Green & N. I. Inglis. 1962. Organ-specific behavior exhibited by rat intestine and liver alkaline phosphatase. Biochim. Biophys. Acta **62:** 363–375.
43. Griffin, M. J. & R. P. Cox. 1967. Studies on the mechanism of substrate induction and L-cyst(e)ine repression of alkaline phosphatase in mammalian cell cultures. J. Cell Sci. **2:** 545–555.
44. Cox, R. P. & M. J. Griffin. 1968. Relations between the chemical and physical properties of mammalian alkaline phosphatase and its mode of regulation in cell culture and *in vivo.* Bull. N. Y. Acad. Med. **44:** 1109–1110.
45. Griffin, M. J. & R. P. Cox. 1966. Studies on the mechanism of hormonal induction of alkaline phosphatase in human cell cultures I. Effects of puromycin and actinomycin D. J. Cell. Biol. **29:** 1–9.
46. Griffin, M. J. & R. P. Cox. 1966. Studies on the mechanism of hormone induction of alkaline phosphatase in human cell cultures, II. Rate of enzyme synthesis and properties of base level and induced enzymes. Proc. Nat. Acad. Sci. U.S.A. **56:** 946–953.
47. Elson, N. & R. P. Cox. 1968. (Unpublished observation.)
48. Griffin, M. J. & R. H. Bottomley. 1969. Regulation of alkaline phosphatase in HeLa lines of differing modal chromosome number. Ann. N. Y. Acad. Sci. (This annal.)
49. Cox, R. P. & M. J. Griffin. 1967. Translational control of gene expression regulated by a hormone. Bull. N. Y. Acad. Med. **43:** 399.
50. Komma, D. J. 1968. Glucose 6-phosphate dehydrogenase in Drosophila: sexual effects on structure. Biochem. Genetics **1:** 337–346.
51. Endo, T. & D. Schwartz. 1966. Tissue-specific variations in the urea sensitivity of the E_1 esterase in maize. Genetics **54:** 233–239.
52. Bottomley, R. H., C. A. Lovit, R. Holt & M. J. Griffin. 1968. Purification & properties of alkaline phosphatase from normal and leukemic leukocytes. Clin. Res. **16:** 299.
53. DeCarli, L., J. J. Maio & F. Nuzzo. 1963. Alkaline phosphatase activity and chromosomal variation in human cells in culture. J. Nat. Cancer Inst. **31:** 1501–1509.

Discussion of the Paper

Dr. N. K. Ghosh: (*Brown University, Providence, R.I.*): If I remember correctly, the enzyme activity of the antigen-antibody complexes was entirely different from the antigen. Was it higher or lower than the original enzyme you used?

Dr. Cox: No, that's not true. This antibody precipitates the enzyme quantitatively, and all the activity can be recovered in the antigen-antibody complex.

Dr. Ghosh: But if you express the enzyme activity per milligram of protein, is the specific activity the same in the antigen activity complex?

Dr. Cox: No, it's markedly different.

Dr. Ghosh: Well is it lower or higher? I'd like to know.

Dr. Cox: Well, the control, of course, is very low, and the induced is high. The data are very similar between the leukocyte and HeLa cell situation, and I might add that the complex brings down a contaminating protein, but this contaminating protein constitutes probably no more than fifteen percent of the antigen-antibody complex, so that the antibody is pretty good for this kind of study.

R. H. Bottomley: I might mention some recent data we have on the leukocyte alkaline phosphatase. In addition to the antigen antibody results, we've also had some more purified enzyme which we've placed on a disc-gel electrophoresis and could show, even without the antigen-antibody precipitation, a marked difference in the specific activity of the enzyme from the three cell types, i.e., very low specific activity in the chronic ascitic leukemic leukocytes, a very high specific activity in the patients with either leukemoid reaction or reactive granulocytosis. These two methods seem to confirm this difference in specific activity.

REGULATION OF ALKALINE PHOSPHATASE IN HELA CLONES OF DIFFERING MODAL CHROMOSOME NUMBER*

M. J. Griffin and R. H. Bottomley

Cancer Section, Oklahoma Medical Research Foundation, and the Department of Biochemistry, University of Oklahoma School of Medicine, Oklahoma City, Okla.

Introduction

HeLa cells were originally isolated and adapted to cell culture from a case of squamous cell carcinoma of the cervix by Gey, Coffman and Kubichek,[1] and since then have been used for a variety of biochemical and cytological studies. Recent papers have described both an increase[2] and a decrease[3] in alkaline phosphatase upon the cultivation of "HeLa S_3" clones in monolayer culture with hydrocortisone. We have previously suggested a nomenclature for HeLa cell clones (variants) based on modal chromosome number.[4,5] In this system, the two "HeLa S_3" clones described above are named $HeLa_{65}$ and $HeLa_{75}$.

The present report deals with the biochemical characteristics and response to hydrocortisone of alkaline phosphatase from three clones that have major modal chromosome numbers, two being $HeLa_{65}$ and $HeLa_{75}$, and a third with high alkaline phosphatase activity, $HeLa_{71}$. One of the alkaline phosphatase isoenzymes of $HeLa_{71}$ is missing in preparations from cells cultured continuously with hydrocortisone. The isoenzyme pattern of the other two clones are very similar when obtained from cells in the control and the hydrocortisone-regulated states. Differences in the number and types of G group chromosomes are also present, and these differences might be related to alkaline phosphatase characteristics.

Methods

Cell Culture

Cells were grown in monolayer culture in MEM (Minimal Essential Medium, Eagle's) containing 10% calf serum, 50 U/ml penicillin, and 50 μg/ml each of streptomycin and kanamycin. Medium supplemented with 1.75 μg/ml hydrocortisone was used to grow cells in the hydrocortisone-regulated state (Hcr). Unless otherwise stated, cells had been maintained in the Hcr state with routine subculturing for at least two weeks before being used for studies.

Enzyme Preparation

Alkaline phosphatase was partially purified from cell cultures by a modification of Morton's procedure using *n*-butyl alcohol extraction.[6] The final purification of the enzyme after dialysis was approximately 25- to 40-fold from all three clones. The yield of enzyme using this method varied between 60 and 80 percent of the amount of activity present in a sonicated preparation.

Assay Techniques

Alkaline phosphatase was assayed as previously described[2] using *p*-nitrophenyl phosphate as substrate in 0.15 M Tris-HCl, pH 10.0. After an appropriate period,

* Supported in part by grant GB–6043 from the National Science Foundation and grants CA–10614 and CA–06420 from the National Cancer Institute, National Institutes of Health, Bethesda, Md.

the reaction was stopped with 1 ml of 0.25 N NaOH, and the O.D at 410 mμ was determined. Protein was estimated by the method of Lowry *et al.*[7]

Starch Gel Electrophoresis

Vertical starch gel electrophoresis was carried out at 22 ma constant current (5 to 6 volts/cm) for four to five hours at 4°.[8] Zones of alkaline phosphatase were developed directly on the starch gel slice at room temperature using Kaplow's histochemical staining method for alkaline phosphatase.[9]

Heat Stability Characteristics

A dialized, *n*-butyl alcohol enzyme preparation in 0.025 M Tris-HCl, pH 7.4 (200 to 400 μg/ml) was diluted with one volume of 1.0 M Tris-HCl, pH 10.2, and the pH (9.8) was checked before and after heating. The diluted enzyme was heated at 56 ± 0.5° C, and aliquots were removed at various times thereafter, immediately cooled in ice and heated samples were assayed for enzyme activity.

Methods of Chromosome Preparation

HeLa cells in the log growth phase were used for the preparation of chromosomes. After the addition of colcemid (0.4 μg/ml), the cells were incubated at

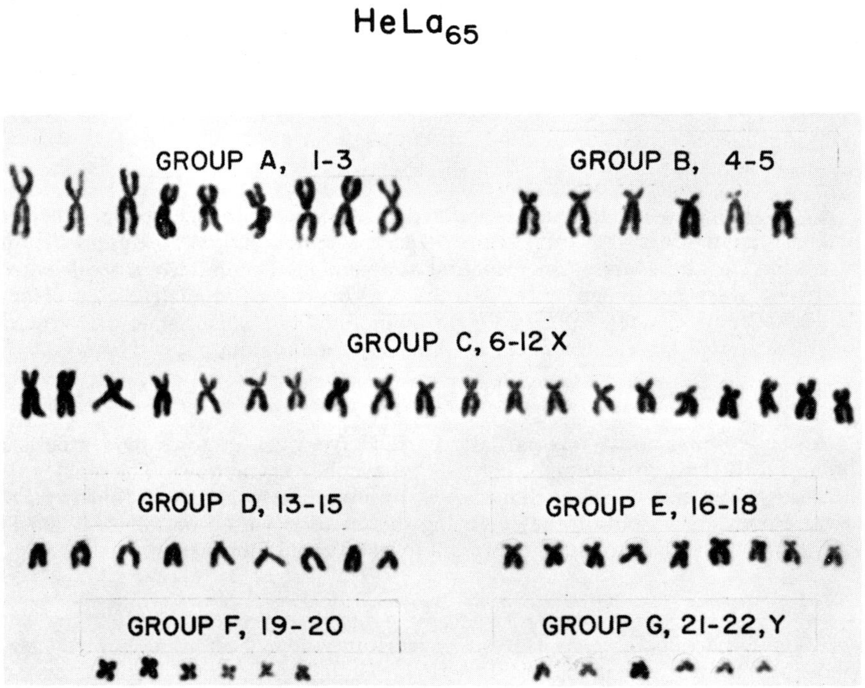

FIGURE 1. Karyogram of a representative cell from $HeLa_{65}$ using the Denver-London classification. Four group C chromosomes are missing in comparison with a theoretical triploid cell.

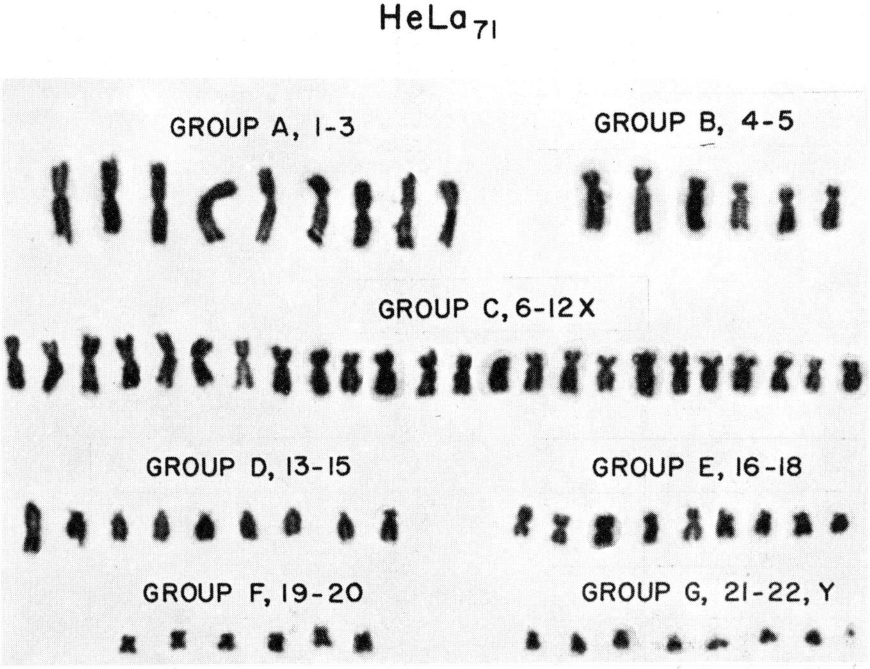

FIGURE 2. Karyogram of $HeLa_{71}$ arranged as in FIGURE 1. The two additional chromosomes greater than theoretical triploid are in group G, and one is small (minute).

37° for four hours, and chromosome spreads were prepared.[5] A minimum of 40 spreads from each preparation were examined under oil immersion, and each spread was counted twice. If the counts were not identical, the spread was recounted until consistent results were obtained. Representative spreads of the modal chromosome number from each preparation were photographed using an oil immersion lens (100×) on 4″ x 5″ Polaroid positive/negative film, type 55. After enlargement, the final magnification was 4000X. Karyotyping was carried out by cutting out the chromosomes and arranging them into groups according to the Denver classification.[10] Five karyotypes were made of each chromosome mode, and a representative karyotype is presented.

RESULTS

Karyology

The three clones studied exhibited a single major mode of chromosome number. $HeLa_{65}$ had a mode of 65 (in 77 out of 100 counted); $HeLa_{71}$ had a mode of 71 (65 of 100), and $HeLa_{75}$ had a mode of 75 (67 of 100). Chromosome analysis of cells adapted to cortisol for periods of up to six months show no change in the percentage of cells in the stemline.

Karyotypes were performed on five cells of the major modal chromosome number from each clone (FIGURES 1, 2 and 3 and TABLE 1). The karyotype of the cells from the major mode of $HeLa_{65}$ (FIGURE 1) has 4 chromosomes less than the human triploid number. This karyotype deviates from the normal triploid in group C (−4), but there are 6 normal-appearing G group chromosomes in this clone (FIGURE 1). $HeLa_{71}$ possesses two chromosomes more than human triploid, and its karyotype is illustrated in FIGURE 2. Both additional chromosomes are in group G, and one of them is abnormally small (henceforth designated as a minute chromosome). There are two abnormal chromosomes in group D, one with the long arms increased in length compared to other chromosomes in the same group,

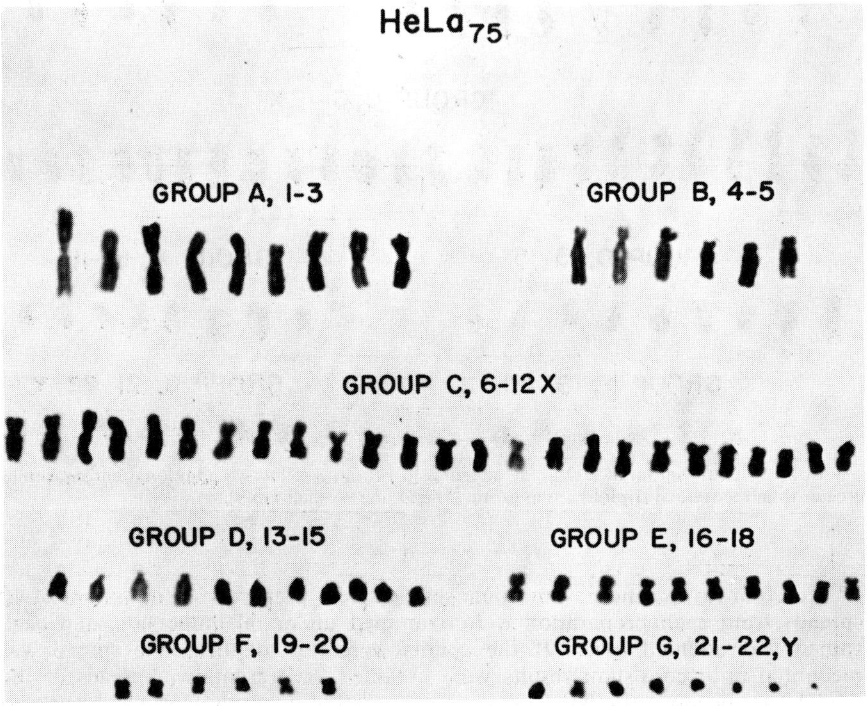

FIGURE 3. Karyogram of $HeLa_{75}$ arranged as in FIGURE 1. The extra chromosomes occur in group C (+1), group D (+2), group E (+1) and group G (+2). The latter group contains three minute chromosomes.

TABLE 1

KARYOTYPE VARIATIONS IN HELA CLONES

Group	$HeLa_{65}$					$HeLa_{71}$					$HeLa_{75}$				
A	9	9	9	9	9	9	9	9	9	9	9	10	9	9	9
B	6	6	6	6	6	6	6	6	6	6	6	8	6	6	7
C	21	20	20	21	20	21	24	20	24	24	27	24	24	25	22
D	9	9	9	8	9	12	9	12	9	9	9	10	11	11	14
E	9	9	9	9	9	9	9	10	9	9	10	9	11	10	9
F	5	6	6	6	6	6	6	6	6	6	6	6	6	6	6
G	6	6	6	6	6	8	8	8	8	8	8	8	8	8	8
Number of Chromosomes	65	65	65	65	65	71	71	71	71	71	75	75	75	75	75

TABLE 2

ALKALINE PHOSPHATASE SPECIFIC ACTIVITY OF CLONES IN CONTROL AND HCR STATES

Clone (State)	Alkaline Phosphatase*	Acid Phosphatase*‡	β-Glucuronidase†‡
$HeLa_{65}$	0.008	0.052	0.034
$HeLa_{65}$ Hcr	0.02	0.050	0.055
$HeLa_{71}$	0.64	0.045	0.025
$HeLa_{71}$ Hcr	0.23	0.063	0.032
$HeLa_{75}$	0.16	0.035	0.024
$HeLa_{75}$ Hcr	0.04	0.038	0.031

* Activities expressed as μmoles of *p*-nitrophenyl phosphate hydrolyzed/min/mg of protein.

† Activities expressed as μmoles of phenolphthalein glucuronide hydrolyzed/min/mg of protein.

‡ Assayed at pH 5.1 in 0.1 N acetate buffer using *p*-nitrophenyl phosphate and phenolphthalein glucuronide, respectively. Phenolphthalein color was developed with 0.2 N glycine buffer at pH 10.2, and the O.D. at 540 mμ was determined immediately.

and another "marker" chromosome with one arm longer than the other plus a secondary constriction toward the end of the longer arm. $HeLa_{75}$ has six chromosomes more than the human triploid number (FIGURE 3). Deviations from triploid are as follows: group C (+1); group D (+2); group E (+1); and group G (+2). Group G, however, contains five normal-appearing acrocentric chromosomes and three minute chromosomes (FIGURE 3).

As TABLE 1 shows, some variation in karyotype has been found within the major mode of these three clones. However, almost all the variation occurs in groups C, D and E, the groups whose similarities result in difficulty of chromosome position assignment. Moreover, the G groups that are compared below, seem to be a constant set and, thus, representative of the clone.

Alkaline Phosphatase

TABLE 2 shows the alkaline phosphatase specific activity of all three clones in the control state and of the clones cultured continuously with added hydrocortisone (Hcr). The enzyme value for cells grown in control medium varies from 0.008 in $HeLa_{65}$ to 0.64 for $HeLa_{71}$, a 75-fold range. The activity in the Hcr state is decreased in $HeLa_{71}$ Hcr, and in $HeLa_{75}$ Hcr, but is increased in $HeLa_{65}$ Hcr. The steady-state Hcr alkaline phosphatase levels were obtained from cells cultured at least two weeks with hydrocortisone. As TABLE 2 indicates, two other enzymes – acid phosphatase and β-glucuronidase – showed little variation from clone to clone or from state to state. FIGURE 4 illustrates the kinetics of change in alkaline phosphatase specific activity for these three HeLa clones. Although $HeLa_{71}$ and $HeLa_{75}$ both have decreased levels of alkaline phosphatase activity in the Hcr state, the latter decreases within 50 hours to its new minimum value, whereas $HeLa_{71}$ undergoes an initial increase in activity for the first 75 hours and then falls to a new steady-state level after seven days (FIGURE 4). $HeLa_{65}$, on the other hand, shows a persistent five- to six-fold elevation in alkaline phosphatase in the Hcr state, and this level is reached by 75 hours.

The phosphatase preparations possessed two extremes of heat stability at 56° C, pH 9.8 (FIGURE 5). $HeLa_{75}$, with three minute G group chromosomes, produces an alkaline phosphatase that is completely inactivated by heating at 56° C for 20 minutes. $HeLa_{75}$ Hcr has 20% of its alkaline phosphatase activity stable to heat at 56° C. The alkaline phosphatase enzyme preparations from the other two clones, whether from cells in the control or Hcr state, have much more complex heat kinetics at 56° C, but generally can be described as almost completely heat stable for at least four hours. This experiment has been repeated twice, and each time some activity was apparently lost and regained in $HeLa_{65}$ and $HeLa_{71}$, both in control and Hcr states.

The starch gel electrophoretic pattern of histochemically stained alkaline phosphatase from the three clones in both the control and Hcr states are illustrated in FIGURE 6. $HeLa_{65}$ had activity in a fast-moving anodal band (isoenzyme) and also a closely spaced triplet near the origin. Little activity can be seen between these groups. $HeLa_{71}$ had a somewhat similarly appearing electrophoretic pattern with an additional very fast anodally moving isoenzyme, which appears as a weak band in both $HeLa_{71}$ and $HeLa_{65}$ (25 mm from the origin). $HeLa_{75}$ has most of its activity in two bands near the origin (3 to 5 mm from the origin) with no appreciable activity in the area of the highly active anodal isoenzyme (20 mm from the origin) seen in the other two clones. In $HeLa_{65}$ and $HeLa_{71}$, growth with hydrocortisone results in the disappearance of the fastest moving isoenzyme (25 mm from the origin—FIGURE 7).

The different isoenzymes could be due to variations in the sialic acid residues

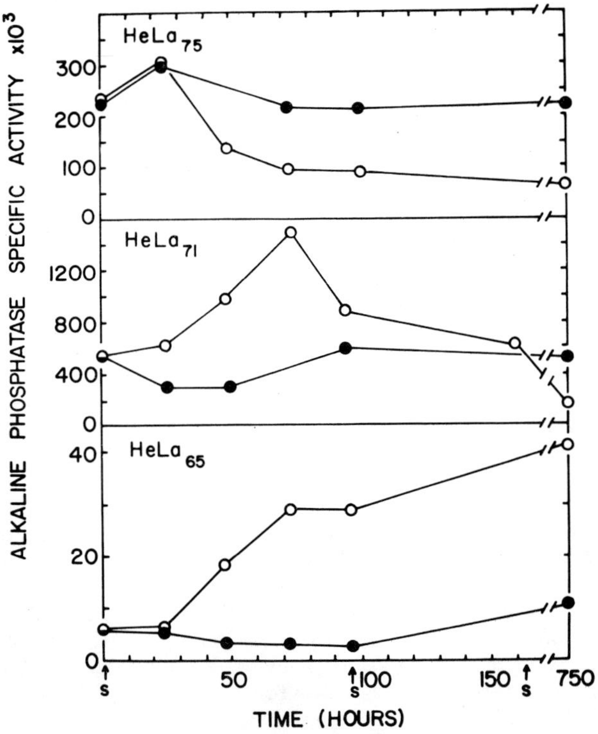

FIGURE 4. The kinetics of hydrocortisone regulation of alkaline phosphatase in three HeLa clones. Open circles represent cultures containing hydrocortisone; closed circles are controls. Replicate cultures were sacrificed near confluency, and subculturing (S) was performed on confluent cultures using the standard procedure of treatment with EDTA (0.7 mM) and versine (0.025%). Alkaline phosphatase specific activity is μmoles p-nitrophenyl phosphate hydrolyzed/min/mg of total culture protein in a sodium deoxycholate cell lysate.

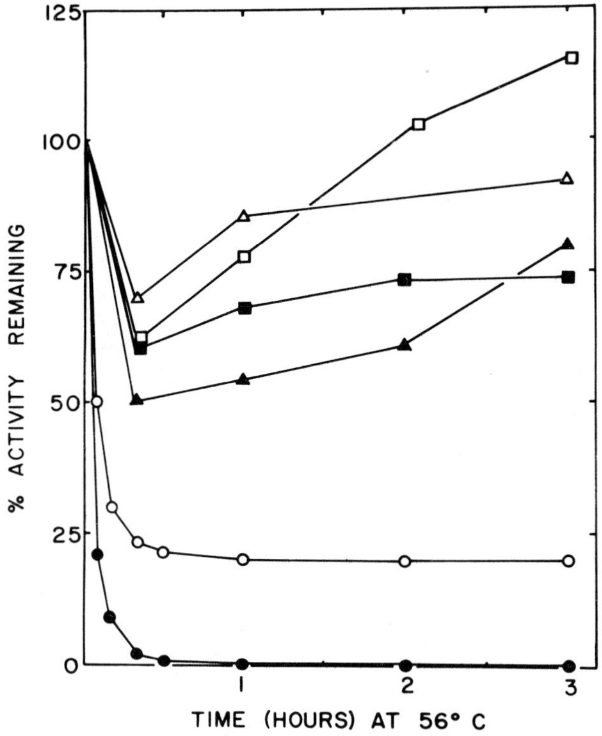

FIGURE 5. Kinetics of heat inactivation of *n*-butyl alcohol lysates of three HeLa clones performed at pH 9.8 and 56.0 ± 0.5° C. $HeLa_{75}$ is designated by -●-●-; $HeLa_{75}$ Hcr, -○-○-; $HeLa_{71}$ control, -▲-▲-; $HeLa_{71}$ Hcr, -△-△-; $HeLa_{65}$ control, -■-■-; $HeLa_{65}$ Hcr, -□-□-.

of a single phosphatase protein. That this is not the case is shown by FIGURE 8. *Clostridium perfingens* neuraminidase (NANAase) treatment retarded all anodally migrating alkaline phosphatase isoenzymes an equivalent percentage of their total migration distance, suggesting the presence of at least one enzymatically hydrolyzable sialic acid residue for all the alkaline phosphatase enzyme molecules.

The variation in enzyme activity in $HeLa_{71}$ through the adaptation period and into the new steady-state period of continuous growth with hydrocortisone (Hcr) is probably due to variation in the specific activities of the individual isoenzyme molecules. FIGURE 9 illustrates a polyacrylamide disc-gel electrophoretogram of *n*-butyl alcohol extracts of control cells (C), cells grown with hydrocortisone for 72 hours (I), and cells cultured continuously with hydrocortisone (H). The left gel of each pair (AP) illustrates the variation in alkaline phosphatase activity from C (medium) through I (intense) to H (low). The protein-stained gel to the right of each pair (labeled P) shows similarly appearing weak protein bands for the main isoenzymes plus a faster moving "contaminant" protein that has no phosphatase activity.

The new isoenzyme, which appears in $HeLa_{71}$ Hcr, midway between the other main bands (about 11 mm from the origin, FIGURE 6), is not simply a function of growing cells with hydrocortisone, but rather is probably a function of the

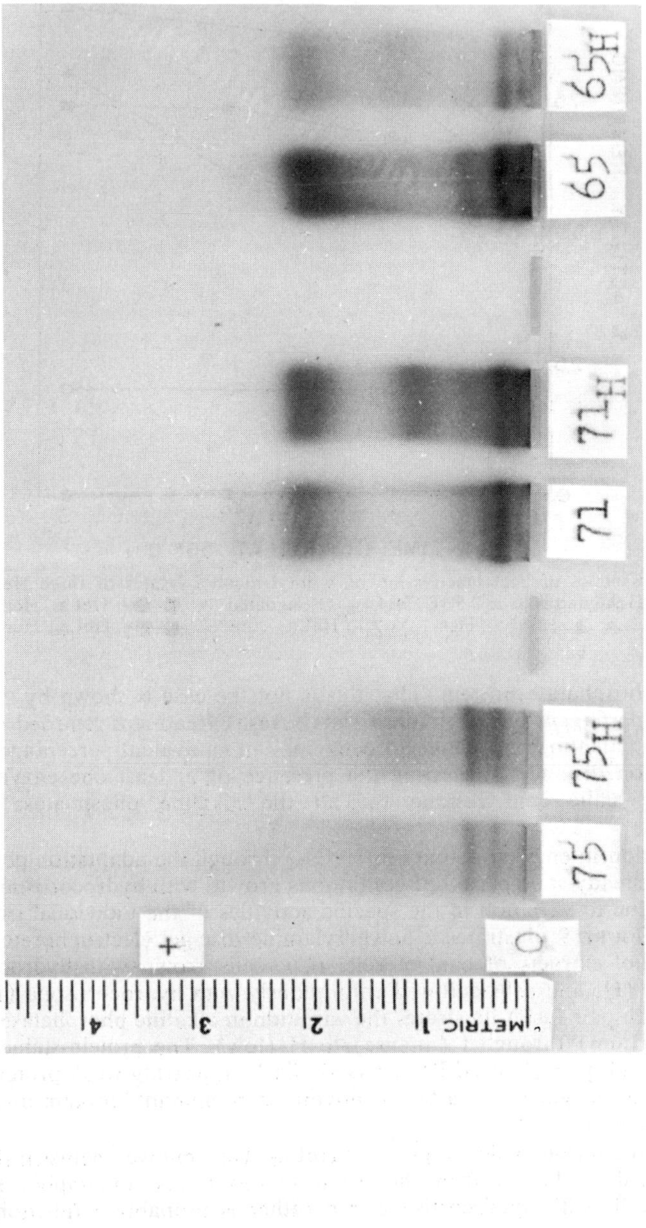

FIGURE 6. Starch gel electrophoretogram of *n*-butyl alcohol lysates of three HeLa clones stained for alkaline phosphatase activity at pH 10.0 with α-naphthyl phosphate as substrate and Fast Blue BB as coupling dye. The H to the lower right of the modal number designation indicates that cells were cultured continuously with hydrocortisone (Hcr state). Controls are un-numbered and to the left. Direction of migration is toward the top.

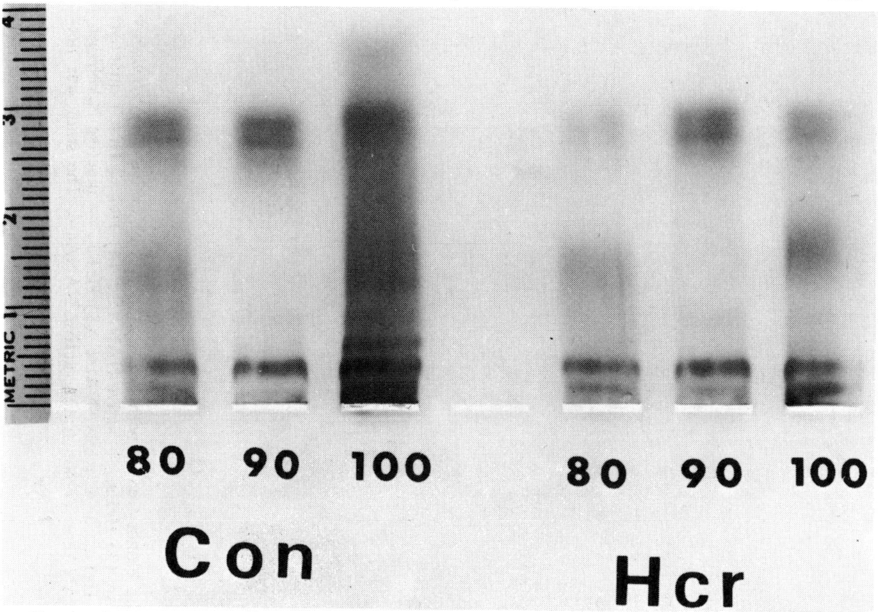

FIGURE 7. Starch gel electrophoretogram of *n*-butyl alcohol lysates of $HeLa_{71}$ cells in the control (Con) and hydrocortisone-regulated (Hcr) states stained for alkaline phosphatase as in FIGURE 6. The numbers refer to the percent of the glass surface that was covered by the cells as estimated by inspection of the monolayer with a Unitron binocular phase-contrast inverted microscope. From cell counting, these confluency estimates represent 4.0×10^5 cells/ml for control 80%, 4.5×10^5 cells/ml for control 90%, and 5×10^5 cells/ml for control 100%. Hcr 80% represents about 3.0×10^5 cells/ml; 90%, about 3.5×10^5 cells/ml; and 100%, about 4.0×10^5 cells/ml. Direction of migration is toward the top (anode).

state of confluency of the cell culture. FIGURE 7 shows three isoenzyme patterns from $HeLa_{71}$ cells in the control state and in the Hcr state. As shown, when the cell monolayer was 80% confluent, both control and Hcr cultures contain appreciable amounts of the isoenzyme 11 mm from the origin. This species is absent in extracts from both type cultures when the cells have covered 90 to 95% of the available surface, but the isoenzyme reappears in completely confluent cultures when little or no glass surface is available for growth. Nevertheless, all control cultures possess the fastest moving isoenzyme, while the Hcr cultures do not.

DISCUSSION

The method of classifying HeLa clones employed in this study, although an improvement over previous nomenclature, is still not completely descriptive. Theoretically, several karyotypes may exist with the same modal chromosome number and, thus, an abbreviated notation of karyotype also should be included in HeLa clonal classification. Moreover, gene mutation within a given karyotype could produce a mutant clone with identical karyotypes, although proving this for human aneuploid clones will be difficult.[11] Our observations on the base level activity of alkaline phosphatase in HeLa clones are in agreement with a previous report[12] that showed a nonlinear gene-dose response of alkaline phosphatase to G group chromosome number in the EUE cell strain. Thus, $HeLa_{65}$ has six G

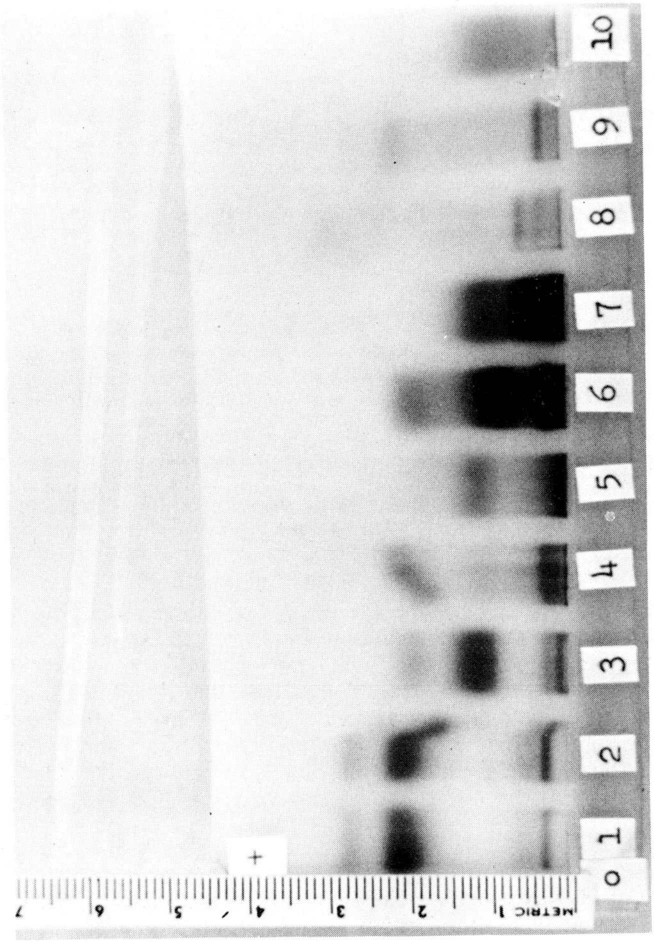

FIGURE 8. Starch gel electrophoretogram of alkaline phosphatase from various HeLa clones treated with heat-inactivated or active *C. perfringens* neuraminidase. Positions listed as follows: (1) $HeLa_{71}$, (2) $HeLa_{71}$ + inactive NANAase, (3) $HeLa_{71}$ + active NANAase, (4) $HeLa_{71}$ Hcr + inactive NANAase, (5) $HeLa_{71}$ Hcr + active NANAase, (6) $HeLa_{65}$ + inactive NANAase, (7) $HeLa_{65}$ + active NANAase, (8) $HeLa_{75}$ + inactive NANAase, (9) $HeLa_{75}$ + active NANAase, and (10) rat kidney alkaline phophatase + active NANAase, demonstrating active NANAase. The stain was performed as in FIGURE 6, and the direction of migration is toward the top.

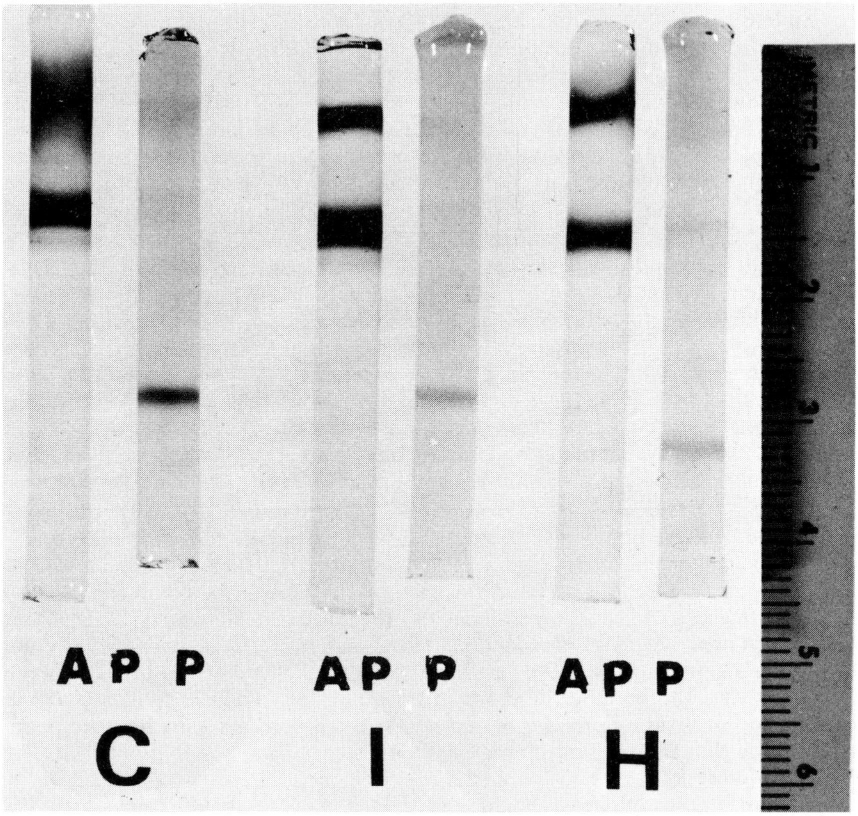

FIGURE 9. Polyacrylamide disc-gel electrophoretogram of *n*-butyl alcohol lysates of $HeLa_{71}$ cells in the control state (C), in the state 72 hours after the cells first received hydrocortisone (intermediate state-I), and in the Hcr state (H). The gels to the left of each pair were stained for alkaline phosphatase as in FIGURE 6 (labeled AP), whereas the gels to the right of each set were stained for protein with Amido-Schwartz and destained electrophoretically (labeled P). The direction of migration at pH 8.8 was from the top toward the bottom (anode).

chromosomes and 1/100 the activity of $HeLa_{71}$ with eight G chromosomes.* Moreover, in general, these HeLa clones respond to hydrocortisone as Maio and DeCarli have reported for EUE cells,[13] namely the clones with lower chromosome number and lower enzyme activity have increased phosphatase activity when cultured in medium containing hydrocortisone. Furthermore, the present study indicates that HeLa clones with greater than triploid number of G group chromosomes eventually have decreased alkaline phosphatase levels in response to hydrocortisone.

This study also suggests that the type of G group chromosomes may have an effect on the type of alkaline phosphatase isoenzyme produced. The phosphatase enzyme from the clone with three minute chromosomes ($HeLa_{75}$) was qualitatively different from the other two clones in three respects: (a) a rapid initial decrease in enzyme activity upon cultivation of the cells with hydrocortisone;

* Since one of the additional chromosomes is a minute one, the 100-fold increase may be due to one additional normal acrocentric chromosome.

(b) an enzyme that was 100% heat labile from control cells and 80% heat labile from Hcr compared to heat-stable enzyme from the other two clones; and (c) an isoenzyme pattern on starch gel electrophoresis that had little or no major anodally moving band, unlike the other two clones. Whether the alkaline phosphatase from $HeLa_{75}$ represents a molecule altered by the presence of regulatory subunits produced by the minute chromosomes, or represents some alteration of the phosphatase molecule in its primary, secondary or tertiary structure, cannot be stated at this time.

$HeLa_{65}$ and $HeLa_{71}$ have different alkaline phosphatase kinetic responses to growth with hydrocortisone (FIGURE 4). $HeLa_{65}$ has an increased alkaline phosphatase activity that is maximal at 72 hours and remains elevated thereafter. $HeLa_{71}$ shows an initial increase in enzyme activity when grown with hydrocortisone, reaching a maximum value at 72 to 96 hours, after which the activity falls below the control level. In this respect, $HeLa_{71}$ is similar to $HeLa_{75}$ (the other minute G group-carrying clone) in that the long term result of cultivation with cortisol is to decrease total phosphatase activity. The delayed decrease in activity in $HeLa_{71}$ as compared to $HeLa_{75}$ may be a balanced response to number and type of G group chromosomes, but this must be tested in other HeLa clones.

It appears that conditions of culture affect the isoenzyme pattern of (especially) $HeLa_{71}$. At or near confluency, the isoenzyme 11 mm from the origin disappears, only to reappear again after the cell monolayer is completely confluent (24 hours later). The disappearance of this isoenzyme could be due to a block in the cell cycle near confluency with collection of most cells in either the G_1 or G_2 phases of the cell cycle. Cells in either phase of the cycle may not have this isoenzyme. On the other hand, a strengthening of the bond between this isoenzyme and its subcellular site in cells cultured in nearly confluent monolayers may result in differential extraction of the isoenzymes. Finally, the possibility exists that this isoenzyme may be converted to one of the other forms by medium deficiencies after 72 hours in culture, and this might also explain its reappearance after 96 hours, when further nutritional deficiencies might be present.

$HeLa_{65}$ and $HeLa_{71}$ have a similar qualitative response of alkaline phosphatase isoenzymes when cultured with hydrocortisone, in that the rapidly migrating isoenzyme disappears in both clones. This may be due to a decrease in the activity of the weakly staining phosphatase below the level detectable on starch gel. Moreover, the evidence obtained with polyacrylamide disc-gel electrophoresis indicates that cells cultured with hydrocortisone contain alkaline phosphatase isoenzymes with altered activities rather than varying amounts of the phosphatase protein, each possessing activities the same as the isoenzyme in the control cell.

The present data show a multiplicity of phosphatase proteins in both $HeLa_{71}$ and $HeLa_{65}$, and suggest that the molecular regulation of alkaline phosphatase in cells cultured with hydrocortisone results from alterations in the enzyme activities of the isoenzyme by apoenzyme-holoenzyme conversion or conformational changes. This is in agreement with results using radio-tracer and immunochemical techniques on the mechanism of induction of this enzyme in $HeLa_{65}$ cells.[14] The cellular significance of the various modes of alkaline phosphatase regulation in these HeLa clones will be better understood when the physiological functions of these enzymes are elaborated.

The effect of the karyotypic variation in the three clones of HeLa cells on the regulation of alkaline phosphatase cannot be explained at the present time, but the data presented do suggest that karyotypic variations may have more subtle effects on the control of alkaline phosphatase than would be expected from a simple gene-dose relationship. We feel that the study of the influence of karyotypic variation on the control of enzyme activity may give some insight into possible action mechanisms of chromosomal control of cellular function.

SUMMARY

The alkaline phosphatase enzymes from three HeLa clones of differing modal chromosome number have been studied. Each clone has greater than 63% of the cells demonstrating the modal chromosome number, and this stemline number is used as a subscript to identify each clone. The modal chromosome numbers of all three clones were stable during six months of continuous subculturing. In two clones ($HeLa_{71}$ and $HeLa_{75}$), the total alkaline phosphatase activity is eventually decreased in the hydrocortisone-regulated state, but one of the two clones ($HeLa_{71}$) evidences an initial increase in total enzyme activity while adapting to hydrocortisone. Growth of the third clone ($HeLa_{65}$) in the presence of added hydrocortisone results in a cell population that continuously shows an elevated enzyme activity. Chromosome analysis of cells adapted to hydrocortisone showed no change in the percentage of cells in the stemline. Polyacrylamide disc-gel electrophoresis indicates that cells cultured with hydrocortisone contain alkaline phosphatase isoenzymes with altered enzyme activities rather than varying amounts of the phosphatase proteins. When cells are grown without added hydrocortisone, the two clones with the greater number of G group chromosomes (eight total G chromosomes in $HeLa_{71}$ and $HeLa_{75}$) possess the highest enzyme activity, but the one that possesses three minute G group chromosomes ($HeLa_{75}$) has less activity than the other clone with only one such chromosome. Moreover, the clone with three minute G group chromosomes has a set of alkaline phosphatase proteins that are different from the enzymes of the other two clones in their early kinetic response to hydrocortisone (decrease), heat stability (labile at 56° C) and isoenzyme pattern on starch gel electrophoresis.

ACKNOWLEDGMENTS

We wish to acknowledge the technical assistance of A. L. Trainer, J. A. Page and C. L. Lovig.

REFERENCES

1. GEY, G. W., W. D. COFFMAN & M. T. KUBICHEK. 1952. Tissue culture studies of the proliferative capacity of cervical carcinoma and normal epithelium. Cancer Res. **12:** 264.
2. GRIFFIN, M. J. & R. P. COX. 1966. Studies on the mechanism of hormonal induction of alkaline phosphatase in human cell cultures. I. Effects of puromycin and actinomycin-D. J. Cell Biol. **29:** 1.
3. MELNYKOVICH, G., C. F. BISHOP & M. B. A. SWAYZE. 1967. Fluctuation of alkaline phosphatase activity in synchronized heteroploid cell cultures: Effects of prednisolone. J. Cell Physiol. **70:** 231.
4. GRIFFIN, M. J., J. A. PAGE, A. L. TRAINER & R. H. BOTTOMLEY. 1968. Hydrocortisone regulation of alkaline phosphatase in HeLa clones with differing modal chromosome numbers. Fed. Proc. **27:** 403.
5. BOTTOMLEY, R. H., A. L. TRAINER & M. J. GRIFFIN. 1969. Enzymatic and chromosomal characterization of HeLa variants. J. Cell Biol. **41:** 806.
6. MORTON, R. K. 1954. The purification of alkaline phosphatase of animal tissues. Biochem. J. **57:** 595.
7. LOWRY, O. H., N. J. ROSEBOROUGH, A. L. FARR & R. J. RANDALL. 1951. Protein measurement with the folin phenol reagent. J. Biol. Chem. **193:** 265.
8. COX, R. P. & M. J. GRIFFIN. 1967. Alkaline phosphatase. I. Comparison of the physical and chemical properties of enzyme preparations from mammalian cell cultures, various animal tissues, and *Escherichia coli*. Arch. Biochem. **122:** 552.

9. KAPLOW, L. 1955. A histochemical procedure for localizing and evaluating leukocyte alkaline phosphatase activity in smears of blood and marrow. Blood **10:** 1023.
10. HUMAN CHROMOSOME STUDY GROUP. 1960. A proposed standard system of nomenclature of human mitotic chromosomes. J. Hered. **51:** 214.
11. HSU, T. C. 1961. Chromosomal evolution in cell populations. Int. Rev. Cytol. **12:** 69.
12. SANTACHIARA-BENERECETTI, S. A., I. CESARI & L. DECARLI. 1967. Some properties of alkaline phosphatase from a human cell strain and from a clonal derivative with low activity. J. Cell Physiol. **69:** 169.
13. MAIO, J. J. & L. DECARLI. 1963. Induction and repression of alkaline phosphatase in human cultured cells by prednisolone, hydrocortisone, and organic monophosphate. Biochem. Biophys. Res. Comm. **11:** 335.
14. GRIFFIN, M. J. & R. P. COX. 1966. Studies on the mechanism of hormone induction of alkaline phosphatase in human cell cultures. II. Rate of enzyme synthesis and properties of base level and induced enzymes. Proc. Nat. Acad. Sci. U.S.A. **56:** 946.

DISCUSSION OF THE PAPER

DR. BECKMAN: We have been trying to study isozymes in different heteroploid cell lines, and we found it rather difficult because in different cell lines one can find many different components. FIGURE 1 shows alkaline phosphatase isozymes in an amnion line called RA which was studied by James Regan and myself. You can see two main components here, called A and B. Samples number 1 and 2 are standard cultures that have both components. Number 3 is a clone and number 4 shows the pattern that we regularly found after a cortisone treatment. After cortisone treatment, one component disappears and the other becomes stronger.

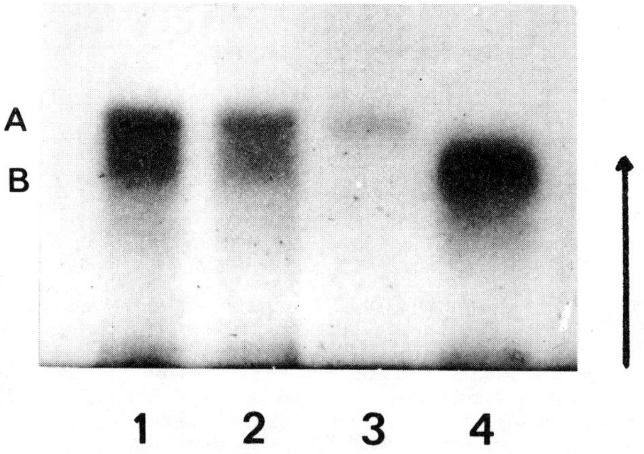

FIGURE 1. Starch gel electrophoresis at pH 8.6 showing variations in alkaline phosphatase isozymes of the RA amnion line. 1 = cells derived from survivors of 800 r; 2 = untreated culture; 3 = subcloning of RA; and 4 = cortisone-treated cells. The arrow points toward the anode. (Reproduced, with permission of the publisher and the authors, from Beckman, L. & J. D. Regan. 1964. Isozyme studies of some human cell lines. Acta Path. Microbiol. Scand. **62:** 567–574.

HeLa cells look very much the same as the RA line, but in the KB line we found a different isozyme pattern. There is one electrophoretically fast-moving component that has sialic acid and is rather heat-resistant, and some slow-moving ones with high activity that are heat-sensitive and lack sialic acid. With this heterogeneity, an important point is that treatment with steroids could take away one enzyme and give you another.

DR. GRIFFIN: Yes, that's very pertinent! As a matter of fact, Dr. Bottomley has observed that one of the two isoenzymes in leukocyte alkaline phosphatase stains very intensely with oil red 0, a lipid stain. So it does look like this enzyme still has the lipid attached, and this would indicate, therefore, that the methods of extraction are important.

DR. GHOSH: I would like to add to your interesting finding that there is a great difference between the electrophoretic mobility of $HeLa_{75}$ and $HeLa_{71}$. Now I was wondering whether this difference in electrophoretic mobility is due to the difference in the presence of a larger or different amount of sialic acid. It has been known that this increased growth rate of tumor cells, including HeLa, is associated with the presence of large amounts of sialic acid. Would you kindly comment on that?

DR. GRIFFIN: Well, your first point I can't answer until we do some quantitative starch gel electrophoretic isolations of the various isoenzymes. Your second point is much more difficult to answer. The nutritional parameters in this system are far from being understood. For instance, only 65 percent of the cells showed the major modal number in Eagles minimal essential medium, but if you employ a rich medium, 100 percent of the cells showed this major modal number.

DR. GHOSH: The doubling time is the same in the $HeLa_{75}$ and the $HeLa_{71}$.

DR. GRIFFIN: Yes it is, under our conditions of culture.

DR. BECKMAN: We found also that there is a very great difference between using Eagles and Parker, and, in fact, Parker may be initially a little bit toxic.

DR. GRIFFIN: You mean that when you convert from MEM to Parker, you go through an adaption phase?

DR. BECKMAN: Yes, in the beginning you can see toxicity.

DR. GRIFFIN: A very interesting paper to read and to give due credit where credit is due is the paper by Dr. Margarita Vogt in Genetics (**44**:1257, 1959) where this problem was attacked most intelligently and showed that serum adaptations occur, resulting in chromosomal variants.

DR. BECKMAN: Do you get any variation in pattern depending upon whether or not human or animal serum is used?

DR. GRIFFIN: We have not investigated that sir. In earlier studies in Dr. Cox's lab, when I was a graduate, we did have cells grown in a really rich medium and in essential mineral medium for comparison, and there didn't appear to be much difference there.

G. MARTIN: Did I understand your last comment that if you use a Parker's medium or a rich medium you get 100 percent of the cells with the modal number?

DR. GRIFFIN: I'll take that back. It's about 96, plus or minus 3 or 4 percent.

DR. MARTIN: Is it fairly consistent with transfers?

DR. GRIFFIN: Well, we've only done this through about a hundred subcultures.

DR. MARTIN: How about macrochromosomes?

DR. GRIFFIN: Dr. Bottomley picked up one interesting macrochromosome in $HeLa_{71}$ and in the D group, one of the chromosomes had exceptionally longer arms and the chromosome right next to it occasionally had one of two long arms deleted, translocated to a site unknown to us, or it may even have been missing.

DR. MARTIN: In your original studies, when you tried to pick out some clones for some reasonable stability, did you come across any near-diploid ones?

DR. GRIFFIN: There does seem to be near-diploid clones as very small percentages in what a microbiologist would consider some wild-type cultures.

DR. MARTIN: On the electrophoretic differences that you found between the two lines, what about simple mixing of extracts?

DR. GRIFFIN: We haven't done that. I will say one thing. I did use the Garen-Leventhal-Schlesinger reduction reactivation to try to compare the base level of the induced and control enzymes. I didn't find any difference. You can reduce the activity of both to zero in urea with thioglycolate, and you can reoxidize the activity back to the exact same level with the conditions for reoxidation of *E. coli* enzymes. That wasn't the answer, at least not for these enzymes.

ALKALINE PHOSPHATASE CONSTITUTIVITY: A MARKER FOR THE ESTIMATION OF SOMATIC CELL "MUTATION" IN MAN

George M. Martin, Mary Ann Derr and Curtis A. Sprague
Department of Pathology, University of Washington School of Medicine, Seattle, Wash.

Dr. Cox has described the system of alkaline phosphatase repression and induction operative in established cultures of essentially diploid human skin fibroblasts.[1-3] If one examines a series of clones from such cultures grown under conditions of relative enzyme repression–i.e., well-fed cultures in the absence of added substrate–one finds that about one in a thousand clones gives a distinctly positive reaction for alkaline phosphatase using naphthol AS-MX as a substrate and fast blue RR as diazonium salt.[4] Alkaline phosphatase-positive clones cannot be regenerated, however, if a series of subclones are obtained from randomly selected alkaline phosphatase-negative cells.[4] On the basis of these and other observations from both our laboratory[5] and the laboratories of P. Farnes[6] and R. DeMars,[7] we conclude that, with respect to alkaline phosphatase, mass cultures of the "fibroblasts" that can be established from skin biopsies include a minor class of alkaline phosphatase-positive cells that are not responsible under the conditions employed *in vitro.* We have referred to such cells as "constitutive" with respect to the synthesis of alkaline phosphatase.[4] This type of constitutive cell appears to be present *de novo* and, presumably, represents maintenance of the state of differentiation that had been achieved *in vivo.*

While we have never observed a subclone of alkaline phosphatase-positive cells from a clone of nonconstitutive cells, rare alkaline phosphatase-positive cells have been seen. TABLE 1 shows some hard-won data that involved microscopic screening of individual cells at a magnification of 100x. The frequencies of these cells are of the order of $0.5 - 6 \times 10^{-6}$. The result, which is marked with an asterisk at the top of the table, is of interest in that these cells were grown in the presence of 1 mM phenylphosphate without change of medium, while the others were regularly fed with the same medium* in the absence of substrate. This particular clone appears to be "super-repressed" with regard to the synthesis of alkaline phosphatase, similar to other such clones that we have previously isolated and characterized.[5] It is, therefore, especially suitable for studies attempting to demonstrate mutation to enzyme constitutivity; most of the subsequent studies have been carried out with this clone, which was derived from the foreskin of a normal newborn. This clone had the further advantage of a comparatively long lifespan *in vitro.*[10]

The first preliminary experiments with a putative mutagen, the thymidine analogue 5-bromodeoxyuridine (5BUdR), gave striking increases in the frequencies of alkaline phosphatase-positive cells. The results appeared to depend upon the cell density at the time of treatment with 5BUdR. Cultures started with an initial inoculum of 50,000 cells/ml, and having patches of contact inhibition at the time of treatment, gave frequencies of positive cells of about 1 to 3×10^{-3}. Subconfluent cultures, starting from an inoculum of 25,000 cells/ml, gave frequencies of up to 4×10^{-2}. The effect of 5 BUdR was not clone-specific, since

* Dulbecco-Vogt modification of Eagle's medium[8,9] supplemented with 16% heat-inactivated newborn calf serum, cysteine (24 mg/l), 0.1 mM amounts of nonessential amino acids and 1 mM Na pyruvate; the concentration of bicarbonate was reduced to permit a pH of 7.3 in an atmosphere of 5% CO_2 in air.

TABLE 1

FREQUENCIES OF ALKALINE PHOSPHATASE CONSTITUTIVE CELLS AMONG CLONES OF HUMAN NEWBORN FORESKIN FIBROBLASTS GROWN UNDER CONDITIONS OF ENZYME REPRESSION

Strain	Clone	No. Cells	No. +	Freq. $\times 10^{-6}$
DEYM*	87	173,888	1	5.8
DEYM	87	408,672	2	4.9
DEYM	87	716,144	3	4.2
DEYM	94	115,104	0	< 8.7
MOTE	35	2,156,024	1	0.46
MOTE	6	89,056	0	<11

* Cells were grown in the presence of 1 mM phenylphosphate without change of medium.

four different clones from three individual donors gave comparable results, as shown in TABLE 2. In these experiments, six-ounce bottles were seeded with 350,000 cells in 10 ml of medium. After an overnight period of attachment, the medium was replaced and 48 hours later, the cultures were again refed with medium containing 0.05 mM 5BUdR. After a 24-hour incubation, the monolayers were rinsed three times with 15 ml of Hank's solution (buffered with 0.02 M tris, pH 7.4, at 37° C), and fresh medium was added. Forty-eight hours later, the monolayers were trypsinized[11] and plated onto glass slides in plastic petri dishes (700,000 cells in 10 ml of medium). After an additional 48 hours, the slides were rinsed twice in warm saline, fixed in neutral phosphate-buffered formalin for 60 minutes at 4° C, rinsed in cold running water for 15 minutes and stained for alkaline phosphatase as previously described,[4] with an incubation time of 40 minutes.

Quantitative assays for alkaline phosphatase using *p*-nitrophenyl phosphate as substrate[12] revealed a five- to six-fold increase in the specific activity of a lysed monolayer after 5BUdR treatment (24 hours, 0.05 mM) compared to a control treated with thymidine. Mixing experiments failed to reveal evidence of enzyme activation or inhibition (TABLE 3). Assuming that the frequency of constitutive cells in the 5BUdR lysate was of the order of three per hundred, one can calculate that the average specific activity in a constitutive cell is somewhat more than a hundred times the average specific activity of a cytochemically negative cell. There is, however, significant variation in the intensity of the staining reaction among the positive cells.

Starch gel electrophoresis of such 5BUdR-treated cultures revealed the same two bands observed in cultures that are derepressed and substrate-induced (FIGURE 1). Dr. Douglas Jackson has shown in our laboratory[13] that traces of these bands can also be detected in some cultures that are not derepressed and sub-

TABLE 2

FREQUENCIES OF ALKALINE PHOSPHATASE CONSTITUTIVE CELLS AMONG CLONES OF HUMAN NEWBORN FORESKIN FIBROBLASTS TREATED WITH 0.05 mM 5BUdR FOR 24 HOURS DURING SUBCONFLUENT GROWTH

Strain	Clone	Freq. $\times 10^{-2}$
DEYM	87	3.3
DEYM	74	2.4
AM	28	2.8
ARCH	2	1.5

TABLE 3

SPECIFIC ACTIVITIES (S.A.) OF DESOXYCHOLATE LYSATES OF MONOLAYERS OF A CLONE OF NEWBORN FIBROBLASTS TREATED WITH 0.05 mM 5BUdR FOR 24 HOURS AS COMPARED TO A CONTROL TREATED WITH 0.05 mM THYMIDINE

Thymidine	5BUdR	S.A.
0.10	—	1.5
—	0.10	8.2
0.09	0.01	2.0
0.01	0.09	7.0
0.05	0.05	4.5

Simple additive effects were found when various proportions of the two lysates were mixed together and assayed. For method of assay, see Reference no. 12.

strate-induced, and that their mobilities appear to be distinct from those of the various isoenzymes in extracts of liver, kidney, bone, intestine, skin, white blood cells, placenta and serum, being closest, but probably not identical, to that of skeletal muscle. We conclude that 5BUdR treatment does not result in expression of a phosphatase locus not already expressed in such cultures.

In order to seek evidence for heritability of the property of constitutivity, a clone treated with 5BUdR for 25 hours were recloned at the time of plating for alkaline phosphatase stains; no alkaline phosphatase-positive clones were found among more than 2,500 examined after 18 days in culture, although at least 75 might have been expected on the basis of the frequency of alkaline phosphatase-positive cells. On only one occasion has an alkaline phosphatase-positive cell been seen in unambiguous mitosis (FIGURE 2); the daughter cells appeared identical in terms of the intensity of the enzyme reaction. Occasionally, two or three alkaline phosphatase-positive cells can be seen to be contiguous, or nearly contiguous, with each other. We conclude that the type of alkaline phosphatase constitutive cells that are observed after 5BUdR treatment are incapable of sustained sequential replication or, alternatively, have exceedingly long cell cycles or are usually blocked at some stage of the cell cycle. The cells appear to be viable, since they apparently persist in culture for long periods of time (at least two to three weeks); after trypsinization, they reattach to glass.

If we assume that the spontaneously appearing "constitutive" cell also replicates rarely, slowly, or not at all, yet persists in culture, and that such cells do in fact represent *de novo* dominant mutations, then the frequency of such cells gives a convenient estimate of the spontaneous mutation rate for this marker in normal human somatic cells. As we have seen, it may be of the order of 0.5 to 6 per million. Obviously, much more data must be accumulated to establish this important point. Treatment with our putative mutagen, thus, may raise the mutation rate some 10,000-fold.

It is important to point out that among the clones examined after 5BUdR treatment, at least one unquestionable morphologic variant was discovered, suggesting that a stable, heritable event can result from such treatment. This distinctly epithelioid clone is shown in FIGURE 3 next to a typical fibroblast clone. Epithelioid clones, or patches of epithelioid cells, have never been observed to arise spontaneously among numerous mass diploid fibroblast cultures and clones examined in our laboratory over the past seven years, despite the fact that we have been especially alert for the occurrence of spontaneous "malignant transformation" *in vitro.*

The fact that contact inhibition appeared to inhibit the 5BUdR effect supported

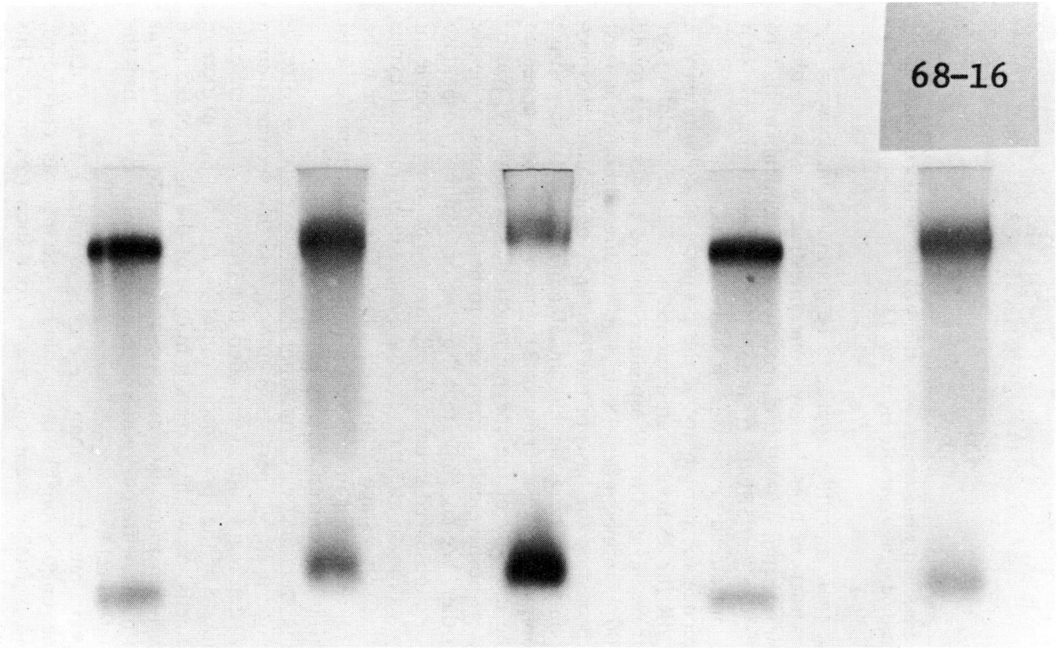

FIGURE 1. Photograph of cut section of starch gel electrophoresis slab stained with α-naphthyl phosphate (0.05%) and fast red TR (0.05%) Borate buffer, pH 9.7. Horizontal electrophoresis was carried out for six hours at pH 8.6. Bridge buffer: 0.3 M Borate; gel buffer: 0.076 M tris-citrate. Initial voltage 150 v and 12 mA. Butanol extracts of tissues and monolayers were lyophilized and redissolved in water. Direction of anodal migration was from top to bottom. From left to right: fetal liver; DEYM clone 87 treated with 5BUdR, 0.05 mM for 24 hours; mass culture of derepressed (unfed) and substrate-induced (1 mM phenylphosphate) newborn foreskin fibroblasts; fetal liver; DEYM clone 87. Consistent differences between relative intensities of the two major bands are not observed. This gel was overloaded with samples for purposes of photography. No differences in mobilities of bands of 5BUdR-treated and untreated cultures were observed with more dilute samples; faintly detectable bands from parental DEYM mass culture were identical in mobilities to those of 5BUdR-treated DEYM clone 87.

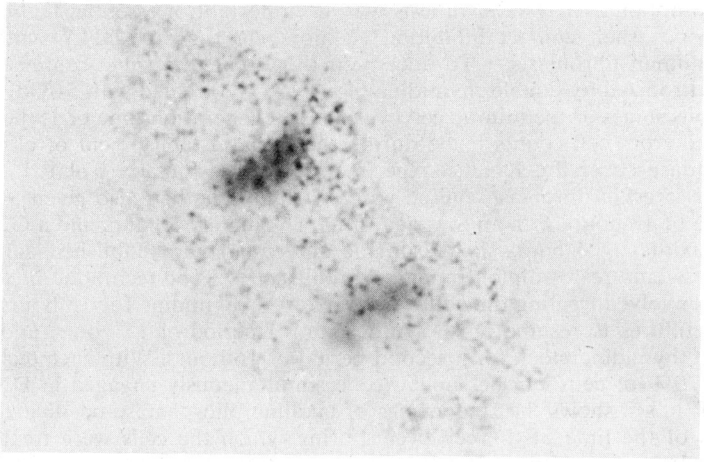

FIGURE 2. Constitutive cell in late stage of mitosis stained for alkaline phosphatase and counterstained with Feulgen reaction. Note that the intensity of staining for the cytoplasmically localized enzyme is identical in the two daughter cells. Note also the alkaline phosphatase-negative cell, in which only the nucleus is stained (for DNA); × 640.

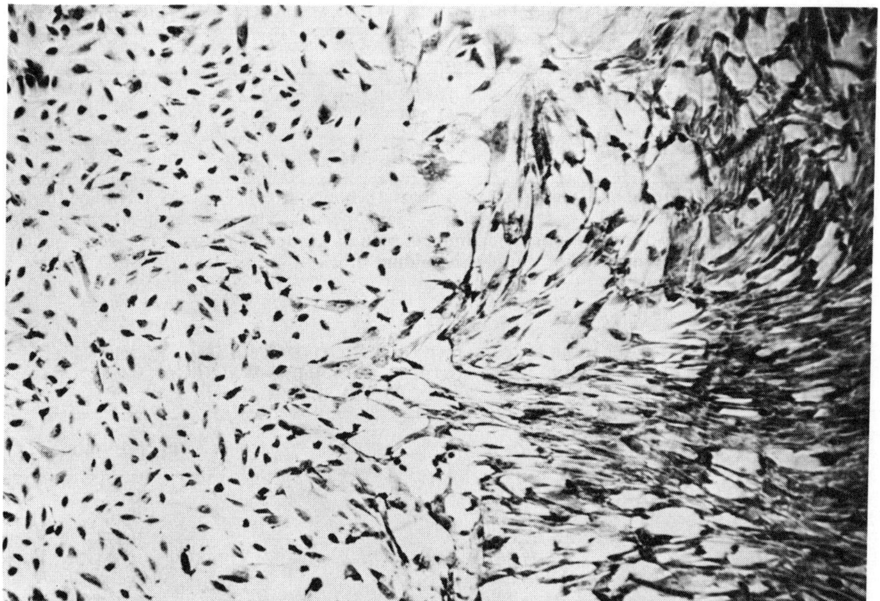

FIGURE 3. Epithelioid clonal variant (left) adjacent to typical fibroblast clone, appearing among approximately 2,500 subclones of DEYM clone 87 after treatment with 0.05 mM 5BUdR for 24 hours. One percent aqueous neutral red stain, after negative cytochemical reaction for alkaline phosphatase. (Orig. mag. × 48.)

the presumption that DNA synthesis was an important or essential feature of its action, since such contact inhibition is known to turn off DNA synthesis in diploid human fibroblasts.[14] To document this point, the super-repressed clone was synchronized by double thymidine block[15-20] and treated with 5BUdR during the various stages of the mitotic cell cycle. A cell generation time of 18 hours was calculated from cell counts made during the initial establishment of clone on a 3-mm-square coverslip. Kinetic experiments with a similarly isolated clone of newborn foreskin fibroblasts pulsed with ^{3}H-thymidine had also given a generation time of 18 hours with an S period of approximately 8 hours and a G2 period of approximately 4 hours, in reasonable agreement with published data based upon mass cultures of diploid human fibroblasts.[21-23] The technique of synchronization involved treating the cultures with 2 mM thymidine for 16 hours, allowing the cultures to resume DNA synthesis for a period of 13 hours, and reinitiating the thymidine block for a second period of 16 hours. With such techniques, at least 70% of cells can be shown to be simultaneously engaged in DNA synthesis. TABLE 4 shows the frequencies of alkaline phosphatase-positive cells as a function of the time of the cell cycle during which the cells were treated with 5BUdR. It is quite clear that the striking increase in constitutives is related to treatment of the cells during the S period, although there is also a smaller but significant increase related to treatment during G1.

Fractionation of the S period with pulses of 5BUdR gave clear evidence that

TABLE 4

FREQUENCIES OF ALKALINE PHOSPHATASE CONSTITUTIVE CELLS AS A FUNCTION OF THE STAGE IN THE MITOTIC CELL CYCLE DURING WHICH 0.05 MM 5BUdR WAS GIVEN

Stage	Hrs Rx	No. Cells	No. +	Freq. $\times$ 10^{-3}
G.T.	18	41,008	282	6.9
S	7.5	61,234	284	4.6
G2	4.0	118,096	6	0.05
G1	6.5	245,520	150	0.61

G.T. = treatment during entire generation time of 18 hours; S = period of DNA synthesis. G2 = post-S "gap" period; G1 = post-mitosis "gap" period. The estimated 30 to 60 min period of peak mitosis was not separately examined, being included as parts of G1, G2 or both. DEYM clone 87 synchronized with double thymidine block.

TABLE 5

FREQUENCIES OF ALKALINE PHOSPHATASE CONSTITUTIVE CELLS AS A FUNCTION OF THE PERIOD DURING DNA SYNTHESIS (S) DURING WHICH CELLS WERE TREATED WITH 0.05 MM 5BUdR

(Hrs) Period of S	No. Cells	No. +	Freq. $\times$ 10^{-3}
0–7.5	152,768	89	0.582
0–5.0	44,000	18	0.409
2.5–7.5	61,600	23	0.373
0–2.5	95,568	0	$<$0.011
2.5–5.0	46,640	19	0.407
5.0–7.5	189,200	10	0.053
0–7.5 (Thymidine)	51,920	2	0.038

A control culture received 0.05 mM thymidine for the 7.5-hour period of S. DEYM clone 87 synchronized with double thymidine block.

TABLE 6

FREQUENCIES OF ALKALINE PHOSPHATASE CONSTITUTIVE CELLS AS A FUNCTION OF THE PERIOD OF MID-S DURING WHICH CELLS WERE PULSED WITH 0.05 MM 5BUdR

(Min) Period of S	No. Cells	No. +	Freq. $\times 10^{-3}$
150–200	456,720	19	0.041
200–250	736,384	0	<0.0014
250–300	243,056	0	<0.0041
200–250 (Thymidine)	289,520	1	0.0035

A control culture received 0.05 mM thymidine for the period of 200 to 250 min after the onset of S. DEYM clone 87 synchronized with double thymidine block.

the effect was maximal during the mid-period of S (TABLE 5). TABLE 6 shows results obtained upon subfractionation of mid-S. In this experiment, a peak of constitutives was found in cultures treated during the first part of mid-S, between 150 and 200 minutes after the release of the second thymidine block. Replicate monolayers from this experiment were pulsed with tritiated 5BUdR (specific activity, 12.7 c/mM, 2 μc/ml). Cultures treated with both cold and hot 5BUdR were post-treated with a cold thymidine chase (0.2 mM). At the end of the S period, metaphases from the radioactive cultures were accumulated by overnight treatment with low doses of colcemide (0.004 μg/ml) and examined cytologically[24] after dipping with Kodak NTB-2 nuclear track emulsion followed by a seven-day exposure time. Thus, we could identify at the chromosomal level those segments of DNA that were incorporating 5BUdR at a time corresponding to the peak frequency of presumptive mutagenesis. In order to obtain more precise chromosomal localization, the following scheme was used (FIGURE 4). In each cell, one of the number 1 homologues was chosen as an "internal standard" upon which all other chromosomes could be superimposed. The number 1 chromosome was divided into nine segments: the centromeric region (labeled C); four equal segments of the short arm (labeled S1 through S4); and four equal regions of the long arm (labeled L1 through L4). The centromere of a given chromosome was superimposed on the centromere of the standard number 1 and subdivided into segments according to the extent of overlap with the standard regions. Thus, the human haploid genome was subdivided into 128 segments, all of which, with the exception of the somewhat smaller centromeric segments, were of approximately equal size.

FIGURE 5 shows a karyotype of a labeled metaphase plate from the first portion of mid-S, illustrating the comparatively light density of grains, permitting unambiguous grain counts over the various segments. While it is recognized that unambiguous identification of all chromosomes is not possible, definite or tentative assignments were made in all cases according to the criteria of the Denver, London and Chicago conferences.[25] Twenty-two such karyotypes have so far been prepared and analyzed. The data of homologues was pooled and is summarized in TABLE 7. Six sites are comparatively heavily labeled, having grain counts in excess of 25: 2L2, 3L2, 14L1, 17L2, 19L1 and 22L1. Identification of three of these is always unambiguous in our material, but it is obvious that chromosome number 14 can be confused with numbers 13 and 15, chromosome 19 with 20, and 21 with 22. It is remarkable, however, that the grain counts for the L1 regions appear to differentiate, 19 from 20 and 21 from 22. The comparatively low labeling throughout the X chromosome is also of interest, indi-

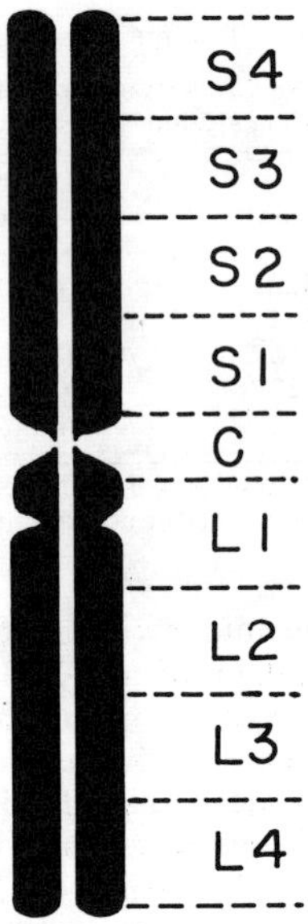

FIGURE 4. Diagram of chromosome number 1 of normal human karyotype, illustrating the nine segments used as "internal standards" in scoring for localization of silver grains throughout karyotypes of cells treated with ^{3}H 5BUdR (See text).

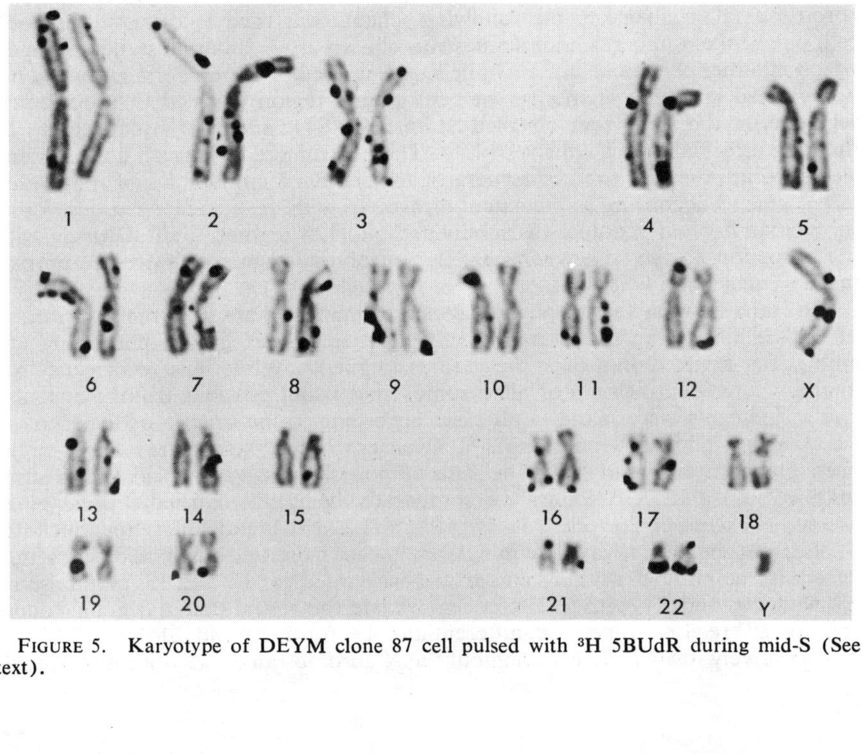

FIGURE 5. Karyotype of DEYM clone 87 cell pulsed with ^{3}H 5BUdR during mid-S (See text).

TABLE 7

SUMMARY OF DISTRIBUTION OF SILVER GRAIN COUNTS AMONG 128 CHROMOSOME SEGMENTS OF KARYOTYPES PREPARED FROM CELLS PULSED WITH ^{3}H 5BUdR DURING THE 150 TO 200-MIN PERIOD OF S

	1 (43)	2 (43)	3 (44)	4 (44)	5 (44)	6 (44)	7 (44)	8 (44)	9 (44)	10 (44)	11 (43)	12 (44)	X (42)	13 (44)	14 (44)	15 (43)	16 (44)	17 (44)	18 (44)	19 (44)	20 (44)	21 (44)	22 (44)	Y (42)
S4	16																							
S3	16	20	13										6											
S2	15	12	20	15	12	22	13	15	13	5	11	7	3											
S1	18	10	11	11	10	19	14	14	17	10	13	8	9	5	7	11	19	12	9	16	12	3	9	2
C	1	6	8	10	1	5	5	2	6	5	8	2	4	6	1	6	2	7	3	9	4	4	6	0
L1	11	15	14	18	15	15	17	8	19	21	15	12	8	21	28	16	12	15	12	31	18	8	25	4
L2	20	27	25	19	18	20	19	17	21	17	15	19	11	15	19	18	17	27	19					
L3	15	19	20	13	20	16	17	18	14	14	10	20	9	12	9									
L4	22	16		17	9																			

Data from homologues were pooled from 22 metaphase plates, giving a total of 42 to 44 samples for each linkage group.

cating that we have successfully differentiated this chromosome from the numbers 6 and 7 pairs. However, it is also evident from this table that there are large numbers of segments that become moderately heavily labeled during the 50-minute pulse period. Much shorter pulses and improved synchronization will be required to obtain more discrete labeling patterns. By increasing the concentration of 5BUdR from 0.05 mM to 0.2 mM, we have been able to narrow the pulse to a 25-minute period; more than three times as many constitutives appear after treatment during the 150- to 175-minute period of S than appear during the 175- to 200-minute period of S. No cytogenetic studies have as yet been carried out with this material, however.

It should be emphasized that while our findings are consistent with the interpretation of locus-specific mutation, they certainly do not prove such an interpretation. A simple alternative explanation is that, as a result of nonspecific chromosomal damage, alkaline phosphatase is *induced* to appear in a proportion of cells, perhaps as an enzyme that participates in the DNA repair process.[26] Against this interpretation, however, is the fact that, in our material, enzyme localization is always cytoplasmic. It is also conceivable that what we have observed results from enzyme induction independent of effects upon DNA. The finding of a discrete single peak of presumed mutation may merely be related to the time of peak uptake of 5BUdR. The use of the thymidine block technique results in an abnormally large intracellular pool of thymidine, so that maximum labeling may not be evident until the mid-period of S.[27] Average grain counts of cells pulsed with tritiated thymidine during the mid-150 minutes of S are in fact about 2.6 times those of cells pulsed during the first 150 minutes of S (203.2 vs. 76.9). However, this difference hardly seems sufficient to account for the striking preponderance of constitutives in mid-S. Furthermore, the average grain count of thymidine-pulsed cells in late-S was not significantly different from that in mid-S (217.8 vs. 203.2). Finally, the average grain count (71.8) of metaphase plates pulsed with tritiated 5BUdR during the period of peak "mutagenesis" (150 to 250 minutes of S) was not significantly different from the mean of 68.8 per metaphase plate in the contiguous pulse period of 200 to 250 minutes, and only slightly higher than the mean of 57.0 found at 250 to 300 minutes.

The frequency of constitutive cells clearly does not parallel the frequency of random chromatid and chromosomal breaks, which in our control material involved about 1 to 5 percent of cells. The frequency of Feulgen-positive "micronuclei" in interphase cells, a convenient index of the extent of gross chromosomal damage,[28] is unaffected in the 5BUdR treated monolayers, averaging 0.5 to 0.7 percent in both control and treated cultures. We have, in fact, been successful in carrying out Feulgen reactions on monolayers first stained cytochemically for phosphatase; it is quite clear that cells containing micronuclei are not alkaline phosphatase-positive, and cells that are alkaline phosphatase-positive do not contain micronuclei. It also seems clear that the level of visible light present in our laboratory does not influence the frequency of constitutive cells, at least not as we presently handle these cultures. 5BUdR-treated monolayers handled in a dark hood gave frequencies of constitutives identical to those obtained after deliberate exposure to the hood florescent lights at a distance of 10 cm (but with plastic lids on the petri dishes) for periods of up to 30 minutes. Finally, preliminary cytogenetic studies of a small sample of cells have failed to provide evidence of a significantly increased freqeuncy of chromosomal aberrations attributable to 5BUdR under the conditions in which it was employed. We tentatively conclude that gross chromosomal mutation is not a major explanation for the enhanced frequency of constitutives. Further work is necessary to document this conclusion, especially in view of the evidence for preferential breakage at secondary constrictions attributable to 5 BUdR treatment.[29] All of our "hot" segments are at or near secondary constrictions, or could be confused with chromosomes having secondary constrictions in the specific long arm segments.[30] Deletion of a segment of a chromosome could conceivably eliminate a regulatory locus, resulting in constitutive expression of a structural gene even in the heterozygous state. One such regulator could be a Jacob-Monod type operator.[31]

Point mutation via a base transition is an accepted mechanism of base analogue mutagenesis.[32] In the case of the r II cistron of phage T4, the probability of mutation at a specific site was raised by a factor of 10^4 following 5BUdR treatment.[33] While such a highly mutable locus may be responsible for the comparatively high frequency of "mutant" cells observed in our experiments, there are possible alternative explanations. A dominant mutation occurring within a highly redundant set of genes[34,35] is one possibility, although one might also expect a comparatively high frequency of spontaneous mutation in this situation. Mitochondrial DNA is such a redundant set, but it is an unlikely candidate in view of the recent evidence that the mitochondrial DNA of cultured human cells replicates mainly in G2.[36] Other genetic mechanisms could contribute to the observed results, such as somatic segregation,[37] mitotic nondisjunction[38] and mitotic crossing over.[39] Finally, an effect of 5BUdR at the phenotypic level should also be seriously considered.[40]

The techniques that have been described might prove useful as a novel and fruitful approach to the formal genetic analysis of man. Significant improvements in synchronization can undoubtedly be obtained, and it would be important to explore other methods of synchronization in conjunction with 5BUdR and to examine the effects of other base analogues. A model system suitable for testing the validity of this approach might involve the enzyme glucose-6-phosphate dehydrogenase, which is expressed in cell culture,[41] can be scored cytochemically[42] and is known to be X-linked.[43] Staining subclones under conditions that inhibit wild-type enzyme might reveal the presence of structural gene mutations that result in the synthesis of a protein no longer responsive to inhibition.

Summary

When mass cultures of human diploid skin fibroblasts are grown under conditions of enzyme repression, alkaline phosphatase can be demonstrated in about 1 in 10^3 clones. However, when mass cultures are first purified by cloning, the frequency of "constitutive" cells falls to about 0.5 to 6×10^{-6}. Exposure of such clones to 0.05 mM 5-bromodeoxyuridine (5BUdR) for 24 hours raises the frequency to from $>10^{-3}$ to $>10^{-2}$, depending upon the conditions of treatment. Such constitutive cells, while apparently viable, replicate rarely or have prolonged generation times and do not form clones. Thus, a measure of their frequency may give a direct estimate of the frequency of what is presumed to be a dominant mutation involving a locus regulating the synthesis of the enzyme. The enzymes affected appear to be the same as those that appear after derepression (unfed cultures) and substrate induction, as judged from electrophoretic properties.

Exposure of a synchronized clone (double thymidine block) to 5BUdR at various stages of the mitotic cycle indicated that the peak frequency of constitutives occurred during a discrete period of S (150 to 200 minutes after the onset of DNA synthesis). Autoradiographic cytogenetic studies with ^{3}H 5BUdR during this time period revealed comparatively heavy labeling in discrete long arm segments of chromosomes members 2, 3, 17, and what are presumed to be numbers 14, 19 and 22, implicating one or more of these sites as a possible regulatory locus for alkaline phosphatase. A variety of alternative interpretations are considered.

The experiments described, when employed with a variety of enzymatic cytochemical markers, preferably those compatible with clonal growth, may prove useful as a new approach to the formal genetic analysis of man.

References

1. Cox, R. P. & C. M. MacLeod. 1964. Regulation of alkaline phosphatase in human cell cultures. Cold Spring Harbor Sympos. Quant. Biol. **29:** 233.
2. Martin, G. M. 1964. Alkaline phosphatase of human skin fibroblast cultures. II. Kinetics of various "inductions." Exp. Molec. Path. **3:** 634.
3. Cox, R. P. 1969. Activity and regulation of alkaline phosphatase in cells from patients with abnormal chromosome complements. Ann. N. Y. Acad. Sci. (This annal)
4. Papayannopoulou, T. G. & G. M. Martin. 1967. Alkaline phosphatase "constitutive" clones: evidence for de-novo heterogeneity of established human skin fibroblast strains. Exp. Cell Res. **45:** 72.
5. Martin, G. M. 1966. Clonal variation of derepressed phosphatase in chromosomally mosaic cell cultures from a child with Down's syndrome. Exp. Cell Res. **44:** 341.
6. Farnes, P. 1967. Histochemical approaches to cell characterization in vitro. Nat. Cancer Inst. Monogr. **26:** 199.
7. DeMars, R. 1967. Discussion of paper by P. Farnes. Nat. Cancer Inst. Monogr. **26:** 225.
8. Ginsburg, H. 1965. Growth and differentiation of cells of lymphoid origin in embryo cell monolayers. Methodological approaches to the study of leukemia. V. Defendi, Ed., Wistar Inst. Symp. Monogr. No. **4:** 21.
9. Ginsburg, H. & D. Lagunoff. 1967. The *in vitro* differentiation of mast cells. J. Cell Biol. **35:** 685.
10. Hayflick, L. 1965. The limited *in vitro* lifetime of human diploid cell strains. Exp. Cell Res. **37:** 614.
11. Martin, G. M. 1964. Use of tris (hydroxymethyl) aminomethane buffers in cultures of diploid human fibroblasts. Proc. Soc. Exp. Biol. Med. **116:** 167.
12. Martin, G. M. 1964. Alkaline phosphatase of human skin fibroblast cultures. I. A microassay demonstrating strain variation. Exp. Molec. Path. **3:** 622.
13. Jackson, D. W. 1966. Electrophoretic studies of human alkaline phosphatase. M.S. Thesis. University of Washington. Seattle, Wash.
14. Levine, E. M., G. Burleigh, C. W. Boone & H. Eagle. 1965. Contact inhibition, macromolecular synthesis and polyribosomes in cultured human diploid fibroblasts. Proc. Nat. Acad. Sci. U.S.A. **53:** 350.
15. Bootsma, D., L. Budke & O. Vos. 1964. Studies on synchronous division of tissue culture cells initiated by excess thymidine. Exp. Cell Res. **33:** 301.
16. Drew, R. M. & B. L. Commerford. 1967. Radionucleoside incorporation by thymidine synchronized cells. Radiat. Res. **30:** 455.
17. Morris, N. R. & G. A. Fischer. 1963. Studies concerning the inhibition of cellular reproduction by deoxyribonucleosides. I. Inhibition of the synthesis of deoxycytidine by a phosphorylated derivative of thymidine. Biochim. Biophys. Acta **68:** 84.
18. Morris, N. R., P. Reichard & G. A. Fischer. 1963. Studies concerning the inhibition of cellular reproduction by deoxyribonucleosides. II. Inhibition of the synthesis of deoxycytidine by thymidine, deoxyadenosine and deoxyguanosine. Biochim. Biophys. Acta **68:** 93.
19. Firket, H. & P. Mahieu. 1966. Synchronisme des divisions induit dans des cellules HeLa par un exces de thymidine. Exp. Cell Res. **45:** 11.
20. Xeros, N. 1962. Deoxyriboside control and synchronization of mitosis. Nature (London) **194:** 682.
21. Moorhead, P. S. & V. Defendi. 1963. Asynchrony of DNA synthesis in chromosomes of human diploid cells. J. Cell Biol. **16:** 202.
22. Defendi, V. & L. A. Manson. 1963. Analysis of the life-cycle in mammalian cells. Nature (London) **198:** 359.
23. Comings, D. E. 1967. Sex chromatin, nuclear size and the cell cycle. Cytogenetics (Basel) **6:** 120.

24. Martin, G. M. & C. A. Sprague. 1966. Chromosomal analysis of "leukocyte" cell lines. Lab. Invest. **15:** 692.
25. Bergsma, D., J. L. Hamerton & H. P. Klinger, (Eds.) 1966. Chicago Conference: Standardization in human cytogenetics. Birth Defects: Original Article Series 2.
26. Weiss, B., T. R. Live & C. C. Richardson. 1968. Enzymatic breakage and joining of deoxyribonucleic acid. V. End group labeling and analysis of deoxyribonucleic acid containing single strand breaks. J. Biol. Chem. **243:** 4530.
27. Cleaver, J. E. & R. M. Holford. 1965. Investigations into the incorporation of [3H] thymidine into DNA in L-strain cells and the formation of a pool of phosphorylated derivatives during pulse labeling. Biochim. Biophys. Acta **103:** 654.
28. German, J. & L. Pugliatti Crippa. 1966. Chromosomal breakage in diploid cell lines from Bloom's syndrome and Fanconi's anemia. Ann. Genet. (Paris) **9:** 143.
29. Hsu, T. C. & C. E. Somers. 1961. Effect of 5-bromodeoxyuridine on mammalian chromosomes. Proc. Nat. Acad. Sci. U.S.A. **47:** 396.
30. Ferguson-Smith, M. A., M. E. Ferguson-Smith, P. M. Ellis & M. Dickson. 1962. The sites and relative frequencies of secondary constrictions in human somatic chromosomes. Cytogenetics (Basel) **1:** 325.
31. Jacob, F. & J. Monod. 1961. Genetic regulatory mechanisms in the synthesis of proteins. J. Molec. Biol. **3:** 318.
32. Stahl, F. W. 1964. *In* The mechanics of inheritance. **:** 53. Prentice-Hall, Inc., Englewood Cliffs, N. J.
33. Benzer, S. & E. Freese. 1958. Induction of specific mutations with 5-bromouracil. Proc. Nat. Acad. Sci. U.S.A. **44:** 112.
34. McCarthy, B. J. & B. L. McConaughy. 1968. Related base sequences in the DNA of simple and complex organisms. I. DNA/DNA duplex formation and the incidence of partially related base sequences in DNA. Biochem. Genetics **2:** 37.
35. Britten, R. J. & D. E. Kohne. 1968. Repeated sequences in DNA. Science **161:** 529.
36. Koch, J. & E. L. R. Stokstad. 1967. Incorporation of [3H] thymidine into nuclear and mitochondrial DNA in synchronized mammalian cells. European J. Biochem. **3:** 1.
37. Martin, G. M. & C. A. Sprague. 1968. A parasexual cycle in cultivated human somatic cells. Proc. Twelfth International Cong. of Genetics. Tokyo.
38. Martin, G. M., C. Sprague & J. S. Bryant. 1967. Mitotic nondisjunction in cultivated human cells. Nature (London) **214:** 612.
39. Shaw, M. & M. M. Cohen. 1965. Chromosome exchanges in human leukocytes induced by mitomycin C. Genetics **51:** 181.
40. Abbott, J. & H. Holtzer. 1968. The loss of phenotypic traits by differentiated cells. V. The effects of 5-bromodeoxyuridine on cloned chondrocytes. Proc. Nat. Acad. Sci. U.S.A. **59:** 1144.
41. Gartler, S. M. 1961. Maintenance of genetically determined glucose-6-phosphate dehydrogenase differences in human cell cultures. Proc. 2nd Intern. Cong. Human Genetics **1:** 622.
42. Wajntal, A. & R. DeMars. 1967. A tetrazolium method for distinguishing between cultured human fibroblasts having either normal or deficient levels of glucose-6-phosphate dehydrogenase. Biochem. Genetics **1:** 61.
43. Davidson, R. G., H. M. Nitowsky & B. Childs. 1963. Demonstration of two populations of cells in the human female heterozygous for glucose-6-phosphate dehydrogenase variants. Proc. Nat. Acad. Sci. U.S.A. **50:** 481.

Discussion of the Paper

Dr. Beckman: Dr. Martin, do you have any significant population of floating cells?

Dr. Martin: These are all attached cells, so that there aren't any floating cells evaluated in the staining procedure.

Dr. Beckman: But do you grow them in bottles? If so, some of them are floaters.

Dr. Martin: Oh yes, that's right.

Dr. Beckman: Well, what would be the distribution of alkaline phosphatase among the floaters.

Dr. Martin: We don't have data on that point. At the low concentration of

5-Bromo UdR, there's not a substantial decrease in growth, but we have no quantitative information.

DR. BECKMAN: We have been doing some experiments with adhesion of cells, making up fifty-fifty mixtures of nonstaining and staining cells and maintaining them in chambers, letting them attach, and counting the attached ones and the unattached ones. At least with the heteroploid cell lines, the alkaline phosphatase-positive ones come off.

DR. MARTIN: You mean, after you trypsinize them and allow them to reattach, there's an enrichment of the alkaline phosphatase-positive cells in the unattached? That's very interesting. Which cell lines are they?

DR. BECKMAN: Well, these are not fibroblasts. This is a mixture of heteroploid clones.

DR. MARTIN: Mixture of known positives, heteroploid known to be positive?

DR. BECKMAN: Yes, One very high and one completely diploid, so you can see the origin of the two, but immediately, if you allow them to attach you're far away from the initial fifty-fifty mixture out. So there could be a possibility that there is a selection going on. It seems unlikely, though.

DR. MARTIN: In our earlier studies with mass cultures, there was, in fact, selection against the constitutive cell; that seemed pretty clear.

PART II. DEVELOPMENT AND PHYSIOLOGY

THE DIFFERENTIATION OF ALKALINE PHOSPHATASE IN THE SMALL INTESTINE*

Florence Moog, Marilynn E. Etzler,† and Robert D. Grey‡

Department of Biology, Washington University
St. Louis, Mo.

The small intestine of vertebrates has long been recognized as a rich source of a nonspecific phosphomonoesterase active at alkaline pH. The pioneering histochemical studies of Gomori (1941) indicated many years ago that the enzyme might be localized in what was then called the striated border of the epithelium. In recent years, this finding has been abundantly supported, not only by histochemical techniques adapted to the ultrastructural level (Hugon & Borgers, 1966), but also by studies on isolated and fractionated microvilli. The enzyme is found with the microvilli if these are stripped away from the bulk of the epithelial cells (Miller & Crane, 1961; Holt & Miller, 1962). If the microvilli are further separated by sonication and density gradient centrifugation into fibrous cores and covering membranes, it is the latter component that retains the phosphatase activity (Overton *et al.*, 1965). The enzyme also remains with the continuous phase of the membrane after dipeptidases and disaccharidases have been removed by papain (Oda & Seki, 1966). Evidently alkaline phosphatase is an integral part of the outer membrane of the microvilli.

In the duodenum of the mouse, phosphatase assumes its localization in the microvilli in prenatal stages (Moog, 1951). Specific activity rises just before birth, then falls somewhat, and near the end of the second postnatal week begins a brief upsurge to a maximum that is more than 20 times higher than at birth (Moog, 1951). Determination of activity with different substrates has revealed that the enzyme changes qualitatively at the same time that it is rising to its maximal level. Up to 12 days, it hydrolyzes phenylphosphate (PhP) less rapidly than beta-glycerophosphate (bGP), but after 16 days the reverse is true (Moog, 1961). This alteration in characteristics is conveniently expressed as the ratio of phosphorus split from one substrate to that split from the other by the same amount of enzyme in the same time (PhP/bGP ratio); this ratio rises from about 0.7 at 12 days to 2.5 or more at 20 days.

The period during which phosphatase activity increases in the duodenum is one of far reaching change in the intestines of both mice and rats. Within the same period, sucrase activity rises from very low levels (Doell & Kretchmer, 1964; Denes & Moog, unpublished); leucyl naphthylamidase rises to adult levels in the jejunum (Birkenmeier & Moog, unpublished); the epithelial surface acquires the ability to bar the passage of large molecules (Clark, 1959); and the microvilli change from the short, broad form of infancy to the long slender form characteristic of the adult intestine (Overton, 1965). All these differentiative alterations can be elicited precociously by corticosteroids, and appear to be dependent on the outflow of secretions from the adrenal cortex (Moog, 1953; 1969).

* Supported by research grant 03490 and training grant HD 00012 from the National Institutes of Health.

† Present address: Department of Microbiology, College of Physicians and Surgeons, Columbia University, New York, N. Y. 10032

‡ Present address: Department of Zoology, University of California, Davis, Calif. 95616

THE SPATIAL DISTRIBUTION OF PHOSPHATASE ON THE DUODENAL VILLI

Histochemical studies have long suggested that phosphatase activity may be maximal at the villi tips. Recently, this suggestion has been verified by a new technique involving the sectioning of frozen villi at right angles to their length (Dahlqvist & Nordstrom, 1966). Quantitative determination of phosphatase activity in small groups of sections from villi tips to crypts shows that in the intestines of both mice (Moog & Grey, 1967) and rats (Nordstrom, Dahlqvist and Joseffson, 1967), activity is highest at the tips and declines steadily through more proximal levels. In the duodenum of the mouse, moreover, Moog and Grey (1967) have shown that activity is graded in character as well as in intensity, with the PhP/bGP ratio being substantially higher at the tips of the villi than at their bases (FIGURE 1). It is well known that the epithelial cells clothing the villi are in continual transit from the crypts, where new cells are proliferated, to the tips, where the mature cells are extruded (Leblond & Messier, 1958). As the cells glide upward, therefore, the phosphatase invested in their microvillar membranes must undergo not only enhancement of activity, but also alteration of its properties.

In the infant mouse, as previously pointed out, phosphatase activity is low and has a PhP/bGP ratio below 1. FIGURE 2 shows that this activity is uniformly distributed along the length of the villi, with no difference in ratio from tip to base (Moog & Grey, 1968). By 14 days, activities are elevated in all areas of the villi, but the ability to hydrolyze PhP is more strongly affected, so that the PhP/bGP ratio rises above unity at all levels, including the crypts (FIGURE 2). Between 14 and 16 days, activity approximately doubles with both substrates, so that PhP/bGP ratios remain almost unchanged. After 16 days, however, a new phase is entered, one in which only PhP-splitting ability is strongly enhanced, particularly in the distal regions of the villi; in consequence, PhP/bGP ratios at 20 days are above 5 at the villi tips, and gradients of both activity and ratio

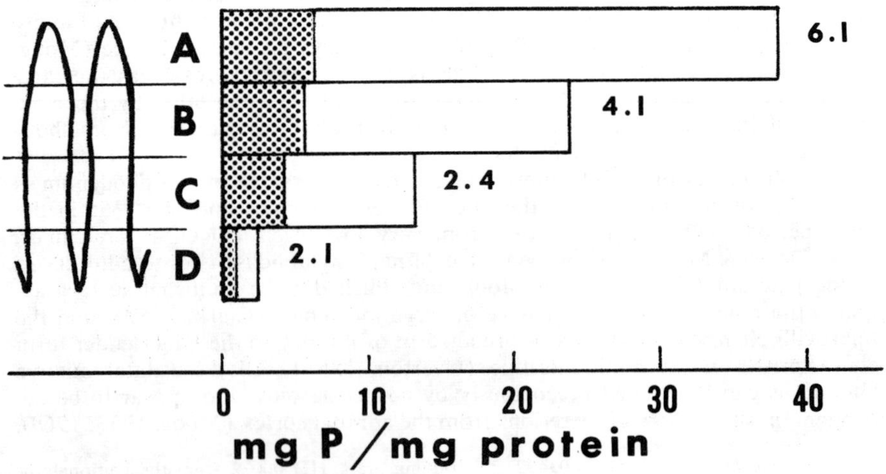

FIGURE 1. Distribution of phosphatase activity and PhP/bGP ratio in groups of sections from the villi tips to the crypts. Clear columns show activity per 30 min. with PhP; stippled columns show activity with bGP. Small figures near the ends of the bars are the ratios. (Adapted from Moog & Grey, 1967.)

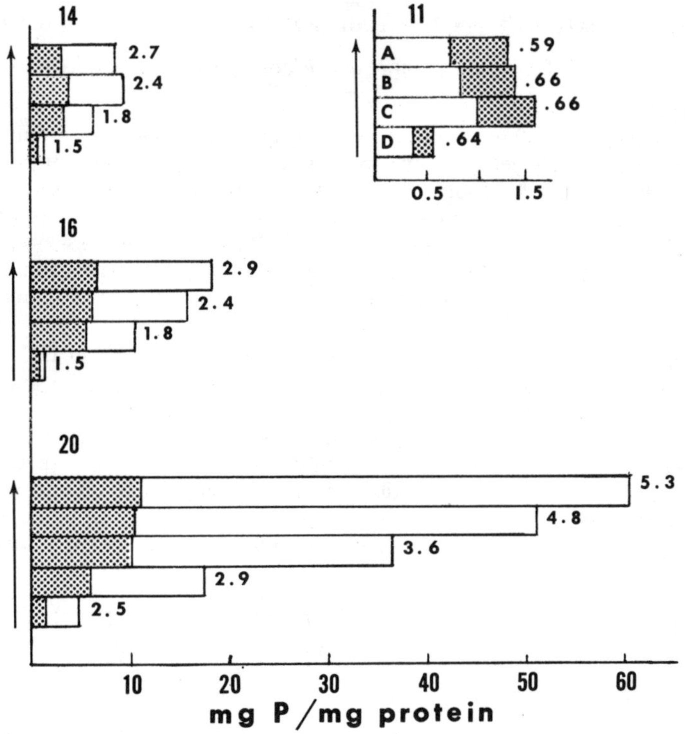

FIGURE 2. Development of the distribution pattern of phosphatase activity and PhP/bGP ratio from 11 to 20 days of age. Arrows indicate the direction from crypt to villus tip; clear columns show activity per 30 min. with PhP; stippled columns, activity with bGP. (Adapted from Moog & Grey, 1968.)

become well established. Throughout the period under consideration, activity with bGP remains fairly uniform from base to tip, and shows only a slight gradient even in the adult (FIGURES 1 and 2). Thus, it appears that at about 16 days, the epithelial surface acquires the ability to cleave PhP (or other aromatic phosphomonesters) at a rate that increases as the cells pass up the sides of the villi.

The acquisition of this new property cannot be attributed to a change in migration rate that might alter the capacity of the cells to express inherent potentialities. Grey (1968) has shown that the time required for a cell to pass from crypt to tip at 11 and 16 days is only slightly longer than that required in the adult. A change in villus length is probably not an important contributory factor either, for the average length is only about 20 percent greater at 20 days than at 11 (O'Connor, 1966; Grey, 1968). It may, however, be significant that the appearance of the high-ratio phosphatase that achieves maximal activity at the villi tips coincides with an apparent reorganization of the microvilli. Between 16 and 18 days, the microvilli shift from a short, broad form to a long, slender form, without change of total volume (Overton, 1965); the lengthening of the microvilli is most pronounced near the villi tips, and in adult life a similar morphogenetic change goes on continuously as the cells migrate up the villi (Brown, 1962).

Differentiation of the Molecular Forms of Ducdenal Phosphatase

1. Chromatographic and Electrophoretic Patterns

That the phosphatase of the mouse duodenum is heterogeneous at all stages has been decisively demonstrated by investigations employing column chromatography and starch gel electrophoresis (Moog, Vire & Grey, 1966; Nayudu & Moog, 1967; Etzler & Moog, 1968b). All this work has been based on homogenates of whole duodenal (or sometimes jejunal) wall, in which the phosphatase has been solubilized with butanol (Morton, 1954). The results have confirmed and extended the inferences concerning phosphatase heterogeneity that have been derived from the previously discussed studies of the development of phosphatase activity and its spatial distribution.

When butanol extracts of 11-day duodenum are eluted from DEAE-cellulose in a rising concentration of acetate, the greater part of the activity appears as a single peak (FIGURE 3) with a uniform, low PhP/bGP ratio in all fractions (Etzler & Moog, 1968b). Extract of 20-day duodenum similarly yields a single peak (FIGURE 3), but this proves to be strongly asymmetrical with respect to activity on the two substrates, the fractions at the leading edge of the peak having PhP/bGP ratios of 6 or occasionally higher, those at the trailing edge falling to 2.0, but rarely lower. In addition, some activity with ratios above 6 fails to bind to

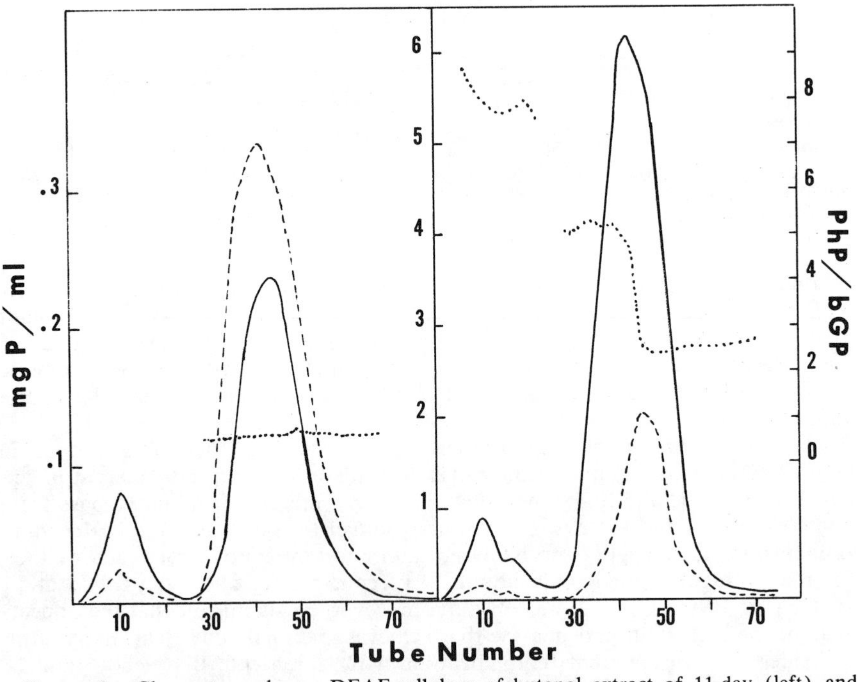

FIGURE 3. Chromatography on DEAE-cellulose of butanol extract of 11-day (left) and 20-day (right) duodenum. The column was equilibrated with 0.05M tris acetate buffer at pH 7.4. Gradient elution with sodium acetate rising to 0.4M was begun at tube 21; the eluate was collected in 5 ml portions. Solid line indicates activity on PhP; short dashes, activity on bGP; dotted line, PhP/bGP ratio. (Adapted from Moog *et al.*, 1966; Etzler & Moog, 1968b.)

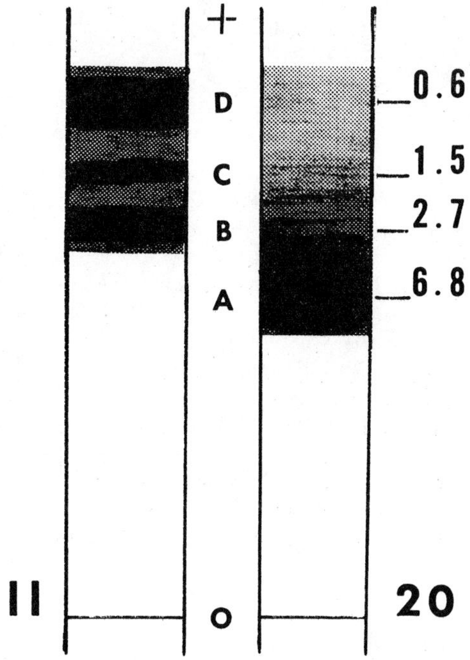

FIGURE 4. Electrophoresis on starch gel of butanol extract of 11-day and 20-day duodenum. "O" indicates origin, migration being toward the anode. Numbers at the right represent PhP/bGP ratios of phosphatase eluted from the regions indicated. (Sketch adapted from Moog *et al.*, 1966.)

the column, and is collected before the acetate gradient is applied (Moog, Vire & Grey, 1966; Etzler & Moog, 1968a; 1968b).

When 11-day extract is electrophoresed in starch gel, three distinct bands appear; whether these differ in catalytic properties is not known. FIGURE 4 shows that 20-day extract yields a zymogram differing from that produced by 11-day material in three important respects: (1) a large part of the 20-day activity is less mobile than that from 11 days, and forms a broad new (A) band behind the others; (2) a portion of the 20-day activity appears in the region occupied by the 11-day bands, but it does not form distinct bands (FIGURE 4); (3) a very small part of the 20-day activity is of the highly mobile type, represented by the most mobile (D) band at 11 days. That the intermediate (B and C) bands of 11-day duodenum cannot be identical with isozymes migrating to the same region in 20-day preparations was revealed by cutting out the bands from unstained strips of gel and eluting the phosphatase for quantitative determination of activity (Moog, Vire & Grey, 1966). The A and B bands contained 90 percent of the recoverable activity; the former had a PhP/bGP ratio of 6.8, the latter of 2.7 (FIGURE 4). Only a trivial amount retained a ratio below 1.

These results indicate that during the course of postnatal development, duodenal phosphatase comprises three families of isozymes. The first group is the trio of bands that can be resolved from 11-day extract by electrophoresis, but not separated from each other by any chromatographic technique that we have used; in aggregate these make up what we have designated as "low-ratio phosphatase" (LRP; PhP/bGP$<$1). The second type is "intermediate ratio phosphatase"

(IRP; PhP/bGP ≅ 2), abundant at 20 days, which resembles LRP in electrophoretic mobility. The third type is "high-ratio phosphatase" (HRP; PhP/bGP ≅ 6), predominant at 20 days, which is separable from IRP by both chromatographic and electrophoretic means. The distribution pattern shown in FIGURES 1 and 2 suggests that HRP and IRP are, to some extent, spatially separated in the living state.

2. *Immunochemical Studies of HRP and LRP*

Immunochemical investigations of the forms of phosphatase just identified have revealed that these forms are antigenically distinct, but cross-reactive (Etzler & Moog, 1968a; 1968b). In these investigations, we prepared antisera to LRP derived from 11-day duodena, and to HRP from 20-day duodena. Both antigen preparations were purified by chromatography on DEAE-cellulose, with HRP fractions being separated from those of lower ratio, rechromatographed, and, in some cases, also passed through Sephadex G-200.

When a series of 11-day LRP or 20-day HRP preparations of different ratios were adjusted to the same initial activity and combined with antisera of increasing concentration, both kinds of activity were precipitated by both antisera (the activity being recoverable in the precipitates). FIGURE 5 shows, however, that the slopes of the titration curves differ, each antiserum removing its own antigen at lower concentration (Etzler & Moog, 1968a). When the two enzyme prepara-

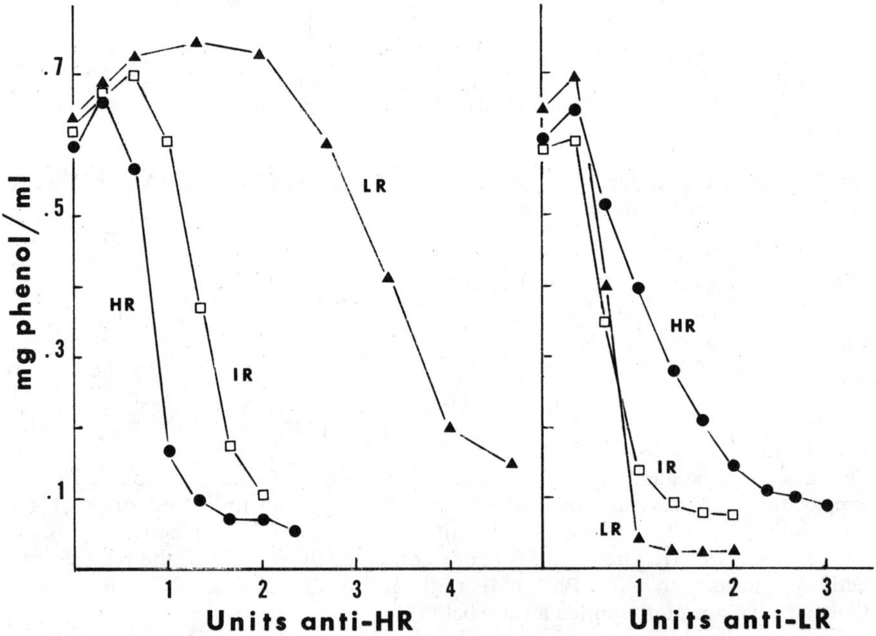

FIGURE 5. Titration of high-, intermediate-, and low-ratio phosphatases with antiserum to high-ratio and low-ratio phosphatase. One unit of antiserum = 0.3 ml of a 1/20 dilution of whole serum. Enzyme preparations were adjusted to the same initial activity, allowed to stand in the presence of antiserum for 36 hours at 4°, and then centrifuged. Ordinate indicates the activity (measured with PhP) remaining in the supernatant fraction. (Adapted from Etzler & Moog, 1968a.)

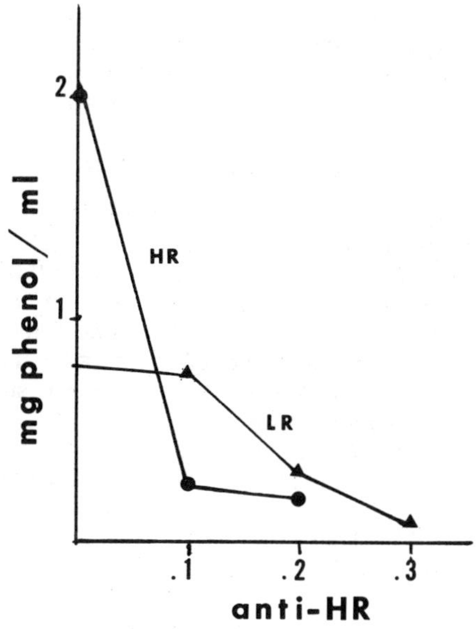

FIGURE 6. Titration of 20-day, high-ratio phosphatase and 11-day, low-ratio phosphatase with antiserum to high-ratio phosphatase. Procedure is same as for FIGURE 5, except that enzyme preparations were adjusted to the same initial protein content (9.6 μg protein per tube). (Adapted from Etzler & Moog, 1968a.)

tions were adjusted to the same initial protein content, and then mixed with antiserum to Sephadex-purified HRP, the titration curves crossed, thus confirming the inference that anti–HRP has higher specificity for its own isozyme than for LRP (FIGURE 6). These results, together with those obtained from absorption and immunodiffusion experiments (Etzler & Moog, 1968a), support the conclusion drawn from chromatography and electrophoresis that 11-day LRP is a different molecule from 20-day HRP; but they also reveal that the two forms do have antigenic resemblances.

3. The Nature of IRP

When 20-day IRP is titrated with antiserum to either HRP or LRP, it reacts readily with both (FIGURE 5). In immunochemical terms, at least, this isozyme appears to embody characteristics of both of the others. If the supernatant and precipitant fractions obtained on titration of 20-day IRP with anti-HRP serum are assayed with both PhP and bGP, the precipitates show higher PhP/bGP ratios than the controls with normal serum, but the supernates show lower ratios, falling below 1 (TABLE 1). Apparently the IRP preparation is not homogeneous. It is, however, significant that the precipitates do not have ratios much above 2; evidently, IRP is not simply a mixture of high- and low-ratio forms.

The results do suggest, on the other hand, that the IRP fraction obtainable from the 20-day duodenum includes two or more isozymes with PhP/bGP ratios ranging from below 1 to above 2. These isozymes have several interesting resemblances to LRP. Both IRP and LRP, as previously noted, migrate to the same region in starch gel, though only the latter forms distinct bands within that region. In immunodiffusion studies with anti-LRP serum, LRP and IRP yield a confluent precipitation line, indicating identity (Etzler & Moog, 1968a). Further, both groups of isozymes bind to DEAE-cellulose equilibrated with 0.05M tris acetate at various pH's, and can be eluted only by increasing the concentration of acetate (Etzler & Moog, 1968b). In all these respects, LRP and IRP both differ from 20-day HRP.

4. The Nature of HRP

In butanol extracts of 20-day duodenum, HRP is distinguished from IRP by the fact that the former migrates more slowly in starch gel and is eluted from DEAE-cellulose at lower concentrations of acetate. In 0.05 M tris acetate at pH 7.0, HRP scarcely binds to DEAE-cellulose at all, so that the extract is, by this treatment, separated into two discrete fractions, one with PhP/bGP ratios rising above 8, and the other with ratios of about 2 (FIGURE 7). The heterogeneity that is suggested by the spread of ratios in the first fraction is supported by the results obtained when 20-day extract is eluted by a series of buffers of decreasing pH (Etzler & Moog, 1968b). Each drop in pH is followed by the elution of a phosphatase peak of lower ratio than the preceding one (FIGURE 8). The series of peaks thus obtained may, in part, be artifacts caused by the sudden shifts of pH (Peterson & Sober, 1962). That they are more than merely artifactual, however, is shown by two findings: (1) If a single peak is rechromatographed under the original conditions, it appears as a new peak with the same pH range and PhP/bGP ratios that characterized the first peak (Etzler & Moog, 1968b); (2) If individual eluates resulting from stepwise pH elution are condensed and electrophoresed, they show increasing mobility corresponding with their decreasing PhP/bGP ratios (FIGURE 9).

HRP thus appears to be made up of a series of forms not sharply delimited by the separation techniques we have used. Hog kidney phosphatase has similarly been resolved into a large series of stable isozymes by step-wise elution with increasing concentrations of acetate (Nüske & Venner, 1966). The intestinal forms may differ slightly in molecular size, since molecular exclusion chromatography of 20-day duodenum extract with Sephadex-G-200 yields a single peak of activity in which, however, PhP/bGP ratios drop continuously from the first-eluted fractions to the last (Etzler & Moog, 1968b). Although the indicated differences are probably not great enough to be accounted for by differences in numbers of subunits constituting the various molecular forms, it does appear that within the high-ratio class of isozymes, increase of ratio is by some means associated with increase in molecular size.

TABLE 1

PhP/bGP RATIOS OF SUPERNATANT AND PRECIPITANT FRACTIONS OBTAINED ON TITRATION OF IRP WITH ANTI-HRP SERUM

Units Anti-HR Serum*	PhP/bGP Supernatant	PhP/bGP Precipitate
0	1.45, 1.60†	
0.33	1.40, 1.45	
0.67	1.40, 1.45	
1.00	1.28, 1.35	1.90, 2.05
1.33	1.10, 1.15	1.92, 2.05
1.67	0.95, 1.00	1.75, 2.05
2.00	0.82	1.72, 1.95

* In three controls with normal serum, ratios were 1.35, 1.45, and 1.45.
† Ratios in duplicate titrations.

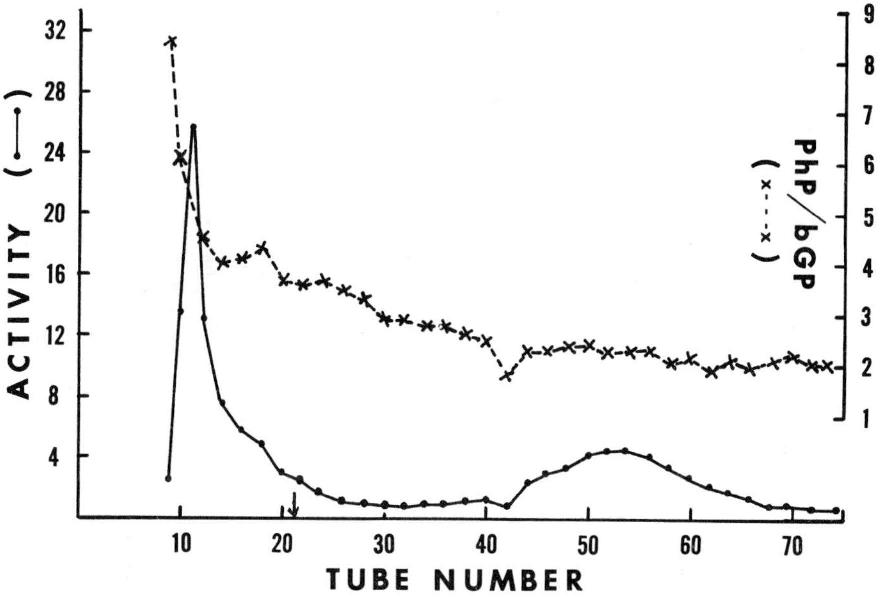

FIGURE 7. Chromatography of butanol extract of 20-day duodenum on DEAE-cellulose equilibrated with 0.05 M trisacetate buffer at pH 7.0. Elution with increasing concentration of acetate was begun at tube 21 (arrow). (Adapted from Etzler & Moog, 1968b.)

Although chromatography of 11-day duodenal extracts does not yield any activity with ratios above 3, the low-ratio activity eluted from the DEAE-cellulose column is, nevertheless, accompanied by a material that cross-reacts with anti-HRP serum. This is indicated by the fact that when LRP is combined with anti-HRP serum, a precipitate appears that has no phosphatase activity. For example, in the titration of 11-day LRP shown in FIGURE 4, 2 1/3 units of anti-HRP serum, though removing no phosphatase activity from the supernatant, clearly caused the formation of a precipitate that was enzymatically inactive; subsequent addition of HRP to the supernatant fraction revealed that the anti-serum had virtually lost the ability to combine with its own antigen (Etzler & Moog, 1966). The indicated conclusion that an enzymatically inactive molecule antigenically similar to HRP is present in the 11-day duodenum is further supported by the results of agar diffusion tests between anti-LRP serum and its own antigen (Etzler & Moog, 1968a). In this case, two precipitant lines are formed, only one of which stains for phosphatase activity; the inactive line is continuous (identical) with a single phosphatase-active line that forms between anti-LRP serum and HRP (FIGURE 10).

In addition to this inactive component, 11-day extracts also contain a small amount of activity with ratios above 1 (Etzler & Moog, 1968b). The quantity of such phosphatase, and its ratio, differs between mouse strains, being relatively abundant and having ratios as high as 3, in our high-activity strain (Nayudu & Moog, 1967). This activity resembles HRP in that it does not bind the DEAE-cellulose equilibrated with 0.05 M tris acetate at pH 7.4; thus, it is completely separable from the major fraction (used in the titration experiments described in the preceding paragraph), which appears as a peak with ratios below 1 through-

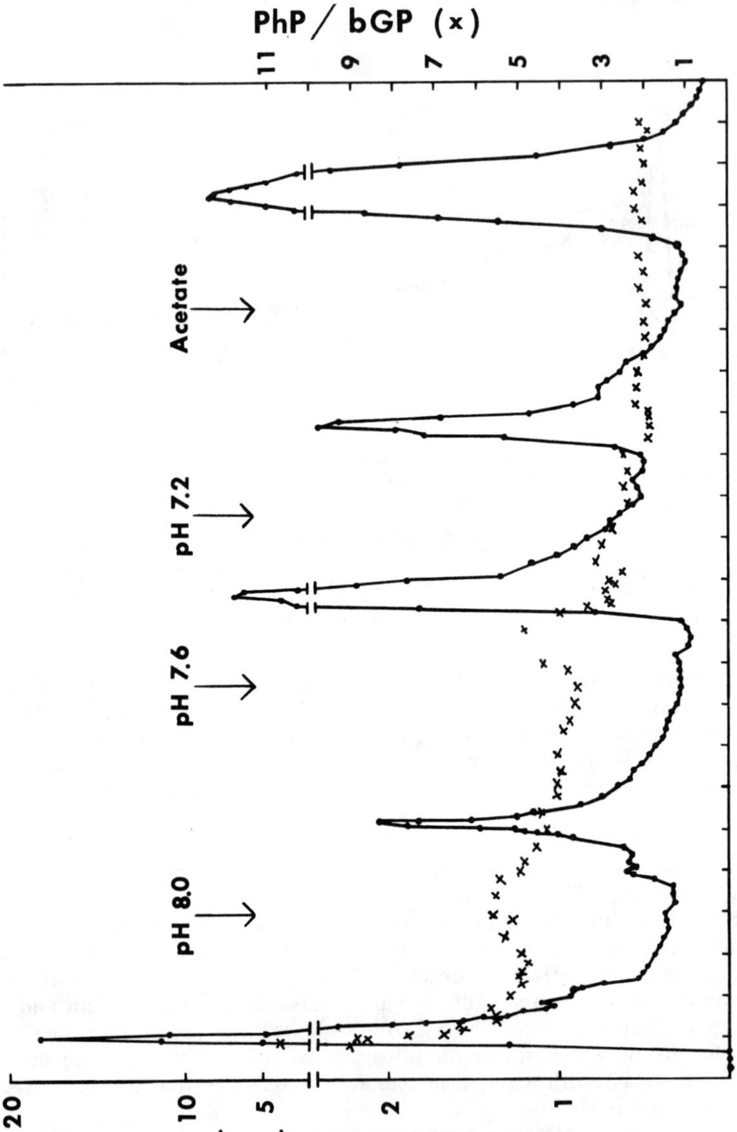
PhP / bGP (x)
11
9
7
5
3
1
ACTIVITY (•—•)
20
10
5
2
1
pH 8.0
pH 7.6
pH 7.2
Acetate
40
80
120
160
200
240
280
320
360
400
440
TUBE NUMBER

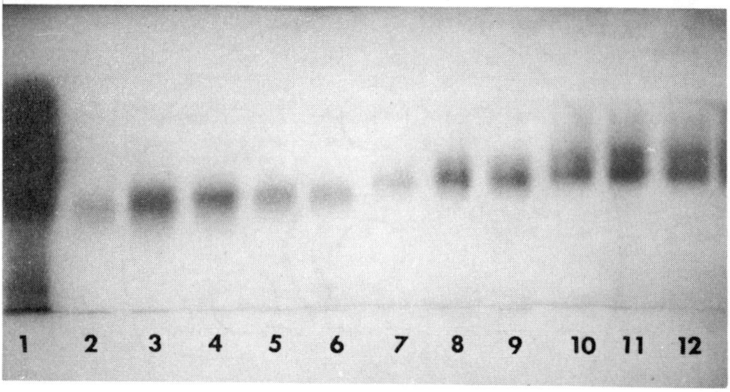

FIGURE 9. Starch gel electropherograms showing mobility of duodenal extract and of individual eluates from the column shown in FIGURE 7. The gel was stained for phosphatase activity with sodium alpha-naphthol and diazo blue B. Sources of samples and their PhP/bGP ratios are as follows: slot (1) adult duodenal extract; (2) tube 17 in FIGURE 7, ratio 10.80; (3) tube 20, ratio 8.97; (4) tube 21, ratio 7.71; (5) tube 22, ratio 6.83; (6) tube 23, ratio 6.71; (7) tube 123, ratio 4.48; (8) tube 232, ratio 2.99; (9) tube 235, ratio 3.02; (10) tube 314, ratio 1.88; (11) tube 424, ratio 2.44; (12) tube 426, ratio 2.28; (13) tube 430, ratio 2.01.

out. The relationship between the nonbinding phosphatase obtained from 11-day extracts to that obtained under similar conditions at later stages has not been determined.

DUODENAL PHOSPHATASE ISOZYMES IN DEVELOPMENT: INTERRELATIONS AND CONTROLLING MECHANISMS

That the high level of phosphatase activity present in the duodenum of the mature mouse is achieved in a brief critical period has been known for many years (Moog, 1951). Preliminary evidence that this period comprises two distinct, if partly overlapping, phases (Moog, 1961) has been decisively supported by recent studies that have elucidated the characteristics of the two phases (Moog & Grey, 1968; Etzler & Moog, 1968b). In the first phase, which is over by 16 days, phosphatase activity increases with relation to both PhP and bGP, though to a somewhat greater extent with the former; in effect, the isozymes with PhP/bGP ratios below 1 give way to a new group with ratios rising to 2 or above. At this stage, the isozymes show only a slight tendency toward spatial segregation on the villus (FIGURE 2). The second phase, which begins after 14 days, differs from the first in two important respects. First, the large increase of phosphatase activity that continues up to 19 or 20 days substantially affects hydrolysis of PhP only, a result that has now been shown to be due to the appearance of a new class of isozymes with increasingly high preference for PhP (Etzler & Moog, 1968b). Second, this new HRP is graded along the villi from the time of its initial appearance, the highest ratios being confined to the tips of the villi (Moog & Grey, 1968). Since the epithelial cells are in continuous transit up the villi, the isozymes of the high-ratio class must undergo some alterations

FIGURE 8. Chromatography of butanol extract of adult duodenum on DEAE-cellulose equilibrated with 0.05 M tris acetate buffer at pH 8.2. After the completion of the first peak elution was continued with a series of buffers of decreasing pH, as indicated. Gradient elution with sodium acetate was begun at tube 370. (From Etzler & Moog, 1968a; reproduced by permission of Academic Press, Inc., New York, N. Y.)

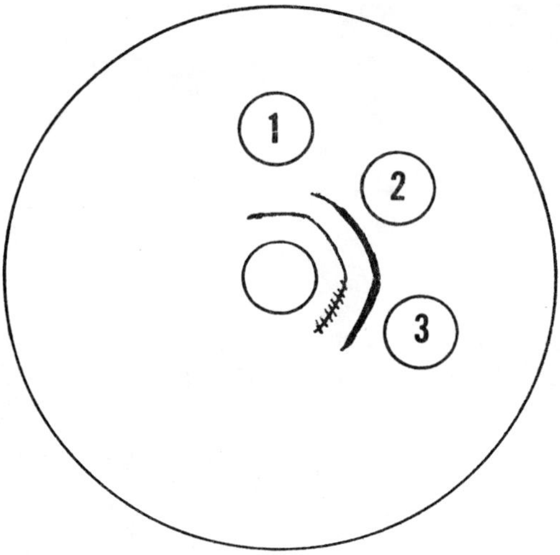

FIGURE 10. Immunodiffusion with anti-LR serum. Well No. 1, 20-day HRP; No. 2, 20-day IRP; No. 3, 11-day LRP.

or replacement as the cells of which they are a part travel toward the extrusion zone.

Although the sequence of developmental events affecting phosphatase activity in the duodenum is clear, the interrelations of the isozymes is still open to question. New molecular forms might be produced by conversion or transformation of preexisting types, or they might arise by *de novo* synthesis at the appropriate time. The numerous resemblances of 20-day IRP and 11-day LRP suggests that the former might be converted from the latter. Similarly, the presence at 11 days of an enzymatically inactive material that cross-reacts with anti-HRP suggests that the high-ratio isozymes might originate from the activation of an inactive precursor.

The question raised by these observations may be explored in terms of the factors known to influence that pattern of phosphatase development. The secretions of the adrenal cortex are essential (Moog, 1953; 1962). In mice adrenalectomized at 12 days, the infant condition persists, whereas exogenous corticosteroid elicits a precocious rise in phosphatase activity, whether administered *in vivo* (Moog, 1953) or added to (chick embryo) duodenum in organ culture (Moog & Kirsch, 1955). In both cases, the effect is slow, requiring more than 24 hours for a significant increase to occur. If cortical hormone is added directly to duodenal homogenates or extracts, however, phosphatase activity is not affected. These results might suggest that the role of the corticoid is to stimulate the synthesis of new enzyme molecules; this appears to be the mechanism by which corticoids elevate glutamine synthetase activity in the developing retina (Moscona *et al.*, 1968; Reif-Lehrer & Amos, 1968) or tyrosine transaminase activity in the liver (Kenney, 1962). On the other hand, the effects that actinomycin D, puromycin, cycloheximide and ethionine exert on duodenal phosphatase activity militate against this interpretation in the present case. These drugs cause a marked increase of phosphatase activity and shift in isozyme population when administered to normal young mice, and they act additively with cortisone in producing the same effects (Moog, 1964; 1966). Although it has not been demonstrated that these drugs depress synthesis of RNA or protein in the intestine at the dose levels employed, the fact that the one property they have in common is the ability to interfere with protein synthesis suggests that the alterations in duodenal phosphatase activity during the critical period of development are not primarily a matter of *de novo* synthesis.

The alternative view that new isozymes arise in development from precursors that may or may not have phosphatase activity is compatible with the demonstration that prednisolone (Δ'-hydrocortisone) elicits in HeLa cell cultures an increase in activity that is not accompanied either by increase of enzyme protein or decrease in degradation rate (Griffen & Cox, 1966). Although the authors have attributed this result to a configurational change induced during the synthesis of the enzyme, they also recognize the possibility that prednisolone might act by way of some other substance that interacts with alkaline phosphatase in such a manner as to enhance its activity. The corticoid-induced increase of phosphatase in HeLa cells is correlated with protection against lysis of deoxycholate (Melnykovych, 1966), a fact suggesting that the configurational change induced in the enzyme is linked to a change in the character of the cell membrane. When purified phosphatase is allowed to spread on artificial membranes, its activity is raised as much as six times that in homogeneous solution (Poltorak & Vorobeva, 1966).

In the duodenum, the surface membrane expands during the period that has been identified here as the second phase of phosphatase increase. Since this expansion involves no change in volume of the microvilli, Overton (1965) suggested that "the maturation of these structures may involve reorganization rather than synthesis." Probably the membrane changes in character as well as in extent, for in rats (in which intestinal differentiation is very similar to that in mice) microvilli (brush border particles) are less stable in 10-day-old animals than in adults (Noack *et al.*, 1966). In the light of these observations, it seems reasonable to suggest that at least the second phase of phosphatase differentiation in the duodenum is associated with the expansion of the microvillar surface, with the topographical seriation of isozymes that becomes established in this period being also linked to the continued expansion of the surface that goes on throughout life as cells migrate up the villi (Brown, 1962). Whatever the nature of the change affecting phosphatase during cell transit, it is interesting that its dimensions are not fixed. If adult mice are given actinomycin D, the PhP/bGP ratios of their duodenal phosphatase rise abnormally, with ratios as high as those ordinarily associated with villus tips being found at their bases (Moog & Grey, 1968). This result supports the view that in the normal duodenum, the differentiation of phosphatase goes on under the control of some restraining mechanism (Moog, 1966).

Summary

Alkaline phosphatase is an integral part of the outer surface of the microvillus border of the epithelial cells that line the small intestine. In the duodenum of the infant mouse, phosphatase activity is relatively low and is uniformly distributed over the surfaces of the villi. The enzyme at this stage hydrolyzes beta-glycerophosphate more rapidly than phenylphosphate; the PhP/bGP ratio is about 0.7. Between 11 and 14 days, activity increases, particularly with PhP, so that PhP/bGP ratios rise above 1. The distribution of activity on the villi remains fairly uniform from tip to base. After 16 days, activity with PhP increases sharply, especially toward the tips of the villi, so that by 20 days a gradient of activity and ratio rising from base to tip becomes established.

The low-ratio phosphatase (LRP) of the infant stage yields three bands on electrophoresis in starch gel; it is eluded from DEAE-cellulose as a single peak in which all fractions have the same PhP/bGP ratio. Phosphatase extracted from duodena of 20-day-old mice contains activity that shows the same mobility in starch gel as the 11-day bands, but it also has a large amount of more slowly migrating activity that has a PhP/bGP ratio of about 6. By chromatography on DEAE-cellulose, 20-day phosphatase can be divided into two fractions, one that does not bind to the column with 0.05 M tris acetate at pH 7.2 or below, and one that can be eluted by raising the concentration of acetate. The former fraction has PhP/bGP ratios of about 6, the latter of about 2; these are designated "high-ratio phosphatase" (HRP) and "intermediate-ratio phosphatase" (IRP), respectively.

Immunochemical studies made with antiserum to purified 11-day LRP and 20-day HRP have shown that the three types of phosphatase are distinct but have antigenic similarities. The 11-day duodenum has also been shown to contain enzymatically inactive material that cross-reacts with anti-HRP serum.

Further examination of HRP by ion exchange and molecular exclusion chromatography indicates that this material consists of an indeterminate series of forms that differ slightly in molecular size. These forms, which have ratios ranging from about 2.5 to 10, seem to be differentially distributed on the villus, those of highest ratio being concentrated toward the tip. Since the epithelial cells continually migrate from the crypts, where they arise, to the tips, where they are extruded, it appears that the phosphatase invested in their surface membrane differentiates as migration proceeds.

References

Birkenmeier, E. H. & F. Moog. (Unpublished.)

Brown, A. L. 1962. Microvilli of the human jejunal epithelial cell. J. Cell Biol. **12:** 623–627.

Clark, S. L. 1959. The ingestion of proteins and colloidal materials by columnar absorptive cells of the small intestine in suckling rats and mice. J. Biophys. Biochem. Cytol. **5:** 41–50.

Dahlqvist, A. & C. Nordstrom. 1966. The distribution of disaccharidase activities in the villi and crypts of the small intestinal mucosa. Biochim. Biophys. Acta **113:** 624–626.

Denes, A. E. & F. Moog. (Unpublished.)

Doell, R. G. & N. Kretchmer. 1964. Intestinal invertase; precocious development of activity after injection of hydrocortisone. Science **143:** 42–44.

Etzler, M. & F. Moog. 1966. Inactive alkaline phosphatase in the nursing mouse duodenum: immunological evidence. Science **154:** 1037–1038.

Etzler, M. & F. Moog. 1968a. Immunological characterization of alkaline phosphatase isozymes of the mouse duodenum. Biochim. Biophys. Acta **154:** 151–161.

Etzler, M. & F. Moog. 1968b. Biochemical identification and characterization of the multiple forms of alkaline phosphatase in the developing duodenum of the mouse. Develop. Biol. **18:** 515–535.

Gomori, G. 1941. The distribution of phosphatases in normal organs and tissues. J. Cell. Comp. Physiol. **17:** 71–83.

Grey, R. D. 1968. Epithelial cell migration in the intestine of the young mouse. Develop. Biol. **18:** 501–514.

Griffen, M. J. & R. P. Cox. 1966. Studies on the mechanism of hormonal induction of alkaline phosphatase in cell cultures. Proc. Nat. Acad. Sci. USA **56:** 946–953.

Holt, J. H. & D. Miller. 1962. The localization of phosphomonoesterases and aminopeptidase in brush borders isolated from intestinal epithelial cells. Biochim. Biophys. Acta **58:** 239–243.

HUGON, J. & M. BORGERS. 1966. Ultrastructural localization of alkaline phosphatase in the absorbing cells of the duodenum of mouse. J. Histochem. Cytochem. **14:** 629–640.

KENNEY, F. T. 1962. Induction of tyrosine-alpha-keto-glutarate transaminase in rat liver. IV. Evidence for an increase in the rate of protein synthesis. J. Biol. Chem. **237:** 3495–3498.

LEBLOND, C. P. & B. MESSIER. 1958. Renewal of chief cells and goblet cells in the small intestine as shown by radioautography after injection of thymidine-H^3 into mice. Anat. Rec. **132:** 247–259.

MELNYKOVYCH, G. 1966. Glucocorticoid induced resistance to deoxycholate lysis in HeLa cells. Science **152:** 1086–1087.

MILLER, D. & R. K. CRANE. 1961. The digestive function of the epithelium of the small intestine. I. An intracellular locus of disaccharide and sugar phosphate ester hydrolysis. Biochim. Biophys. Acta **52:** 281–293.

MOOG, F. 1951. The differentiation of alkaline phosphomonoesterase in the duodenum of the mouse. J. Exp. Zool. **118:** 187–208.

MOOG, F. 1953. The influence of the pituitary-adrenal system on the differentiation of phosphatase in the duodenum of the suckling mouse. J. Exp. Zool. **124:** 329–346.

MOOG, F. 1961. Regional differences in the alkaline phosphatases of the small intestine of the mouse from birth to one year. Develop. Biol. **3:** 153–174.

MOOG, F. 1962. Developmental adaptations of alkaline phosphatases in the small intestine. Fed. Proc. **21:** 51–56.

MOOG, F. 1964. Intestinal phosphatase activity: acceleration of increase by puromycin and actinomycin. Science **144:** 414–416.

MOOG, F. 1966. The regulation of alkaline phosphatase activity in the duodenum of the mouse from birth to maturity. J. Exp. Zool. **161:** 353–368.

MOOG, F. 1969. Corticoids and the Enzymic Maturation of the Intestinal Surface: Alkaline Phosphatase, Leucyl Naphthylamidase, and Sucrase. *In* Hormones and Development. M. Hamburgh & E. C. Barrington, Eds. The National Foundation. (In press.)

MOOG, F. & R. F. GREY. 1967. Spatial and temporal differentiation of alkaline phosphatase on the intestinal villi of the mouse. J. Cell Biol. **32**(2)**:** C1–C6.

MOOG, F. & R. D. GREY. 1968. Alkaline phosphatase isozymes in the duodenum of the mouse: attainment of pattern of spatial distribution in normal development and under the influence of cortisone or actinomycin D. Develop. Biol. **18:** 481–500.

MOOG, F. & M. H. KIRSCH. 1955. Quantitative determination of phosphatase activity in chick embryo duodenum cultured in fluid media with and without hydrocortisone. Nature **175:** 722.

MOOG, F., H. R. VIRE & R. D. GREY. 1966. The multiple forms of alkaline phosphatase in the small intestine of the young mouse. Biochim. Biophys. Acta **113:** 336–349.

MORTON, R. K. 1954. The purification of alkaline phosphatases of animal tissues. Biochem. J. **57:** 595–603.

MOSCONA, A. A., M. H. MOSCONA & B. SAENZ. 1968. Enzyme induction in embryonic retina: the role of transcription and translation. Proc. Nat. Acad. Sci. **61:** 160-167.

NAYUDU, P. R. V. & F. MOOG. 1967. The genetic control of alkaline phosphatase activity in the duodenum of the mouse. Biochem. Genetics **1:** 155–170.

NOACK, R., O. KOLDOVSKY, M. FRIDRICH, A. HERINGOVA, N. JIRSOVA & G. SCHENK. 1966. Proteolytic and peptidase activities of the jejunum and ileum of the rat during postnatal development. Biochem. J. **100:** 775–778.

NORDSTROM, C., A. DAHLQVIST & L. JOSEFSSON. 1967. Quantitative determination of enzymes in different parts of the villi and crypts of rat small intestine. J. Histochem. Cytochem. **15:** 713–721.

NUSKE, R. & H. VENNER. 1966. Die Isoenzymefraktionen der unspezifischen alkalischen Phosphomonoesterase. Biochem. Z. **346:** 226–243.

O'CONNOR, T. M. 1966. Cell dynamics in the intestine of the mouse from late fetal life to maturity. Amer. J. Anat. **118:** 525–536.

ODA, T. & S. SEKI. 1966. Molecular basis of structure and function of the plasma membrane of the microvilli of intestinal epithelial cells. Program of the Sixth International Congress Electron Microscopy, Kyoto, Japan. : 387.

OVERTON, J. 1965. Fine structure of the free surface in developing mouse intestinal mucosa. J. Exp. Zool. **159:** 195–201.

OVERTON, J., A. EICHHOLZ & R. K. CRANE. 1965. Studies on the organization of the brush border in intestinal epithelial cells. J. Cell Biol. **26:** 693–706.

PETERSON, E. A. & H. A. SOBER. 1962. Column chromatography of proteins: Substituted celluloses. *In* Methods in Enzymology **5:** 3–27. S. P. Colowick & N. O. Kaplan, Eds. Academic Press, N. Y.

POLTORAK, O. M. & E. S. VOROBEVA. 1966. Adsorption models of biological membranes and alkaline phosphatase activitation in different types of adsorption layers. Z. Fiz. Khim. **40:** 1665–1667.

REIF-LEHRER, L. & H. AMOS. 1968. Hydrocortisone requirement for the induction of glutamine synthetase in chick embryo retinas. Biochem. J. **106:** 425–430.

DISCUSSION OF THE PAPER

C. L. MARKERT: Do you consider neuraminic acid is possibly being related to some of these changes?

DR. MOOG: Yes. Dr. Etzler has studied the effect of neuraminidase. There is no effect.

R. PHILLIPS (*University of Pennsylvania, Philadelphia, Pa.*): I wonder, Dr. Moog, if you could tell us what sort of considerations went into your choice of substrates in your assays, the beta-glycerophosphate and the phenylphosphate.

DR. MOOG: Well, I hate to answer that question because no particular consideration went into it at all. Many years ago, I began the studying of phosphatase using phenylphosphate because, at that time, which really is back in the early renaissance of this kind of work I suppose, the King-Armstrong technique was relatively new, and it seemed much easier than using beta-glycerophosphate, and I used it. Then some years later, one of my students, Dr. Yoshihiro Kato, was interested in finding out whether he could induce phosphatase in the chick embryo by the administration of substrate, and he found that, although intestinal phosphatase in the chick embryo is nonspecific, the only substrate that induced it was phenylphosphate. He was therefore curious to see whether what he had induced was specifically active on phenylphosphate, and this led to the discovery of this difference in ratio of substrate hydrolysis in the chick embryo. We then extended it to the mouse. Essentially, the difference here, I think, is the presence or absence of an aromatic structure in the substrate, because we have examined a variety of other substrates and they fall into these classes.

S. POSEN: Dr. Moog, does this ratio between phenylphosphatase activity and beta-glycerophosphatase activity hold true at all substrate concentrations or have you had the opportunity of studying it at a number of substrate concentrations?

DR. MOOG: Yes, this is a matter of the optimal substrate concentration. It doesn't necessarily reflect any light whatsoever on the physiological situation. This is a means for differentiating the phosphatases. Actually, when you get this shift to a preference of phenylphosphate, the K_m value increases rather considerably. So one is using a relatively high substrate concentration, but these are optimal activities as far as you can get optimal activities with phosphatase.

W. H. FISHMAN: I'd like to introduce a concept that might merit some consideration in relation to Dr. Moog's paper, and I'm sure that it will relate to some of the other papers that will be presented. Briefly stated, enzymes may simply be units of the structure of membranes, and their catalytic function is nonoperative. We recognize that by measuring alkaline phosphatase activity, we are recognizing a few amino acids of a polypeptide chain perhaps linked with a metal, located in some fortunate spatial configuration, so that when the substrate reaches that area in the enzyme molecule, it undergoes hydrolytic cleavage. Now, the rest of the molecule from the point of view of the biochemist might just as well not exist, but I think from the point of view of biologists, the noncatalytically active region may be even more important or equally important to the catalytically active sites. The location of alkaline phosphatase on the microvilli is not unique, there being other enzyme activities that can be demonstrated on the microvilli, but for which no role in active transport has been formulated. We can believe that alkaline phosphatase could be hydrolyzing in the middle of the intestinal lumen, when the pH might perhaps be at 8.0 or higher, but it would take a lot of imagination to conjure up the circumstances under which alkaline phosphatase in the microvilli of placenta would hydrolyze at pH 10.7, which is its optimum. So, just to crystallize the idea, the observation of enzymes for which the environment provides no opportunity for activity, together with proteins that have activities but for which one cannot at all imagine a purpose in digestion or in transport, all in the same cellular site, makes it easier to interpret phenomena if we forget about the catalytic site except as a marker for a particular protein in the biological system under study.

DR. MOOG: Well I think I would agree with that. What we're saying in this case is that some alteration of the nature of the catalytic site is the consequence of an alteration probably of the rest of the molecule. Our guess would be that it may be the carbohydrate region in the molecule that is being changed and that consequently exerts an effect on the catalytic properties of the molecule and of the active cell.

Dr. MARKERT: Dr. Moog, do you believe that you're probably dealing with a single polypeptide, or more than one? In other words, do you have more than one gene involved in the initial formation of the isoenzymes of alkaline phosphatase? Do you want to hazard a guess?

DR. MOOG: Dr. Etzler might like to say something on that subject.

DR. ETZLER: I really don't think that we have enough information to say whether or not there would be one or more genes involved, but I think the finding that there are these two really distinct classes of isoenzymes would probably require more than one gene. But I would like to make an additional comment, and I wonder if, perhaps, this is why you raised the question. Dr. Moog stated that the high-ratio isozymes differ from the lower-ratio isozymes in molecular weight. This difference in molecular weight is very, very slight, which rules out additional subunits. Actually, very preliminary estimations on Sephadex G-200 columns indicates that the molecular weight may be in the range of 180,000, which perhaps might suggest about four subunits or more.

DR. MARKERT: You never have found a mutant variety. That, of course, will give you the answer.

DR. MOOG: No, we are working with high- and low-phosphatase mouse strains, but the situation is quite complex in that a number of factors enter into the difference in the low-phosphatase strain; the villi are shorter and probably the microvilli are also shorter. So it's really the morphology which, to a certain extent, dictates the type of a phosphatase. It's rather interesting that the rate of transit is the same between the high- and low-phosphatase strain, which means that in the low strain, apparently, the cells spend less time on the villus and, consequently, they don't get as far in developing a high-ratio, high-activity phosphatase as they do in the high strain, where they simply survive longer because the villi are longer.

DR. AMINOFF (*University of Michigan, Ann Arbor, Mich.*): To continue the discussion that Professor Markert raised at a point of the two isozymes where you get the ratio to two substrates differing, would you not expect to have two different species of enzyme there, perhaps made up of the same polypeptide chain but in different proportions?

DR. ETZLER: This was our first thought when we were doing these experiments, but the fact is that we have such a spectrum of forms with the pH alteration of the column, i.e., a ratio of 10, a ratio of 8, a ratio of 6. We could make any ratio we want by simply altering the pH more gradually. A little more is being done here than just simply an alteration in the number or in the type of subunits.

DR. AMINOFF: Did you do an electrophoretic analysis of those different ratio samples?

DR. ETZLER: In one of Dr. Moog's slides, you saw that the samples with the different ratios differed very slightly in their electrophoretic mobility. The ones with the higher ratio were closer to the origin than the lower ratio ones were.

R. C. NORDLIE: I was wondering whether you had ever been tempted to change these ratios by detergents or mild heating.

DR. MOOG: Yes, we have made such attempts, with negative results.

DR. NORDLIE: We have seen quite an interesting change in patterns with fairly mild heating of a bacterial alkaline phosphatase (commerial preparation) at about 30 degrees or so; the activity with phenylphosphate compared with glucose-6-phosphate or beta-glycerophosphate was quite different in the first 10 minutes and then the ratio remained constant over a period of 45 minutes after this. A change in conformation due to the mild heating may have been responsible for this.

DR. MOOG: When you try heat inactivation the ratio does not change.

DR. BECKMAN: We've noticed that even placental alkaline phosphatase in an alkaline pH 8.5 has one major zone and one minor. If you electrophorese that at lower pH (pH 5.6), you will see five zones in a homozygous individual. The same thing applies to acid phosphatase in tissues. So, apparently, many of these descriptions of a whole ladder of isoenzymes of acid phosphatase are artifacts. Yet acid phosphatase can't stand an acid pH, for example, which is shocking. So you can easily get a number of different molecular forms with different pH's through some sort of recombination.

DR. MOOG: Yes, this is quite true, and this, I think, is why the constant assaying of activity on two different substrates and the demonstration of predictable and constant ratios tends to militate against the interpretation that we're merely dealing with artifacts in these cases. These are real differences in characteristics other than electrophoretic mobility.

DR. FISHMAN: I just rise very briefly to challenge the word *artifacts* being used to describe these varieties of phosphatase of Dr. Moog's study. I think the better word, and I'm sure Dr. Beckman would agree, would be the word *variants,* that is, these are variants made evident by the hydrogen concentration of the medium. At a previous isoenzyme conference, a whole collection isozyme bands on starch gel has been demonstrated, but these can be identified as members of the same family of isoenzymes since they have the same biochemical properties, e.g., molecular weight variants. So I think we will learn something by doing the starch gels at two different pH's and finding out how these variant forms are produced and learning about their significance. So I'd like you to avoid the use of the word *artifacts* here.

DR. BECKMAN: In a case where you can back your results with genetic analysis and can show that the individual in question is homozygous, you should make one molecular population of cells. If you can, in fact, show that there are pieces of a mutilated enzyme, then these are not variants to me. These are broken pieces and artifacts in a sense. Sorry.

DR. FISHMAN: Well, if they're broken inside of the cell, you wouldn't call them artifacts. It's only if the investigator is doing the breaking that you would call them artifacts. The proper term for the degraded isoenzyme might be "metabolic variant."

W. L. SIMPSON (*Detroit Institute of Cancer Research, Detroit, Mich.*): Dr. Moog, you've mentioned that different strains of mice have high- and low-phosphatase levels. I wonder if you could tell us whether the work that you've reported has been on one pure strain, and whether, in examining other strains that are high and low in alkaline phosphatase in the intestine, they show the same general ratios or whether the ratios also vary.

DR. MOOG: Well, this work covers such an interval of time that it involves work with more than one strain. Most of the work I reported probably was done with a noninbred strain. Since we've become interested in genetically controlled differences, we have screened a number of strains from Bar Harbor, Maine. Right now we are working with a high-phosphatase strain that we have screened out of the SWR strain from Bar Harbor, which had the highest activity we could find, but we've still been able to raise that considerably, although that strain has a hundred generations of inbreeding behind it, by selecting for phosphatase.

PHYSIOLOGY OF PROSTATIC PHOSPHOHYDROLASE SECRETION*

Harris Rosenkrantz
Mason Research Institute, Worcester, Mass.

In 1935, Kutscher and Wolbergs reported that the human prostate contained high activities of acid phosphatase and that the preferred substrates were α- and β-phosphoglycerol and not diphosphofructose or pyrophosphate.[1] It soon became evident that the measurement of acid phosphatase activity in serum and prostatic secretion could be used as a biochemical indicator of prostatic function. That the activity of the phosphomonoesterase was hormone-dependent was established by Gutman and Gutman, who described a rapid increase in activity from a low level in childhood to a high level at puberty.[1] Similar findings were observed for the monkey and dog.

The lack of seminal vesicles and bulbo-urethral glands in the dog afforded earlier and recent investigators with a necessary *in vivo* model for studying prostatic function. The major contribution of Huggins[2] and coworkers on the physiology and biochemistry and of Farrell and Lyman[3] on the pharmacology of the prostate were attained in the dog. In addition, it was known that prostatic tumors occurred spontaneously only in man and dog, with some tumors being hormone sensitive. Construction of a suitable prostatic fistula in the dog provided workers with an *in vivo* system amenable to the estimation of phosphohydrolase activity in the prostatic outflow.

Although little histochemistry was carried out on dog prostate, extensive determinations of phosphatase localization has been performed in rat and man.[5] Acid phosphatase activity was visualized as discrete cytoplasmic granules most often concentrated in the supranuclear region of the secretory cells. Positive reactions could be elicited in the luminal secretion. Development of cancer cells in the human prostate resulted in loss of acid phosphatase activity, which made its appearance in the serum.[6]

Anatomy of the Prostate

The relatively extensive organogenesis of the prostate gland and its contribution to the complex secretion of the seminal plasma would lead one to infer some importance of its function in reproductive physiology. Although a definitive biological assignment for the various components of prostatic fluid has not as yet been attained, the prostate gland has unfortunately endowed mankind with serious clinical hardships.

Five discrete groups of epithelial cords originating from the entodermal lining of the urethra and urogenital sinus develop into five lobes of the human prostate.[5] The sensitivity of this gland to sex hormones becomes evident in the newborn male when prostatic hypertrophy may be observed. In the fetal prostate, squamous metaplasia and focal hyperplasia of the acini due to estrogen activity has long been recognized. Localization of hormone influence suggested that the dorsal (posterior) lobe is predominantly androgen-sensitive; the middle (median) lobe, strongly estrogen-sensitive; the lateral lobes, androgen- and estrogen-responsive; and the ventral (anterior) lobe, least responsive to sex hormones.[5]

In the dog, three pairs of symmetrical buds arise from the urethral wall, two

* Supported largely by contract PH43–65–6 from the Endocrine Evaluation Branch, General Laboratories and Clinics, National Cancer Institute, D. H. E. W.

dorsal and one ventral, which eventually form a compact prostate completely encircling the urethra at the neck of the bladder.[5] Dorsal and ventral regions remain distinct in their histological staining and response to estrogen.

The prostate is innervated by parasympathetic (nervi erigentes) and sympathetic (hypogastric nerve) fibers from the pelvic plexus.[7,8] Stimulation of the hypogastric nerve partially empties the stored secretions of the prostate lumina, but parasympathetic stimulation evokes an increased output of prostatic secretion.

Recently Connolly *et al*[9] employed India ink and an iron compound (Imferon) to demonstrate a functional intraprostatic lymphatic system in the dog. They confirmed the earlier work of classical anatomists who described the fine capillaries arranged in a delicate network around each acinus. The periacinar capillaries become larger vessels that radiate toward the periphery of the gland via the trabeculae. After passing the capsule of the prostate, a second network, the periprostatic lymphatic plexus, feeds into the collecting lymph channels and reaches the regional lymph nodes. Prostatic blood flow in the dog has also been recently measured and found to be between 0.31 and 0.79 ml/g of tissue/min.[10] min.[10]

The size of the canine prostate in puppies and adult dogs has been investigated by Berg[11] and Lebeaux.[12] Correlation of acid phosphatase activity with canine prostatic size was not performed.

Preparation of Standardized Animals

The utilization of pharmacologic stimulation in dogs with prostatic fistula opened the way for biochemical studies on phosphohydrolase activity. Farrell and Lyman[3] utilized cholinergic drugs such as pilocarpine to evaluate their effect on prostatic secretion in dogs with ligations between the neck of the bladder and the urethra. The innovation of prostatic fistulas by Huggins[2] afforded a physiologically functional system for repeated studies on the same animal. Newer surgical modifications have permitted the healthy maintenance of dogs for more than five years.[13]

Is is very desirable to standardize an *in vivo* model for the study of enzyme production and activity. The castrated prostatic fistula dog with its anatomical advantage due to the lack of seminal vesicles provided a suitable model for the present investigation. Initially, masturbation was employed to obtain seminal plasma samples in order to evaluate prostatic function. Occasionally, wedge biopsies were performed during laparotomy. By and large, the technique of rectal palpation was routinely used for selecting animals with desirable, normal prostate glands.[12] A very good correlation between rectally estimated prostate size, actual size determined at autopsy and prostatic secretion production has been found. These approaches with a large number of dogs have indicated that the best animals can be selected between the ages of two to five years.

In a study of different modes of prostatic stimulation, masturbation, electroejaculation and pilocarpine, it was found that similar levels of acid phosphohydrolase activity could be achieved by each type of stimuli.[14] Pilocarpine yielded the most consistent results and was the stimulus of choice.

Construction of a proper prostatic fistula concerned us next. Huggins' original methods separated the bladder from the prostate and either translocated the gland to a more superficial position or left it undisturbed. Urinary flow was diverted through the abdominal wall by a brass cannula. Because of the high incidence of ascending urinary infections and the desire to retain the prostate in its normal orientation, the cystopreputiostomy fistula was devised.[13] The proximal end of the prepuce sheath is dissected and passed through the abdominal wall, and attached to an opening in the fundus of the bladder. The intact urethral canal serves the prostate gland in a normal fashion. The prostate is separated from the neck of the bladder.

In order to select a desirable dose of pilocarpine, several dogs were titrated with 0.30 to 7.50 mg pilocarpine/kg administered intravenously. Increases in pilocarpine induce increments in both volume and acid phosphohydrolase activity. Experience with a large number of dogs has led to standardization of the pilocarpine dose at 0.7 mg/kg. This dose evokes a copious flow of prostatic secretion with minimum discomfort regarding salivation and micturition. Volumes achieved in ten minutes were equivalent to those obtained by masturbation, suggesting a nearly physiological response.

Previously, Huggins had shown that a single intravenous injection of pilocarpine (12 to 18 mg/dog) elicited maximal secretion rates of volume and phosphohydrolase activity in the first 15 minutes of an hourly collection.[2] A progressive decline in three succeeding quarter-hour periods was observed for these parameters. Recent work has confirmed optimal enzyme activity in the first quarter-hour, but a remarkably constant level of acid phosphohydrolase activity was found in the subsequent intervals.[15] For example, in a group of four dogs the mean values ± S.E. for acid phosphohydrolase activity were 13.2 ± 1.40 (0 − 15 min), 7.7 ± 1.9 (15 − 30 min), 7.5 ± 1.6 (30 − 45 min) and 7.9 ± 0.5 (45–60 min) mg of phosphate released per ml. Intramuscular administration of pilocarpine displaced the greater enzyme activity to the second and third periods.[2]

In the human, Eliasson[16] has found that daily consecutive ejaculations decrease the volume of seminal plasma but not the activity of acid phosphatase. Also in the human, Clark and Treichler[17] reported variation of acid phosphatase activity in relation to the extent of psychic excitement. In both man and dog, pharmacologic or hormonal stimulation of prostatic secretion can result in a marked rise in acid phosphohydrolase activity.[2]

Our standard procedure of biweekly collections on cystopreputiostomy dogs using 0.7 mg pilocarpine/kg body weight provides relatively stable levels of acid phosphohydrolase activity characteristic for each dog. Using a β-glycerophosphate substrate-buffer medium, normal enzyme values vary from 1.19 ± 0.09 to 11.02 ± 0.81 mg of phosphate released per ml of prostatic fluid.[18,19] No correlation of enzyme activity with age or body weight has been detected.

Endocrine-Maintenance of the Castrate

Our attention was directed toward selection of a proper maintenance dose of testosterone so that support therapy would be in the physiologic range. The earlier workers employed testosterone propionate, but in the present investigation the nonesterified steroid was studied in order to be closer to the usual metabolic processes encountered by endogenous hormone. Finally, levels of testosterone were kept down in order to have acceptable testosterone: test-compound ratios in attempts to modify prostatic function.

By comparing prostatic output of acid phosphohydrolase activity before castration with that obtained on known levels of testosterone after castration on the same animals, a near physiologic testosterone level could be estimated for the maintenance of normal prostatic function. These data are shown in TABLE 1,

TABLE 1

ESTIMATION OF TESTOSTERONE LEVELS TO MAINTAIN PHYSIOLOGICAL PROSTATIC FUNCTION IN THE DOG

Dog No.	Age (Yr)	Total Acid Phosphohydrolase Activity* ($mg\ PO_4$ released/hr)		Testosterone Per Castrate (mg/kg)
		Intact	Castrate & Testosterone	
640	3	115	125	0.12
433	2	18	14	0.14
440	3	48	43	0.15
444	5	41	67	0.18
682	2	84	80	0.20
834	3	55	58	0.24

* The values represent the mean of three to four determinations.
Hourly volumes were between 13 and 28 ml.

and they suggest that a range of 0.12 to 0.24 mg of testosterone/kg body weight approaches physiological hormone levels in the dog.

Several workers have reported the noticeable decline in acid phosphatase activity in man between the ages of 40 and 60 years.[20,21] Despite this evidence, serum testosterone levels are not markedly changed in this age group.[22] In the age group (two to seven years old) of dogs studied in the present investigation, 0.12 to 0.24 mg of testosterone/kg was adequate to elicit 10 to 20 ml of prostatic secretion/hour.[23] In order to maintain maximum prostatic tone and secretory capability, our colony of prostatic fistula dogs are actually given 5 mg (approximately 0.4 mg/kg) testosterone subcutaneously daily in a carboxymethylcellulose medium. This dose assured relatively stable volumes between 20 and 50 ml/hr.

Testosterone titrations have been carried out by diminishing the daily 5-mg dose in a stepwise fashion or by stabilizing prostatic performance at approximately 0.1 mg/kg in dogs that were originally maintained on 5 mg testosterone daily, and then increasing the testosterone dose.[23,24] Representative results of such testosterone titrations are given in TABLE 2. Four to six determinations were made at each testosterone dose, which meant that each dog was maintained at a particular hormone level for two to three weeks before a change in the quantity of testosterone was initiated. Two collections of prostatic fluid were made

TABLE 2

THE RESPONSE OF PROSTATIC ACID PHOSPHOHYDROLASE ACTIVITY TO TESTOSTERONE TITRATION*

Testosterone (mg/kg)	Dog No. 440		Dog No. 649		Dog No. 135		Dog No. 149	
	No. of Days	Total PO_4 (mg/hr)	No. of Days	Total PO_4 (mg/hr)	No. of Days	Total PO_4 (mg/hr)	No. of Days	Total PO_4 (mg/hr)
0.4	30	289	30	251	28	154	28	214
0	0		0		44	0.01	44	0.02
0.01	0		0		10	0.04	10	0.02
0.02	0		0		13	0.04	13	0.02
0.1	14	39	14	25	10	0.08	10	0.03
0.2	14	42	14	37	0		0	
0.3	14	107	14	98	0		0	
0.4	17	214	17	188	24	180	52	248
0.5	28	298	28	253	0		0	

* Results are mean of four to six determinations; prostatic fluid was collected twice weekly.

weekly for each dog. As expected, increments in enzyme activity paralleled increases in hormone dose.

When animals were kept on a low androgen maintenance dose, (dogs No. 440 and 649), the concentration (mg/ml) of phosphohydrolase activity increased in a gradual fashion as the level of testosterone was raised. Volume gains were more dramatic. On the other hand, when animals received no testosterone (dogs No. 135 and 149) before titration was begun, the concentration of enzyme activity rose rapidly and exceeded physiologic levels as exogenous hormone was increased. This response is depicted in the data of TABLE 3, and clearly demonstrates stimulation of enzyme secretion and probably enhancement of enzyme synthesis, since fluid mobilization for secretion followed behind. Decrements in hormone replacement usually initiate a decline in the acid phosphohydrolase activity before alterations in volume, also suggesting a dependency of enzyme synthesis on testosterone.[23]

In earlier studies Huggins *et al.*[25] determined the rate of prostatic atrophy after castration and observed a cessation of prostatic secretion within 7 to 23 days. Daily injections of large amounts of testosterone propionate restored prostatic function, and once secretion was normal, the exogenous androgen could be greatly reduced without causing a decrease in prostatic volume. These investigators also observed a transient testicular atrophy with a corresponding decline in prostatic activity when dogs were caged for several months. Pazos and Huggins[26] found that starvation in the dog resulted in a reduction in prostatic volume that could be restored by administration of androgen. In the rat, Bialy and Pincus[27] did not detect a stimulation of acid phosphohydrolase activity, total or tartrate-sensitive, in ventral prostate tissue. Our own work has demonstrated a testosterone-induced increase in acid phosphohydrolase activity in canine prostatic secretion in castrated and intact dogs[23] as well as increased histochemical staining of this enzyme in the ventral prostate of castrated rats.[28] The histochemical reaction may be more apparent that real when testosterone is given to the castrated rat because the atrophied condition of the columnar secretory cells tends to concentrate the localization of enzyme.

The Effect of Hypophysectomy

In 1946, Huggins and Russel[29] reported that histological examination showed that a greater degree of epithelial atrophy occurred in hypophysectomized dogs than in comparable prostate preparations from gonadectomized dogs. Further-

TABLE 3

PATTERNS OF PHOSPHOHYDROLASE ACTIVITY AFTER HORMONE DEPLETION AND RESTORATION

Treatment (Days)	Testosterone (mg/kg)	Dog No. 649		Dog No. 149	
		Volume (ml)	Enzyme Activity (mg/ml)	Volume (ml)	Enzyme Activity (mg/ml)
30	0.4	20.7	12.1	34.2	6.29
44	0	—*	—*	0.1	0.20†
14	0.1	6.3	4.05	0.1	0.30†
14	0.4	18.1	6.60	6.7	10.4
10	0.4	18.8	10.0	17.0	17.1
14	0.4	19.7	9.75	28.0	8.94
14	0.4	20.5	10.1	34.0	7.30

* Not studied in the absence of testosterone.
† At limit of detection.

more, they announced that prostatic acid and alkaline phosphatase was more depressed in hypophysectomized than in gonadectomized dogs. Van der Laan[30] and Grayhack *et al.*,[31] using the growth of the ventral prostate as an index, found greater growth in testosterone-treated hypophysectomized-gonadectomized rats as compared to testosterone-treated gonadectomized animals. All three studies suggested some direct influence of pituitary hormones on the prostate gland.

Our approach was to measure prostatic secretion and acid phosphohydrolase activity in hypophysectomized, cystopreputiostomy dogs. To circumvent irreversible atrophy of the prostate gland and a possible harmful immunological response, experiments were planned carefully regarding removal of testosterone, employment of relatively low quantities of protein hormone and the supplementing of the prostate with androgen as soon as possible after a test was run. This approach permitted utilization of the same animals for evaluating more than one pituitary hormone. The transbuccal approach for hypophysectomy in the cystopreputiostomy dog was carried out successfully in 12 animals, but this only represented a 50 percent success by this surgical technique.

Animals were selected in the 10 to 15 kg body-weight range, and an age range between two and four years. Rectal palpation was employed to insure normal prostate size. Approximately half the animals were castrated and maintained on daily testosterone. The noncastrated, hypophysectomized, cystopreputiostomy dogs were put on routine collection to determine the extent of testicular and prostatic atrophy due to hypophysectomy. It has been found that properly hypophysectomized dogs undergo testicular atrophy in two to three weeks, at which time their prostate secretion is virtually zero. This preliminary testing of prostatic function has proven to be a reliable test for the success of the hypophysectomy operation.

The pituitary hormones tested were NIH preparations. The proteins were of bovine, ovine or porcine origin. Prostatic secretion volumes and acid phosphatase activity were determined on three pre-test, three test and several post-test samples. The protein hormone was given subcutaneously daily in saline for 10 days.

In the instance of noncastrated, hypophysectomized dogs, prostatic volumes were near or approaching zero, as all exogenous testosterone was deleted before the test compound was administered. Castrated, hypophysectomized animals were maintained on 0, 1, 2.5 or 5 mg testosterone daily throughout a test. Whenever an intact or hormone-untreated castrate hypophysectomized dog was exposed to a test substance, some testosterone was administered after sufficient collections during the recovery phase in order to check whether the prostatic gland was still responsive. Some of the noncastrated, hypophysectomized dogs were subsequently castrated and used for additional trials.

The results obtained with pituitary hormones in hypophysectomized, cystopreputiostomy dogs are outlined for noncastrates in TABLE 4 and for castrates in TABLE 5. Where no exogenous testosterone was used, the last pre-test value is given as the base line to follow the effect of the protein hormone. This arbitrary selection was necessary because prostatic secretion progressively fell during testicular atrophy or withdrawal of exogenous testosterone and could reach zero.

Stimulation of enzyme activity was elicited by prolactin when low levels of exogenous or endogenous testosterone were present (dogs No. 173 and 178 in TABLE 4 and dogs No. 164 and 186 in TABLE 5). Deletion of testosterone prevented the stimulatory action of prolactin (dogs No. 186, 171 and 192, TABLE 5). A similar finding was observed for leutinizing hormone (LH), in that testosterone plus LH (dogs No. 171, 192 and 197, TABLE 4) increased enzyme activity, while the absence of testosterone prevented the stimulation of LH (dogs No. 190 and 192, TABLE 5). High doses of testosterone could inhibit the effect of prolactin (dog No. 165, TABLE 5) or LH (dogs No. 163 and 165, TABLE 5). The negative effect seen in dog No. 190 (TABLE 4) for LH suggested that this animal was more depleted of endogenous testosterone than the other three non-castrated dogs on this protein hormone.

The other pituitary hormones studied, follicle-stimulating hormone (FSH), growth hormone (GH) and adrenocorticotropic hormone (ACTH), showed either little influence or an inhibitory influence on enzyme activity or prostatic secretion. The castrated dogs No. 163 and 165 (TABLE 5) given one mg testosterone with FSH responded with a depression of enzyme activity, while little effect was seen in the noncastrate dog No. 171 (TABLE 4). A similar result was obtained with ACTH. In testosterone-maintained castrates (dogs No. 164 and 186, TABLE 5) ACTH was inhibitory and, although in one noncastrate receiving testosterone (dog No. 190[c], TABLE 4), ACTH seemed to be stimulatory, removal of testosterone eliminated this effect (dog No. 190[e], TABLE 4). It is possible that dog No. 190 was showing a residual testosterone effect during this trial because it had been on exogenous testosterone before the ACTH trial. The results with GH were somewhat variable but in the main did not support prostatic secretion or enzyme activity.

The data on all the pituitary hormones tested did not indicate a direct influence on the prostate. Prostatic function could be improved by prolactin or LH in the presence of small amounts of testosterone. This result would suggest an effect of prolactin or LH on the testis and/or a potentiating effect on the prostate gland.

TABLE 4

THE EFFECT OF PITUITARY HORMONES ON PROSTATIC ACID PHOSPHOHYDROLASE ACTIVITY IN NONCASTRATED, HYPOPHYSECTOMIZED, CYSTOPREPUTIOSTOMY DOGS

Dog No.	Hormone Tested	Daily Dose For 10 Days (mg)	Volume (ml)		Total Phosphate Released (mg)	
			Pre-Test	Greatest Effect	Pre-Test	Greatest Effect
173	prolactin†	2.5	0.3	2.8	0.27	5.26
178	prolactin†	2.5	0.4	1.0	0.06	0.51
171	NIH–LH–S11	2.5	0.5	7.8	0.48	42.82
190	NIH–LH–B5	2.5	0.1	—*	—*	—*
192	NIH–LH–B6	2.5	0	0.1	0	0.03
197	NIH–LH–B6	2.5	0.3	0.7	0.07	0.24
171	NIH–FSH–S3	2.5	0.1	—*	0.50	—*
171	NIH–GH–S8	2.5	0.6	0.2	0.26	0.16
192	NIH–GH–S8	2.5	0.1	0.3	—*	—*
190[c]	ACTH‡	10 IU	0.7	2.3	2.09	6.10
190[e]	ACTH	10 IU	0.1	0.1	0.01	$<$0.01
197	ACTH + prolactin†	10 IU + 2.5	0.2	0.4	0.02	0.16

* Volumes too low to determine enzyme activity; exogenous testosterone did restore prostatic function.

† Armour Panliter, 1 mg = 30 IU.

‡ Armour Acthar.

Dog No. 190[c]: maintained on 1 mg testosterone daily throughout test.

Dog No. 190[e]: no testosterone given.

TABLE 5

THE EFFECT OF PITUITARY HORMONES ON PROSTATIC ACID PHOSPHOHYDROLASE ACTIVITY IN CASTRATED, HYPOPHYSECTOMIZED, CYTOPREPUTIOSTOMY DOGS

Dog No.	Daily Testosterone (mg)	Hormone Tested*	Volume (ml)		Total Phosphate Released (mg)	
			Pre-Test	Greatest Effect	Pre-Test	Greatest Effect
165	5	prolactin	17.7	11.5	52.57	44.62
166	5	prolactin	32.3	41.5	144.38	223.27
164	1	prolactin	2.5	3.3	3.18	5.41
186	1	prolactin†	1.3	2.1	0.88	2.39
186	0	prolactin†	0.3	0	0.18	0
171	0	prolactin†	0.7	0.4	0.11	0.16
192	0	prolactin†	0.2	0	0.08	0
163	5	NIH–LH–B5	15.7	12.8	84.94	65.41
165	5	NIH–LH–S11	23.6	19.7	75.76	53.78
190	0	NIH–LH–S13	<0.1	<0.1	—‡	—‡
192	0	NIH–LH–S13	0.2	0.2	0.34	0.34
163	1	NIH–FSH–S3	6.4	4.0	20.22	7.52
165	1	NIH–FSH–P1	11.1	3.8	17.43	2.93
163	1	NIH–GH–B	3.4	4.4	8.37	14.70
165	1	NIH–GH–B	3.1	1.5	2.67	1.01
164	1	ACTH	2.5	0.4	4.95	0.89
186	1	ACTH	8.8	2.9	9.68	5.05

* Same preparations and doses used as given in TABLE 6.
† NIH–P– S7 or S8.
‡ Volume too small to analyze.

Prostatic secretion in hypophysectomized animals has been studied by other investigators. Goodwin *et al.*[32] have shown a depression of prostatic volume by estrogen in the androgen-maintained, hypophysectomized dog. Such an affect was not surprising in light of the earlier work of Huggins' group on estrogen-androgen balance in castrated dogs.[33] However, the latter investigators reported no influence of estrogen on acid phosphohydrolase activity in canine prostatic fluid, but this has been demonstrated not to be the case.[24,34,35] Although Kato *et al.*[36] did not use hypophysectomized animals, they did report that 0.1 g daily thyroid hormone decreased the total volume and the concentration of acid phosphatase activity in prostatic fistula dogs.

In hypophysectomized-orchiectomized rats, Tullner observed an increase in ventral prostate weight during treatment with ACTH or prolactin-ACTH, but he did not estimate phosphatase activity.[5] Other investigators studied the effect of pituitary hormones on hypophysectomized rats, but estimates of acid phosphatase activity were not included in their studies.[37,38] Injections of 50 IU bovine prolactin per day for seven days increased acid phosphatase activity between 20 and 50 percent in intact adult, rats but the presence of the testis precluded interpretation of a direct effect of prolactin on the prostate acid phosphohydrolase.[38]

Histochemical Localization of Acid Phosphohydrolase

Although Huggins and Clark[39] performed a detailed study of the histology of normal and hyperplastic canine prostates, little data was collected on localization of enzymes. Recently, Neri *et al.*[40] reported a loss in acid phosphatase content in hormone-suppressed canine prostate. In our own histochemical investigation, prostatic acid phosphatase activity was determined in cystopreputiostomy dogs that were intact, hormone-maintained castrates or hypophysectomized animals.

Freshly autopsied prostate glands were frozen in dry ice, and frozen sections were fixed with cold, absolute acetone. Naphthol AS-TR-phosphate was employed as the substrate,[41] and serial sections from the anterior, middle and posterior portions of the prostate were examined. The details of the histochemical findings, and photomicrographs, will be published elsewhere.

Intact and castrated animals receiving near-physiologic levels of daily testosterone yielded a similar picture of uniform staining of acini with the fine granules distributed in the Golgi region. When dogs were given a ten-day administration of pharmacologic (5 mg/kg) dose of testosterone immediately before sacrifice, an intensification of the acid phosphatase reaction was discerned. On the other hand, castration without hormone replacement, hypophysectomy (of three months duration) or ten-day estrogen treatment (17β-estradiol or stilbestrol 0.1 mg/kg) in the presence of physiologic doses of testosterone initiated a decrease in acid phosphatase-staining granules with a disrupted pattern of distribution. There appeared to be some attempt by some sections of the gland to compensate for the atrophy occurring in other sections.

The histochemical picture seen for the dog was similar to that reported for mouse, rat and the human prostate. In the normal mouse, prostate acid phosphatase gave a positive reaction exclusively in the epithelium and mostly in the region of the Golgi apparatus.[5] Castration or stilbestrol treatment decreased the intensity of the reaction, and the discrete granules became scarcer with time. Testosterone re-established a normal picture.[5] Maggi, Franks and Carbonell[42] have histochemically demonstrated two acid phosphatases in mouse ventral prostate. One was a lysosomal acid phosphatase while the other could not split β-glycerophosphate. In cancer of the human prostate, many cancer cells retained acid phosphatase activity,[43] but loss of this enzyme into the blood was evident.[6] A recent localization of human prostatic acid phosphatase by electron microscopy has associated this enzyme with the Golgi vesicles, Golgi vacuoles, secretory vacuoles, lysosomes and within the acinar lumen.[44] Wolman[45] has suggested that acid phosphatase molecules are bound to polar lipids, which can form droplets (lysosomes) that prevent intracellular enzyme action.

Cellular Secretion of Acid Phosphohydrolase

The release of acid phosphohydrolase from the secretory cells of the canine prostate gland takes place at the apical end of the epithelial cell into the acinar lumen. The secretory granules enter the collecting ducts probably by a process of pinocytosis. The regulation of the secretion in general must be dependent on the health of the gland, endocrine factors, neural stimulation and pharmacologic intervention. By and large, the major secretion of enzyme is directed into the prostatic ducts. In the absence of common histochemical localization of acid phosphatase activity near blood vessels, it would appear that serum prostatic acid phosphatase originates through acinar leakage, reabsorption from prostatic ducts and, in part, from nonprostatic sources. In the human with prostatic carcinoma, it seems clear that marked leakage does occur, and the enzyme appears in the blood probably via the lymphatics.[6] Wojnas and Bester[46] have reported that serum prostatic acid phosphatase activity is related to the age and size of the prostate in rats.

That health and disease of the prostate play a role in secretion is more discernable by measuring volume than acid phosphatase activity. The data outlined

TABLE 6

PHOSPHOHYDROLASE LEVELS IN CANINE PROSTATIC SECRETION IN HEALTH, DISEASE AND AFTER ABLATIVE PROCEDURES*

Treatment	Histology of Prostate	Prostate Wt. (g)	No. of Dogs	Prostatic Vol. (ml/hr)†	Acid Phosphate (mg PO_4 release/ml)†
None	Normal	7–15	10	10–41	0.9– 9.2
Castrate + Testosterone‡	Normal	12–29	23	20–130	1.9–12.5
None	Prostatitis	10–15	4	1–6	0.3– 6.5
Castrate + Testosterone‡	Prostatitis	10–20	16	1–10	2.0– 8.3
None	Atrophy	7–23	6	1–5	0.1– 3.5
Castrate + Testosterone‡	Atrophy	4–8	7	1–2	0.1– 1.5
Castrate + Testosterone† 17 β-Estradiol§	Stages of Atrophy	12–42	7	0–10¶	0 – 2.2¶
Hypophysect.‖	Stages of Atrophy	6–9	7	0–3**	0 – 2.1**

* Body weights ranged from 9 to 16 kg and ages were between two and five years.
† Values given are the range of mean values obtained on three to six individual analyses on each dog.
‡ Daily maintenance dose of testosterone was between 0.25 and 0.45 mg/kg.
§ A daily dose of 1 mg 17 β-estradiol/kg was given for 10 days in the presence of daily testosterone.
¶ Pretreatment volumes were between 9 and 75 ml and acid phosphatase activity between 0.2 and 10.4 mg of phosphate released/ml of prostatic secretion.
‖ Hypophysectomized for two to six months.
** Prehypophysectomy volumes were between 15 and 50 ml and acid phosphatase activity between 1.8 and 7.6 mg/ml.

in TABLE 6 indicate that volumes are greater for the normal dog than for those suffering from prostatitis or prostatic atrophy. Despite the reduced secretory activity of diseased prostates, significant quantities of acid phosphatase activity are elaborated. This finding would suggest that functional portions of the gland are capable of sustaining production and release of acid phosphohydrolase. Endogenous atrophy or atrophy induced by castration, hypophysectomy or estrogen-treatment suppress both volume and enzyme secretion.

In most instances, inhibition evoked by estrogen could be overcome if treatment with the estrogen was suspended. Both the dose and route of estrogen administration determined the extent of inhibition. In fact, subcutaneous or oral administration of either stilbestrol or 17 β-estradiol at low doses caused a stimulation of volume and enzyme activity. Estrogen: testosterone ratios of 1:50 were stimulatory via the subcutaneous route, while ratios of 1:10 yielded stimulation by the oral route. Increasing amounts of estrogen caused a progressive and marked inhibition of both endpoints.[35,47]

The pharmacologic control of prostatic secretion has been evaluated on the basis of volume secreted by the dog,[3,48–50] by the rat[51] and by weight changes of the prostate gland in the mouse.[52] Although acid phosphatase activity was not determined, it would be expected that pharmacologic agents that inhibit prostate secretion would also prevent release of acid phosphohydrolase. This would also be true of stimulating agents that cause contraction of the muscular elements of the prostate with a net result of expression of enzyme into prostatic fluid.

In dogs with cystopreputiostomy fistulas, Smith *et al.*[48] found that atropine, hexamethonium and pronethalol decreased the secretion elicited by pilocarpine, while Dibozane, phenoxybenzamine, reserpine, morphine and cocaine did not inhibit the response. A comparison of sympathomimetic amines, norepinephrine, isoproterenol, tyramine and ephedrine with pilocarpine showed that the former were much less effective.[49] The pharmacological investigations indicate that the hypogastric nerve is largely responsible for the neural control of prostatic secretion through cholinergic fibers that can be blocked by atropine. This interpretation suggests that the innervation of the prostate is similar to the sweat gland where post ganglionic fibers of the sympathetic chain also release acetylcholine.

A few analyses of prostatic fluid from Smith's study on atropine and reserpine were carried out. Atropine was administered i.v. one hour before pilocarpine, while reserpine was given i.p. for two days and pilocarpine used on the third, seventh, tenth and fourteenth day for routine collections of prostatic fluid. In general, in those dogs that were particularly sensitive to the higher doses of atropine, marked inhibition of enzyme release was discerned. That the effect was on secretion and not synthesis may be deduced by the rapidity of the response. A two-day treatment with reserpine also evoked an inhibitory response, and recovery in the absence of drug proceeded over a period of weeks.

The function of the canine prostate regarding production and secretion of acid phosphohydrolase has also been influenced by immunological techniques. Macalagag and Prout[53] and Peel[54] have prepared rabbit antiserum to canine prostatic acid phosphatase and, upon injection of the immunoglobulins to normal dogs, induced prostatic degeneration. Peel[54] has found little or no acid phosphatase in the prostate of those dogs responding to the antibodies.

Testing of Compounds on Prostatic Function

The earlier work of the Huggins and Scott groups utilized the volume of prostatic secretion as the sole endpoint for evaluating test compounds.[5] Subsequently, Rosenkrantz and Mason[34] found that the acid phosphatase activity of prostatic fluid afforded a parameter capable of differentiating certain biological effects of test compounds. For example, some compounds would primarily influence water metabolism and cause a concentration or dilution of enzyme activity, while others would actually influence enzyme activity. When volume and acid phosphatase activity are handled as distinct endpoints, an opportunity is available to assess synthesis, secretion and water metabolism, respectively. With two parameters, nine possible responses may be evoked: one parameter increases or decreases with the other unchanged, each parameter varies oppositely to the other, both parameters change in the same direction and, finally, no change occurs for both parameters. In over 100 steroid and nonsteroid compounds tested, compounds have been found for each category[35,47] (also unpublished data).

Because of the extensive use of our standardized fistula animals for the evaluation of compounds, we present some representative substances that influence the synthesis and secretion of prostatic acid phosphohydrolase (TABLE 7). The extent of stimulation or inhibition of enzyme activity was estimated by dividing the enzyme activity of the sample of greatest change by the mean enzyme activity of three pretest prostatic fluids and multiplying by 100. Inhibition (−) and stimulation (+) were expressed as the difference from 100 percent. An effect on synthesis was assigned if enzyme activity varied with minimum changes

TABLE 7

THE INFLUENCE OF STEROIDS ON THE SYNTHESIS AND SECRETION OF PROSTATIC ACID PHOSPHOHYDROLASE IN CASTRATED CYSTOPREPUTIOSTOMY DOGS

Chemical Name	NSC No.	Testosterone (mg/kg)	Compound (mg/kg)	Mean Effect on Volume (%)	Mean Effect on Phosphatase Activity (%)	Mode of Action
5(10)-Estren-3-one, 17 β-hydroxy-	37320	0.43	4.22	+18	+165	synthesis stimulation
Androsta-1,4-dien-3-one, 7 α, 17 β-dihydroxy-17-methyl	51181	0.50	1.00	± 0	+ 36	synthesis stimulation
Estra-1,3,5(10), 16-tetraene, 3-methoxy-	71305	0.40	0.08	+ 8	− 30	synthesis inhibition
5 α-Androstane-3 β, 17 β-diol, 5-bromo-6 β, 19-epoxy	85413	0.31	3.14	+ 9	− 32	synthesis inhibition
Androst-5-en-17-one, 3 β, 19-dihydroxy-3-acetate	72259	0.50	5.02	+58	+ 56	secretion stimulation
4-Androstene-3 α, 17 β-diol, diacetate	11250	0.25	2.53	+54	+ 74	secretion stimulation
17 β-Estradiol, 17-(chloro-ethynyl)	57429	0.24	0.05	−99	− 82	secretion inhibition
Estradiol-17 β	9895	0.60	0.08	−95	− 87	secretion inhibition
Androstane, 11 β, 17 β-diol	19986	0.39	3.93	+36	− 40	water stimulation
Testololactone, 1-dehydro-16 α-hydroxy	69537	0.38	3.79	+43	− 43	water stimulation
Progesterone, 11-keto-6 α-methyl-	17256	0.36	0.73	−45	+ 45	water inhibition
Cortisol, 2 α-methyl-, 21-acetate	12602	0.40	0.81	−48	+ 51	water inhibition

in volume; the action was on secretion if the parameters varied in the same direction and on water metabolism if they varied equally but in opposite directions.

Three collections of prostatic fluid were obtained in a control period, three during a ten-day treatment period and several during the recovery phase. The compounds were administered subcutaneously as a suspension in a steroid-suspending vehicle.[35] At least two dogs were used for each compound, and mean results are given in TABLE 7. Generally potent estrogens inhibit both parameters, potent androgens stimulate both parameters, and corticoids decrease volume while increasing enzyme activity.

These interpretations are not intended to infer a single activity since biologically active steroid hormones are known to have relatively wide effects (e.g., androgens may have a uterotrophic effect). It should not be surprising that corticoids effect water metabolism since their activity may overlap with 11-deoxycorticosterone or aldosterone and decrease prostatic volume by inducing retention of sodium. Determinations of electrolyte balance in prostatic secretion should clarify this point. That potent androgens can initiate biosynthesis of acid phosphohydrolase may be deduced from their known stimulation of nucleic acid and protein synthesis in the rat prostate.[55] This point may be directly established by investigating acid phosphohydrolase activity in hormone-maintained prostate tissue exposed to inhibitors of nucleic acid (e.g., actinomycin D) or of protein synthesis (e.g., puromycin).

Summary

The lack of seminal vesicles and bulbo-urethral glands, plus the construction of a cystopreputiostomy prostatic fistula in the dog, have provided a relatively stable *in vivo* model for studying the secretion of prostatic phosphohydrolase. It has been shown that 0.7 mg of pilocarpine/kg closely mimics the physiological secretion of the enzyme in castrate dogs maintained on testosterone. Comparison of enzyme activity before and after castration has permitted an estimate of endogenous testosterone that was between 0.1 and 0.3 mg/kg. Under standardized conditions of pilocarpine and testosterone, healthy dogs between two and five years of age generally secreted a quantity of enzyme activity capable of releasing 3 to 7 mg of phosphate from β-glycerophosphate per ml prostatic solution collected for one hour. Two to three weekly collections of prostatic fluid yielded relatively stable levels of enzyme activity characteristic for each dog. Cessation of exogenous hormone to the castrate, hypophysectomy, severe prostatitis or atrophy due to disease abolished synthesis and secretion of prostatic acid phosphohydrolase. Neither age nor body weight has been found to correlate with enzyme activity. Hormone replacement therapy in the hypophysectomized dog has not revealed a direct influence of prolactin, LH, FSH, ACTH or GH on the prostate; LH and prolactin were stimulatory if physiological levels of testosterone were present. Depletion of testosterone decreased the intensity of histochemical localization of prostatic acid phosphohydrolase. A similar result was induced with potent estrogens that also inhibit the secretion of the enzyme. Anticholinergic agents like atropine prevented enzyme secretion, while certain steroids affected synthesis, secretion or water metabolism.

Acknowledgments

We wish to express our gratitude to Drs. Vladimir R. Illievski and Andras Fabry for preparation of prostatic fistulas and hypophysectomized dogs; to Dr.

Alexandros Gouvelis and Mr. John R. Baker for the histochemistry; to Dr. Erwin P. Vollmer for helpful suggestions; and to Dr. Marcus M. Mason and Arthur G. Hilgar for their support of the project.

Our sincere thanks go to Mr. Morris Graff of the Endocrinology Study Section of the National Institute of Arthritis and Metabolic Disease, D. H. E. W., for providing samples of pituitary hormones through the Pituitary Hormone Distribution Program at Emory University and to Dr. D. Jane Taylor for samples of prolactin.

References

1. MANN, T. 1964. *In* The Biochemistry of Semen and of the Male Reproductive Tract. : 41, 74, 113, 182, 308. Metheun & Co., London.
2. HUGGINS, C. 1947. The prostatic secretion. Harvey Lect. **42:** 148.
3. FARRELL, J. I. & Y. LYMAN. 1937. A study of the secretory nerves of, and the action of drugs on, the prostate gland. Amer. J. Physiol. **118:** 64.
4. HUGGINS, C. 1967. Endocrine induced regression of cancer. Science **156:** 1050.
5. VOLLMER, E. P. & G. KAUFFMAN. 1963. Biology of the prostate and related tissues. Nat. Cancer Inst. Monogr. **12:** 1.
6. PARKIN, L., G. BYLSMA, A. V. TORRE, W. DREW & R. J. MADDEN. 1964. Acid phosphatase in carcinoma of the prostate in man. J. Histochem. Cytochem. **12:** 288.
7. PRICE, D. & H. G. WILLIAMS-ASHMAN. 1961. The Accessory Reproductive Glands of Mammals. *In* Sex and Internal Secretion. William C. Young. **1:** 366. The Williams and Wilkins Co., Baltimore, Md.
8. MISLAWSKY, N. 1927. Innervation de la prostate. C. R. Soc. Biol. (Paris) **97:** 101.
9. CONNOLLY, J. G., A. THOMSON. M. A. S. JEWETT, N. HARTMAN & M. WEBBER. 1968. Intraprostatic lymphatics. Invest. Urol. **5:** 371.
10. ANDERSSON, L., I. DAHN, C. NELSON & A. NORGREN. 1967. Method for measuring prostatic blood flow with xenon^{133} in the dog. Invest. Urol. **5:** 140.
11. BERG, O. A. 1958. Effect of stilbestrol on the prostate gland in normal puppies and adult dogs. Acta Endocr. (Kobenhaun) **27:** 155.
12. LEBEAUX, M. I. 1966. Rectal palpation for the estimation of the size of the canine prostate. Invest. Urol. **4:** 208.
13. MASON, M. M., F. KEEFE & T. BORIA. 1961. Specialized surgery of the canine bladder and prostate gland. J. Amer. Vet. Med. Ass. **139:** 1007.
14. BORIA, T., M. M. MASON & H. ROSENKRANTZ. 1963. A volumetric and biochemical study of canine prostatic fluid using mechanical and pharmacologic stimuli. Amer. J. Vet. Res. **24:** 343.
15. SMITH, E. R., A. A. PAWLOSKI & H. ROSENKRANTZ. 1964. Secretion of nitrogenous substances by the pilocarpine-stimulated canine prostate gland. Proc. Soc. Exp. Biol. Med. **117:** 815.
16. ELIASSON, R. 1965. Effect of frequent ejaculations on the composition of human seminal plasma. J. Reprod. Fertil. **9:** 331.
17. CLARK, L. C., JR. & P. TREICHLER. 1950. Psychic stimulation of prostatic secretion. Psychosom. Med. **12:** 261.
18. ROSENKRANTZ, H., J. LANGILLE & M. M. MASON. 1961. The chemical analysis of normal canine prostatic fluid. Amer. J. Vet. Res. **22:** 1057.
19. ROSENKRANTZ, H. & J. LANGILLE. 1961. A comparison of canine prostate and wheat germ acid phosphatase. Proc. Soc. Exp. Biol. Med. **108:** 417.
20. KIRK, E. 1948. The acid phosphatase concentration of the prostatic fluid in young, middle aged and old individuals. J. Geront. **3:** 98.
21. GRAYHACK, J. T. & K. KROPP. 1964. Changes with aging in prostatic fluid: citric acid, acid phosphatase and lactic dehydrogenase concentration in man. Trans. Amer. Ass. Genitourin. Surg. **56:** 6.
22. LIPSETT, M. B., H. WILSON, M. A. KIRSCHNER, S. G. KORENMAN, L. M. FISHMAN, G. A. SARFATY & C. W. BARDIN. 1961. Studies on Leydig cell physiology and pathology: Secretion and metabolism of testosterone. Recent Prog. Hormone Res. **22:** 245.
23. ROSENKRANTZ, H. & V. ILIEVSKI. 1964. Estimated testosterone requirements of the castrated male dog. Amer. J. Vet. Res. **25:** 47.
24. MASON, M. M. & H. ROSENKRANTZ. 1968. Influence of steroid hormones on the dog prostate. Twenty-second Ann. Conf., Bureau of Biol. Res., Reproductive Physiology and the Dog. Rutger University. (In press.)

25. Huggins, C., M. H. Masina, L. E. Eichelberger & J. D. Wharton. 1939. Quantitative studies of prostatic secretion. I. Characteristics of the normal secretion, the influence of thyroid, suprarenal, and testis extirpation and androgen stimulation of the prostatic output. J. Exp. Med. **70:** 543.
26. Pazos, R., Jr. & C. Huggins. 1945. Effect of androgen on the prostate in starvation. Endocrinology **36:** 416.
27. Bialy, G. & G. Pincus. 1967. Hormonal influences of phosphatase activity of rat accessory sexual glands. Endocrinology **81:** 1125.
28. Javery, M. H., M. M. Mason & H. Rosenkrantz. 1963. A histochemical study of androgen-dependent succinic dehydrogenase in rat ventral prostate. Lab. Invest. **12:** 422.
29. Huggins, C. & P. S. Russel. 1946. Quantitative effects of hypophysectomy on testis and prostate of dogs. Endocrinology **39:** 1.
30. Van der Laan, W. P. 1953. Observations on the hormonal control of prostate gland. J. Clin. Invest. **32:** 609.
31. Grayhack, J. T., P. L. Bunce, J. W. Kearns & W. W. Scott. 1955. Bull. Hopkins Hosp. **96:** 154.
32. Goodwin, D. A., D. S. Rasmussen-Taxidal, A. A. Ferreira & W. W. Scott. 1961. Estrogen inhibition of androgen-maintained prostatic secretion in the hypophysectomized dog. J. Urol. **86:** 134.
33. Huggins, C. & J. L. Sommer. 1953. Quantitative studies of prostatic secretion. III. Simultaneous measurement of size and secretion of the canine prostate and the interaction of androgenic and estrogenic substances hereon. J. Exp. Med. **97:** 663.
34. Rosenkrantz, H. & M. M. Mason. 1961. The influence of hormones on biochemical constituents of canine prostatic fluid. Cancer Chemother. Rep. **12:** 143.
35. Rosenkrantz, H. & M. M. Mason. 1962. Progress report: bioevaluation of estrogenic compounds by the canine prostatic secretion method. Cancer Chemother. Rep. **20:** 33.
36. Kato, T., Y. Tanabe, F. Ono, K. Kajio, N. Miyao, T. Hirakawa, T. Chabata, M. Mizoguchi, H. Tanaka & T. Ishibe. 1965. Basic studies on the prostatic fluid of dog under various hormonal environments. Endocr. Jap. **12:** 173.
37. Scow, R. O. & S. N. Hagan. 1965. Effect of testosterone propionate and growth hormone on growth and chemical composition of muscle and other tissues in hypophysectomized male rats. Endocrinology **77:** 852.
38. Okamoto, R., K. Kawashima & K. Fujii. 1967. Actions of prolactin on the male sexual organs of the rat. Bull. Tokyo Med. Dent. Univ. **14:** 37.
39. Huggins, C. & P. J. Clark. 1940. Quantitative studies of prostatic secretion. II. The effect of castration and of estrogen injection on the normal and on the hyperplastic prostate glands of dog. J. Exp. Med. **72:** 747.
40. Neri, R. O., C. Casmer, W. V. Zeman, F. Fielder & I. I. A. Tabachnick. 1968. Effects of an anti-androgen, SH 714 (6-chlor Δ^6-1,2α-methylen-17α-hydroxyprogesterone acetate, Cyproterone acetate) on canine prostate hyperplasia. Endocrinology **82:** 311.
41. Barka, T. 1960. A simple azo dye method for histochemical demonstration of acid phosphatase. Nature (London) **187:** 248.
42. Maggi, V., L. M. Franks & A. W. Carbonell. 1966. Histochemical study of a number of hydrolases, including a new acid phosphatase, in various tissues of men and mice. Histochemie **6:** 305.
43. Kirchheim, D., F. Gyorkey, D. Brandes & W. W. Scott. 1964. Histochemistry of the normal, hyperplastic and neoplastic human prostate gland. Invest. Urol. **1:** 403.
44. Mao, P., K. Nakao & A. Angrist. 1966. Acid phosphatase and 5-nucleotidase activities of human nodular prostatic hyperplasia as revealed by electron microscopy. Lab. Invest. **15:** 422.
45. Wolman, M. 1965. The nature of lysosomes and their acid phosphatase. Z. Zellforsch. **65:** 1.
46. Wojnas, R. H. & J. H. Bester. 1963. Relation of prostatic serum acid phosphatase to age and size of the prostate in rats. J. Pharm. Sci. **52:** 475.
47. Rosenkrantz, H., S. S. Gandbhir & M. M. Mason. 1962. The antiprostate activity of a variety of steroid and non-steroid compounds. Cancer Chemother. Rep. **23:** 1.
48. Smith, E. R., V. Ilievski & Z. Hadidian. 1966. The stimulation of canine prostatic secretion by pilocarpine. J. Pharmacol. Exp. Ther. **151:** 59.
49. Smith, E. R. 1967. The stimulation of canine prostatic secretion by sympathomimetric amines. J. Pharmacol. Exp. Ther. **156:** 227.
50. Lebeaux, M. & E. R. Smith. 1966. The secretory response of the canine prostate gland to electrical stimulation of the hypogastric nerves. Invest. Urol. **3:** 625.
51. Farnsworth, W. E. & M. H. Lawrence. 1965. Regulation of prostate secretion in the rat. Proc. Soc. Exp. Biol. Med. **119:** 373.

52. O'Steen, W. K. 1963. Serotonin and histamine: effects of a single injection on the mouse testis and prostate. Proc. Soc. Exp. Biol. Med. **113:** 161.
53. Macalagag, E. V., Jr. & G. R. Prout, Jr. 1967. Anti-canine prostatic fluid serum and prostatic degeneration. Invest. Urol. **4:** 321.
54. Peel, S. 1968. An immunologic study of dog prostate and the effects of injecting anti-dog prostate serum. Invest. Urol. **5:** 427.
55. Lerner, L. J., R. Hilf & D. N. Harris. 1968. The effect of antagonists on androgen- and estrogen-induced changes in the male accessory sex organs of the rat. Trans. N. Y. Acad. Sci. **30:** 783.

DECIDUAL ALKALINE PHOSPHATASE ACTIVITY IN THE PREGNANT AND PSEUDOPREGNANT RAT

John P. Manning, Bernard G. Steinetz* and Thomas Giannina*
Warner-Lambert Research Institute, Morris Plains, N. J.

Introduction

There are well over a thousand studies of the activity and distribution of the phosphohydrolases in the reproductive systems of male and female animals, and it would be an impossible task to review this vast literature. Therefore, the present paper will consider primarily an area of our own work and interests, namely the alkaline phosphatase (ALP) in the female reproductive tract and especially the enzyme associated with decidualization of the uterus of rodents.

ALP activity is found in the oviducts of some lower vertebrates and may be influenced by ovarian hormones.[1,2] Among the mammals, there are interesting species differences in the physiological factors that influence the distribution and activity of uterine ALP. Estrogens increase the activity of the uterine enzyme in the mouse,[3-6] rabbit,[7] rhesus monkey[8,9] and human.[10-20] The rise in enzyme activity may not simply be a corollary of uterine growth, as other uterotrophic agents (e.g. progesterone, testosterone) do not induce the increase.[4-6] In the rat, there are conflicting reports claiming an increase,[21-24] no change, or a decrease[25,26] in ALP following estrogen administration. These seemingly opposite findings may be due to the comparison of animals in differing physiological states.

The effects of estrogens on uterine ALP in ovariectomized mice or rats may be inhibited by administration of actinomycin D[21,27,28] or estrogen antagonists.[29,30] The increase in the endometrial enzyme may be induced by instilling RNA extracted from uteri of estrogen-treated mice into the lumina of uteri of ovariectomized mice.[31,32] These findings suggest that, in the mouse, estrogen stimulates DNA-directed synthesis of RNA which, in turn, is responsible for the synthesis of enzyme protein.[21,27,28,31,32]

Unlike the findings in the above mentioned species, the endometrial ALP activity in the cow[33,34] and hamster[35] appears to be stimulated by progesterone rather than by estrogens. This is curious because progesterone may inhibit or decrease the estrogen-induced increase in uterine ALP in the rat,[22] rabbit,[7] rhesus monkey[8,9] and human.[10]

Endometrial ALP activity is also observed to rise precipitously following implantation of the fertilized ovum in mice and rats.[23,26,36-42] The activity is localized in the decidual cells and the reaction may be duplicated by inducing deciduoma formation in pseudopregnant animals[37,40,43,44] The decidua of other species do not show these dramatic changes in ALP activity. Activity is low or absent in dog, cat and man.[45-48] In the sheep, however, where the decidual reaction is sparse, there is a marked rise in stromal ALP.[49] A similar picture is seen in the guinea pig.[45] In the rabbit, chemically determined endometrial ALP, remains essentially unchanged except for a decrease on the tenth day of pregnancy.[50] However, histochemical studies reveal a decrease from days 5 to 7 in the trophoblastic ALP, followed by a marked increase in the enzyme of the developing syncytiotrophoblast.[51]

From the foregoing investigations, it appeared that only in the rat was there a clearcut correspondence between the implantation process and the rise in

* Present address: CIBA Pharmaceutical Co., Summit, N. J.

uterine ALP activity, uncomplicated by possible indirect hormonal or anatomical influences. The following studies were conducted to characterize the alkaline phosphatase of implantation in the rat.

Materials and Methods

The rats used were 220-gram virgin female albinos (KG Farms). The animals were housed in an air-conditioned, controlled light room in which night and day were reversed (12 hours of light, 12 hours of darkness). Standard rat chow and fresh water were available *ad libitum*. Only animals with normal five-day estrus cycles were used. Surgical procedures (ovariectomy, ligation and section of the oviduct, cardiac puncture, uterine trauma, partial hysterectomy) were carried out under ether anesthesia. Occurrence of mating with fertile males was determined within three hours by the presence of spermatozoa in the vaginal smear; this point in time was designated as day zero of pregnancy. Pseudopregnancy was induced by electrical stimulation (9 volts for 30 seconds) of the cervix uteri at proestrus or estrus and that point in time also designated as day zero. The animals were killed by decapitation. The uterine horns were removed, weighed on an analytical balance and transferred to an ice-cooled ground-glass homogenizer containing precooled distilled water. Nidation and interimplantation sites were separated with a razor blade at 1 mm on either side of the uterine expansion produced by the implanting embryo. The tissue was ground in the homogenizer at 1000 rpm until a uniform suspension was obtained (usually two to three minutes). This stock homogenate was then diluted to the desired concentration for the determination of alkaline phosphatase[52] (0.1%), β-glucuronidase[53] (1%), and acid phosphatase[54] (0.2%). Sera for alkaline phosphatase activity were diluted 1 to 10. Because of differences in water content of the various samples, dry weights were obtained by drying pieces of tissue to constant weight in a vacuum at 60° C for 24 hours.

Results and Discussion

Study 1.[36] *Uterine Enzyme Patterns In the Unilaterally Pregnant Rat*

The animals were prepared with unilateral section and ligation of the oviduct (USLT rats). When mated, they become pregnant in only one uterine horn. They were mated approximately 10 days after operation, and enzyme assays were carried out on uterine tissue on days 2 to 8 of pregnancy. β-glucuronidase was determined in pregnant and nonpregnant horns. Alkaline and acid phosphatase activity was assayed in gravid and nongravid horns on days 2 to 4, and in interimplantation and nidation sites and nonpregnant horns on days 5 to 8.

The results are shown in FIGURES 1 to 3. ALP activity rose precipitously from days 5 to 8 in the implantation area and then declined rapidly. The enzymatic activity remained at a low level in the interimplantation areas and in the sterile horn during this entire period (FIGURE 1). Acid phosphatase activity rose in both the fertile and sterile horns up to the fifth day of gestation, and then rose further in the implantation sites while declining in the interimplantation areas and sterile horns (FIGURE 2) over the ensuing three days. The β-glucuronidase activity declined steadily from the first to the eighth day of pregnancy (FIGURE 3).

The results are in agreement with numerous studies that have shown a rise in ALP following induction of decidualization by implantation or by traumatization.[23,26,36–44] The rise in acid phosphatase activity has not been as extensively

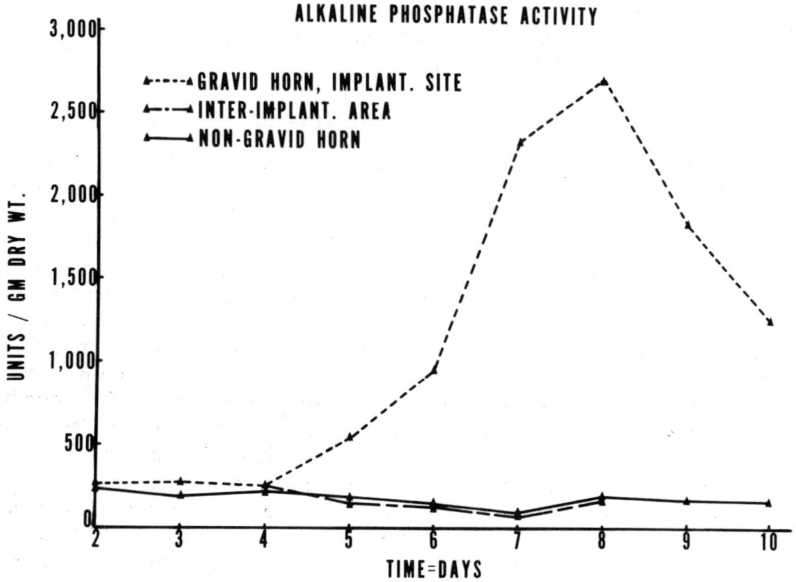

FIGURE 1. ALP activity in the gravid horn (days 2 to 4), implantation site (days 5 to 8), interimplantation area (days 5 to 8), and nongravid horn (days 2 to 8) of pregnant USLT rats. (Based on data from Manning *et al.*[36] Reproduced with permission of J. Endocrinol.)

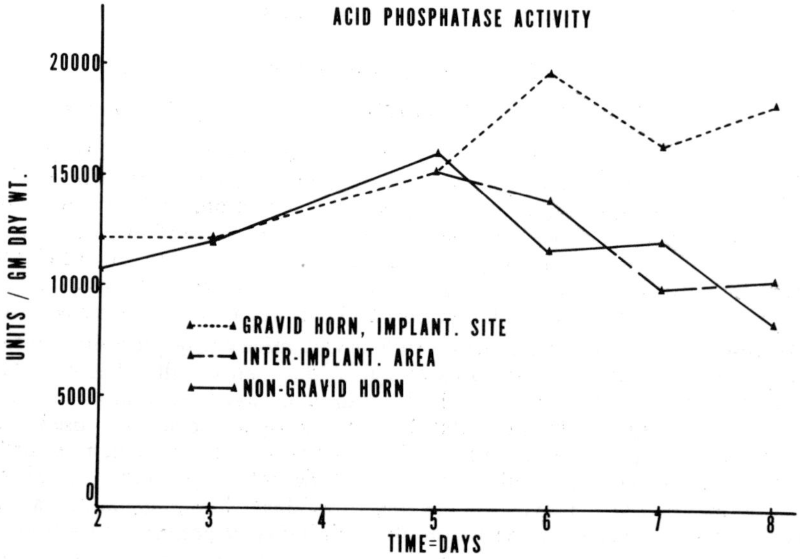

FIGURE 2. Acid phosphatase activity in the gravid horn (days 2 to 5), implantation site (days 6 to 8), interimplantation area (days 6 to 8) and nongravid horn (days 2 to 8) of pregnant USLT rats.

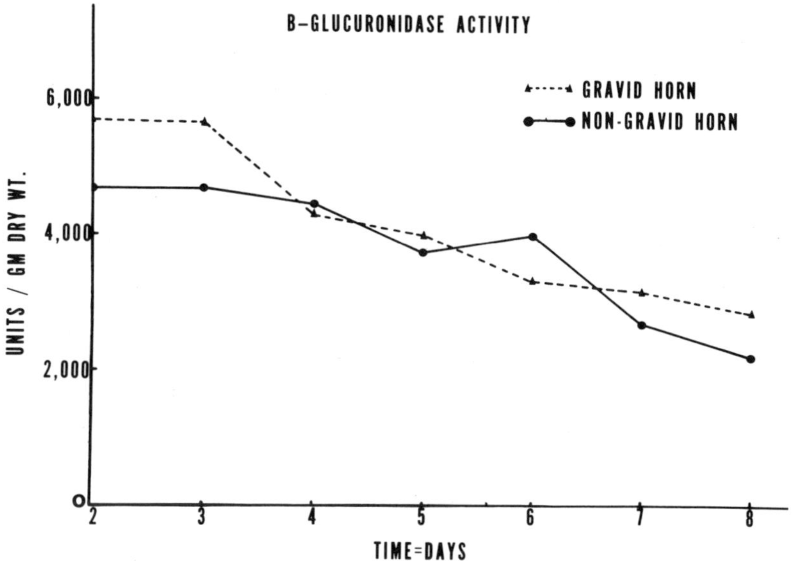

FIGURE 3. β-glucuronidase activity in the gravid and nongravid horn of USLT rats during the first eight days of pregnancy. (Based on data from Manning *et al.*[36]; reproduced with permission of J. Endocrinol.)

studied. The enzyme is probably located within larger decidual cells.[44] The observed decline in β-glucuronidase activity does not agree with the report of Prahlad that there is an increase in the activity of this enzyme on the day of the postulated prenidatory "estrogen surge".[55] We made several attempts to find such a peak with no success.[36] The overall gradual decline in β-glucuronidase activity with advancing pregnancy is, however, common to both studies.

By far the most dramatic change occurred in the ALP activity, and subsequent studies were undertaken to delineate more precisely the factors involved in this increase.

Study 2.[23] *Uterine Alkaline Phosphatase In Ovariectomized, Hormone-Treated Unilaterally Pregnant Rats*

USLT rats were bilaterally ovariectomized one or four days after proven mating. 17β-estradiol (0.1 or 1.0 μg/0.25 ml sesame oil) and progesterone (5 mg/0.25 ml sesame oil) were injected subcutaneously alone or in combinations at various times during the first seven days of pregnancy. (See TABLE 1 for exact dose schedule). Uterine ALP was measured in the nidation site, interimplantation area and sterile horn on the eighth day of pregnancy. Rats that were ovariectomized on the first or fourth day after mating but not treated with steroids showed no evidence of implantation of embryos and no rise in ALP activity (TABLE 1). When rats were ovariectomized on the first day and treated daily for seven days with 1.0 μg 17β-estradiol alone or in combination with 5 mg progesterone, or the progesterone alone, no implantation sites were found, and ALP did not rise. However, implantation occurred in all rats that were ovariectomized on the first day and then treated with 0.1 μg 17β-estradiol from the first to the third day, followed by 1.0 μg of the estrogen from the fourth to the

TABLE 1*

INFLUENCE OF 17β–ESTRADIOL AND/OR PROGESTERONE ON UTERINE ALKALINE PHOSPHATASE ACTIVITY IN MATED OVARIECTOMIZED USLT RATS ON THE EIGHTH DAY OF PREGNANCY

Group	Day of Ovariectomy	17β–Estradiol		Progesterone 5 mg/Day on Days Numbered	Rats With Implantation Sites†/Rats Per Group	Alkaline Phosphatase‡ (U/G Dry Wt)		
		0.1 μg/Day on Days Numbered	1.0 μg/Day on Days Numbered			Implantation Sites	Nonligated Horn	Ligated Horn
1	none	—	—	—	5/5	2545†	220	230
2	day 1	—	—	—	0/5	—	249	213
3	day 1	—	1–7	—	0/6	—	320§	336§
4	day 1	—	—	1–7	0/5	—	195	237
5	day 1	—	1–7	1–7	0/5	—	110§	173
6	day 1	1–3	4–7	1–7	5/5	2578†	188	150
7	day 4	—	—	—	0/5	—	217	193
8	day 4	—	4–7	—	0/5	—	311	393
9	day 4	—	—	4–7	8/8	2475†	256	246
10	day 4	—	4–7	4–7	9/9	2486†	150	172
±	SD					336	73	82

* Data from Manning *et al.*[23]; reproduced with permission of Proc. Soc. Exptl. Biol. Med.
† = $p < 0.05$ as compared to ovariectomized controls.
§ = $p <$ 0.05–0.01 as compared with LT and NLT from same rats.
‡ 10 units of alkaline phosphatase activity liberate 1 mg of phenolphthalein in 1 hr at pH 9.6 and 37°C from phenolphthalein diphosphate under standard conditions.

seventh day along with 5 mg progesterone daily. The rise in uterine ALP activity was similar to that seen in intact pregnant control rats. When ovariectomy was performed on the fourth day, daily injections of 5 mg progesterone were sufficient to permit implantation, and the anticipated rise in ALP activity was observed.

These experiments supported the view that the rise in ALP depended upon the interaction between the blastocyst and the progestationally conditioned endometrium, and not upon the hormonal environment *per se*. Estrogens appeared to have no direct role in the ALP reaction. Further studies were designed to test these views.

Study 3.[26] *Influence Of Implantation Inhibitors And Embryocidal Agents On Uterine Alkaline Phosphatase In Unilaterally Pregnant Rats*

Uterine ALP was determined in intact, mated USLT rats that were treated with the following drugs known to interfere with implantation in different ways: 1. large doses of estrogen (disrupts hormonal balance); 2. medroxyprogesterone acetate (MAP, delays implantation); 3. ethamoxytriphetol (MER-25, antagonizes endogenous estrogen); 4. ergocornine (inhibits decidualization); 5. amethopterin (antagonizes folic acid, kills embryo). The steroid hormones (17β-estradiol, estrone, progesterone), MAP, MER-25 and ergocornine were injected subcutaneously in 0.5 ml volumes of sesame oil. Amethopterin was injected as 0.5 ml aqueous suspension. Doses and durations of treatments are specified in TABLES 2 and 3.

As in the previous study, the ALP activity was not influenced *per se* by the hormonal and nonhormonal agents tested. In group 5 and groups 8 to 12 (TABLE 2), treated with 17β-estradiol and/or progesterone, the rise in ALP at the implantation sites was entirely comparable to that of the untreated control animals. When implantation failed to occur, there was no rise in ALP. MAP delayed implantation (TABLE 2, group 2), and no increase in ALP occurred unless estrone was administered to induce nidation (TABLE 2, group 4). Only 4 of 10 rats treated with estrone alone showed implantation sites (TABLE 2, group 3). The ALP rose in the uterus of the implanted, but not the unimplanted, animals. Of the animals receiving threshold doses of MER-25 or amethopterin (TABLE 3, groups 13, 14, 16 and 17), some had normal implantation sites while others had resorbing embryos. In the former cases, the ALP rose as expected, in the latter cases the enzyme activity of the implantation sites was only slightly higher than that of the interimplantation areas or sterile horns. These data not only supported our previous hypothesis that the ALP rise depends upon the interactions of the blastocyst with a progestationally conditioned endometrium, but also demonstrated that the embryo had to retain its invasiveness and viability to induce the rise. Thus the presence of living, but noninvading, blastocysts in the uterine lumen of MAP-treated rats did not induce a rise in ALP activity. Nor did dying or dead implanted embryos (MER-25, amethopterin) sustain a high level of ALP. That the compounds themselves had no direct influence on the enzyme was demonstrated by the rise in ALP observed in some rats in each group in which normal implantation occurred.

Study 4. Uterine Alkaline Phosphatase in Rats in Which Implantation was Delayed and Then Induced by Various Steroids

In Study 2, we had observed that when rats were ovariectomized on the fourth day, progesterone was the only substitution therapy required to induce implanta-

TABLE 2*

INFLUENCE OF ESTROGENS AND PROGESTAGENS ON UTERINE ALKALINE PHOSPHATASE IN USLT RATS ON THE EIGHTH DAY POST COITUM

Group No.	Treatment			No. Rats Implanted/ Mated	Appearance of Implanta- tions	No. of Rats	Uterine Alkaline Phosphatase† (U/G Dry Wt)					
							Implanted			Not Implanted		
	CPD#	Daily Dose	Days Treated				IS	NLT	LT	No. of Rats	NLT	LT
1	O	—	—	10/10	Normal	10	2373 ± 110	221 ± 18	220 ± 11	0	—	—
2	MAP	2.4 mg	1–7	0/4	—	0	—	—	—	4	209 ± 9	218 ± 20
3	E_1	1.0 μg	4–7	4/10	Normal	4	1972 ± 83‡	170 ± 28	169 ± 71	6	180 ± 9	186 ± 13
4	MAP	2.4 mg	1–7	5/5	Normal	5	2578 ± 174	239 ± 14	257 ± 37	0	—	—
	E_1	1.0 μg	4–7									
5	P	5.0 mg	1–7	7/7	Normal	7	1942 ± 164‡	159 ± 17‡	183 ± 12‡	0	—	—
6	E_2	1.0 μg	1–7	0/6	—	0	—	—	—	6	80 ± 7§	75 ± 5§
7	P	5.0 mg	1–7	0/5	—	0	—	—	—	5	91 ± 14§	92 ± 15§
	E_2	1.0 μg	1–7									
8	E_2	0.1 μg	1–3	5/5	Normal	5	2681 ± 352	149 ± 20‡	123 ± 11§	0	—	—
	E_2	1.0 μg	4–7									
9	E_2	0.1 μg	1–3									
	E_2	1.0 μg	4–7	4/4	Normal	4	2615 ± 157	74 ± 16§	75 ± 2§	0	—	—
	P	5.0 mg	1–7									
10	P	5.0 mg	4–7	7/7	Normal	7	2023 ± 186	174 ± 13‡	121 ± 9§	0	—	—
11	E_2	1.0 μg	4–7	7/7	Normal	7	3283 ± 212§	144 ± 27‡	126 ± 10§	0	—	—
12	P	5.0 mg	4–7	6/6	Normal	6	2859 ± 285	104 ± 12§	141 ± 19§	0	—	—
	E_2	1.0 μg	4–7									

* Data from Steinetz *et al.*[26]; reproduced with permission of Enzymologia.

† 10 units of alkaline phosphatase activity liberates 1 mg of phenolphthalein in 1 hr at pH 9.6 and 37°C from phenolphthalein diphosphate under standard conditions.

‡ $P < 0.05$ versus corresponding tissue from untreated pregnant control rats.

§ $P < 0.01$ versus corresponding tissue from untreated pregnant control rats.

O = No treatment
MAP = Medroxyprogesterone acetate
E_1 = Estrone
E_2 = 17β–Estradiol
P = Progesterone
IS = Implantation sites
NLT = Horn with non-ligated tubes (exclusive of implantation sites when these are present)
LT = Horn with ligated tubes

TABLE 3*

INFLUENCE OF DRUGS THAT INTERFERE WITH NIDATION ON UTERINE ALKALINE PHOSPHATASE IN USLT RATS ON THE EIGHTH DAY POST COITUM

Group No.	Treatment			No. Rats Implanted/Mated	Appearance of Implantations	Uterine Alkaline Phosphatase† (U/G Dry Wt)						
						Implanted				Not Implanted		
	CPD	Daily Dose	Days Treated			No. of Rats	IS	NLT	LT	No. of Rats	NLT	LT
1	O	—	—	10/10	Normal	10	2510 ± 103	290 ± 51	304 ± 78	0	—	—
13	MER 25	0.5 mg	1–7	11/17	Normal	7	2193 ± 101	221 ± 21	198 ± 10	6	215 ± 26	185 ± 16
					Underdeveloped	1	1016	196	201			
					Resorbing	3	213 ± 20‡	240 ± 2	213 ± 7			
14	MER 25	1.0 mg	1–7	3/8	Underdeveloped	1	1380	205	196	5	236 ± 27	211 ± 21
					Resorbing	2	223 ± 25‡	322 ± 126	338 ± 97			
15	Ergocornine	0.5 mg	Day 4	1/8	Normal	1	2358	115	124	7	395 ± 60	297 ± 46
16	Amethopterin	0.5 mg	5–7	2/7	Resorbing	2	446 ± 75‡	186 ± 5	216 ± 17	5	225 ± 21	247 ± 15
17	Amethopterin	1.0 mg	5–7	4/11	Resorbing	4	453 ± 105‡	226 ± 8	224 ± 4	7	222 ± 15	185 ± 19

* Data from Steinetz *et al.*[26]; reproduced with permission of Enzymologia.

† 10 units of alkaline phosphatase activity liberates lmg of phenolphthalein in 1 hr at pH 9.6 and 37° C from phenolphthalein diphosphate under standard conditions.

‡ $P < 0.01$ versus corresponding tissue from untreated pregnant rats.

IS = implantation sites

NLT = Horn with nonligated tubes (exclusive of implantation sites when these are present)

LT = horn with ligated tubes

MER 25 = Ethamoxytriphetol

tion and a rise in ALP activity. This finding did not preclude the prior action of an "estrogen surge" on the third day of pregnancy. To find if such a "surge" was in fact required, additional USLT rats were ovariectomized on days one or two after mating. No pregnancies ensued in the absence of any substitution therapy, nor did progesterone alone support pregnancy in rats that were ovariectomized on the first day (TABLE 4). However, more than half of the rats that were ovariectomized on the second day and maintained on progesterone alone exhibited normal implantation sites and elevated uterine ALP levels when examined on the eighth day (TABLE 4). This result may be at variance with that of Cochrane and Meyer,[56] who found that implantation was delayed in progesterone-treated rats that were ovariectomized 45 to 60 hours after detection of sperm in the vagina. However, the experimental designs were quite different in the two studies.

Our findings still did not rule out an early effect of estrogen, although they are contrary to the generally accepted view that an "estrogen surge" is required on day three (day of mating = day zero) to induce implantation.[57,58]

According to Barnes and Meyer, implantation is delayed by means of medroxyprogesterone acetate (MAP), but is then inducible by the subsequent administration of an estrogen.[59]

In our experiments, mated intact rats were treated with daily doses of MAP, 2.4 mg for 13 to 18 days. No implantations were found at autopsy on day 19 (TABLE 5, groups 1 and 3). However, when similarly delayed rats received daily injections of 5 mg progesterone on days 14 to 18 post coitum, implantation usually occurred, and this was accompanied by the anticipated rise in ALP activity (TABLE 5, groups 2 and 4). The progesterone was just as effective as 17β-estradiol in this regard (compare groups 4 and 5). These findings suggested either that progesterone was converted to an estrogen, that progesterone induced release of pituitary LH in the blocked animals (which would in turn induce ovarian secretion of estrogen), or that progesterone itself was capable of inducing implantation in MAP-delayed rats. To segregate these factors, the experiment was repeated in rats that had been ovariectomized on day 2 of pregnancy and then maintained on daily doses of MAP. In these animals, progesterone injections on days 14 to 18 post coitum did not induce implantation, whereas estrogen injections did (TABLE 5, groups 6, 7 and 8). This proved that progesterone required the presence of the ovaries to exert its implantation-inducing effects, and suggested that it somehow induced estrogen secretion.

TABLE 4

INFLUENCE OF TIME OF OVARIECTOMY ON IMPLANTATION AND UTERINE ALKALINE PHOSPHATASE ACTIVITY IN MATED PROGESTERONE–TREATED RATS

Group	Ovariectomy	Progesterone (5 mg) on Days Numbered	No. Rats Implanted/ Mated	Alkaline Phosphatase* (U/G Dry Wt)		
				Implantation Site	Inter-implantation Site	Nonpregnant Horn
1	Day 1	—	0/5	—	249	213
2	Day 1	1–7	0/5	—	195	237
3	Day 2	—	0/5	—	212	—
4	Day 2	2–7	31/54	2190	213	—
5	Day 4	—	0/5	—	217	—
6	Day 4	4–7	8/8	2475	256	—

* 10 units of alkaline phosphatase activity liberates 1 mg of phenolphthalein in 1 hr at pH 9.6 and 37° C from phenolphthalein diphosphate under standard conditions.

TABLE 5

INDUCTION OF IMPLANTATION BY PROGESTERONE, 17β–ESTRADIOL OR OVARIECTOMY IN PREGNANT RATS IN WHICH NIDATION WAS DELAYED BY MEDROXYPROGESTERONE ACETATE (MAP)

Group	Operation	MAP (2.4 mg) on Days Numbered	Prog. (5 mg) on Days Numbered	E_2 (1.0 μg) on Days Numbered	No Rats Implanted/ Mated	Alkaline Phosphatase* (U/G Dry Wt)			
						Implantation Sites	Inter-implantation Areas	Nonpregnant Horn	Deciduomata
1	None	1–13	—	—	0/5	—	—	244 ± 21	—
2	None	1–13	14–18	—	15/15	1933 ± 170	276 ± 27	—	—
3	None	1–18	—	—	0/5	—	—	229 ± 17	—
4	None	1–18	14–18	—	11/14	1913 ± 102	238 ± 21	—	—
5	None	1–18	—	14–18	8/8	1973 ± 161	118 ± 21	—	—
6	Ovariex day 2	0–18	—	—	0/10	—	—	280 ± 10	—
7	Ovariex day 2	0–18	14–18	—	0/10	—	—	260 ± 35	—
8	Ovariex day 2	0–18	—	14–18	3/13	1780 ± 199	276 ± 129	—	—
9	Ovariex day 14	1–18	—	—	5/9	1127 ± 146†	310 ± 74	—	—
10	Ovariex day 14	1–18	14–18	—	11/13	1900 ± 274	290 ± 45	—	—
11	Trauma day 14	1–18	—	—	0/5	—	—	216 ± 26	1628 ± 133
12	Ovariex day 10 + trauma day 14	1–18	—	—	0/8	—	—	272 ± 41	1586 ± 384

* 10 units of alkaline phosphatase activity liberate 1 mg of phenolphthalein in 1 hr at pH 9.6 and 37° C from phenolphthalein diphosphate under standard conditions.

† These implantation sites were viable but underdeveloped.

MAP = Medroxyprogesterone acetate

PROG. = Progesterone

E_2 = 17β–Estradiol

Further experiments revealed that simple removal of the ovaries on day 14 of MAP-delayed implantation likewise induced nidation, whether or not progesterone was administered (TABLE 5, groups 9 and 10). However, the rise in ALP was significantly greater in the progesterone-treated group, (with MAP, group 9, the sites were viable but underdeveloped). The cause of implantation was not clear unless the mechanical manipulations released estrogens from the ovaries. Trauma alone was not responsible, as deliberate traumatization of the uteri did not induce implantation, although it did result in deciduoma formation (TABLE 5, groups 11 and 12). It is of interest that the ALP rise in the deciduomata was similar to that seen in implantation sites.

We have not resolved the question of ovariectomy-induced implantation, but our observations are reminiscent of those by Enders[60] in the armadillo, an animal in which implantation is normally delayed; ovariectomy promptly induces implantation in the armadillo.

Study 5.[37] Alkaline Phosphatase Activity Following Deciduoma Formation

The purpose of this experiment was to evaluate whether the requirements for the rise in decidual ALP activity were comparable in the pregnant and pseudopregnant animal.

Pseudopregnant rats were subjected to bilateral ovariectomy, unilateral uterine trauma (multiple pinching of one uterine horn from the oviduct to approximately 1 cm above the cervix), or to both procedures. The 17β-estradiol (1.0 μg/0.25 ml sesame oil) and/or progesterone (5.0 mg/0.25 ml sesame oil) were injected subcutaneously. Rats were usually killed at the time of the enzyme determination. However, in some groups, uterine biopsies were obtained on days 5 and 6 under ether anesthesia. Such rats were killed on day 8 for observation of the deciduomata (see TABLE 6 for the exact treatment and killing schedule for experimental groups 1 to 9). Deciduomal ALP was compared with the ALP activity in implantation sites and nonpregnant horns of mated USLT rats (TABLE 6, group 10). Additionally, the nidation sites of other pregnant USLT rats were split into mesometrial and antimesometrial halves and assayed separately in comparison with the contralateral nongravid horn (TABLE 6, group 11).

On the eighth day of pseudopregnancy in intact or progesterone-maintained ovariectomized rats, the ALP activity in the traumatized horn was increased twelve-fold, while that of the contralateral nontraumatized horn was unaltered (TABLE 7, groups 6, 7 and 8). The enhanced ALP reaction in the traumatized horn was not a function of circulating hormone, since the enzyme was not increased in the nontraumatized horn of the same animals. Similarly, no deciduoma formation or rise in ALP was observed in untreated ovariectomized rats or castrated animals receiving injections of 17β-estradiol and/or progesterone (TABLE 7, groups 1 to 4).

The physical irritation of the endometrium was not alone responsible for the stimulated ALP because we were unable to elicit an enzyme response in pseudopregnant rats ovariectomized and traumatized on day 4 (TABLE 7, group 9). Estrogen administration to similar surgically-prepared animals also had no effect on the ALP reaction (TABLE 7, group 5). Intraluminal injection of sesame oil did not increase uterine ALP activity in ovariectomized mice but did so in intact pseudopregnant mice in conjunction with deciduoma formation.[40] Thus, the effects of chemical trauma are similar to those of physical trauma on the progestationally conditioned endometrium. A rise in ALP invariably accompanies

TABLE 6*

TREATMENT AND SACRIFICE SCHEDULE FOR EXPERIMENTAL GROUPS, STUDY 5

Experimental Group	Electrical Cervical Stimulation	Mated	Uterine Trauma	Ovariectomy	17 β-Estradiol (1.0 μg/Day)	Progesterone (5 mg/Day)	Assay Time†
	Time in Days						
1	0	—	—	4	–	–	8
2	0	—	—	4	4 – 7	–	8
3	0	—	—	4	–	4 – 7	8
4	0	—	—	4	4 – 7	4 – 7	8
5	0	—	4	4	4 – 7	–	8
6	0	—	4	4	–	4 – 7	8
7	0	—	4	4	4 – 9	4 – 9	5, 6, 7, 8, 9, 10
8	0	—	4	—	–	–	5, 6, 7, 8, 9, 10
9	0	—	4	4	–	–	5, 6, 7, 8
10	—	0	—	—	–	–	5, 6, 7, 8, 9, 10
11‡	—	0	—	—	–	–	8, 9, 10

* Data from Manning *et al.*;[37] reproduced with permission of Acta Endocrinol.
† Assay Time: days from electrical cervical stimulation or mating that the alkaline phosphatase was determined.
‡ Experimental group 11: Special group of mated intact rats whose implantation sites were split into antimesometrial and mesometrial halves.

TABLE 7*

ALKALINE PHOSPHATASE LEVELS IN DECIDUALIZED AND NONDECIDUALIZED UTERI AND IN NONPREGNANT HORNS AND IMPLANTATION SITES

Experimental Group	Type of Tissue Assayed	Assay Time — Days†					
		5	6	7	8	9	10
		Alkaline Phosphatase‡ (Units/G Dry Weight, Mean ± S.E.)					
1		—	—	—	207 ± 17	—	—
2		—	—	—	306 ± 34	—	—
3		—	—	—	194 ± 17	—	—
4		—	—	—	121 ± 11	—	—
5	TH	—	—	—	276 ± 37	—	—
	NTH	—	—	—	301 ± 31	—	—
6	TH	—	—	—	2576 ± 151	—	—
	NTH	—	—	—	209 ± 11	—	—
7	TH	385 ± 64	1195 ± 188	2439 ± 194	2555 ± 122	1899 ± 212	990 ± 115
	NTH	282 ± 58	397 ± 73	116 ± 13	123 ± 8	109 ± 8	141 ± 10
8	TH	226 ± 17	1023 ± 188	2942 ± 151	2460 ± 93	1707 ± 224	581 ± 53
	NTH	202 ± 14	234 ± 35	235 ± 44	156 ± 10	140 ± 7	184 ± 20
9	TH	178 ± 18	148 ± 18	221 ± 23	124 ± 18	—	—
	NTH	203 ± 9	209 ± 42	227 ± 14	128 ± 30	—	—
10	IS	545 ± 12	960 ± 51	2333 ± 127	2729 ± 153	1862 ± 55	1272 ± 49
	NPH	182 ± 5	158 ± 19	113 ± 6	207 ± 26	185 ± 23	172 ± 15
11	ISM	—	—	—	2806 ± 100	1969 ± 306	1015 ± 60
	ISA	—	—	—	3182 ± 148	2487 ± 72	1400 ± 70
	NPH	—	—	—	285 ± 43	243 ± 6	179 ± 5

* Data from Manning *et al.*;[37] reproduced with permission of Acta Endocrinol.

† Assay Time: days from electrical cervical stimulation or mating that the alkaline phosphatase was determined.

‡ 10 units of alkaline phosphatase activity liberate 1 mg of phenolphthalein in 1 hr at pH 9.6 and 37°C from phenolphthalein diphosphate under standard conditions.

TH = traumatized horn
NTH = nontraumatized horn
IS = implantation site
ISM = implantation site mesometrial
ISA = implantation site antimesometrial
NPH = nonpregnant horn

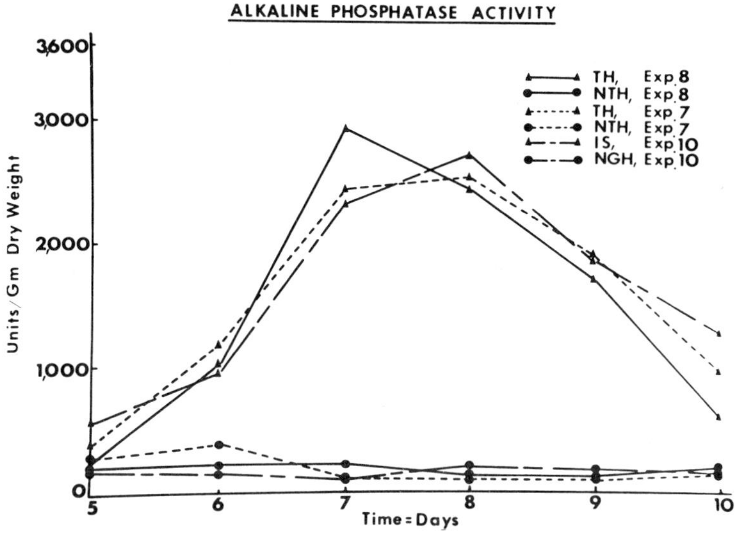

FIGURE 4. Distribution of ALP activity in the uterus of pregnant and intact or ovariectomized pseudopregnant rats. Experiment Group 7: pseudopregnancy, day 0; ovariectomy and uterine trauma, day 4; 17β-estradiol, 1.0 μg/day and progesterone, 5 mg/day, days 4–9. TH = traumatized horn, NTH = nontraumatized horn. Experimental Group 8: pseudopregnancy, day 0; uterine trauma day 4. TH = traumatized horn, NTH = nontraumatized horn. Experimental Group 10: pregnancy, day 0. IS = implantation site, NGH = nongravid horn. (Data from Manning *et al.*,[37]; reproduced with permission of Acta Endocrinol.)

deciduoma formation. Blandau favors the view that localized pressure is the stimulus to the decidual reaction.[61] However, Wilson found that pieces of tumor and muscle introduced into the uterine cavity of the pseudopregnant mouse failed to stimulate the decidual response even though the tissue was implanted below the epithelium.[62] Mouse ova and fixed rat ova and sea urchin eggs placed in the uteri of pseudopregnant rats were also ineffective in stimulating the formation of a decidua.[63] A precise chemical mechanism cannot be defined, since mineral oil (straight-chain hydrocarbons), vegetable oils (triglycerides), agar gel or solution (sulfated polysaccharide) and arachis oil (fatty acid) are all potent deciduoma producing substances.[64] In any event, regardless of the exact mediator of the decidual reaction, it is clear that the requirements for the elevation of uterine ALP in the traumatized horn of rats from days 5 to 8 of pseudopregnancy are similar (if not identical) to those of pregnant rats, i.e., irritation (day 4) of a progestationally conditioned endometrium. The similarity in the changes of this enzyme from days 5 to 10 in intact and hormone-treated ovariectomized, pseudopregnant rats with traumatized uterine horns, and the intact pregnant animals supports this view (FIGURE 4). Based on these results, we would broaden and alter our original proposal for the pregnant rat to include our findings in the pseudopregnant animal as follows: Estrogen may sensitize the endometrium and be a necessary stimulus for nidation, but the enhanced ALP activity is dependent on the interaction of the blastemic irritation (not the presence of the blastocyst *per se*; physical and/or chemical irritation of the uterus is needed in pseudopregnancy) with a progesterone-conditioned endometrium. The decline in endometrial ALP from days 8 to 10 in intact and hormone-treated ovariectomized pseudopregnant rats with traumatized uterine horns, as well as in intact pregnant animals, is difficult to understand. The decreased ALP reaction in the nidation site was generalized, since both the mesometrial and antimesometrial halves showed parallel diminished activity (FIGURE 5). Lobel *et al.* reported similar histochemical findings in intact pseudopregnant rats.[65] A drop in progestagen levels is not a likely explanation, since traumatized, ovariectomized, pseudopregnant rats treated with estrogen and progesterone showed a similar decrease in enzyme activity. The process involved may be synthesis and/or conversion of a quantitative amount of ALP to an active form, after which the enzyme could undergo degradation. Physiologically, this may occur because the fetal placenta is being established at this time and is beginning to produce its own ALP protein. Rat placentae of the 19th and 20th day of pregnancy have approximately 3200 units of ALP activity per gram of dry weight; thus, there appears to have been a shift in the location of the active enzyme from the decidua to the placenta.

The role of ALP under the conditions described above may be one of increased phosphate transfer of phosphorylated substrates (hexose and pentose phosphates, etc.). Danielli emphasized that ALP activity was generally greater at sites of extensive molecular transfer, such as in the endothelium of capillaries and at the cell membrane of secretory cells.[66] Fishman, Goldman and DeLellis suggested that nonlysosomal sites of hydrolases (such as β-glucuronidase, acid phosphatase, etc.) may be ordered in a sequence and in numbers adequate for membrane structure.[67]

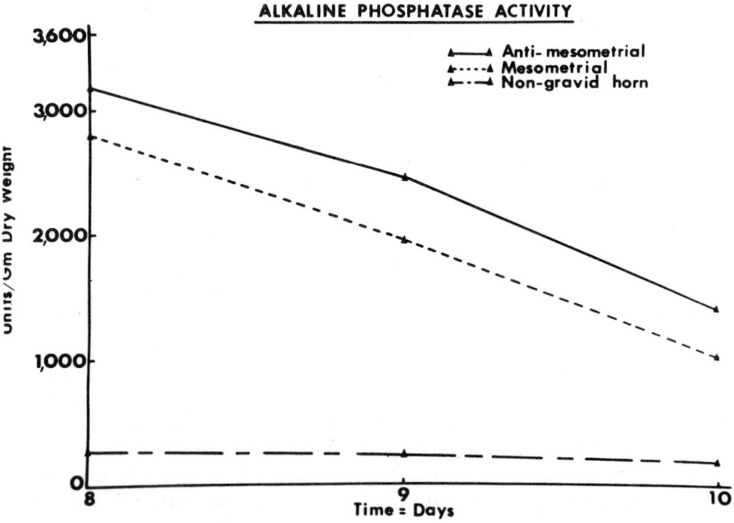

FIGURE 5. Distribution of ALP activity in the pregnant and nonpregnant horn. Experimental Group 11: pregnancy, day 0. Assay of mesometrial and antimesometrial halves of the implantation site. (Data from Manning *et al.*[37]; reproduced with permission of Acta Endocrinol.)

TABLE 8

TISSUE AND SERUM ALKALINE PHOSPHATASE IN PREGNANT AND PSEUDOPREGNANT RATS

Experimental Group	Type of Animal	Treatment: Uterine Trauma	Treatment: Ovariectomy	Treatment: Progesterone (5 mg/Day)	Sacrifice Time†	Alkaline Phosphatase‡ (Mean ± S.E.): Serum (Units %)	Alkaline Phosphatase‡ (Mean ± S.E.): Tissue (U/G Dry Wt)	
		Time in Days						
1	C	—	—	—	—	368 ± 20	226 ± 32	(uterus)
2	P	—	—	—	8	397 ± 37	2801 ± 126	(implantation site)
3	P	—	—	—	9	420 ± 45	1792 ± 96	(implantation site)
4	P	—	—	—	10	352 ± 31	1291 ± 74	(implantation site)
5	P	—	—	—	19	412 ± 42	3197 ± 141	(placenta)
6	P	—	—	—	20	410 ± 26	2910 ± 148	(placenta)
7	Ps	4	—	—	8	324 ± 41	2694 ± 153	(decidua)
8	Ps	4	—	—	9	364 ± 41	1856 ± 148	(decidua)
9	Ps	4	—	—	10	324 ± 47	690 ± 53	(decidua)
10	Ps	4	4	4 – 7	8	294 ± 39	2493 ± 93	(decidua)
11	Ps	4	4	4 – 8	9	363 ± 38	1791 ± 122	(decidua)
12	Ps	4	4	4 – 9	10	293 ± 24	780 ± 49	(decidua)

† Sacrifice Time: days after mating or electrical stimulation of the cervix uteri.

‡ 10 units of alkaline phosphatase activity liberate 1 mg of phenolphthalein in 1 hr at pH 9.6 and 37° C from phenolphthalein diphosphate under standard conditions.

C = Control
P = Pregnant
Ps = Pseudopregnant

Study 6.[38] *Failure to Detect Rat Placental ALP in the Systemic Circulation*

Elevation in human serum ALP during the last trimester of pregnancy has been reported by numerous investigators.[68–73] Subsequently, electrophoretic, heat stability and L-phenylalanine inhibition studies have showed that the origin of this increased serum enzyme is the placenta.[73–80] Since alkaline phosphatase levels are 10 to 15 times greater in pregnant and pseudopregnant rat deciduae than in nonpregnant uterine areas,[23,26,36,37] we were interested to see if any detectable enzyme component "spilled over" into the serum. For this study, pregnant and traumatized pseudopregnant rats (some animals were ovariectomized on day four and received hormone replacement; progesterone, 5.0 mg/0.25 ml. sesame oil) were bled by cardiac puncture according to the sacrifice time indicated in TABLE 8. The sera and tissue (control uteri, implantation site, placentae and deciduae) were assayed for alkaline phosphatase activity. In addition, the sera were subjected to electrophoresis using an EC-470 Vertical Gel Electrophoresis Cell (EC Apparatus Corp., Philadelphia, Pa.). The acrylamide[81] was made to a 5 percent gel, 6 mm thick in 90 parts 15 mM tris-3.3 mM citric acid plus 10 parts 24 mM sodium hydroxide-76 mM boric acid buffer (pH 8.0) containing 17 mM magnesium chloride. The chamber buffer (pH 8.6) consisted of 120 mM sodium hydroxide-380 mM boric acid and 17 mM magnesium chloride.[82] Each cm-gel slot contained 25 μg of serum. The sera were prepared with 15% sucrose to increase the density. A constant voltage of 65 v with an average current of 75

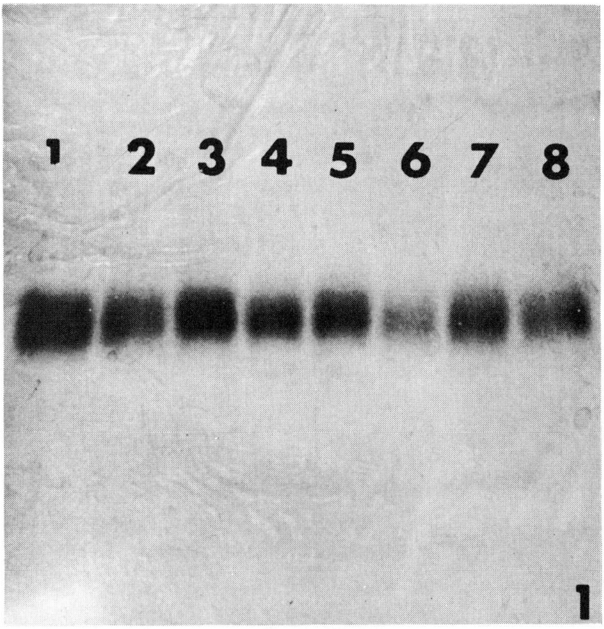

FIGURE 6. Electrophoretic pattern of rat serum ALP activity: (1) Control; (2) 8 days pregnant; (3) 19 days pregnant; (4) 10 days pregnant; (5) 20 days pregnant; (6) 8 days pseudopregnant, uterine trauma, day 4; (7) 9 days pseudopregnant, uterine trauma, day 4; (8) 10 days pseudopregnant, ovariectomy and uterine trauma, day 4, 17β-estradiol and progesterone, days 4 to 9.

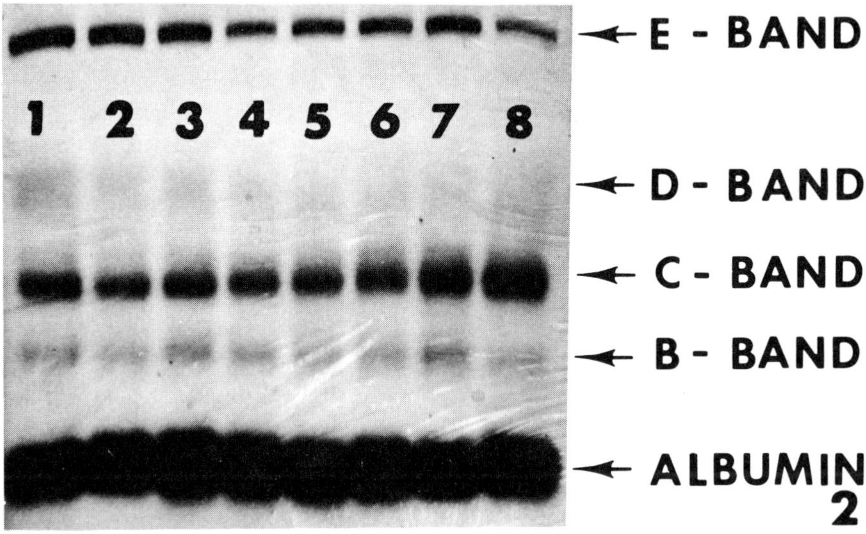

FIGURE 7. Electrophoretic pattern of rat serum proteins stained with amido black 10B: (1) Control; (2) 8 days pregnant; (3) 19 days pregnant; (4) 10 days pregnant; (5) 20 days pregnant; (6) 8 days pseudopregnant, uterine trauma, day 4; (7) 9 days pseudopregnant, uterine trauma, day 4; (8) 10 days pseudopregnant, ovariectomy and uterine trauma, day 4, 17β-estradiol and progesterone, days 4 to 9.

ma was used for 19 hours at 14° C. After separation, the gel was sliced in half and the top segment stained with 0.25% amido black 10B in methanol-acetic acid-water (50:10:50). The bottom gel slab was stained for alkaline phosphatase with sodium α-naphthyl acid phosphate and 4-amino diphenylamine diazonium sulfate at pH 9.8 at 4° C for 4 hours.[83]

In pseudopregnant, intact or castrated rats receiving progesterone replacement, and in pregnant rats, the decidual alkaline phosphatase of traumatized uteri and implantation sites was 12 times more active on day 8 than in uterine horns of control animals (TABLE 8). These results are comparable to previous reports.[23,26,36,37] The placentae of animals obtained on the day 19 or 20 of pregnancy also demonstrated a similarly increased enzyme reaction. Additionally, pregnant and pseudopregnant rats showed diminishing uterine activity from days 8 to 10 (TABLE 8). Regression of histochemical decidual alkaline phosphatase of traumatized uteri in pseudopregnant rats has been described.[65]

The serum alkaline phosphatase activity from all experimental groups did not differ significantly from that of the control animals (TABLE 8). Electrophoretic patterns of control serum showed only one alkaline phosphatase band (FIGURE 6), a fact that would favor the recognition of another isoenzyme, which might enter the circulation under certain conditions. With pregnant and pseudopregnant sera, however, only one alkaline phosphatase band with activity and migration characteristics similar to control was observed (FIGURE 6). This band (of intestinal origin)[84,85] migrated slightly behind the C protein band (FIGURE 7). Thus, unlike in the human, no detectable rat placental alkaline phosphatase "spills over" into the circulation.

TABLE 9*

TREATMENT SCHEDULE FOR UNILATERALLY TRAUMATIZED PSEUDOPREGNANT RATS INJECTED WITH NUCLEIC ACID INHIBITORS AND AMINO ACID ANTAGONISTS (STUDY 7)

Group No.	Compound	Daily Dose	Vehicle	Daily Injection Schedule	Days Treated	Total Dose
1	Control	—	—	—	—	—
2	Control	—	—	—	—	—
3	Control	—	—	—	—	—
4	Control	—	—	—	—	—
1	Actinomycin D	30 μg	Saline	30 μg × 1	0	30 μg
2	Actinomycin D	30 μg	Saline	30 μg × 1	4	30 μg
3	Actinomycin D	30 μg	Saline	30 μg × 1	0; 4	60 μg
4	Actinomycin D	10 μg	Saline	10 μg × 1	4–7	40 μg
5	Actinomycin D	10 μg	Saline	10 μg × 1	0–7	80 μg
1	5-Fluorodeoxyuridine	40 mg	Saline	40 mg × 1	5	40 mg
2	5-Fluorodeoxyuridine	40 mg	Saline	40 mg × 1	1; 5	80 mg
1	Chloramphenicol	30 mg	Saline	10 mg × 3	4–7	120 mg
2	Chloramphenicol	30 mg	Saline	10 mg × 3	0–7	240 mg
3	Chloramphenicol	150 mg	Propyleneglycol	50 mg × 3	4–7	600 mg
4	Chloramphenicol	150 mg	Propyleneglycol	50 mg × 3	0–7	1200 mg
1	Cycloheximide	50 μg	Saline	25 μg × 2	4–7	200 μg
2	Cycloheximide	50 μg	Saline	25 μg × 2	0–7	400 μg
1	DL-*p*-Chlorophenylalanine	25 mg	0.1NHCl	25 mg × 1	4–7	100 mg
2	DL-*p*-Chlorophenylalanine	25 mg	0.1NHCl	25 mg × 1	0–7	200 mg
1	DL-*p*-Fluorophenylalanine	25 mg	Water	25 mg × 1	4–7	100 mg
2	DL-*p*-Fluorophenylalanine	25 mg	Water	25 mg × 1	0–7	200 mg
3	DL-*p*-Fluorophenylalanine	50 mg	Water	25 mg × 2	4–7	200 mg
4	DL-*p*-Fluorophenylalanine	50 mg	Water	25 mg × 2	0–7	400 mg
1	L-Ethionine	25 mg	Saline	25 mg × 1	4–7	100 mg
2	L-Ethionine	25 mg	Saline	25 mg × 1	0–7	200 mg
3	L-Ethionine	50 mg	Saline	25 mg × 2	4–7	200 mg
4	L-Ethionine	50 mg	Saline	25 mg × 2	0–7	400 mg

* Data from Manning *et al.*;[85] reproduced with permission of Enzymologia.

Study 7.[86] *Influence of Nucleic Acid Inhibitors and Amino Acid Antagonists on Deciduomal ALP*

The purpose of this investigation was to determine by the use of nucleic acid inhibitors (actinomycin-D,* 5-fluorodeoxyuridine,† chloramphenicol,‡ cycloheximide§) and amino acid antagonists (DL-*p*-chlorophenylalanine,* DL-*p*-fluorophenylalanine,* L-ethionine*) whether the increased decidual alkaline phosphatase activity represented newly synthesized enzyme protein or activation of an existing latent form. For this study, unilaterally traumatized pseudopregnant rats were injected intraperitoneally with the compounds, and the uterine enzyme activity was determined on the eighth day. (See TABLE 9 for the specific doses and durations of treatment.) Animals dosed on day zero and/or day four received their injection approximately two hours before electrical stimulation and uterine trauma. Not all animals had a decidual reaction; however, all traumatized and nontraumatized uteri of decidualized and nondecidualized animals were assayed.

Neither the nucleic acid inhibitors nor the amino acid antagonists prevented the increased ALP activity in traumatized uteri of pseudopregnant rats (TABLE 10). The maintenance of this high ALP activity was not a function of the aqueous tissue mass, since (a) the enzyme reaction was based on units per gram dry weight, and (b) the percent water was similar in decidualized uteri of control and treated rats (TABLE 11). Some doses of the compounds (actinomycin-D groups 1, 2 and 3; DL-*p*-chlorophenylalanine groups 1 and 2; DL-*p*-fluorophenylalanine groups 2 and 4; and L-ethionine 4) were extremely toxic; however, even in these cases, a full ALP response was observed. The data favor the view that (a) the decidual ALP is released and/or activated from a latent precursor protein, and (b) *de novo* nucleic acid and/or protein synthesis is not necessary for the formation of the active enzyme molecule. The decidual reaction (a process involving hypertrophy and hyperplasia of the endometrial stroma) would thus require a redistribution of the latent enzyme protein between the interstitial cells undergoing mitosis.

Fishman has suggested uterine albumin as a source for the latent precursor protein.[87] In purifying ALP from human placenta, Ghosh and Fishman noted that albumin (a) had a similar molecular weight, 69000; (b) had the same percentage of some amino acids (tyrosine, serine, cysteine); (c) had a similar sedimentation constant, 4S; (d) was the major contaminate of the enzyme-rich fractions, and (e) was the most difficult protein to separate from the enzyme.[88]

Several groups of treated rats (actinomycin-D groups 2 and 3; 5-fluorodeoxyuridine groups 1 and 2; DL-*p*-fluorophenylalanine groups 1, 2 and 3; L-ethionine groups 1 and 2) showed an enhanced ALP reaction (TABLE 10). Similar results were described by Moog for the ALP found in the microvilli of the developing duodenum in the mouse.[89,90] There was a rise in activity that paralleled the appearance of a phenylphosphate-preferring moiety compared to the moiety hydrolyzing glycerophosphate. This increased ALP reaction was enhanced, not prevented, by actinomycin-D, ethionine, cycloheximide, colchicine and puromycin. The lack of inhibition by these compounds was attributed by Moog to the production of a phenylphosphate-preferring enzyme from a latent precursor mole-

* Actinomycin-D, DL-*p*-chlorophenylalanine, DL-*p*-fluorophenylalanine and L-ethionine were provided by Mann Research Laboratories, Inc., New York, N. Y.

† 5-fluorodeoxyuridine came from Hoffmann-LaRoche, Inc., Nutley, N. J.

‡ Chloramphenicol was provided by Parke-Davis and Co., Detroit, Mich.

§ Cycloheximide was obtained from Aldrich Chemicals, Fairfield, N. J.

TABLE 10*
INFLUENCE OF NUCLEIC ACID INHIBITORS AND AMINO ACID ANTAGONISTS ON ALKALINE PHOSPHATASE ACTIVITY OF DECIDUALIZED AND NONDECIDUALIZED UTERINE TISSUE

Group No.		Total No. of Animals	No. of Decidualized Animals	No. of Non-decidualized Animals	Alkaline Phosphatase† (U/G Dry Wt, Mean ± S.E.) Decidualized		Non-decidualized	
					TH	NTH	TH	NTH
1	Control	9	7	2	2685 ± 202	166 ± 10	171 ± 51	248 ± 89
2	Control	6	3	3	2328 ± 175	181 ± 8	138 ± 6	182 ± 42
3	Control	4	4	0	2463 ± 439	137 ± 14	—	—
4	Control	15	5	10	2584 ± 205	229 ± 14	191 ± 22	181 ± 19
1	AD	19	10	9	2535 ± 207	178 ± 8	178 ± 11	224 ± 17
2	AD	16	13	3	3600 ± 362	296 ± 27	183 ± 17	215 ± 13
3	AD	3	1	2	2682	296	207 ± 51	241 ± 23
4	AD	11	7	4	3527 ± 365	219 ± 16	213 ± 29	214 ± 14
5	AD	9	6	3	2562 ± 221	262 ± 18	285 ± 58	231 ± 17
1	FUDR	12	6	6	3150 ± 315	214 ± 27	166 ± 17	201 ± 17
2	FUDR	22	9	13	3310 ± 192	187 ± 11	159 ± 17	169 ± 16
1	CAP	7	5	2	2713 ± 412	197 ± 16	234 ± 57	191 ± 6
2	CAP	13	6	7	2380 ± 218	201 ± 20	160 ± 19	220 ± 27
3	CAP	20	14	6	2922 ± 251	164 ± 27	174 ± 18	182 ± 16
4	CAP	17	8	9	2842 ± 291	276 ± 19	310 ± 43	290 ± 16
1	CY	9	7	2	2139 ± 108	156 ± 7	154 ± 5	160 ± 19
2	CY	13	8	5	2589 ± 386	178 ± 19	334 ± 59	137 ± 7
1	PCP	4	3	1	1938 ± 150	215 ± 10	270	290
2	PCP	3	2	1	2066 ± 98	353 ± 55	393	75
1	PFP	8	5	3	4105 ± 207	240 ± 11	168 ± 42	213 ± 32
2	PFP	10	7	3	3221 ± 188	264 ± 17	149 ± 24	237 ± 42
3	PFP	8	5	3	4397 ± 284	238 ± 34	249 ± 24	246 ± 14
4	PFP	9	7	2	2345 ± 297	275 ± 31	298 ± 33	221 ± 13
1	ET	10	5	5	3864 ± 197	262 ± 23	172 ± 23	228 ± 9
2	ET	19	7	12	3702 ± 405	239 ± 14	289 ± 19	299 ± 17
3	ET	15	10	5	2885 ± 375	264 ± 20	244 ± 44	239 ± 18
4	ET	12	7	5	3069 ± 562	287 ± 45	277 ± 73	320 ± 19

* Data from Manning *et al.*[85]; reproduced with permission of Enzymologia.

† 10 units of alkaline phosphatase activity liberate 1 mg of phenolphthalein in 1 hr at pH 9.6 and 37° C from phenolphthalein diphosphate under standard conditions.

AD = Actinomycin–D
FUDR = 5–Fluorodeoxyuridine
CAP = Chloramphenicol
CY = Cycloheximide
PCP = DL-p-Chlorophenylalanine
PFP = DL-p-Fluorophenylalanine
ET = L-Ethionine
TH = Traumatized horn
NTH = Nontraumatized horn

cule, rather than *de novo* synthesis.[89,90] The present study supports this mechanism, since the various amino acid antagonists and nucleic acid inhibitors failed to depress the decidual phenolphthalein diphosphate-splitting ALP.

Conclusions

These studies lead to the following conclusions:

1. The enhanced decidual ALP of pregnant and traumatized pseudopregnant animals depends on physical and/or chemical irritation of a progesterone-conditioned endometrium.
2. The blastocyst must retain its invasiveness and viability to induce and sustain the rise in ALP.
3. Unlike the effect in the human, no detectable rat placental enzyme "spills over" in the serum near term.
4. Our work with nucleic acid inhibitors and amino acid antagonists favor the view that the decidual ALP is released and/or activated from a latent precursor protein, and *de novo* nucleic acid and/or protein synthesis is not necessary for the formation of the active enzyme molecule.

[Note Added in Proof]: Since submission of this manuscript, further electrophoretic evaluation was made of serum alkaline phosphatase from control, pregnant and pseudopregnant rats (see Study 6 in main text).

The acrylamide was made to a 5% gel, 6mm thick in 90 parts 16mM tris-3.3mM citric acid plus 10 parts 24mM sodium hydroxide-76mM boric acid buffer (pH 8.0). Two electrophoretic separations were done with the following chamber buffers; pH 7.0 (380mM boric acid-19mM sodium hydroxide) and pH 10.6 (120mM boric acid-120mM sodium hydroxide). Additionally, the sera were studied with gel and chamber buffers at pH 9.3 (0.4M tris-glycine) and pH 5.2 (0.2M acetic acid-sodium acetate). Sample application, voltage, staining etc. were similar to that described in Study 6 of the main text.

In agreement with our previous observations (see Study 6), control, pregnant and pseudopregnant sera, regardless of the different pH and buffer systems used, showed only one alkaline phosphatase band with similar activity and migration characteristics.

Acknowledgments

The authors wish to express their appreciation to: Dr. Robert L. Kroc, Director of Physiology, Warner-Lambert Research Institute, Morris Plains, N.J. for his guidance and encouragement; to Dr. Alberto Meli, Vister Labs., Italy, for his assistance in planning some of the experiments; and to Dr. W. H. Fishman, New England Medical Center Hospital, Boston, Mass., for his advice and guidance. We also wish to thank Drs. Jerome Chart and Robert Gaunt, CIBA Pharmaceutical Company, Summit, N.J., for editing the manuscript; Mr. Neil Stasilli for the statistical analyses; and Mrs. Margaret C. Butler, Mrs. Sara Priester, Mrs. Lali Calenti, Mrs. Janet I. Anderson and Miss Shirley G. Carter for their technical assistance.

References

1. Callard, I. & J. Leathem. 1967. Proc. Penn. Acad. Sci. **40**: 59.
2. Callard, I. & J. Leathem. 1965. Proc. Penn. Acad. Sci. **34**: 131.
3. Steplewski, Z. & J. Jonek. 1964. Endokr. Pol. **15**: 127.
4. Atkinson, Wm. B. & H. Elftman. 1947. Endocrinology **40**: 30.
5. Atkinson, Wm. B. & H. Elftman. 1946. Proc. Soc. Exp. Biol. Med. **20**: 148.

TABLE 11*

INFLUENCE OF NUCLEIC ACID INHIBITORS AND AMINO ACID ANTAGONISTS ON WET WEIGHT OF DECIDUALIZED AND NONDECIDUALIZED UTERINE TISSUE

Group No.		Total No. of Animals	No. of Decidualized Animals	No. of Nondecidualized Animals	Percent Wet Weight (Mean ± S.E.): Decidualized, Traumatized Horn	Decidualized, Nontraumatized Horn	Nondecidualized, Traumatized Horn	Nondecidualized, Nontraumatized Horn
1	Control	9	7	2	84.7 ± 0.3	74.1 ± 1.1	77.1 ± 3.4	76.7 ± 0.7
2	Control	6	3	3	84.1 ± 0.2	77.6 ± 0.6	77.8 ± 0.9	78.8 ± 1.7
3	Control	4	4	0	84.1 ± 0.6	78.0 ± 1.4	—	—
4	Control	15	5	10	84.6 ± 0.6	79.4 ± 0.4	80.5 ± 1.0	80.7 ± 0.5
1	AD	19	10	9	83.8 ± 0.4	79.1 ± 0.3	79.2 ± 1.0	80.8 ± 0.8
2	AD	16	13	3	83.8 ± 0.5	79.4 ± 0.3	80.4 ± 0.5	80.1 ± 0.9
3	AD	3	1	2	83.6	80.4	79.3 ± 1.8	79.3 ± 0.1
4	AD	11	7	4	85.5 ± 0.3	80.0 ± 0.4	81.2 ± 1.0	81.1 ± 0.1
5	AD	9	6	3	83.1 ± 1.0	79.1 ± 0.9	80.1 ± 0.8	80.1 ± 0.8
1	FUDR	12	6	6	85.4 ± 0.3	76.4 ± 1.1	80.4 ± 0.7	77.2 ± 0.5
2	FUDR	22	9	13	84.6 ± 0.6	77.8 ±1.2	78.2 ± 0.6	75.8 ± 0.9
1	CAP	7	5	2	83.4 ± 0.7	75.3 ± 0.6	79.3 ± 2.5	77.4 ± 3.3
2	CAP	13	6	7	83.7 ± 0.3	76.2 ± 0.5	78.4 ± 0.5	78.3 ± 0.7
3	CAP	20	14	6	84.6 ± 0.4	76.7 ± 1.7	78.3 ± 0.9	76.2 ± 2.3
4	CAP	17	8	9	83.8 ± 1.5	80.0 ± 0.5	80.5 ± 1.0	80.1 ± 0.7

1	CY	9	7	2	84.8 ± 0.2	79.1 ± 0.2	81.3 ± 0.9	79.2 ± 0.4
2	CY	13	8	5	84.0 ± 0.5	79.2 ± 0.4	80.6 ± 0.5	79.5 ± 0.7
1	PCP	4	3	1	84.3 ± 0.4	78.6 ± 0.6	81.1	77.9
2	PCP	3	2	1	83.6 ± 0.6	79.0 ± 1.6	80.5	80.6
1	PFP	8	5	3	84.6 ± 0.8	78.7 ± 2.1	79.7 ± 3.1	81.5 ± 0.3
2	PFP	10	7	3	83.8 ± 0.7	74.6 ± 2.2	76.9 ± 1.9	78.2 ± 0.7
3	PFP	8	5	3	83.2 ± 0.2	75.3 ± 1.5	76.1 ± 0.5	74.9 ± 1.5
4	PFP	9	7	2	83.5 ± 1.0	75.3 ± 1.1	75.9 ± 1.1	73.1 ± 2.3
1	ET	10	5	5	83.7 ± 0.4	75.6 ± 0.8	76.2 ± 2.6	75.7 ± 1.9
2	ET	19	7	12	83.2 ± 0.6	75.5 ± 2.2	78.8 ± 0.7	77.2 ± 0.8
3	ET	15	10	5	83.7 ± 0.5	77.3 ± 0.7	80.4 ± 0.4	79.7 ± 0.6
4	ET	12	7	5	83.8 ± 0.5	76.2 ± 0.3	78.3 ± 1.7	75.9 ± 0.2

* Data from Manning *et al.*[85]; reproduced with permission of Enzymologia.

AD = Actinomycin-D
FUDR = 5-Fluorodeoxyuridine
CAP = Chloramphenicol
CY = Cycloheximide
PCP = DL-*p*-Chlorophenylalanine
PFP = DL-*p*-Fluorophenylalanine
ET = L-Ethionine

6. Leathem, J. H. 1959. Ann. N. Y. Acad. Sci. **75**: 463.
7. Giering, J. E. & M. X. Zarrow. 1958. Acta. Endocr. **29**: 499.
8. Atkinson, Wm. B. & E. T. Engle. 1947. Endocrinology **40**: 327.
9. Manning, J. P., F. L. Hisaw, B. G. Steinetz & R. L. Kroc. 1967. Anat. Rec. **157**: 465.
10. Mansour, F. S. & A. J. Baradi. 1967. Amer. J. Obstet. Gynec. **97**(3): 109.
11. DiPaola, G., A. F. Mendizabal, N. Gomez Rueda, A. L. Usubiagal & A. J. Monserrat. 1966. Fertil. Steril. Proc., Fifth World Congress.
12. Dass, A. & G. Mookerjea. 1964. J. Indian Med. Ass. **43**: 362.
13. Jonek, J. & F. Glenc. 1963. Endokr. Pol. **14**: 85.
14. Levine, B. 1963. Obstet. Gynec. **22**: 563.
15. Boutselis, J. G., J. C. DeNeef, J. C. Ullery & O. T. George. 1963. Obstet. Gynec. **21**: 423.
16. Connell, E. B., A. Sedlis & M. S. Stone. 1967. Fertil. Steril. **18**: 35.
17. McKay, D. G., A. T. Hertig, W. A. Bardawil & J. T. Velardo. 1956. Obstet. Gynec. **8**: 22.
18. Hall, J. E. 1950. Amer. J. Obstet. Gynec. **60**: 212.
19. Gross, S. J. 1964. Amer. J. Obstet. Gynec. **88**: 647.
20. Arzac, J. P. & E. Blanchet. 1948. J. Chem. Endocr. **8**: 315.
21. Botte, V., S. S. Koide & S. J. Segal. 1968. Endocrinology **82**: 1069.
22. Verlardo, J. T. 1953. Anat. Rec. **120**: 770.
23. Manning, J. P., B. G. Steinetz, T. Giannina & A. Meli. 1967. Proc. Soc. Exp. Biol. Med. **125**: 508.
24. Watanabe, K. & W. H. Fishman. 1964. J. Histochem. Cytochem. **12**: 908.
25. Leathem, J. H., R. Oslapas & C. J. Fisher. 1968. Fertil. Steril. **19**(2): 206.
26. Steinetz, B. G., J. P. Manning, T. Giannina & A. Meli. 1967. Enzymologia **33**: 153.
27. Steplewski, Z. 1966. Bull. Acad. Pol. Sci. **14**(6): 387.
28. Bialy, G. & G. Pincus. 1966. Endocrinology **78**(2): 286.
29. Clitheroe, H. J., D. D. Bonnycastle & L. Kukla. 1966. Proc. Soc. Exp. Biol. Med. **122**: 70.
30. Clitheroe, H. J. & J. H. Leathem. 1965. Endocrinology **76**: 127.
31. Mansour, A. M. 1967. Acta Endocr. **54**: 541.
32. Mansour, A. M. & M. C. Niu. 1965. Proc. Nat. Acad. Sci. **53**: 764.
33. Sykes, J. F., S. Moss & T. R. Wrenn. 1955. Proceedings of the Centennial Symposium on Reproduction and Fertility, Michigan State Univ., East Lansing, Mich.
34. Skjernen, O. 1956. Fertil. Steril. **7**: 31.
35. Hall, K. & H. S. Khaligh. 1968. J. Endocrinol. **40**: 353.
36. Manning, J. P., A. Meli & B. G. Steinetz. 1966. J. Endocr. **35**: 385.
37. Manning, J. P., S. G. Carter & M. C. Butler. Acta Endocr. (In press.)
38. See Note added in proof.
39. Finn, C. A. & A. McLaren. 1967. R. Reprod. Fertil. **13**: 259.
40. Finn, C. A. & J. R. Hinchcliffe. 1964. J. Reprod. Fertil. **8**: 331.
41. Christie, G. A. 1966. J. Reprod. Fertil. **12**: 279.
42. Hall, K. 1968. J. Endocr. **41**(1): 53.
43. Lobel, B. S., L. Tic & M. C. Shelesnyak. 1965. Acta Endocr. **50**: 469.
44. Lobel, B. L., L. Tic & M. C. Shelesnyak. 1965. Acta Endocr. **50**: 517.
45. Christie, G. A. 1967. Histochemie **9**: 93.
46. Vacek, Z. 1965. Acta Histochem (Jena) **20**: 8.
47. Vacek, Z. 1963. Ceck. Gynek. **28**: 438.
48. Wislocki, G. B. & E. W. Dempsey. 1945. Am. J. Anat. **72**: 365.
49. Hafez, E. S. E. & I. G. White. 1968. J. Reprod. Fertil. **16**: 59.
50. Hafez, E. S. E. & I. G. White. 1967. Anat. Rec. **159**: 273.
51. Christie, G. A. 1967. Histochemie **9**: 13.
52. Manning, J. P., B. G. Steinetz, A. L. Babson & M. C. Butler. 1966. Enzymologia **31**: 309.
53. Talalay, P., W. H. Fishman & C. Huggins. 1946. J. Biol. Chem. **166**: 757.
54. Manning, J. P., A. L. Babson, M. C. Butler & S. F. Priester. 1966. Canad. J. Biochem. **44**: 755.
55. Prahlad, K. U. 1962. Acta Endocr. **39**: 407.
56. Cochrane, R. & R. K. Meyer. 1957. Proc. Soc. Exp. Biol. Med. **96**: 155.
57. Psychoyos, A. 1963. J. Endocr. **27**: 337.
58. Shelesnyak, M. C., P. F. Kraicer & G. H. Zeilmaker. 1963. Acta Endocr. **42**: 225.
59. Barnes, L. E. & R. K. Meyer. 1964. J. Reprod. Fertil. **7**: 139.
60. Enders, A. C. 1967. *In* Cellular Biology of the Uterus. Appleton-Century-Crofts, Inc., New York, N. Y.

61. Blandau, R. J. 1949. Anat. Rec. **104:** 331.
62. Wilson, I. B. 1963. Proc. Zool. Soc. Lond. **141:** 137.
63. Alden, R. H. & M. J. Smith. 1959. J. Exp. Zool. **142:** 215.
64. Finn, C. A. & P. M. Keen. 1963. J. Embryol. Exp. Morph. **11:** 673.
65. Lobel, B. L., L. Tic & M. C. Shelesnyak. 1965. Acta Endocr. **50:** 537.
66. Danielli, J. 1958. *In* General Cytochemical Methods. Academic Press, Inc., New York, N. Y.
67. Fishman, W., S. Goldman & R. DeLellis. 1967. Nature **213:** 457.
68. Cayla, J. & P. Fabre. 1935. C. R. Soc. Biol. (Paris) **120:** 748.
69. Coryn, G. 1934. J. Chir. (Paris) **33:** 213.
70. Meranze, T., D. R. Meranze & M. M. Rothman. 1937. Amer. J. Obstet. Gynec. **33:** 44.
71. Young, J., E. J. King, E. Wood & I. D. P. Wooton. 1946. J. Obstet. Gynaec. Brit. Comm. **53:** 251.
72. McMaster, Y., R. Tennant, J. S. Chubb, F. C. Neale & S. Posen. 1964. J. Obstet. Gynaec. Brit. Comm. **71:** 735.
73. Fishman, W. H. & N. K. Ghosh. 1968. In Advances in Clinical Chemistry. Academic Press, Inc., New York and London.
74. Boyer, S. H. 1961. Science **134:** 1002.
75. Clubb, J., F. Neale & S. Posen. 1965. J. Lab. Clin. Med. **66:** 493.
76. Fishman, W. & S. Green. 1967. Enzymologia **33:** 89.
77. Ghosh, N., S. Goldman & W. Fishman. 1967. Enzymologia **33:** 8.
78. Fishman, W., N. Inglis, L. Stolbach & M. Krant. 1968. Cancer Res. **28:** 150.
79. Sussman, H. & E. Cotlove. 1967. Fed. Proc. **26:** 279.
80. Sussman, H., M. Bowman & J. Lewis. 1968. Nature **218:** 359.
81. EC Apparatus Corp., Technical Bulletin 128, Philadelphia, Pa.
82. Fishman, W., N. Inglis & N. Ghosh. 1968. Clin. Chim. Acta **19:** 71.
83. EC Apparatus Corp., Technical Bulletin 146, Philadelphia, Pa.
84. Fishman, W. H., S. Green & N. Inglis. 1962. Biochim. Biophys. Acta **62:** 363.
85. Fishman, W., S. Green & N. Inglis. 1962. Biochim. Biophys. Acta **62:** 429.
86. Manning, J. P., S. G. Carter, L. Calenti & J. I. Anderson. Enzymologia (In press).
87. Fishman, W. H. 1968. (Personal communication.)
88. Ghosh, N. K. & W. H. Fishman. 1968. Biochem. J. **108:** 779.
89. Moog, F. 1965. Advances Enzyme Regulat. **3:** 221.
90. Moog, F. 1966. J. Exp. Zool. **161:** 353.

Discussion of the Paper

N. K. Ghosh: In one of the slides you presented, you have shown that the intensity of the enzyme band increases with the progress of pregnancy in these rats. You also have evidence that placenta is not a contributor in this elevation. Now do you think that during pregnancy in these rats the intestine produces a larger amount of the enzyme that is leaking into the circulation.

Dr. Manning: If I understand your question correctly, we were not able to see any difference in an enzyme activity in the serum enzyme using the standard biochemical assay or doing the electrophoresis.

Dr. Ghosh: Indeed, eight, ten, eleven in different days, the intensity of the band increases. Does it stay the same?

Dr. Manning: It stays the same.

C. L. Markert: There's no doubt in your presentation that you showed dramatically the change in titer of the enzyme with various conditions of the endometrium interacting with the blastocyst, and with hormonal treatment or the absence of it, but among all of these facts, do you see any basis for saying anything about what the enzyme is doing.

Dr. Manning: No, we don't claim that the enzyme is really doing anything. We think it's merely a membrane protein because if it was so important to the metabolism of the fetus, then why don't all animals that show a decidual reaction exhibit a high alkaline phosphatase titer. In the animals that do not show high alkaline phosphatase titer, there is probably another protein doing the same job as the alkaline phosphatase is doing in the rat.

DR. MARKERT: I find it very difficult to accept on biological grounds that that enzyme is synthesized for the entertainment of the cells. It must have some more important meaning than that.

DR. MANNING: Yes, but what I'm driving at is that, at the pH of the cell, the alkaline phosphatase has no activity and is simply a component of the cell in the same way as that shown by Fishman earlier with β-glucuronidase, a dual localization in endoplasmic reticulum and in lysosomes. It is reasonable perhaps to define some type of a transfer mechanism rather than a specific hydrolytic activity occurring within the cell.

M. KAPLAN (*New England Center Hospital, Boston, Mass.*): How much inhibition of nucleic acid and protein synthesis did you achieve with actinomycin D and the amino acid antagonists.

DR. MANNING: We did not measure these.

L. BECKMAN: Early in human pregnancy, there is one kind of alkaline phosphatase that disappears around seven to eight weeks, and then another one makes its appearance. That is the true placental alkaline phosphatase, which is synthesized under the influence of genotype of the fetus. Did you look into the placenti at different stages?

DR. MANNING: Just at 19 and 20 days, as I showed here.

DR. BECKMAN: You did all the work on rats?

DR. MANNING: Yes, we did all the work on rats.

DR. BECKMAN: How are the rat placenti? Are they like the mouse placenti, like little round buttons.

DR. MANNING: Yes.

DR. BECKMAN: Then they're easy to grab in different stages.

DR. MANNING: Yes.

DR. BECKMAN: I mean, if you were following this, it's quite possible that in other form, a truly different molecular species would appear, and it isn't so puzzling that your phosphatase disappears. It could be a true enzyme that is used only at this stage of development, let's say.

DR. MANNING: Well, we have subsequently done studies on the decidual alkaline phosphatase (pregnant and pseudopregnant animals) and compared these with the studies on the placenta of the rat. We found that for the pseudopregnant, or pregnant rat, that they had exactly the same pH optimum and the same K_m. The placental enzyme, on the other hand, although it had the same pH optimum, did not have the same K_m. So it looks like they are two different enzymes. In response to that last question, there was a noticeable drop in the gross decidual reaction in the animals treated with the amino acid antagonists and nucleic acid inhibitors. The water content, however, was exactly the same in the traumatized horn of the treated animals as in that of the nontreated animals. We did not do the protein analysis, but it appeared that we did not get a gross decidual reaction.

W. A. BARDAWIL (*St. Margaret's Hospital, Boston, Mass.*): In human pregnancy, early in initial stages of implantation, the endometrium usually shows a halo of reactivation of the glandular tissue that is beyond any level attributable purely to trauma. I wonder whether the blastocyst contains any significant amount of estrogen or progesterone to account for this local reaction.

DR. MANNING: I can't answer that question. I don't know. Dr. Steinetz?

B. STEINETZ: So far as I know, there is very little evidence that the rat placenta produces any hormones, particularly at these early stages. It's well known that the ovaries are essential to maintain pregnancy, and that if they are removed at any time before parturition the animal will abort.

DR. MARKERT: Any further comments or questions?

F. ROELS (*University of Ghent, Ghent, Belgium*): Concerning the possible role of the enzyme, it would certainly be interesting to look at where it sits in the cell, especially on the microscopic level. I don't know if this has been done, but, for example, one could imagine that this enzyme is sitting in the lysosomes. Alkaline phosphatase has been demonstrated in lysosomes in the intestine. I would like to ask whether, when you measure your enzyme, you are sure that the lysosomes aren't destroyed? I mean, in your medium, is there some detergent, or are you sure that lysosomal enzymes are liberated.

DR. MANNING: Well, we used three standard methods without any increase in the enzyme activity. In fact, there might have been a slight decrease. We also used some of the Tweens detergents, and they also did not increase the alkaline phosphatase activity.

DR. ROELS: There are no morphologic studies about the localization.

DR. MANNING: The activity in the placenta is in the syncytiotrophoblast. In the deciduae it's in what's referred to as the decidual cell, which starts as a crescent shape right in the area of implantation and then appears to expand from a focus. There is very little glandular activity in the area. It all seems to be derived, at least by histological section, from the decidual cells.

MECHANISMS OF PHOSPHOHYDROLASE TRANSPORT AND OF HOMEOSTASIS

R. Keiding

Department of Clinical Chemistry, University of Aarhus
Aarhus, Denmark

This paper is confined to the human alkaline phosphatase. Although much useful information has been gained concerning the transport of alkaline phosphatases in animals, it is known that significant differences exist in concentration, composition and metabolic behavior of the circulating alkaline phosphatases in different animal species, including the rat, cat, ox and dog (Gutman, 1959). Thus, a comparison of the metabolic behavior of alkaline phosphatase between man and animal is considered irrelevant in the present context.

A number of limitations must be considered before experimental results can be discussed.

It is only possible to characterize the concentration of the enzyme in "activity" per volume or per mass unit. Molecular or mass concentration cannot be stated. Differences in conditions, in the assessment of activity, the composition of the fluid in which the enzyme is present, and the "unphysiological" conditions present in the assessment of activity (pH) are obvious factors limiting a parallelism between activity and molecular or mass concentration.

The lack of knowledge about the physiological role of alkaline phosphatase is another limitation. As long as we do not know whether it is the hydrolytic action, the transphosphorylation action, or the pyrophosphatase action that is operative, serious discrepancies may arise, since it is known that there is no parallelism between the different types of activities in the different alkaline phosphatase enzymes found in man. (Ingerslev, 1968).

Only occasionally do we have suitable experimental conditions when we study the metabolic behavior of human alkaline phosphatase. Most often, we are limited to the examination of a variety of disease conditions and, in many of these cases, the assumption is made that only one parameter in the complex of parameters determining the homeostasis of alkaline phosphatases is operative. Most often, however, we are actually dealing with a complex chain of events that ultimately influence a number of mechanisms that bring about changes in the circulating alkaline phosphatase. The tendency to oversimplify the conclusions drawn from clinical experiments with alkaline phosphatase is obvious from the extensive literature on the subject.

Alkaline phosphatase, like many other circulating enzymes, has a low concentration in human serum compared with that found in many tissues. However, the concentration is surprisingly stable. FIGURE 1 shows the concentration of serum alkaline phosphatase in three normal persons over a period of two years. The concentration in the three persons varies within $\pm$ 10%. The phosphatase fractions (electrophoretic fractions) (Nordentoft-Jensen, 1964) also vary little. Dent and Harper (1962) also found a reasonable constancy of serum alkaline phosphatase concentration by repeated determinations over a period of four years. Compared to other serum constituents, this constancy is of the same order as those subjected to homeostatic regulation (Neuman, 1960).

This relative stability of the plasma concentration of alkaline phosphatase does not imply an inert metabolism. From the work of Clubb, Neale and Posen (1965), it seems that the half-life of infused placental phosphatase is of the order of seven

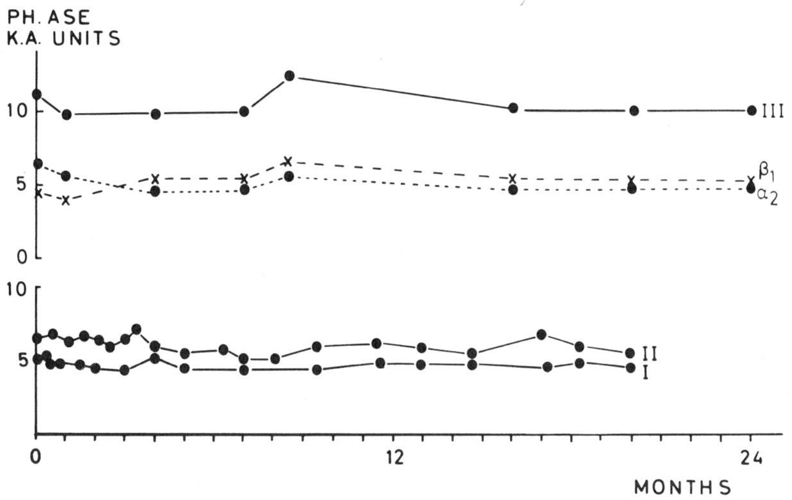

FIGURE 1. Serum alkaline phosphatase (PH.ASE) concentration in relation to time in three persons. The concentration of electrophoretic phosphatase fractions in person III are represented by dotted lines.

days, and that a shorter half-life of "bone phosphatase" is possible. Similar evidence can be found in animal experiments. (Dalgaard, 1950; Le Veen *et al.,* 1950; Armstrong *et al.,* 1934).

Although there are many problems in evaluating data on the disappearance rate of enzymes from the circulation, these data prompt a consideration of the rates of delivery, removal or inactivation of the circulating alkaline phosphatase.

SUPPLY OF ALKALINE PHOSPHATASE TO CIRCULATION

Tissue. Numerous investigations have been published containing indirect or correlative evidence of a constant tissue phosphatase supply to the circulation. Clinical evidence from the study of hyperphosphatasemia, as well as biochemical similarities, make such a theory very likely, especially concerning osseous tissue.

The subject of hepatic tissue phosphatase as a donor of alkaline phosphatase to the circulation is much more controversial (Gutman, 1959; Posen, 1967; Fishman & Ghosh, 1967). It is not surprising, therefore, that we are unable to deal with the quantitative aspect of such a delivery; the qualitative aspect will be considered below.

Lymph. The lymph of the thoracic duct seems to supply a considerable amount of alkaline phosphatase to the circulation. The lymph contains variable quantities of alkaline phosphatase. This has been shown in animals (Flock & Bollman, 1948; Linder & Blomstrand, 1958) and in man by Keiding (1964) and Blomstrand & Werner (1965). The same authors have demonstrated that lymph alkaline phosphatase concentration increases six to eight hours after a fat-rich diet.

The electrophoretic composition of lymph alkaline phosphatase is shown in FIGURE 2. The nine different lymph samples were all taken in the absorptive phase. The main fraction shown is the slow β fraction, which has been identified as intestinal phosphatase (Keiding, 1966). Further details are given about one of the patient in TABLE 1. There is an increase in the intestinal fraction of lymph alkaline phosphatase, whereas the other phosphatase fractions are almost constant. The serum alkaline phosphatase fractions during the same period show no significant variations. During the total examination period of from 10 to 36 hours after cream (400 g), 139 to 1159 units of intestinal alkaline phosphatase are transported through the lymph. Similar values in seven patients are calculated from the work of Blomstrand and Werner (1965) (TABLE 2). The values are of the same magnitude, although stated in other units of activity. From the same investigation, it can be seen that serum alkaline phosphatase is not substantially affected by the deprivation of lymph alkaline phosphatase. On the other hand, in the intact person the addition of high intestinal phosphatase activity is followed only by a slight increase in the intestinal fraction of serum alkaline phosphatase after a fat meal (Beckman, 1964; Langman *et al.*, 1966).

Removal of Alkaline Phosphatase

Urine. It is generally agreed that urinary excretion of alkaline phosphatase is moderate in quantity compared to that of circulating alkaline phosphatase. TABLE 3 shows the ranges of normal urinary excretion of alkaline phosphatase. (The figures given are on dialyzed urine). Disregarding what I have stated in the introduction, it may be calculated that the excreted alkaline phosphatase is roughly 1/10 to 1/5 of the total circulating alkaline phosphatase. Variations in excretion during the day are of the order of ± 50%, and in normals independent of urine volume (Dubach & Padline, 1966). There is no constant correlation between increased serum alkaline phosphatase and the activity excreted in urine; also, the increase of urine phosphatase excretion in renal disease does not influence the

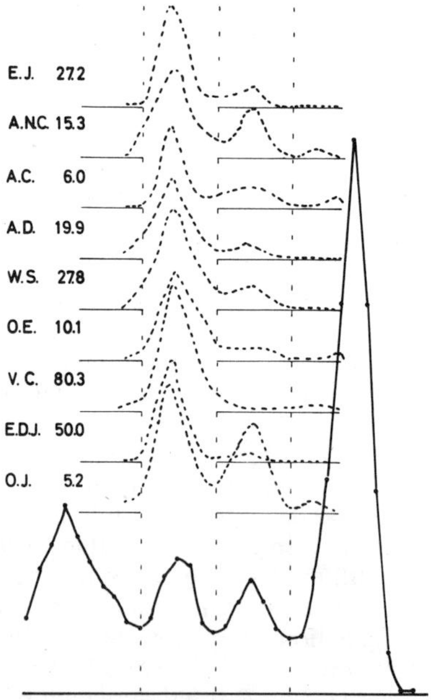

FIGURE 2. Thoracic duct lymph alkaline phosphatase fractions of nine patients determined by polyvinylchloride electrophoresis. Below the protein fractions, from left to right are: γ, β, α_2 and albumin fraction. The dotted curves represent alkaline phosphatase activity.

TABLE 1

ACTIVITY OF THORACIC DUCT LYMPH AND SERUM ALKALINE PHOSPHATASE FRACTIONS (POLYVINYLCHLORIDE ELECTROPHORESIS) FOLLOWED IN A PATIENT OVER 27 HOURS AFTER INGESTION OF 400 G OF CREAM

			Alkaline Phosphatase (K.A. Units)					
			Lymph		Serum			
Procedure	Time in Hours	Vol. (ml)	β_2	$\beta_1 + \alpha_2$	β_2	β_1	α_2	α_1
Cream 200 ml	−4							
Cannulation	0							
Cream (200 ml)	0– 3	166	11.9	4.8	0	3.5	4.8	0.2
	3– 5	221	13.5	5.5				
	5– 7	187	21.2	5.1				
	7– 9	144	21.8	5.4	0.2	4.8	4.4	0.1
	9–11	84	4.7	4.7				
	11–15	270	3.5	4.9				
	15–19	293	1.6	4.7	0	4.6	4.6	0
	19–23	306	0.5	4.9	0.1	4.7	4.6	0
	23–27	290	0.5	4.2	0	4.7	4.8	0

TABLE 2

CUMULATIVE ACTIVITY OF INTESTINAL PHOSPHATASE AFTER CANNULATION OF THORACIC DUCT

Keiding Series*	Sampling Period (Hours)	Intestinal Phosphatase Cumulative (K.A. Units × Vol.)
1	10	566
2	36	129
3	24	280
4	16	1159
5	27	139
6	20	240
Blomstrand & Werner Series (1965)*	**Sampling Period (Hours)**	**(B.L. Units × Vol.)**
1	16	667
2	19.5	—
3	19	977
4	18	1969
5	21	766
6	19	1468
7	12	177

* Intestinal phosphatase was determined by electrophoretic technique in the author's series, and by ℓ-phenylalanine inhibition in the series of Blomstrand and Werner.

TABLE 3

CUMULATIVE ALKALINE PHOSPHATASE ACTIVITY FOUND IN URINE OVER 8 OR 24 HOURS BY DIFFERENT INVESTIGATORS

Investigators	Units/Hours	
Amador *et al.* (1963)	< 7560 U/8 Hr	(Keiding Units)
Dubach & Padlina (1966)	1191–9343 U/8 Hr	(Amador Units)
Allen & Spellberg (1967)	19–90 U/8 Hr	(Gomory Units)
Butterworth *et al.* (1965)	1–11 U/24 Hr	(K.A. Units)

level of serum alkaline phosphatase (Butterworth *et al.*, 1965a). Urinary alkaline phosphatase composition as determined by electrophoresis shows no constant pattern (Butterworth *et al.*, 1965b; Pasternack, 1964). Therefore, there is no evidence to indicate whether or not urine alkaline phosphatase is derived from circulating alkaline phosphatase. The excretion is moderate and highly variable within the same individual.

Bile. It has long been known that alkaline phosphatase is present in bile. (Armstrong *et al.*, 1934; Green *et al.*, 1934). Many physiological studies have since been reported on the character of this excretion in animals, and marked species variations have been observed (Gutman, 1959). The amount of alkaline phosphatase activity present in the bile varies in different reports because of differences in the methods used, the instability of the enzyme and the presence of inhibitors (Peterlik, 1966).

Allen and Spellberg (1967) found the concentration of bile alkaline phosphatase in 14 patients to be from 470 to 8350 Gomori units. In our own series of 20 patients, the concentration was from 29 to 197 K.A. units. Edlund and Christoffersson (1967) found a mean concentration of 40 Buch units in 59 bile samples from the gall bladder in patients without biliary obstruction. In patients with biliary obstruction of long duration, however, they found a lower phosphatase concentration. Alkaline phosphatase concentration in bile seems to vary with the ingestion of food. As shown in FIGURE 3, there is an increase in bile phosphatase concentration after two hours, and in five of the six patients, a late increase 8 to 10 hours after food. The first increase in concentration follows the increase in bile salts and bile volume. The second increase was found in patients examined on the

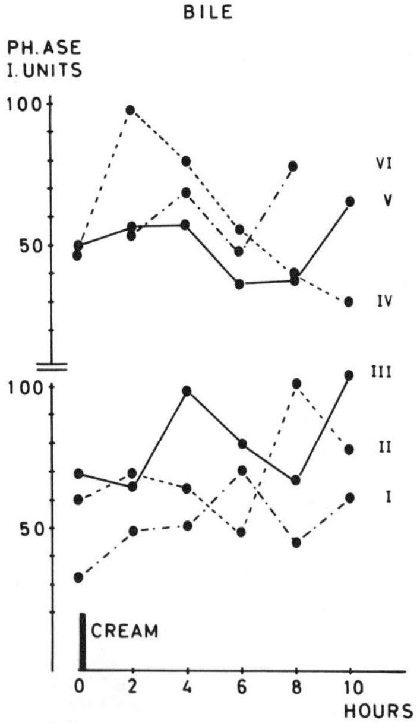

FIGURE 3. The relation between alkaline phosphatase (PH.ASE) concentration in bile and time after ingestion of 200 g of cream in six patients with indwelling T tube in the common bile duct.

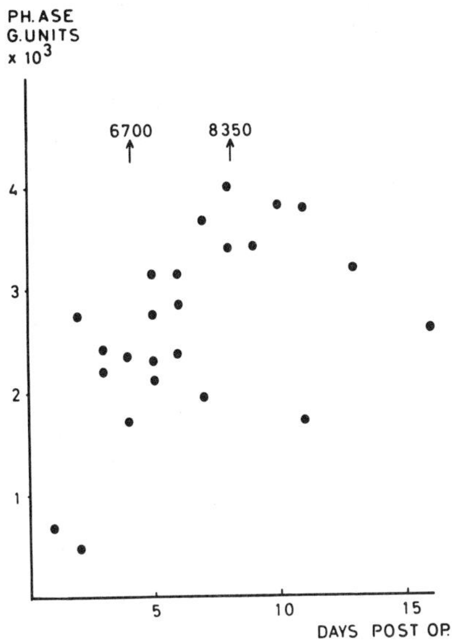

FIGURE 4. Alkaline phosphatase concentration in bile related to time after T tube cannulation of common bile duct. Calculated from Allen & Spellberg (1967).

tenth to fourteenth day after operation, shortly before restoration of normal bile outlet to the duodenum. The patient with no late increase was examined on the fourth day after operation. From the data of Allen and Spellberg (1967) on 14 patients examined on different days after operation, bile alkaline phosphatase concentration can be calculated. FIGURE 4 shows that there is an increase in concentration related to the time after operation. Since bile volume also increases in the same manner, there is a considerable increase in bile alkaline phosphatase output from about the seventh day after operation. A similar finding of a marked increase in bile alkaline phosphatase concentration in patients following cholecystectomy, but without changes in serum alkaline phosphatase, was reported by Keiding (1964). Before reporting on the composition of the bile alkaline phosphatase, the electrophoretic pattern of serum alkaline phosphatase using various techniques must be reemphasized. FIGURE 5 shows the principal phosphatase fractions of five sera in electrophoresis on different supporting media. The so-called main fraction in the α_2 globulin region generally has the same mobility in different media. It is important in the present context that the fraction in Pevikon or starch grain electrophoresis—called the α_1 fraction—moves somewhat slower in cellogel, agarose, and agar, and that, in starch gel, this α_1 fraction occurs in the γ region almost at the application point. The identity between the α_1 fraction in Pevikon and the almost immobile fraction in starch gel has been controlled by electrophoresis of the isolated α_1 fraction from Pevikon on starch gel. This difference in electrophoretic mobility is due to the molecular sieve function of the different media. In gel filtration experiments on G200 Sephadex, this α_1 fraction is found in the first fraction, the so-called high molecular fraction as seen in FIGURE 6.

In FIGURE 7, the different experiences with bile alkaline phosphatase composition from both normal and so-called abnormal bile is shown The dominant fraction of bile alkaline phosphatase is the α_1 fraction. In addition, variable activity of the α_2 fraction (corresponding to the principal serum fraction) and of the slow β fraction (corresponding to the intestinal alkaline phosphatase) is found. Gel filtration on Sephadex G200 shows the main fraction in the "void volume" high molecular fraction.

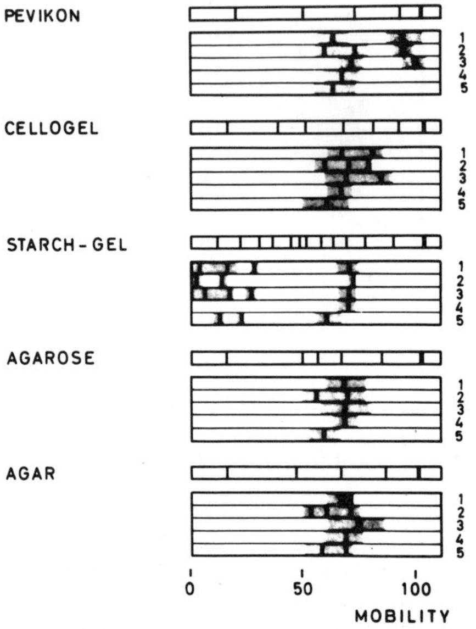

FIGURE 5. Five different sera exposed to electrophoresis on five different supporting media. The protein pattern of each type of electrophoresis is given in the top panel. The patterns of alkaline phosphatase activity are indicated by lines showing the maximal activity of the fractions and by hatching to show the width of the bands.

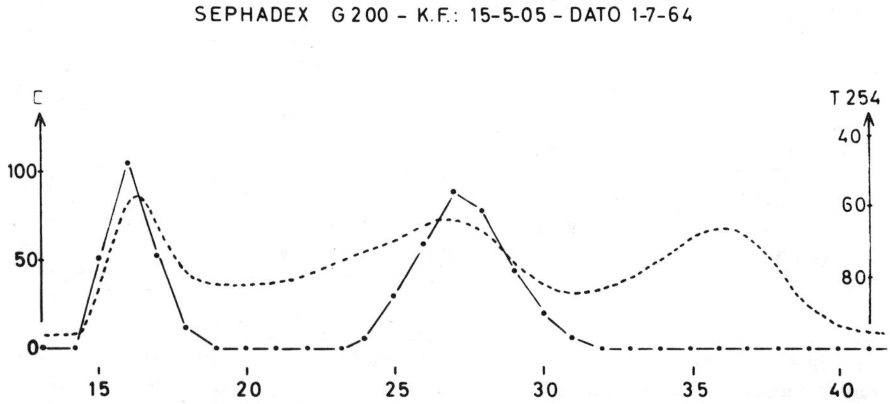

FIGURE 6. Serum alkaline phosphatase activity in the different protein fractions obtained after gel filtration on Sephadex G200. The serum corresponds to serum 1 in FIGURE 5.

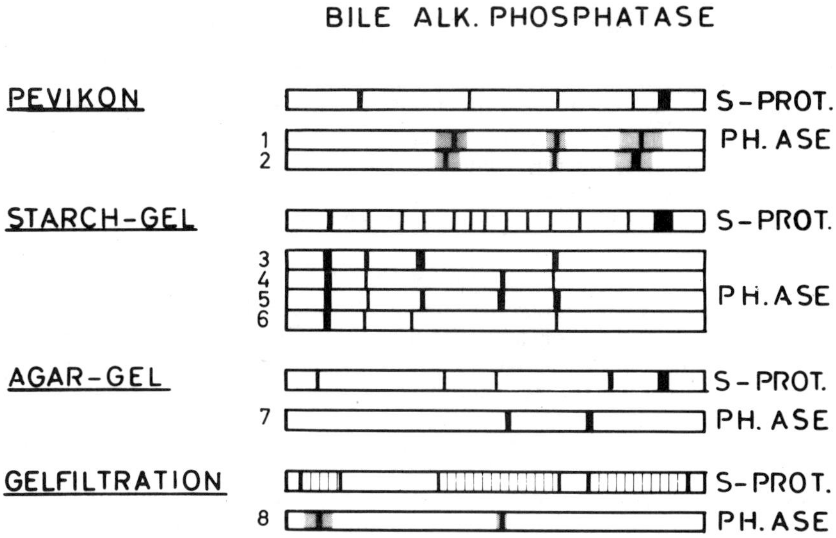

FIGURE 7. Protein and alkaline phosphatase characteristics of bile in electrophoretic and Sephadex G200 fractionation. The figure as drawn corresponds to FIGURE 5. The examples are taken from Keiding (1964); Rosenberg (1959); Chiandussi *et al.* (1962); Gordon (1965); Pope & Cooperband (1966); Hill & Sammons (1967); Haije & deJong (1963); and Estborn (1964).

TABLE 4

CONCENTRATION OF TOTAL ALKALINE PHOSPHATASE AND OF THE ELECTROPHORETIC PHOSPHATASE FRACTION (CELLOGEL) IN BILE OBTAINED EVERY SECOND HOUR FOR 10 HOURS AFTER INGESTION OF 200 G OF CREAM

	Bile Alkaline Phosphatases (K.A. Units)			
Hours	Total	β_2	α_2	α_1
0	50.5	0	2.5	48.0
2	58.0	4.6	8.2	45.2
4	59.5	2.3	14.2	43.0
6	37.0	5.7	6.1	25.2
8	37.2	3.1	4.1	30.0
10	65.0	3.2	8.4	53.4

In TABLE 4, data is shown on one of the patients with a late increase in bile alkaline phosphatase. Here the α_1 fraction is also the dominant one in the sample taken 10 hours after cream.

Feces. It is well known that mammalian feces contain high activities of alkaline phosphatase (Posen, 1967). This excretion is not of chief concern in regard to the homeostasis of circulating alkaline phosphatase because of the intimate relation with the high alkaline phosphatase activity in the intestinal fluid. It is unlikely that the feces phosphatase is derived from bile since α_1 phosphatase immediately disappears when it reaches the duodenum (Keiding, 1968).

Other routes. Through experimental obstruction of the common bile duct in animals, it has been shown that the regurgitation of bile pigments through the liver lymph is followed by a regurgitation of bile alkaline phosphatase (Alikan & Hardy, 1962). Unfortunately, there is no experimental evidence to show that such a mechanism is operative in the normal man.

It has been suggested that intestinal fluid phosphatase might reach the portal circulation after absorption, and that variable amounts of intestinal phosphatase might reach the liver by this route. (Lincheer *et al.*, 1967). Keiding (1964) found no intestinal phosphatase in the portal vein blood, but since the patients were fasting, the possibility of intestinal phosphatase transport through the portal vein is not excluded.

Discussion

The homeostasis of circulating human alkaline phosphatase represents the problem of a small, but constant, circulating enzyme activity surrounded by a huge intracellular enzyme activity, and a transport through the blood of phosphatase activities 5 to 10 times the normal activity in the total plasma volume. From a conventional standpoint, a great deal of chemical and biochemical evidence has been collected to support the view that part of the normal circulating alkaline phosphatase is closely related to bone phosphatase. The fact that we are totally ignorant of the delivery rate of such phosphatase to the circulation should not invalidate the qualitative relation. An important argument for a relation between circulating alkaline phosphatase and tissue phosphatases is the discovery in disease hypophosphatasia, of a low tissue phosphatase activity together with a low but constant, serum alkaline phosphatase level with normal electrophoretic composition (Rasmussen, 1968; Korner, 1962). Low tissue phosphatase is found in this disease in all tissues examined except the intestinal mucosa, where normal phosphatase activity has been reported (McCance *et al.*, 1956; Danovitch *et al.*, 1968). This last finding supports the opinion that intestinal phosphatase plays a minor role in the composition of normal circulating alkaline phosphatase.

The main electrophoretic phosphatase component of normal serum has for many years been related to liver phosphatase. Again, we are without evidence concerning the rate of delivery of such phosphatases to the circulation. However, we have much evidence, especially from clinical findings, to support the opinion that the liver plays an important role in regulating the serum alkaline phosphatase level. Thus, it is reasonable to believe that intestinal phosphatase carried by lymph to the circulation is in some way removed, inactivated, or modified by the liver (Keiding, 1964; Fishman & Ghosh, 1967).

The theory that, in the normal man, intestinal phosphatase delivered to the circulation is removed in the liver and through the bile, is supported by the following evidence: (1) a considerable output of phosphatase, (2) an increase in concentration of alkaline phosphatase after operation at a time when food and bile in the intestinum favor absorption of fat and, consequently, a larger transport of intestinal phosphatase through the lymph, and (3) the finding of an increase in bile alkaline phosphatase concentration 8 to 10 hours after ingestion of fat. This removal cannot take place without a modification of the enzyme that changes its electrophoretic mobility, its L-phenylalanine sensitivity, and its molecular weight.

The presence in serum of α_1 alkaline phosphatase fraction in substantial concentration in a majority of hepatic disorders (Nordentoft-Jensen, 1966) might, consequently be explained as a regurgitation of α_1 phosphatase to the circulation, (possibly via the liver lymph), considering the decreased amount of fat absorbed in such diseases.

Increased serum alkaline phosphatase in liver disorders is not explained by the increase in α_1 fraction alone. Most often, a high increase in the α_2 fraction is seen, an increase not included in the present theory. However, one might make certain assumptions with the aid of animal perfusion experiments that show increased phosphatase activity in the perfusate (Sebesta *et al.*, 1964), and by the discovery of much higher alkaline phosphatase activities in neoplastic hepatic tissue (Inouye & Higashi, 1963). One might speculate that the liver forms an alkaline phosphatase (the α_2 phosphatase fraction) which, in the normal human subject, constitutes the regulated extracellular enzyme, that it does so parallel to the formation in the liver of serum proteins, and, consequently, that the normal pattern of human serum alkaline phosphatase is (1) the regulated fraction (the α_2 fraction), (2) bone phosphatase in quantities dependent on the osteoblastic activity and (3) intestinal phosphatase in quantities dependent on ABO group, secretor status and food intake.

I regret that I have ignored here the limiting statements made at the beginning of this paper. We have only very scanty information on the homeostasis of human serum alkaline phosphatase, and the deductions we can make will only be of some value for those who plan new research on the subject.

Summary

A survey is made of the different routes by which alkaline phosphatase is delivered to the circulation in man, and of the possible routes of excretion. Special emphasis is placed (1) on the addition of intestinal phosphatase to the circulation through the thoracic duct in quantities 5 to 10 times that of the total circulating phosphatase activity, but without major influence on the serum concentration, and (2) on the occurrence of high bile alkaline phosphatase concentrations 8 to 10 hours after ingestion of fat. It is suggested that the output of bile phosphatase (at least the fast-moving fraction of bile alkaline phosphatase) balances the input of intestinal phosphatase to the circulation. Serum alkaline phosphatase concentration in the normal person is assumed to be regulated in the above-mentioned manner together with a regulated output from the liver of "liver phosphatase." The actual osteoblastic activity of the bones seems to determine the concentration of "bone phosphatase in serum."

References

ALIKAN, F. & J. D. HARDY. 1962. Lymphatic transport of bile pigments and alkaline phosphatase in experimental common duct obstruction. Surgery **52:** 366–372.

ALLEN, H. & M. SPELLBERG. 1967. Alkaline phosphatase in bile and urine. Arch. Intern. Med. (Chicago) **120:** 667–671.

AMADOR, E., T. S. ZIMMERMAN & W. E. C. WACKER. 1963. Urinary alkaline phosphatase activity. JAMA **185:** 953–958.

ARMSTRONG, A. R., E. J. KING & R. I. HARRIS. 1934. Phosphatase in obstructive jaundice. Canad. Med. Ass. J. **31:** 14–20.

BECKMAN, L. 1964. Associations between human serum alkaline phosphatase and blood groups. Acta Genet. (Basel) **14:** 286–297.

BLOMSTRAND, R. & B. WERNER. 1965. Alkaline phosphatase activity in human thoracic duct lymph. Acta Chir. Scand. **129:** 177–191.

BUTTERWORTH, P. J., D. W. MOSS, E. PITKANEN & A. PRINGLE. 1965a. Patterns of urinary excretion of alkaline phosphatase in acute renal failure. Clin. Chim. Acta **11:** 212–220.

BUTTERWORTH, P. J., D. W. MOSS, E. PITKANEN & A. PRINGLE. 1965b. Some characteristics of alkaline phosphatase in human urine. Clin. Chim. Acta **11:** 220–226.

CHIANDUSSI, L., S. F. GREEN & S. SHERLOCK. 1962. Serum alkaline phosphatase fractions in hepato-biliary and bone diseases. Clin. Sci. **22:** 425–434.

CLUBB, J. S., F. C. NEALE & S. POSEN. 1965. The behavior of infused placental alkaline phosphatase in human subjects. J. Lab. Clin. Med. **66:** 493–507.

DALGAARD, J. B. 1950. Serumfosfatasestigningen ved obstruktionsicterus. Rosenkilde & Bagger, Copenhagen.

DANOVITCH, S. H., P. N. BAER & L. LASTER. 1968. Intestinal alkaline phosphatase activity in familial hypophosphatasia. New Eng. J. Med. **278:** 1253–1260.

DENT, C. E. & C. M. HARPER. 1962. Plasma alkaline phosphatase in normal adults and in patients with primary hyperparathyreoidism. Lancet **1:** 559–563.

DUBACH, V. C. & P. PADLINA. 1966. Aktivität der alkalischen Phosphatase im Urin. Klin. Wschr. **44:** 180–186.

EDLUND, Y. & E. CHRISTOFFERSSON. 1967. Alkaline phosphatase and transaminases in serum and hepatic duct bile in patients with normal or blocked biliary flow. Acta Hepatosplen. (Stuttgart) **4:** 230–237.

ESTBORN, B. 1964. Separation of phosphatase isoenzymes by gelfiltration. Z. Klin. Chem. **2:** 53–54.

FISHMAN, W. H. & N. K. GHOSH. 1967. *In* Advances in Clinical Chemistry. O. Bodansky & C. P. Stewart, Eds. **10:** 255–370. Academic Press, Inc., New York, N. Y.

FLOCK, E. V. & J. L. BOLLMAN. 1948. Alkaline phosphatase in the intestinal lymph of the rat. J. Biol. Chem. **175:** 439–449.

GORDON, S. 1965. Alkaline phosphatase isoenzymes in serum and tissue. S. Afr. Med. J. **39:** 49–53.

GREEN, C. H., H. F. SHATLUCK & L. KAPLOWITZ. 1934. Phosphatase content of the blood serum in jaundice. J. Clin. Invest. **13:** 1079–1087.

GUTMAN, A. B. 1959. Serum alkaline phosphatase activity in diseases of the skeletal and hepatobiliary system. (Amer.) J. Med. **27:** 875–901.

HAIJE, W. G. & M. DEJONG. 1963. Iso-enzyme pattern of serum alkaline phosphatase in agar-gel electrophoresis and their clinical significance. Clin. Chim. Acta **8:** 620–623.

HILL, P. G. & H. G. SAMMONS. 1967. An interpretation of the elevation of serum alkaline phosphatase in disease. J. Clin. Path. **20:** 654–659.

INGERSLEV, J. 1968. Studies on the transphosphorylation activity of human alkaline phosphatases. (In press.)

INOUYE, M. & K. HIGASHI. 1963. Proporties of acetone insensitive phosphatase from ascites hepatoma of rat. J. Biochem. (Tokyo) **54:** 130–137.

KEIDING, R. 1964. The alkaline phosphatase fractions of human lymph. Clin. Sci. **26:** 291–297.

KEIDING, R. 1966. Intestinal alkaline phosphatase in human lymph and serum. Scand. J. Clin. Lab. Invest. **18:** 134–140.

KEIDING, R. 1968. (Unpublished.)

KORNER, N. H. 1962. Distribution of alkaline phosphatase in serum protein fractions. J. Clin. Path. **15:** 195–205.

LANGMAN, M. J. S., E. LEUTHOLD, E. B. ROBSON, J. HARRIS, J. E. LUFFMAN & H. HARRIS. 1966. Influence of diet on the "intestinal" component of serum alkaline phosphatase in people of different ABO blood groups and secretor status. Nature **212:** 41–43.

LEVEEN, H. H., L. J. TALBOT, M. RESTUCCIA & J. R. BARBERIO. 1950. Metabolism and excretion of alkaline phosphatase. J. Lab. Clin. Med. **36:** 192–202.

LINCHEER, W. G., A. L. BLUM, N. I. INGLIS & W. H. FISHMAN. 1967. Intestinal phosphatase during glucose absorption. Clin. Res. **15:** 238.

LINDER, E. & R. BLOMSTRAND. 1958. Technic for collection of thoracic duct lymph of man. Proc. Soc. Exp. Biol. Med. **97:** 653–657.

MCCANCE, R. A., D. V. I. FAIRWEATHER, A. M. BARRET & A. B. MORRISON. 1956. Genetic, clinical, biochemical, and pathological features of hypophosphatasia. Quart. J. Med. **25:** 523–537.

NEUMAN, W. F. 1960. Enzymic regulations in the bones. *In* Enzyme Regulations in Clinical Medicine. A. Gigon & H. Ludvig, Eds. : 183–192. Schwalbe. Basel.

NORDENTOFT-JENSEN, B. 1964. Differentiation between the electrophoretic pattern of serum alkaline phosphatase in bone disease and in liver disease. Clin. Sci. **26:** 299–305.

NORDENTOFT-JENSEN, B. 1966. The fastmoving fraction of serum alkaline phosphatase in patients with various diseases. Danish Med. Bull. **13:** 175–180.

PASTERNACK, A. 1964. Alkaline phosphatase in urine. Scand. J. Clin. Lab. Invest. **16:** 145–148.

PETERLIK, H. 1966. Bestimmung der Aktivität der alkalischen Phosphatasen in der Galle. Z. Klin. Chem. **4:** 34–35.

POPE, C. E. & S. R. COOPERBAND. 1966. Protein characteristics of serum and bile alkaline phosphatase. Gastroenterology **50:** 631–636.

POSEN, S. 1967. Alkaline phosphatase. Ann. Intern. Med. **67:** 183–203.

RASMUSSEN, K. 1968. Phosphorylethanolamine and hypophosphatasia. Danish Med. Bull. (Suppl. No. 15.)

ROSENBERG, I. N. 1959. Zone electrophoresic studies of serum alkaline phosphatase. J. Clin. Invest. **38:** 630–644.

SEBESTA, D. G., F. J. BRADSHAW & D. J. PROCKUP. 1964. Source of the elevated serum alkaline phosphatase activity in biliary obstruction. Gastroenterology **47:** 166–170.

DISCUSSION OF THE PAPER

DR. NAUGHETY (*Ohio State University, Columbus, Ohio*): Dr. Keiding, do you in your studies on alkaline phosphatase agree with some opinions put forth by Dr. Posen on the origin of the bile enzyme?

DR. KEIDING: I would hate to go into a discussion on that subject. I can only present some indirect evidence of a physiological type. I would hate to say anything about whether the alkaline phosphatase in the bile is newly synthesized or a modification of preexisting phosphatase.

S. KREITZMAN (*Massachusetts Institute of Technology, Cambridge, Mass.*): I was wondering if you care to comment on the possible role of the saliva as a route of excretion or regulation of the homeostasis for alkaline phosphatase. Do you have any information on that?

DR. KEIDING: Of course we have tried to find out to what extent intestinal phosphatase is secreted from the intestine. Some phosphatase in the intestinal fluid should be of bile origin, but this is not true, because as soon as bile phosphatase (the alpha 1 phosphatase from bile) reaches the intestine, it disappears. This is very simple to illustrate. I don't know anything about saliva.

L. BECKMAN: I should like to comment on one point, namely your results when using many different techniques in supporting media. We had similar problems and, in fact, we have seen alkaline phosphatases that do not separate on the acrylamide slabs, nor on agarose, nor on paper, but only on starch gel, and they separate quite a lot. We have shown that they have no difference in molecular weight and, I believe, no difference in charge under those circumstances, and yet there is a fantastic separation that can be completely abolished if the electrophoresis is conducted at the same pH, but with the addition of EDTA. So I think we have to think a little bit about terminology and identification when speaking about different forms of isozymes. It's rather confusing, and we have so many A's, B's and C's, and I myself have been a sinner in that respect, and I think what you did is very important, i.e., giving reference values and comparing techniques. Do you really believe that there is a correspondence between your fast moving component and the starch component?

DR. KEIDING: That's very easy to show because I separate one ml of serum, cut out the fast component and then run it on starch gel. Of course, the reason I showed this picture was that the alpha 1 phosphatase is a high-molecular-weight phosphatase, and it's very, very easy to prepare your starch gel a little differently and show the molecular sieve function of starch gel. Much of the trouble many people have, and we have, is due to the different rates of molecular sieve function in the different supporting medias.

DR. BECKMAN: Do you see the same molecular sieve function in cyonogam?

DR. KEIDING: Oh yes. It depends on how you prepare it.

DR. BECKMAN: Well, you're dealing with a different enzyme, different from ours.

S. POSEN: I wonder if I could comment on one question raised by the audience about salivery alkaline phosphatase. We have actually studied this quantitatively; there isn't a great deal there. The situation is also complicated by the fact that particularly parotid saliva is fairly rich in inorganic phosphate, and one gets a great deal of increase in activity if one dialyzes. It is no greater in patients with elevated serum phosphatase than it is in normal subjects. Also, we have not had much joy out of correlating the saliva phosphatase with blood groups and with the presence or absence of intestinal alkaline phosphatase in the serum of these individuals. The other thing I might comment on is the disappearance of intestinal alkaline phosphatase from the serum of the rat. We have injected purified rat intestinal alkaline phosphatase into the rat and certainly, there, the half life is very much shorter than what we reported for human placental alkaline phosphatase. In humans, it's fairly close to 30 minutes.

DR. KEIDING: Could you bring yourself to examine the bile at the same time?

DR. POSEN: No, we couldn't do that.

SUMMATION OF THE SESSION ON DEVELOPMENT AND PHYSIOLOGY

Clement L. Markert
Yale University, New Haven, Conn.

In listening to the reports this afternoon and this morning, I tried to discern the general questions that workers on phosphatases or phosphohydrolases have been concerned with, questions and problems that carry general significance beyond the realm of phosphatases. It is clear from the work of many investigators that phosphatases are ubiquitous in vertebrate organisms and present in a great many different kinds of cells as well as in extracellular fluids. One important observation that has emerged from these studies is that phosphatases exist in a variety of different molecular forms, that is, as isozymes. This molecular multiplicity raises several very fundamental questions that can be answered in the near future. First, what is the genetic basis for these isozymic systems? How many genes are involved in coding for the proteins that make up the phosphatase repertory of an organism? Second, and perhaps more important, what are the epigenetic mechanisms that modify the polypeptide chains, once synthesized, in order to generate at least some of the different molecular types that appear to be coded by a single gene. In order to obtain useful, even critical, information on either of these points, it is only necessary to analyze a few milligrams of each of several phosphatase isozymes. Of course, the isozyme must be pure and must be subjected to a comprehensive series of chemical analyses. This can be done today by means of relatively routine, though sometimes tedious, laboratory procedures. When a comprehensive analysis has been completed on an adequate number of the separated molecular forms of phosphatase, we will be able to determine the number of genes involved in synthesizing these different isozymes. We will also be able to identify some of the epigenetic mechanisms that may modify the phosphatase polypeptide chain, as, for example, by the addition of sialic acid residues to the protein. Furthermore, if it is demonstrated that more than one gene encodes the phosphohydrolases–which seems probable in view of the data on many other isozymic systems–then it would be important to examine the linkage relationships of these genes. Such studies might provide some insight into the evolutionary relationships of the genes, and might also be useful in examining the nature of the molecular and chromosomal mechanisms that lead to selective activation of genes during cell differentiation. Are the genes activated or inhibited in packages, or is each gene regulated independently? If in packages, what determines membership in any particular package–metabolic relationships, topographic location on the chromosome, or the time of initial function during development? These are questions of significance for many areas of biology, and continued work on phosphohydrolases is a promising avenue of research that may well lead to exciting answers.

One other topic that was tangentially touched on in the report of Dr. Keiding, one that is extraordinarily significant but that has only been slightly investigated, concerns the biochemical and biological mechanisms by which enzymes are selectively degraded and removed from cells. The numerous changes in the pattern of enzymatic activity in cells during the course of their differentiation is obviously a function both of the synthesis of the enzymes and of their degradation. Both processes are equally important in determining whatever steady state may prevail at any particular stage of differentiation. We now know, in theory at least, most of the events on the synthetic side of this equilibrium, that is, the events of transcription, translation, and, later, the control of the level of activity of the completed enzyme. However, we know almost nothing about the mechanisms involved in the degradation of enzymes. If diminished enzyme activity in cell or tissue involves only the export of the protein from the cell, that is, secretion, then the problem is not so mysterious. But the more significant problem is the differential degradation of enzymes within the cell, an exceedingly important aspect about which we know almost nothing. Are proteins degraded within the cell in accord with their own physical-chemical makeup, or do specific cellular mechanisms recognize and attack specific protein molecules in order to remove them? Such questions may be answered by further studies on the phosphatases.

Finally, we come to the question of the physiological role of the isozymic forms of the phosphohydrolases. This has been the major subject of the last three papers this afternoon. Here our understanding is at a discouragingly low level. Despite the enormous number of facts that have been uncovered to link the synthesis, presence and circulation of the various molecular forms of phosphatases to various states of differentiation and to various hormonal states of the organism, it is still not possible to say anything very concrete about the functions of these different isozymes in the organism. I previously worked on phosphatases myself, but I deserted them because of my inability to identify their physiological roles in the cell. Surely an elucidation of the physiological significance of each of the phosphohydrolases will emerge eventually. It is inconceivable to me that they do not have important roles to play in the structure and function of cells. Whatever may be their physiological roles, we can, without knowing these roles, proceed confidently to an analysis of their physicochemical structure. Such an analysis of structure may even lead to an understanding of function.

PART III. INTRACELLULAR LOCALIZATION

PHOSPHOHYDROLASES IN CELL ORGANELLES; ELECTRON MICROSCOPY*

R. E. Smith†

Veterans Administration Hospital, Palo Alto, Calif., and Department of Pathology, Stanford University, Stanford, Calif.

Today, more than ever before, we are prone to think of vital activity as being chemical. Forty-five years ago, Jones (1924) remarked that "So much modern work has progressed upon purely physical or chemical lines of research that we are, maybe, in some danger of regarding the body as a test tube in which chemical reactions occur." Recently, in an introductory paragraph of a review on lysosomes, Novikoff (1967) stated directly and tersely that, with the *Ciba* Foundation Symposium on Lysosomes in 1963, the biochemical concept became a biological concept. During the past five years, investigation has accelerated remarkably in an effort to affirm and define more precisely the function of lysosomes in physiological and pathological processes. The electron microscope and the lead salt procedure for acid phosphatase staining introduced by Gomori deserve considerable credit for bringing about the realization that structure and chemical reaction cannot be dissociated. With the first electron micrographs of the fine structural localization of acid phosphatase, made by Essner and Novikoff (1961) and Holt and Hicks (1961), a new era of biological investigation began. This is the field of subcellular enzymorphology, which now embraces not only enzymes of hydrolase systems and lysosomes, but also more recently, enzymes of the electron transport system and mitochondria (Seligman *et al.*, 1968). It would be improvident, concerning the limited time, for me to attempt a review of the mass of literature relating only to the fine structural localization of acid phosphatase, much less of that relating phosphohydrolases in general. Such compendious reviews are already available (de Duve, 1959; de Duve & Wattiaux, 1966; Novikoff, 1967; 1961; Straus, 1967). Rather, the value of my presence here would certainly be in recounting the progress in our laboratory toward understanding the effects of sex steroid hormones on acid phosphatase activity in target organ cells, and subsequently, to present our views from these observations in an attempt to extend our thinking in relation to sites of acid hydrolase activity and the organization of lysosomes.

Before we proceed to our experimental observations, let us first consider the cytophysiological factors that underlie any hormonal response. Hormones exert their effects by influencing the speed of existing metabolic processes through enzymatic reactions. The action of sex steroid hormones upon target tissues usually results in increased anabolism, which often is expressed by cell secretion hyperplasia, hypertrophy, or a combination thereof. However, it has become evident that sex steroids may exert their metabolic effects not only by accelerating, but also by inhibiting, enzymatic reactions. Furthermore, the hormones may cause an increase in concentration of a given enzyme in a target tissue, or they may activate existing enzymes by changing the physical state of cellular struc-

* This work was supported by grant E-415 from the American Cancer Society, grant NGR 05-020-177 from the National Aeronautics & Space Administration, and by Syntex Research, Palo Alto, Calif.

† Dernham Fellow, California Division, American Cancer Society.

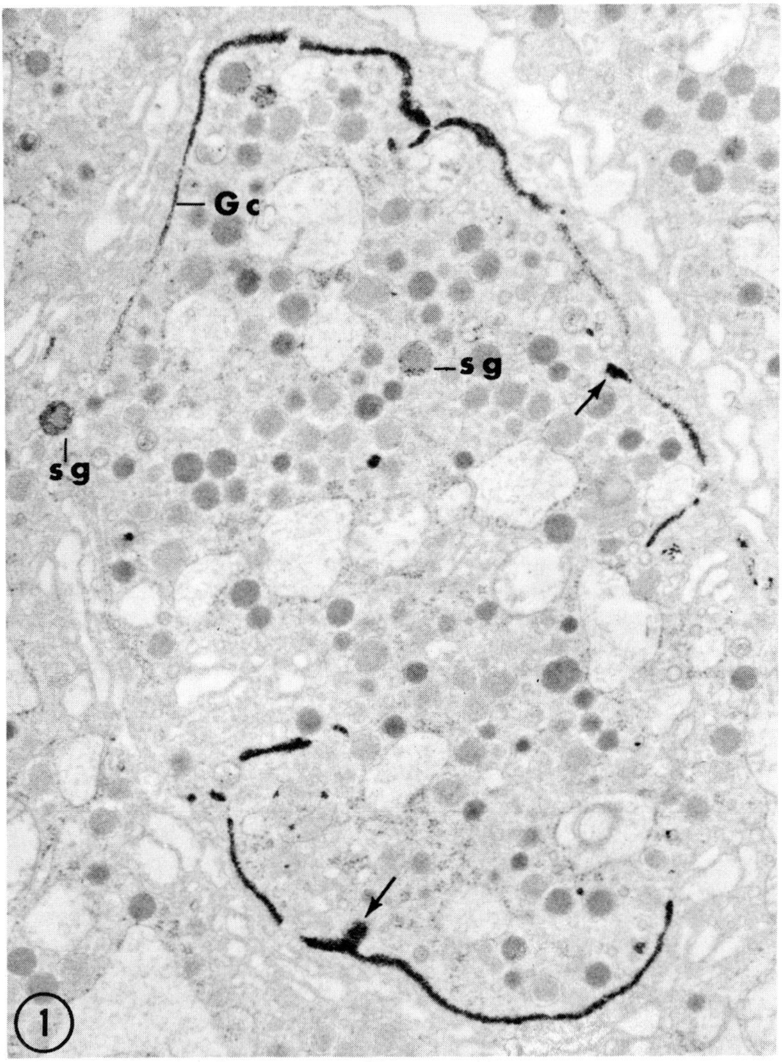

FIGURE 1. Golgi region of a gonadotrophic (GT) cell in the anterior pituitary of an ovariectomized female rat. Preparation incubated 30 minutes in medium for AcPase at 37° C. Note that only the innermost flattened Golgi cisterna is stained (Gc) with the budding of Golgi vesicles (arrows). There is also staining of "free" vesicles and of some secretion granules (sg) within the cytoplasmic core of the Golgi apparatus. Stained with uranyl acetate and lead citrate (×23,000).

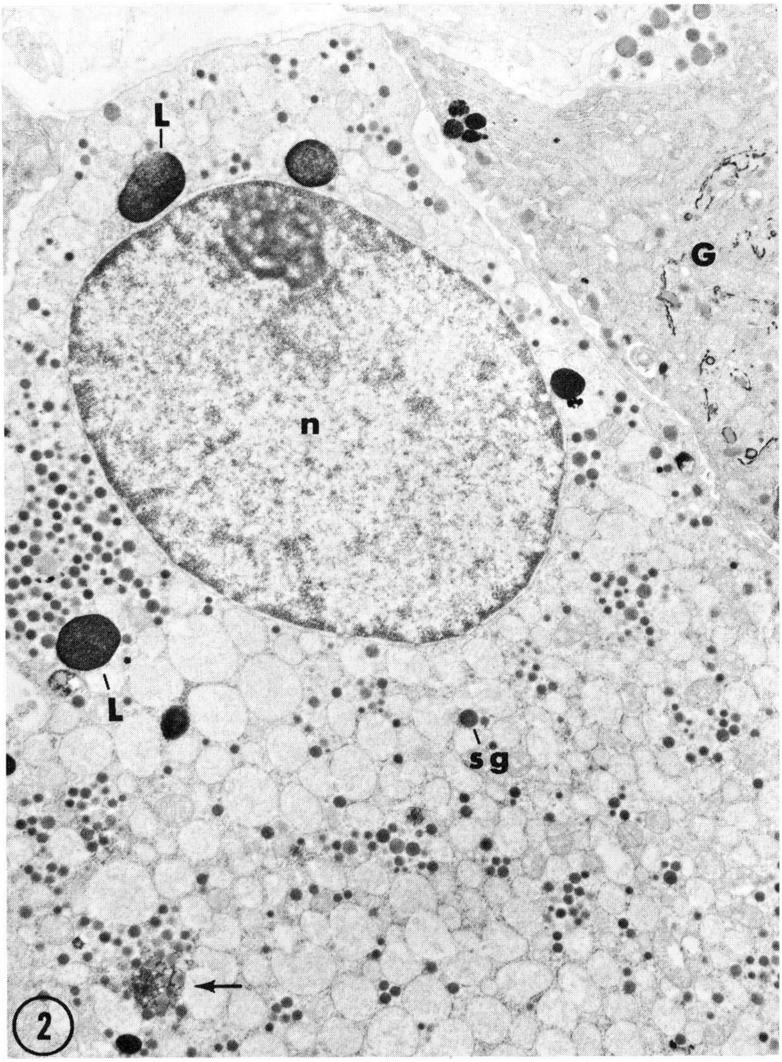

FIGURE 2. Portion of a GT cell showing four dense-body-type lysosomes (L) stained for AcPase. In the upper left is a part of the Golgi complex (G) of a mammotrophic (MT) cell. Preparation from the anterior pituitary of an animal ovariectomized for 20 days and sacrificed after nine additional days of estrogen treatment. Arrow points to a collection of secretion granules staining for enzyme, but not contained within a membrane delimited structure. Staining of section as for FIGURE 1. ($\times$9,000)

tures, for example increasing the permeability of membranes (Weissman, 1965). In the past six years, we have investigated similarities and differences in the effects of estrogens and progestogens in this regard upon the acid hydrolase system in three steroid-dependent tissues, i.e., cells of the anterior pituitary, breast and uterine mucosa.

Anterior Pituitary—Trophic Hormone Synthesis and Degradation

Removal of the gonads from sexually mature mammals results in involution of the uterus and mammary glands and a gradual decrease in the gross weight of these organs. However, gonadectomy usually results in an increase in size and weight of the anterior pituitary. In the rat, this increase has been identified as a result of intensified anabolism, principally in those cells synthesizing and releasing gonadotrophic hormones. Results of early studies for acid phosphatase staining in cells of the anterior pituitary contained some discrepancies (Abolins & Abolins, 1949; Samorajski & Fitz, 1960), which were obviously caused primarily by the emphasis being placed more on the identity of the cell type stained (i.e., acidophils or basophils) than on the functional state of the cells. Furthermore, these investigations were conducted before the biological concept of the lysosome was developed.

Sobel (1961a; 1961b) realized the value of altering the endocrinological state of an animal in order to define more clearly the relation of acid phosphatase activity to cell function. He studied the effects of testosterone and thyroxine treatment, castration and exposure to cold, and observed that states of increased secretory activity were paralleled by an increase of acid phosphatase staining. He found a correlation: that specific cell types of the anterior pituitary of the rat respond to certain stimuli with increased acid phosphatase staining as well as with hormone secretion. For example, castration of the male or female rat resulted in an increase of acid phosphatase staining in those cells which, by morphologic or tinctorial criteria, have been associated with the gonadotrophic hormones (FSH or LH). Whether the increase in enzyme staining was more directly related to hormone synthesis or to hormone release could not be determined at the light microscopic level.

Our first studies extended to the electron microscopic level the staining of acid phosphatase in gonadotrophic (GT) cells after varying periods subsequent to castration. It was observed that, for a short period of time, stimulated trophic cells rapidly formed secretion granules, this activity being paralleled by an intense localization of acid phosphatase staining in elements of the Golgi apparatus (FIGURE 1). After a period, following castration, of about two weeks, morphological observations indicated a slowing of secretion granule formation, and there was a diminishing of acid phosphatase staining within the Golgi. With increased vesiculation of castration cells, we observed a translocalization of enzyme staining from the Golgi to randomly distributed lysosomes (FIGURE 2). Signet-ring castration cells showed virtually no evidence of secretion granule formation or acid phosphatase staining within the Golgi complex, while lysosomes could be seen as intensely staining dense bodies in the peripheral band of cytoplasm. It is generally considered that these hypertrophic cells release hormone; whether the hormone is in the form of secretion granules or is the result of some other mechanism has not been established. From our study of castration cells, a point of uncertainty was clarified: that acid phosphatase activity related to cell secretion is morphologically associated with secretion granule formation and not with secretion, granule release or other processes. In addition, we observed that

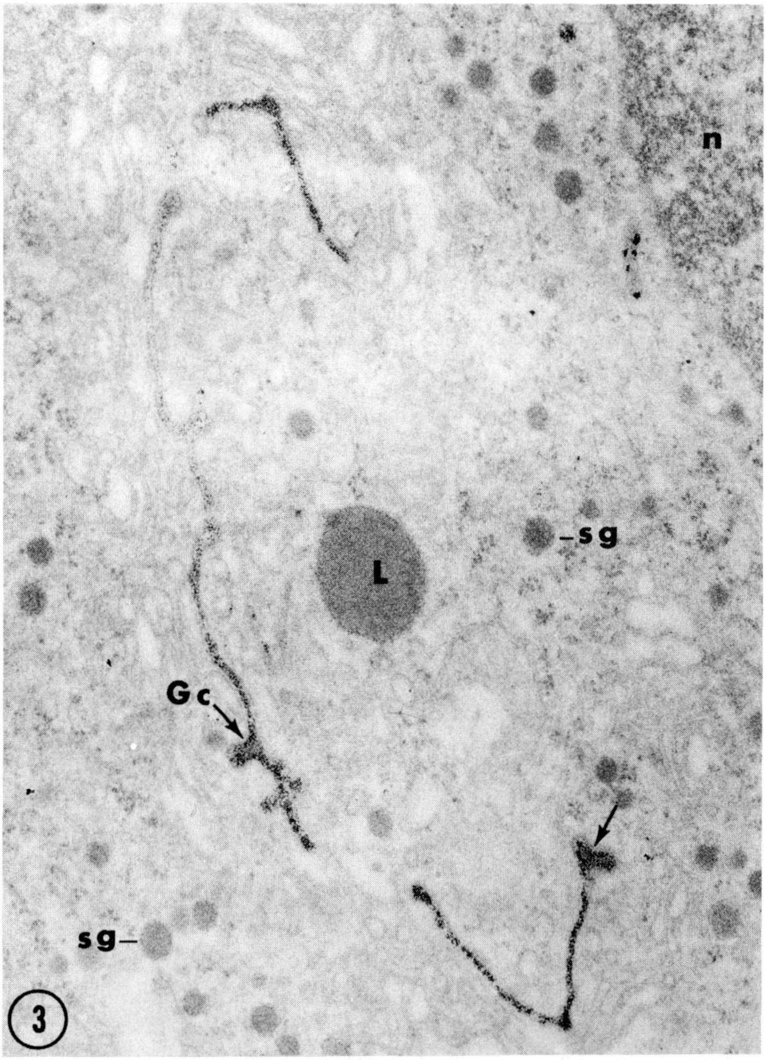

FIGURE 3. Golgi region of a thyrotrophic (TT) cell from the anterior pituitary of a control female rat. Once again, only the innermost flattened Golgi cisterna (Gc) is stained for AcPase. Localization of reaction product is also found around hormone condensing into secretion granules (arrows) within the innermost Golgi cisterna. (×25,000)

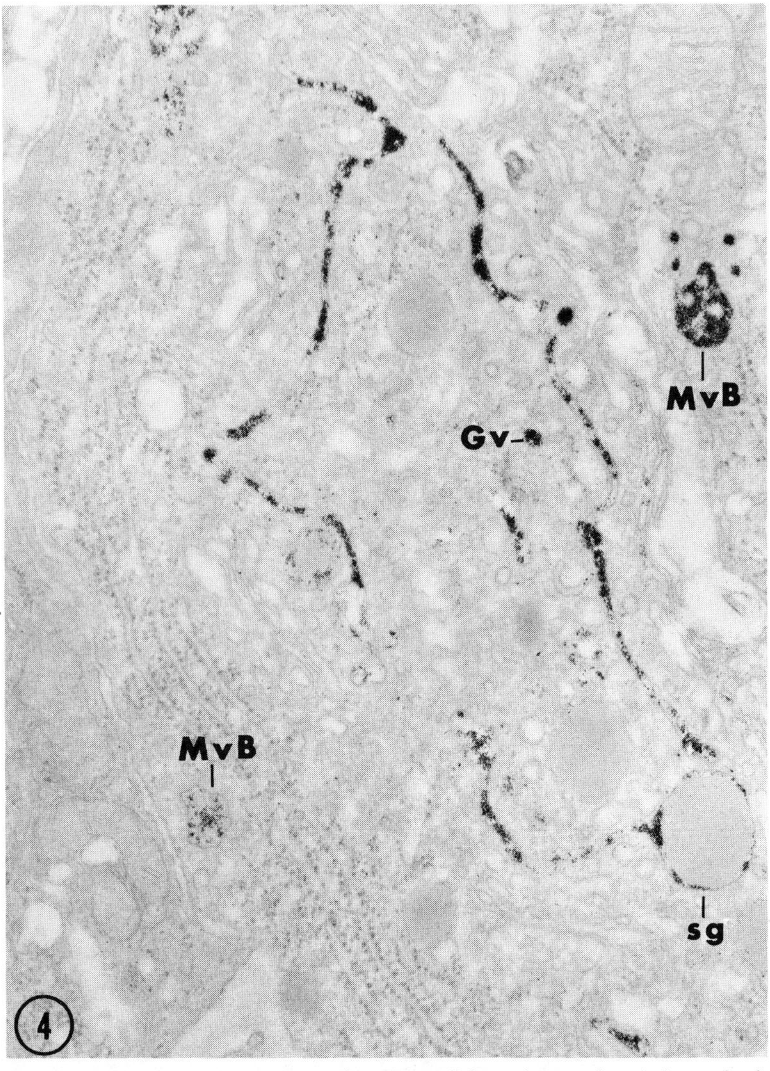

FIGURE 4. Golgi region of a somatotrophic (ST) cell from the anterior pituitary of a female rat. AcPase staining is not confined to, but is most intense within, the innermost Golgi cisterna. A forming secretion granule (sg), located in the labeled Golgi cisterna, is rimmed by reaction product. There is also staining of Golgi vesicles (Gv) and multivesicular bodies (MvB). (×35,000)

an interrelationship exists between the formation of secretion granules, acid phosphatase activity in elements of the Golgi, and the origin of lysosomes. Subsequent study of thyroidectomy cells provided essentially the same information (FIGURE 3). However, these studies did not provide clear-cut information regarding the function of lysosomes. This lack may be due to the fact that castration and thyroidectomy are experimental conditions initiating hypersynthesis and hypersecretion of hormones, whereas lysosomal function is related to cellular autophagy, i.e., to catabolic, not to anabolic, processes (cf. Novikoff *et al.*, 1964).

Studies of enzymatic action in the anterior pituitary of the control rat, in which the parenchymal cells are in various stages of functional activity, suggested that lysosomes, observed in a variety of forms, may be involved with secretion granules in some metabolic process other than their formation. In an attempt to define more clearly the relationship of lysosomes to changes in secretory activity, Dr. Marilyn Farquhar and I carried out a comprehensive physiologic study of the functional activity of those cells to which is ascribed the secretion of the lactogenic or mammotrophic hormone (Smith & Farquhar, 1966). We reasoned that the study of mammotrophic (MT) cells—so termed because of their response to suckling of the mammary gland—from the pituitary of lactating and postlactating rats would offer conditions where enzymorphologic activities could be evaluated with respect to physiologically normal events rather than to those that were the result of experimental alteration. The electron microscope reveals in MT cells large (600 to 900 mm), often elliptically-shaped, secretion granules. In the gland of the lactating animal, the majority of MT cells present a cytologic picture indicative of a cell actively synthesizing and releasing a secretory product. These cells are large, and contain numerous peripheral arrays of rough-surfaced endoplasmic reticulum and an enlarged Golgi complex consisting of five to eight stacks of concentrically arranged cisternae. The cytoplasmic core of the Golgi contains condensing secretory images of various sizes and shapes. The cells contain few large, mature secretion granules. Acid phosphatase (AcPase) staining is essentially limited to the innermost cisterna and to structures within the Golgi arsenal (FIGURE 5). The condensing of secretory material into aggregating granules takes place within the innermost cisterna only. The matured granule resulting from this aggregation is delimited by a membrane from the Golgi cisternae (cf. Bainton & Farquhar, 1966; Beams & Kessel, 1968). A morphological propinquity therefore exists between condensation of secretory material and localization of AcPase reaction product within the innermost Golgi cisterna (FIGURE 6). The rimming of secretion granules by enzyme staining is a reflection of this interrelationship, the possible significance of which will be discussed later. Let it suffice here to state that the same relationship exists within all secretory cell types of the anterior pituitary and in the secretory cells of many other glandular structures (Behnke & Moe, 1964; Holtzman & Dominitz, 1968; Hopkins & Baker, 1968; Novikoff & Essner, 1962; Osinchak, 1964). The staining of the innermost Golgi cisterna only for AcPase in cells of the anterior pituitary is independent of incubation time, i.e., an increase from 20 minutes to 2 hours, in the time that tissue sections are in substrate does not result in an increase in the number of cisternae stained.

Lysosomes were found to originate only after the development of an enlarged Golgi complex with intense AcPase staining of the innermost Golgi cisterna. Although the mechanism of lysosome formation is not established, some facts about lysosome origin seem to be clear. Novikoff (1963) suggested that small vesicles arising from Golgi saccules or cisternae are the "pure lysosomes" and

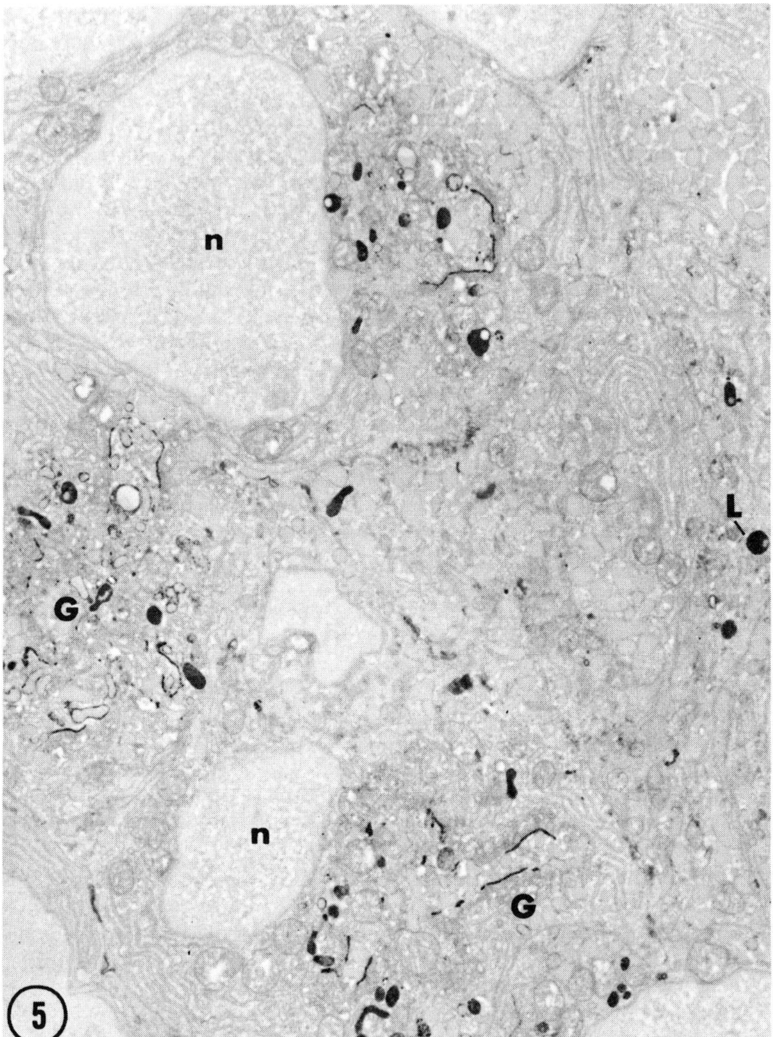

FIGURE 5. An electron micrograph showing the Golgi region (G) of several MT cells (preparation histochemically stained for AcPase) from the anterior pituitary of an animal suckling young for five days. Staining of section as for FIGURE 1. (×7,000)

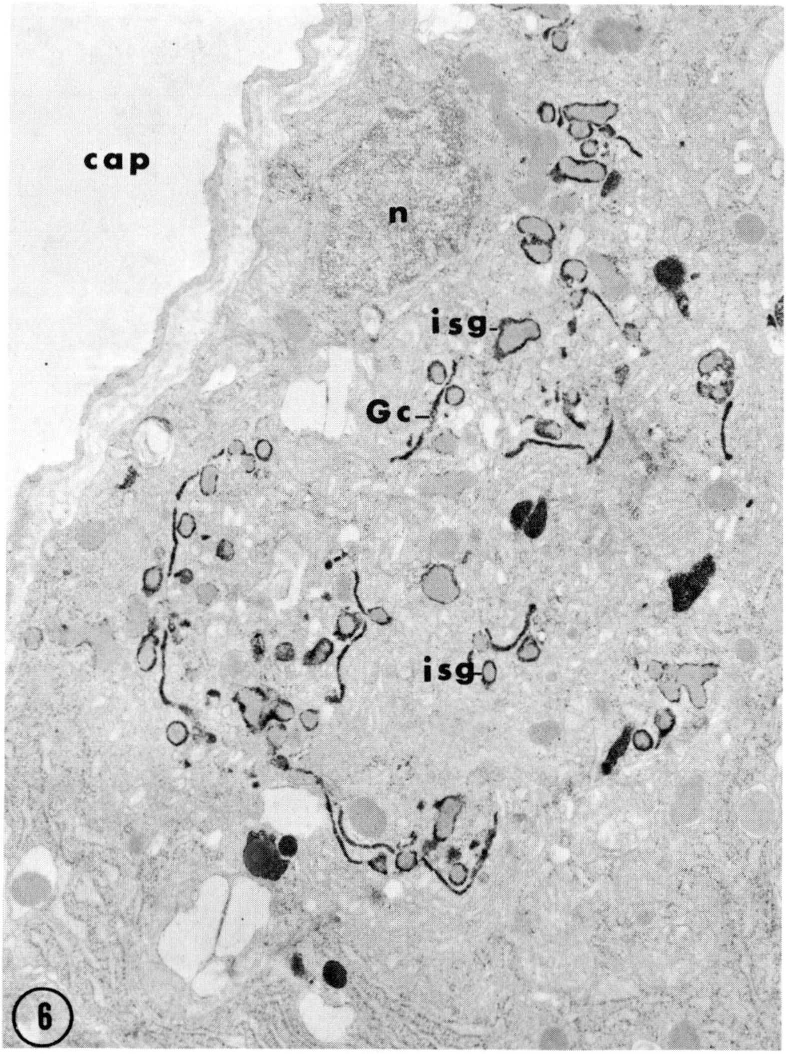

FIGURE 6. Golgi region of a MT cell from the anterior pituitary of a five-day lactating rat. AcPase staining of immature secretion granules (isg) and innermost layer of Golgi cisternae (Gc). Lumen of capillary (cap). (×20,000)

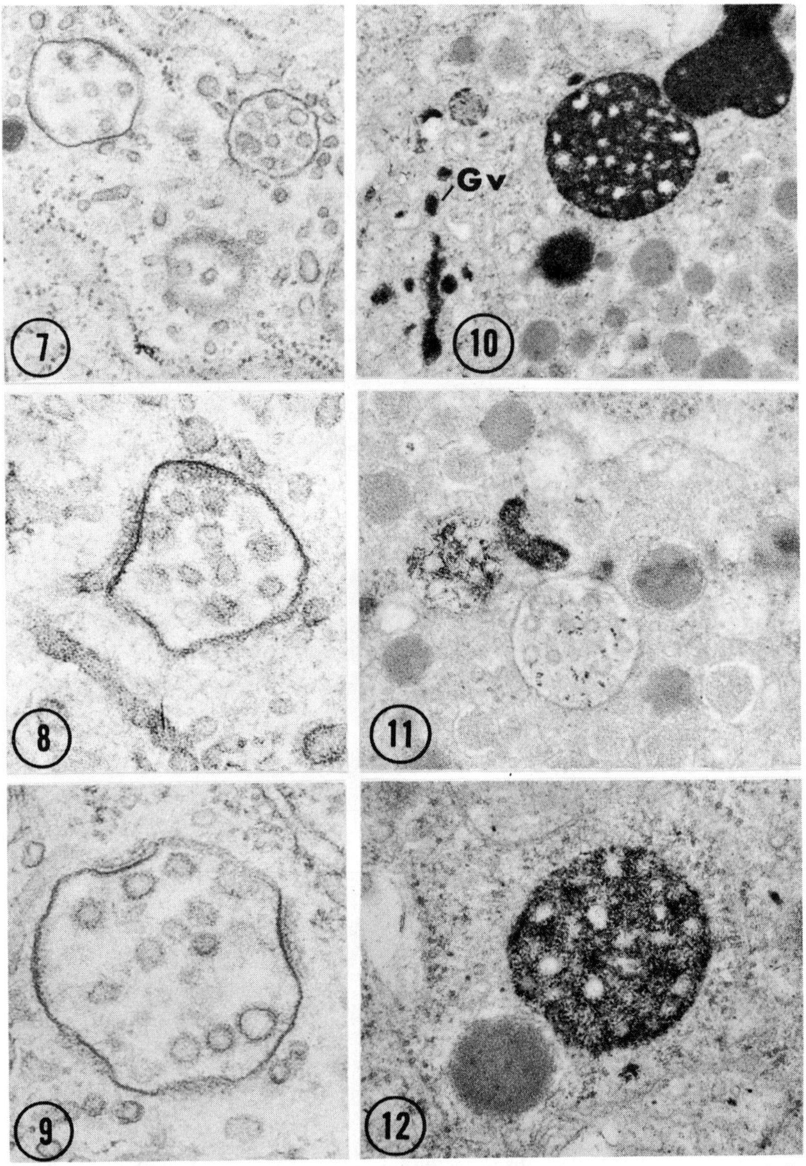

FIGURES 7-9. Various structural forms of multivesicular bodies found in cells of the rat anterior pituitary. (7) ×48,000; (8) ×71,000; (9) ×76,000.

FIGURES 10-12. AcPase staining of Golgi vesicles (Gv) and multivesicular bodies in cells of the rat anterior pituitary. (10) GT cell, ×31,000; (11) TT cell, ×46,000; (12) MT cell, ×40,000.

the principal entities of the structures defined as dense bodies. Numerous independent investigators have demonstrated that this is the case in a variety of cells, and not a biological phenomenon limited only to cells of mammalian or even vertebrate tissue (Brandes *et al.,* 1964; Elliott, 1965). Early in our studies (Smith 1963) we observed in the anterior pituitary of the rat that AcPase-staining vesicles do arise from the Golgi, and that they appear to originate by a "budding off" process that is limited to the innermost cisterna of the Golgi (FIGURES 1–6). More recently, it has been suggested that enzyme-staining vesicles may, under certain conditions, also arise from the endoplasmic reticulum (Elliott, 1965; Goldfischer *et al.,* 1963; Novikoff, 1967). To date, we have not observed this in any cell type of the anterior pituitary. How Golgi vesicles containing AcPase and, presumably, other acid hydrolases, contribute to the formation of dense bodies remains an enigma. There is evidence in a variety of cells (Brandes, 1966; Daems, 1962; Friederici; 1967; Gordon *et al.,* 1965; Lane, 1968; Maunsbach, 1966) that multivesicular bodies change into dense bodies, and that the vesicles that multivesicular bodies contain are of Golgi derivation. Such information has led several investigators to suggest that multivesicular bodies in their various forms are sequential structures in the development of dense-body lysosomes (Friend & Farquhar, 1967; Lane, 1968; Holtzman & Dominitz, 1968). In our studies of MT cells, we have found that after removal of the suckling young, multivesicular bodies were always more prominent before the appearance of dense bodies. The localization of the product of AcPase reaction might be expected within the vesicles of the multivesicular body by virtue of their presumed Golgi origin. However, our findings (Smith & Farquhar, 1966), and those of others (Friend & Farquhar, 1967; Holtzman & Dominitz, 1968; Lane, 1968), the deposition of reaction product to be commonly within the matrix (FIGURES 10 through 15). To conclude we can state with reasonable confidence that, in cells of the anterior pituitary, the principal pathway of lysosome origin is via elements of the Golgi complex.

Lysosomes were found to be dramatically involved in the regulation of the secretory process in cells of the anterior pituitary in rats. MT cells from postlactating animals, sacrificed at selected intervals up to 96 hours after removal of suckling young, showed, with progressive involution of their synthetic apparatus, an incorporation of secretion granules into lysosomes (FIGURE 25). This was followed by a sequence of morphological events that suggested that secretion granules taken up by multivesicular or dense bodies were degraded, resulting in the formation of residual bodies in accordance with the functional classification of lysosomes by deDuve and Wattiaux (1966). In our observations, we have also identified the process of degradation of secretion granules in somatotrophic (ST) cells and in gonadotrophic (GT) cells (FIGURES 22–24); however, after removal of their respective stimuli, the process in the growth-hormone-producing cells seems to differ in some degree and to be more rapid than in MT cells (FIGURES 19 through 21). Thus, within at least four of the distinct morphologically functional cell types in the anterior pituitary of the rat, the principal pathway of secretion granule degradation under reasonably normal conditions appears to be through dense-body-type lysosomes. However, this is not necessarily the only route of granule degradation. It should be emphasized that, concurrent with secretion granule degradation, there is generally cell regression with the formation of autophagic bodies, which sequester cell organelles. We have also observed that secretion granules are included within these lytic structures. The study of MT cells in progressive intervals of regression related

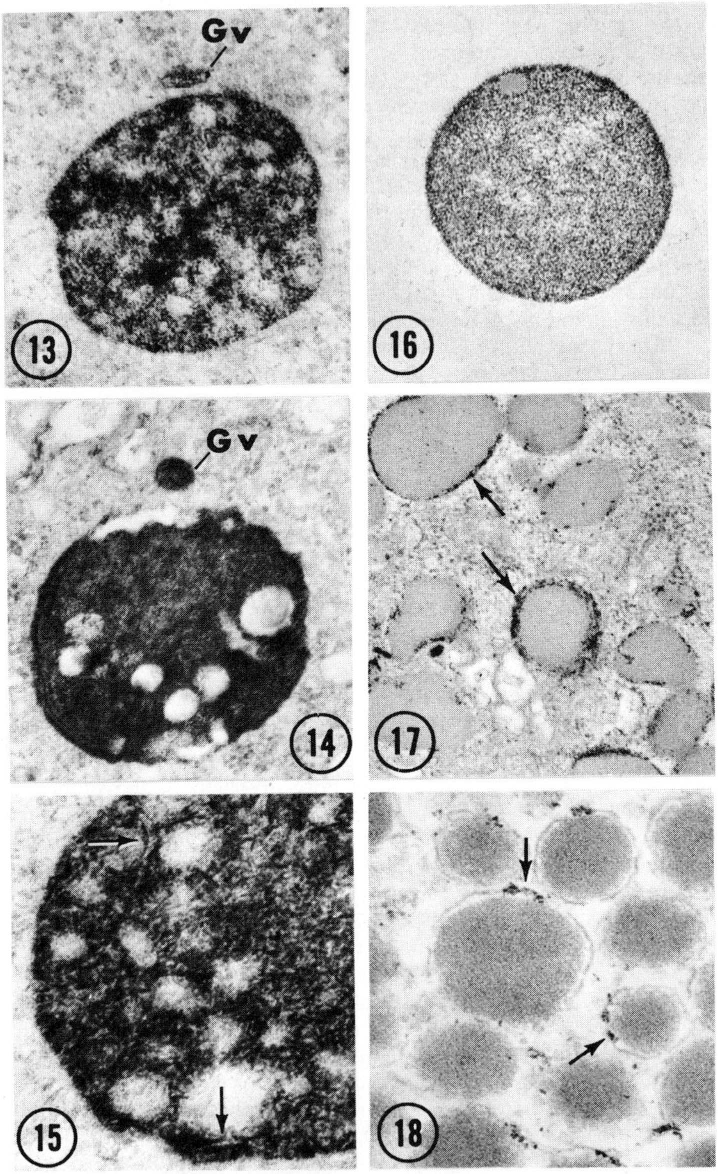

FIGURE 13. AcPase staining of Golgi vesicle (Gv) and multivesicular body in epithelial cell of the endometrium from an ovariectomized rabbit stimulated by estrogen treatment, ×60,000.

FIGURE 14. AcPase staining of Golgi vesicle (Gv) and multivesicular body in epithelial cell of mouse mammary gland 12 hours after removal of suckling young. Arrow points to an area where reaction product is deposited in a concentric layered arrangement. (×50,000)

FIGURE 15. Portion of a multivesicular body stained for AcPase in epithelial cell of human

TABLE 1

RELATIVE DETERMINATION OF DEGREE OF ORGANELLE DEVELOPMENT IN MAMMOTROPHIC CELLS OF THE RAT ANTERIOR PITUITARY

	Anabolic				Catabolic			
		Golgi			Lytic Structures			
Intervals	Endo-plasmic Reticulum	Cisterna	Vesicles	MV Bodies	Dense Bodies	Vacuoiate Dense Bodies	Myelin Figures	Free Lipid Inclusions
5 Days Lact.	xxxxx	xxxxx	xxx	x	x	x	x	0
12 Hrs Post Lact.	xxxxx	xxxxx	xxxx	xx	x	x	x	0
24 Hrs Post Lact.	xxxx	xxxx	xxxxx	xxxx	xx	x	x	0
48 Hrs Post Lact.	xxx	xxx	xxxx	xxx	xxxx	xx	xxx	xx
72 Hrs Post Lact.	xx	xx	xxx	x	xxxx	xxxxx	xxxx	xxx
96 Hrs Post Lact.	x	x	0	x	xx	xxx	xxx	xxxx

to a sequence of normal physiologic events established the principle that lysosomes represent the protein-degrading apparatus for the overproduction of secretory product by an anterior pituitary cell (see also TABLE 1).

Although substantial progress was made in defining and clarifying the role of acid hydrolases in secretory regulation, the reason why certain sites stained for AcPase remained obscure. Most interesting to us were the reasons why a random few mature secretion granules stained for enzyme (Hopkins & Baker, 1968: FIGURE 3) Novikoff and Essner (1962) had observed a similar staining pattern of secretion granules in alpha cells of pancreatic islands in rats. This pattern is characterized by an intense rimming of early (immature) secretion granules by AcPase reaction product, with the apparent dilution or loss of enzyme activity as granules mature. These authors suggested that lysosomal hydrolases may be involved in the condensation of secretory material, "and that the granule membrane plays a metabolic role in the process." Our observations led us to the same conclusion (Smith & Farquhar, 1966), which was altered as reported in a later communication (Smith, 1967). As for the origin of secretion-granule AcPase, Novikoff and Essner (1962) suggested that lysosomes (presumably meaning

secretory endometrium. Arrows point to reaction product as though on membrane of vesicles. (×100,000)

FIGURE 16. Dense-body-style lysosome characteristic in structure and staining to those found in cells of the anterior pituitary, mammary gland and endometrium. Note more intense localization of reaction product around limiting membrane. Preparation from rabbit uterus, no staining of thin section with uranyl or lead. (×56,000)

FIGURE 17. AcPase reaction product rimming mature secretion granules (arrows) in MT cell in the anterior pituitary of an ovariectomized rat; MT cells stimulated to form secretion granules by exogenous estrogen and progesterone. (×30,000)

FIGURE 18. Secretion granule membrane staining for AcPase. Specimen preparation after osmium fixation of 40-micra-thick section was dehydration through warm (35° C) graded ethanols; this shrinks the granule content more than is usual in dehydration and makes the granule membrane discernible. Remaining reaction product appears on secretion granule membrane only. (×50,000)

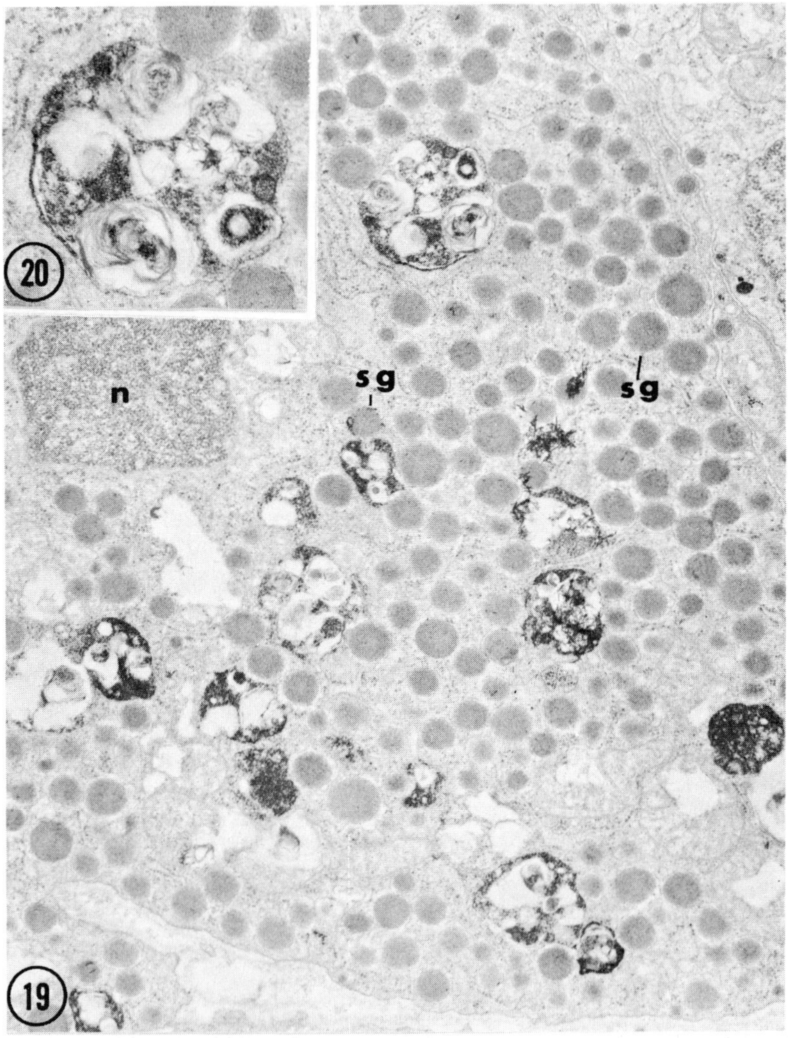

FIGURE 19. Portion of a somatotrophic (ST) cell from a male rat thyroidectomized for four days. AcPase staining of lysosomal structures and secretion granules (sg). It appears that these lysosomal structures are formed by the coalescence of secretion granules and their membranes, forming the limiting membrane of the lysosomal structure. In the anterior pituitary of the thyroidectomized rat, there is rapid degranulation of ST cells, apparently by a process not dependent upon secretion granules being taken up by dense-body-type lysosomes. (×17,000)

FIGURE 20. Enlargement of AcPase-stained lysosome of ST cell from FIGURE 19. (×35,000)

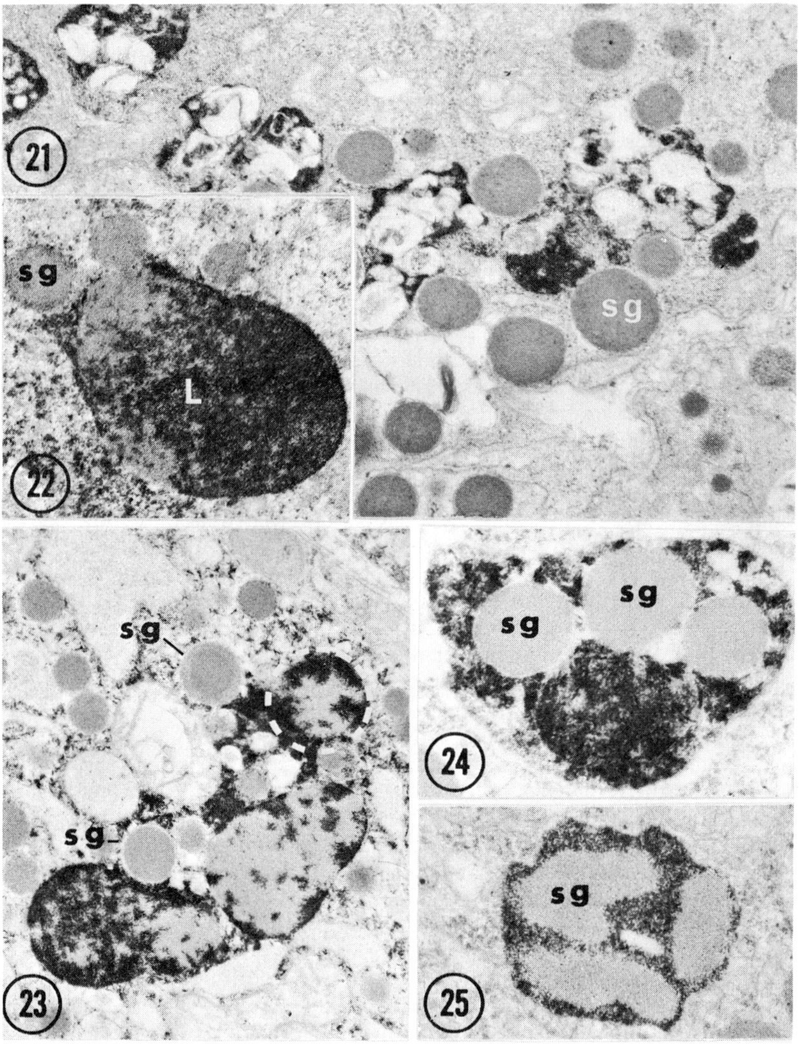

FIGURE 21. AcPase staining and probable secretion-granule degradation. From the anterior pituitary of a starved male rat. (×24,000)

FIGURE 22. AcPase staining of lysosomal structure with secretion granule uptake in a GT cell. Note apparent diffusion of enzyme and/or reaction product. From the anterior pituitary of a rat ovariectomized for 15 days and given a single injection of progesterone one day before the animal was sacrificed. (×38,000)

FIGURE 23. AcPase staining of lysosomal structure in GT cell of a rat ovariectomized for 15 days and given estrogen for nine days before sacrifice. Lysosome may be formed by the coalescence of secretion granules (circle) rather than by the uptake of secretion granules by dense-body-type lysosome. (×25,000)

FIGURE 24. AcPase staining of lysosome containing three GT cell secretion granules. From the anterior pituitary of a control female rat. (×45,000)

FIGURE 25. AcPase staining of lysosome containing three MT cell secretion granules. From the anterior pituitary of a five-day lactating female from which suckling young had been removed for two days before sacrifice. (×42,000)

Golgi vesicles) must empty into secretion granules as the latter are being formed. Our studies of secretion granule formation in four cell types of the anterior pituitary suggest a different means of enzyme acquisition other than the means proposed by Novikoff and Essner (FIGURES 1 through 6).

MT cells, like ST cells, are unique in that they do not participate in the usual endocrine feedback system. As the suckling stimulus from the mammary gland accelerates rather than inhibits mammotrophin secretion, so does exogenous estrogen, and probably progesterone (Greep, 1961)

To understand more fully the hormone-enzyme mechanism in the regulation of the secretory process, and the significance of AcPase staining of "free" mature secretion granules, we studied MT cells in the anterior pituitary of ovariectomized rats. The MT cells were subjected to various levels of exogenous estrogen, combinations of estrogen and progesterone, and estrogen followed at varying time intervals by progesterone (FIGURE 44). In the animal treated with estrogen only, MT cells present a secretory pattern of hormone synthesis and condensation into secretion granules much like that observed in cells of the lactating animal (Smith & Farquhar, 1966). However, in estrogen-stimulated MT cells, there are generally more immature secretion granules–i.e., granules in the process of formation–and numerous mature secretion granules. Nearly all of the condensing images within the innermost Golgi cisterna, and immature secretion granules within the cytoplasmic core of the Golgi, are rimmed by AcPase reaction product. There is a staining also of some mature secretion granules, the number in most cells not appearing significantly different from that found in MT cells of an animal sacrificed 12 to 24 hours after lactation ceases. Regardless of the dosage or length of time that estrogen was administered, AcPase staining was rarely observed in more than the innermost Golgi cisterna.

The evidence that led us to conclude that dense-body-type lysosomes have their principal origin through the activation of multivesicular bodies by Golgi vesicles is accentuated in estrogen-stimulated MT cells. Although more vesicles may not be formed, there is, at least, enzyme staining of many more. The clear increase in the number of multivesicular bodies observed appears to be related to the level and duration of estrogen treatment. The bodies vary in shape, number of vesicles contained, density of matrix, and intensity of enzyme staining; however, their sizes are much the same, 400 to 500 mμ in diameter (FIGURES 7 through 9). We observed that dense bodies, staining with a strong uniform intensity, became progressively more numerous from six hours to six days after the last injection of estrogen. The presence of dense-body lysosomes containing a secretion granule, of multivesicular bodies with secretory material, or of autophagic vacuoles was rare, even six days after the withdrawal of estrogen only. Yet, even as late as six days after estrogen withdrawal, Golgi elements of numerous MT cells stained intensely for AcPase. If progesterone was given in combination with estrogen on the last day before withdrawal, or as a single injection at varying intervals after the last administration of estrogen, the cytological picture of MT cells was considerably different from that when estrogen only was given. Lysosomal structures (with attention to secretion granule degradation) became common, and their appearance was synchronous with progesterone withdrawal. Regardless of the time that a single 10-mg aqueous injection of progesterone was given, the events of secretion granule degradation could be correlated to time intervals between progesterone injection and sacrifice. Any time lapse between the administration of estrogen and progesterone did not significantly alter the pattern, except, perhaps, to intensify it. In animals sacrificed

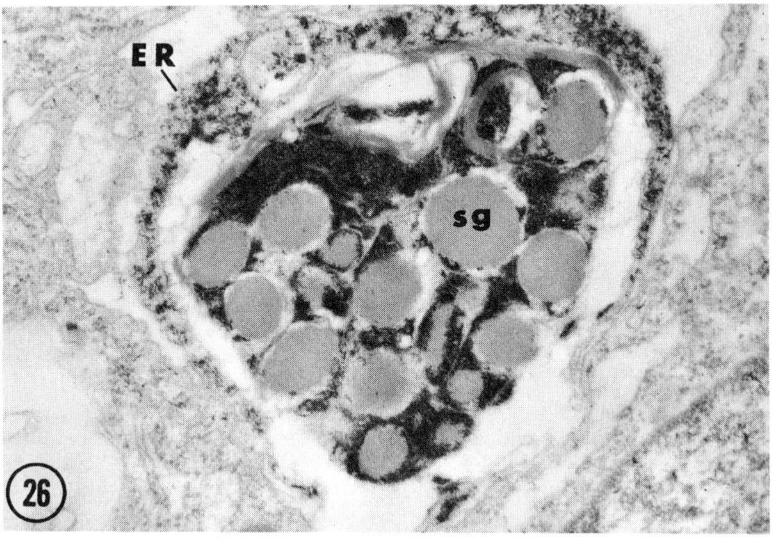

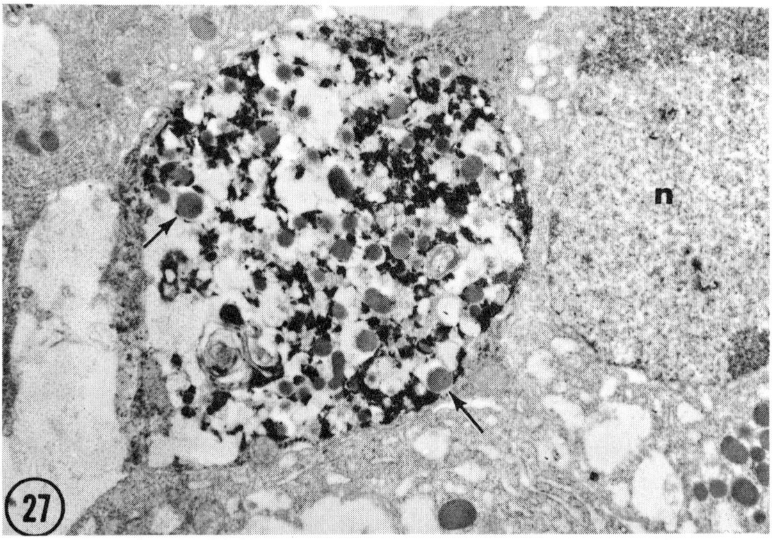

FIGURE 26. An autophagic body in an MT cell of an animal ovariectomized, given estrogen and progesterone, and sacrificed 48 hours after last hormone injection. The lysosomal structure contains several secretion granules (sg), AcPase reaction product, and parallel membranous arrays, delimited from the cytoplasm by a distention of the endoplasmic reticulum (ER), which also contains reaction product. Size of the structure, about 1.5 μ. ($\times$33,000)

FIGURE 27. An autophagic body in a MT cell from an ovariectomized animal given estrogen and then progesterone 48 hours after the last injection of estrogen, and subsequently sacrificed 48 hours after the single injection of progesterone (see TABLE 1). Numerous secretion granules (arrows), AcPase reaction product, and membranous material, a product of granule degradation, are the only contents. It is a large structure about 5 μ in diameter. ($\times$10,000)

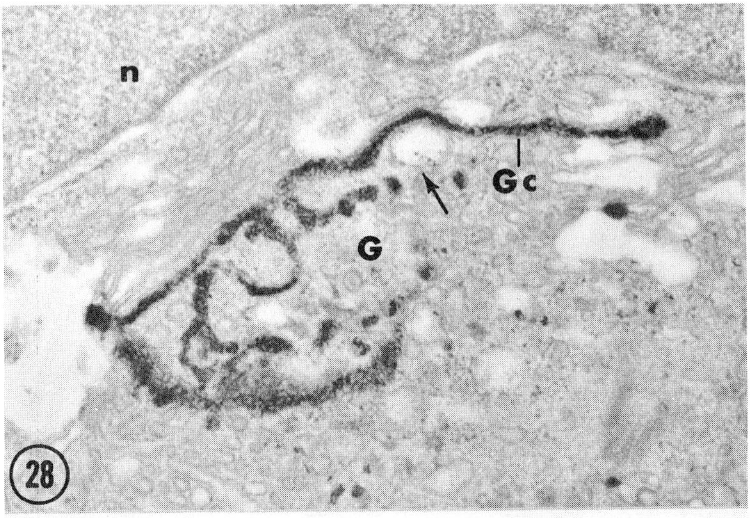

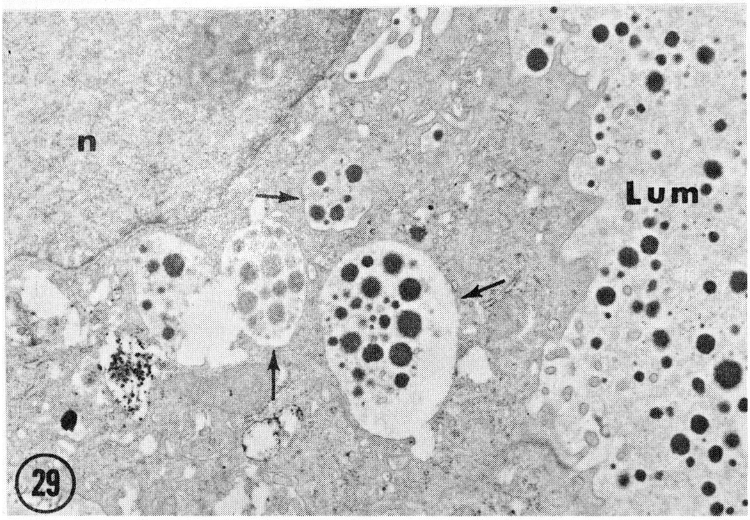

FIGURE 28. Golgi region (G) of a mammary gland epithelial cell stained for AcPase. Tissue from a Balb/C mouse where the breast was sucked for five days, the young removed and the animal sacrificed 24 hours later. (×33,000)

FIGURE 29. Portion of an alveolar epithelial cell two days after initiation of mammary gland involution. Vacuoles within the cell contain milk-protein droplets. Protein droplets are numerous in the lumen (Lum). (×11,000)

24-hours after injection of progesterone, the predominant number of MT cells showed a cytological picture also exemplified in the pituitary of the rat from which suckling young had been removed for one day. The cytological picture 48 hours after withdrawal of progesterone was reminiscent of that 48 hours after lactation ceased, but with the presence of many more lysosomal structures. Observations were made during the following sequence: administration of estrogen; a lapse of 48 hours; administration of progesterone; another lapse of 48 hours; sacrifice. Under these conditions, the lytic events were more closely parallel to those observed 48 hours after lactation ceased. Three to six days after the withdrawal of progesterone, the events of hormone degradation in MT cells can be defined only as massive (FIGURES 26 and 27).

One aspect of the hormone replacement and withdrawal study was the dramatically clear observation of the increased number of mature secretion granules staining for AcPase after progesterone administration (FIGURES 17 and 18). Efforts to establish the significance of this observation have consequently altered our thinking regarding (1) the degradation of overproduced secretory material and (2) the validity of accepting generally recognized sites of enzyme location (not reaction product localization) and the reorganization into residual bodies of dense-body lysosomal structures composed of Golgi vesicles.

There are differences of opinion about whether or not fractions of anterior pituitary secretion granules assay significantly for AcPase (Perdue & McShan, 1962; Schreiber & Lojda, 1967). Our results for assay of secretion granules from MT cells of the anterior pituitary suggest that they do (McDonald *et al.*, 1968). The cytochemical staining of MT secretion-granule fractions has demonstrated that AcPase reaction product localizes around most granules and is applied more closely to the granule membrane than was observed of granules within the cell. This suggested to us that the enzyme may actually be a component of the membrane rather than of the granule content. With regard to progesterone, the hormone probably does not act to promote the movement of enzyme to existing mature secretion granules; it seems more likely that progesterone affects the membrane either to make more sites accessible to substrate for staining of enzyme, or to make more sites accessible to activation of enzyme (Weissman, 1965). Using tissue sections to examine these ideas, we made certain elementary, controlled revisions in the processing of sections 40 μ thick after enzyme staining. The revised processes either shrank or extracted secretion granule content without appreciable damage to granule membranes. Some sections were dehydrated through warm (35° C) graded ethanols or through acetone (24° C) rather than ethanols. Other sections were previously treated with graded percents of trichloroacetic acid (Barrnett *et al.*, 1961). With the shrinkage or extraction of secretion granules, the remaining reaction product for AcPase was deposited on the granule membrane (FIGURE 18).

Interesting lysosomal structures, commonly observed three to six days after progesterone withdrawal, but not identified in physiological conditions of postlactation, are structures apparently formed by the coalescing of varying numbers of secretion granules which are usually segregated by a limiting membrane (FIGURE 26). The structures vary in size, and may become as large in mass as the nucleus (FIGURE 27). They contain only secretion granules, heavy deposits of AcPase reaction product and membranous residue. We have found no enzymorphological evidence to suggest that Golgi vesicles contribute AcPase to these lytic structures, as is frequently observed with autophagic vacuoles in the sequestering of cell organelles. This is not to say that enzyme-containing vesicles cannot contribute;

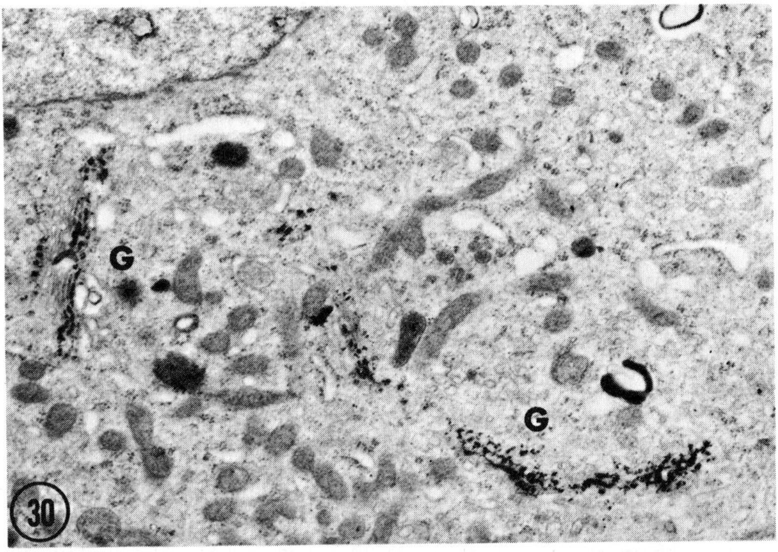

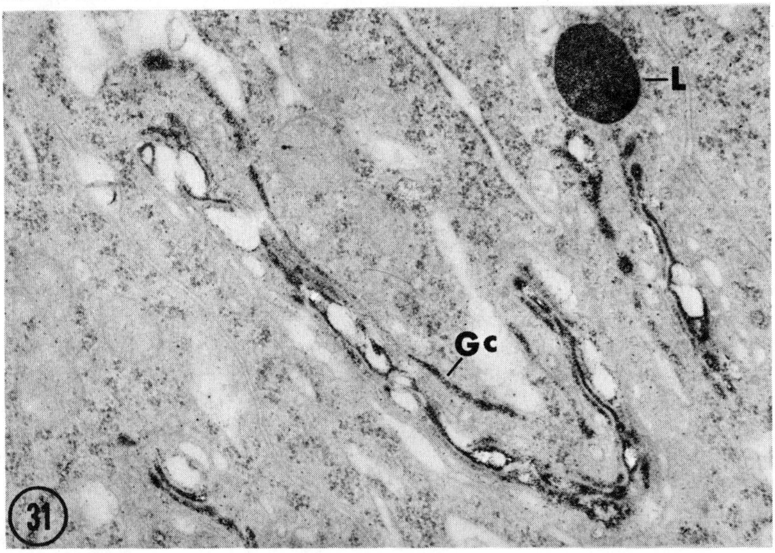

FIGURE 30. Portion of an epithelial cell of the endometrium from a castrate rabbit treated for five days with 1 μg/kg estradiol each day. AcPase staining of three parallel layers of Golgi cisternae. (×12,000)

FIGURE 31. Golgi complex of epithelial cells of castrate rabbit endometrium. Animal treated with estradiol and chlormadinone acetate (see FIGURE 45, group 3) and sacrificed 12 hours after both hormones were withdrawn. AcPase staining of Golgi cisternae (Gc) and lysosome (L). (×27,000)

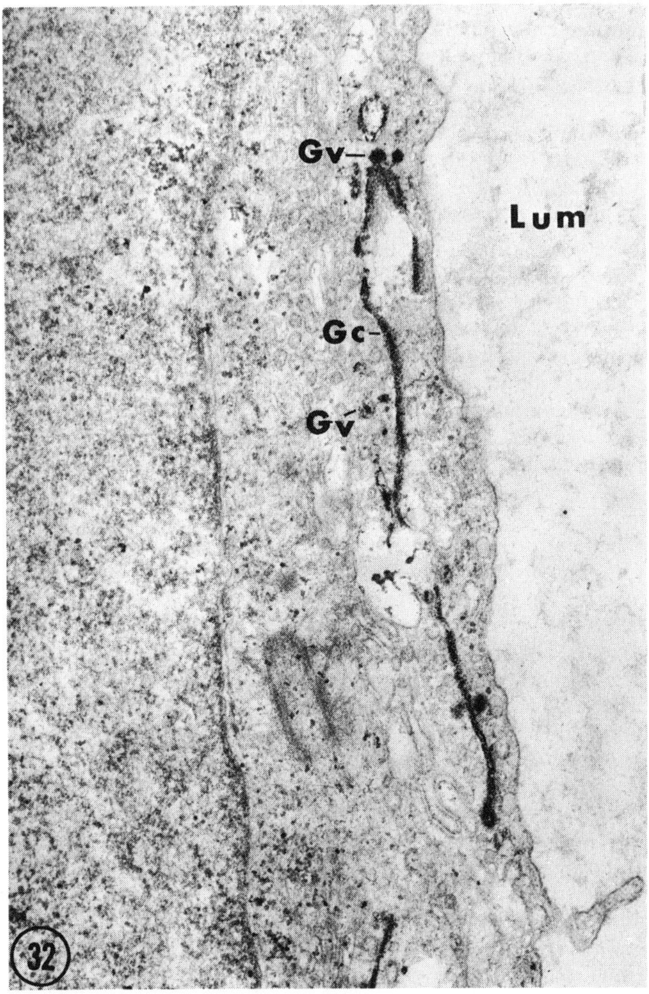

FIGURE 32. Golgi region in an endothelial cell of a small arteriole, in the endometrium of a castrate rabbit. The animal was treated with estradiol and chlormadinone acetate (FIGURE 45, group 3) and sacrificed 12 hours after withdrawal. AcPase staining of one layer of Golgi cisternae (Gc) and several Golgi vesicles (Gv). Lumen of arteriole (Lum). (×37,000)

it simply seems more likely that the enzyme used in the degradation of these secretion granules is contributed by the limiting membrane of the structure and by membranes of the secretion granules it contains.

In conclusion, after observing the effects of hormone replacement and withdrawal on MT cells, we would restate our opinion as follows: the rimming of forming secretion granules with reaction product during condensation of secretory material within the innermost Golgi cisterna is the rule, not the exception; and the incorporation of a secretion granule into a dense-body-type lysosome for degradation may not always be necessary. Self-degradation must be considered an alternate, at least under some conditions. It seems more likely to us that self-degradation happens in ST cells when there is a rapid loss of secretion-granule content rather than that secretion granules are incorporated into dense bodies (FIGURES 19 and 20).

Mammary Gland Secretory-Cell Involution and Destruction of Secretory Products

As part of our investigations into the significance of acid hydrolase activity in hyperplastic alveolar nodules (Smith *et al.* in preparation), it was necessary to evaluate the enzymorphologic events that occur with mammary gland involution. It is through the clear-cut biochemical studies of Greenbaum and associates (1965) that we relate acid hydrolase activity to mammary gland involution. These workers demonstrated that, while there was a general decrease in enzyme amount or activity with removal of the suckling young from a rat, there was no decrease in the amount of those lysosomal acid hydrolases being investigated. The cytomorphologic studies of mammary gland involution by Wellings *et al.,* (1960), and the more recent studies of Sekhri, *et al.* (1967a; 1967b), identify structural changes that parallel the biochemically defined sites of enzyme activity.

Concurrent with some of our studies of the anterior pituitary, we have carried out a cytochemical program in which we investigated AcPase activity in mammary tissue from both rats and mice during late pregnancy and lactation, and, at twelve hour intervals, during the three days following removal of suckling young. Although several aspects of these studies remain to be clarified, certain enzymorphological events can be identified with the genesis of lysosomes. Furthermore, enzyme staining patterns are similar to those observed in cells of the anterior pituitary. There is, however, a distinct difference between pituitary and mammary gland cells in the occurrence of staining of the Golgi cisternae. Whereas the Golgi cisternae of MT cells of the pituitary stain intensely for AcPase in the glands of lactating and early postlactating animals, the Golgi cisternae in mammary gland secretory cells stain intensely only for 12 to 24 hours after suckling young have been removed (FIGURE 28). In mammary tissues from lactating and early postlactating animals, 5 to 12 days postpartum, glandular cells have a highly developed Golgi complex composed of several crescent-shaped parallel layers of cisternae. Circumscribed by the smooth-surfaced stacks of Golgi cisternae, and contained within the cytoplasmic core, single randomly oriented smooth- and rough-surfaced cisternae can frequently be observed (i.e., the GERL of Novikoff, 1964). These "freely oriented" cisternae of the Golgi cytoplasmic core, as well as the innermost layer of the stacked Golgi cisternae, generate vesicles that stain for AcPase. Enzyme-staining Golgi vesicles are commonly observed throughout the supranuclear region in secretory alveolar cells up to about 36 hours after lactation ceases. The origin, structure, shape and contour of multivesicular bodies as entities in cells of mammary tissue and in cells of the anterior pituitary show no difference. Dense-body-type lysosomes are rarely observed in the glandular cells of the lactating animal; their appearance is most common 24 to 48 hours after the end of lactation. Our cytochemical studies corroborate the biochemical studies of Greenbaum *et al.* (1965) regarding the involvement of acid hydrolytic enzymes in mammary gland involution. At the same time, enzymorphologic evidence indicates that the same basic pattern of cell regression, by sequestration of organelles into autophagic bodies, occurs there as occurs in cells of the anterior pituitary. The degradation process of secretory material in

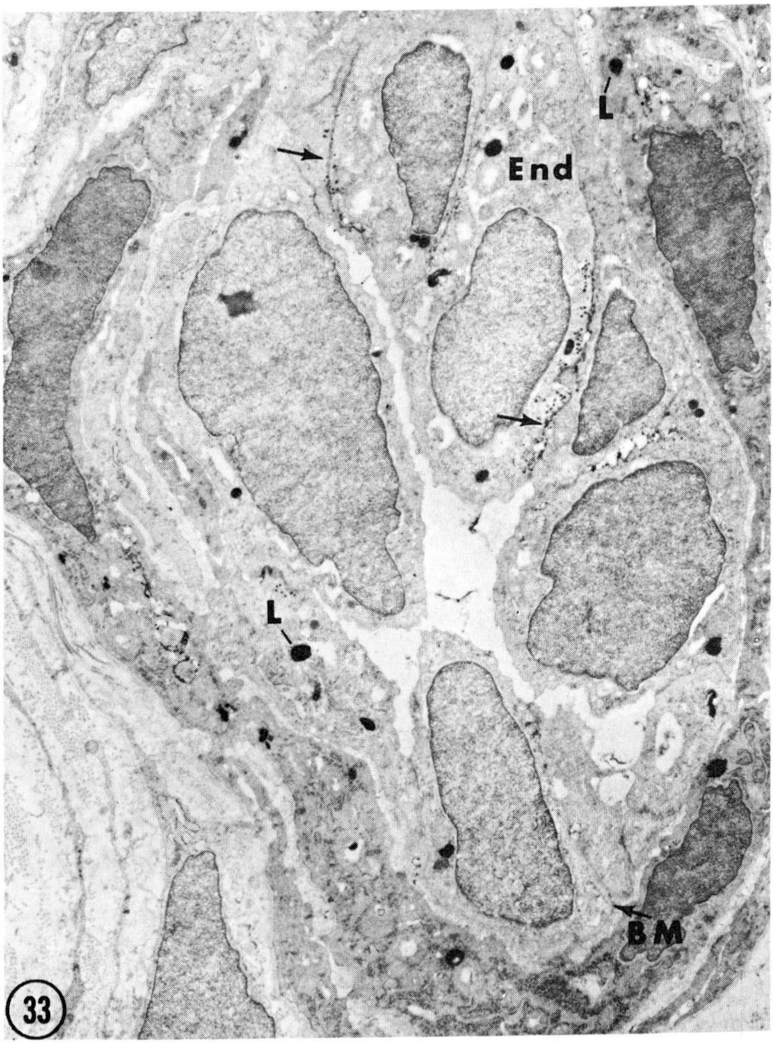

FIGURE 33. Degenerating small arteriole in the endometrium of the rabbit four days after withdrawal of estradiol and chlormadinone. Arrows point to membrane sites of AcPase staining. Enzyme staining also of lysosomes (L) in the endothelium (End) and perithelium. (×7,800)

the mammary gland is somewhat different and more involved than that in the anterior pituitary (FIGURE 29). First, two independent secretory products result—protein and fat; second, the packaging of protein secretion granules is different; and third, secretory product is resorbed by secretory cells, a phenomenon not occurring in the anterior pituitary.

The condensing of protein into secretion granules within Golgi cisternae of mammary gland epithelial cells results in a vacuole usually containing more than one electron-dense granule (Hollmann, 1968; Kurosumi *et al.,* 1968; Wellings & DeOme, 1963). Approximate maximal diameter of the vacuoles varies from 500 mμ to 900 mμ; and the maximal diameter of the protein-secretion granules they contain is about 250 mμ. In the cells of the anterior pituitary, the membrane of the Golgi cisterna becomes the limiting membrane of one secretion granule. In secretory cells of the mammary gland, the membrane of the cisterna becomes the membrane of the vacuole, and the intravacuolar-condensing secretion gran-

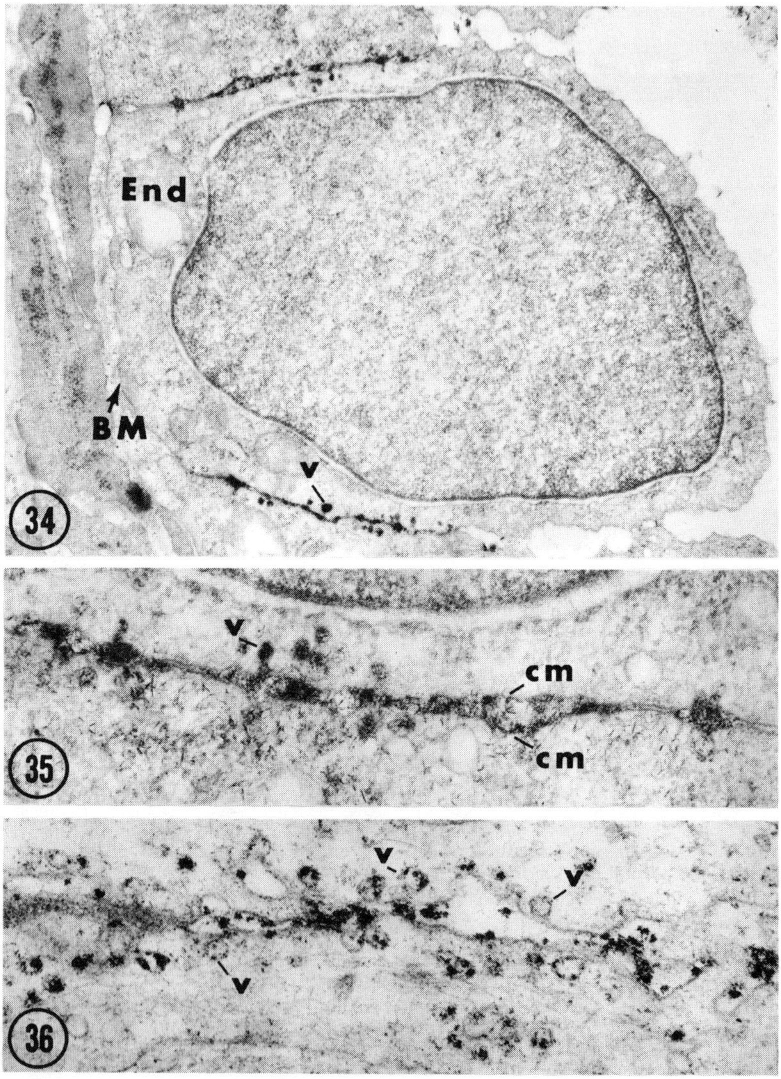

FIGURES 34–36. AcPase staining of cell membranes (cm) and pinocytic vesicles (v) of opposed endothelial cells of degenerating small arterioles after 48 to 96 hours' hormone withdrawal (FIGURE 45, group 3). (34) $\times$15,000; (35–36) $\times$44,000.

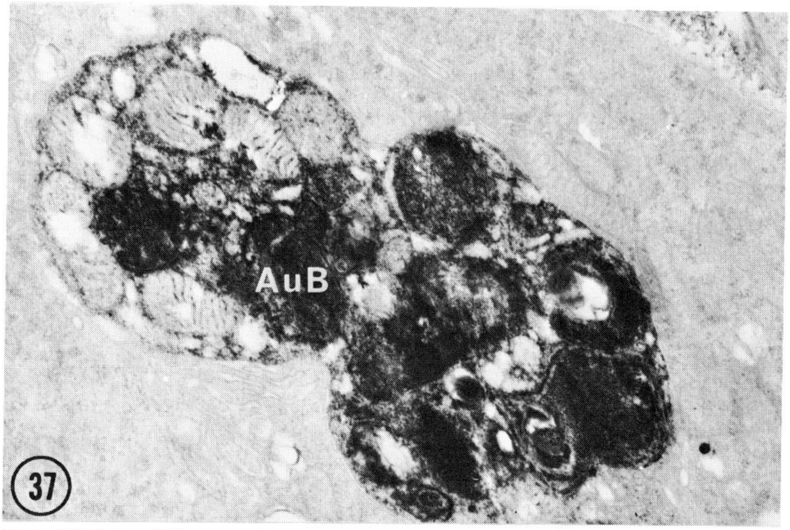

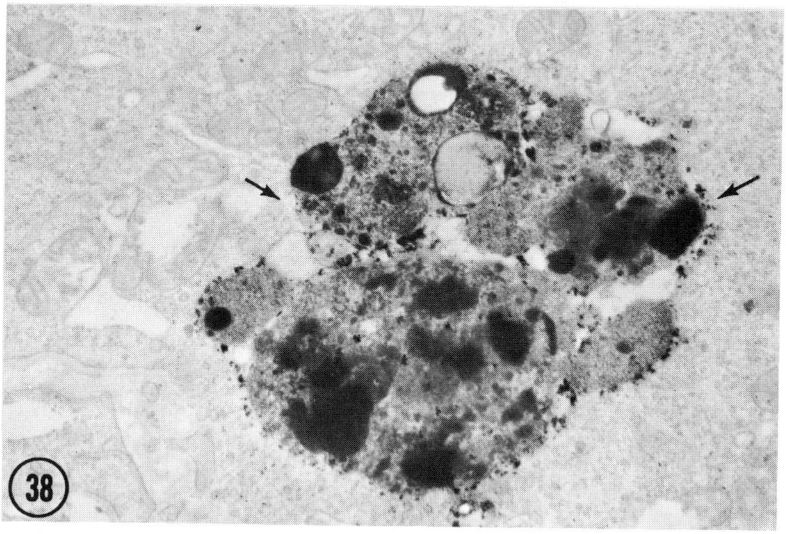

FIGURES 37 AND 38. Detailed structure of membrane-limited autophagic bodies stained for AcPase. From the endometrium of a castrate rabbit treated with estradiol and chlormadinone and sacrificed four days after last hormone administration. In FIGURE 38, arrows point to limiting membrane. (×16,000)

ules have no definable membrane. AcPase staining of mammary gland protein-secretion granules has not been observed, and the staining of a vacuole membrane is infrequent. The absence of enzyme staining may be accounted for by the fact that secretion-granule formation occurs during lactation, and our observations indicate AcPase activity in Golgi cisternae is low at that time. Thus, at least in the mammary gland, condensation of secretory protein into granules appears to be independent of acid hydrolase involvement.

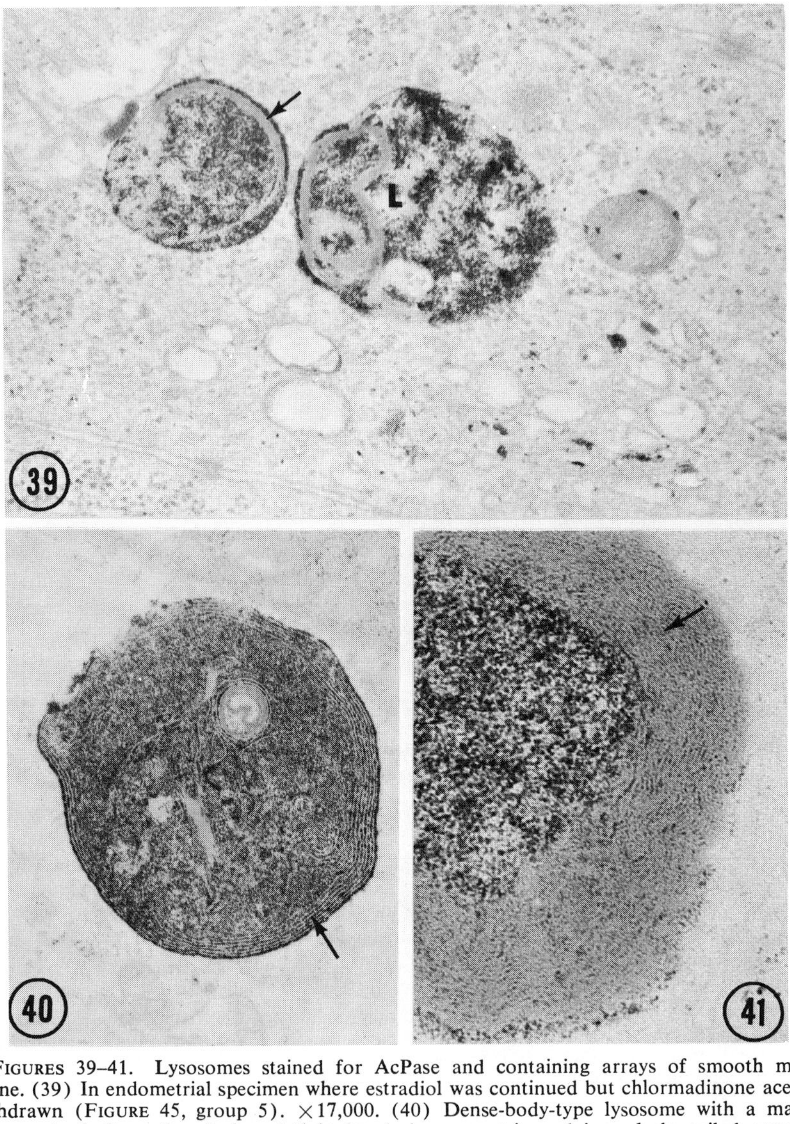

FIGURES 39–41. Lysosomes stained for AcPase and containing arrays of smooth membrane. (39) In endometrial specimen where estradiol was continued but chlormadinone acetate withdrawn (FIGURE 45, group 5). ×17,000. (40) Dense-body-type lysosome with a matrix composed of alternating dark and light bands in concentric and irregularly coiled arrangements. The darker bands stain for AcPase. Such structures are numerous in epithelial cells of the rabbit endometrium where estradiol was continued, but chlormadinone acetate was withdrawn for 48 hours. Stained with lead citrate, ×19,000. (41) A lysosome, the outer structure of layered material, phospholipid in appearance, with light lead salt deposition on the dark bands. The center of the structure has a heavy deposition of AcPase reaction product. (×106,000)

Much less is known about the formation of fat droplets within the secretory cells. Identification of reaction product at the periphery of fat droplets in cells of the lactating gland suggests, at first evidence, a site of AcPase activity. More conclusive data, however, suggest that this may be an artifact of either enzyme diffusion or of the affinity of reaction product for lipid (Smith & Fishman, 1969). In the postlactating animal, the evidence of acid hydrolase involvement with the breakdown of milk fat is more clear-cut since dense-body-type lysosomes are frequently observed in contact with fat droplets. These aspects of secretory product degradation are presently part of a more detailed study of enzyme involvement in mammary gland involution, published since this conference (Helminen, H. J., J. L. E. Ericsson, S. Orrenius. 1968. Studies on mammary gland involution. IV. Histochemical and biochemical observations on alterations in lysosomes and lysosomal enzymes. J. Ultrastruct. Res. **25:**240–252).

Effects of Hormone Administration and Withdrawal on Acid Phosphohydrolase of the Endometrium

In an era when numerous synthetic estrogens and gestagens are widely used for control of reproduction, it becomes increasingly important to understand the action of steroid hormones on cell organelles (Harpel *et al.*, 1968; Shimizu & Okazaki, 1967). During the past two years, Dr. Henzl and I, with the assistance of several persons at Syntex Research, Palo Alto, Calif., have investigated the effects of estradiol and chlormadinone acetate on hydrolytic enzymes of the endometrium of the ovariectomized rabbit (Henzl, Smith, Magoun & Hill, 1968; Smith & Henzl, 1969), and on the endometrium of women using chlormadinone acetate as an oral contraceptive (Henzl, Smith & Tyler, 1968).

In cells of the low columnar epithelium of the endometrium in the untreated castrate rabbit, the Golgi complex is simple and usually has little AcPase reaction product deposited within its cisternae. Exogenous estrogen promotes development of the Golgi complex as an organelle within epithelial and endothelial cells. After five days of estrogen influence, there was a significant increase in the number of cells containing Golgi complexes that stain for enzyme, as well as in the number of cisternae labeled, and in the intensity of staining. It is common in epithelial cells to observe several parallel layers of cisternae labeled by a continuous deposition of reaction product (FIGURE 30). In endothelial cells, generally only one layer of cisternae stain for AcPase. Golgi vesicles identified by staining for AcPase have their origin in epithelial cells of the estrogen-stimulated endometrium much as they do in secretory cells of the mammary gland. In endothelial cells, enzyme staining vesicles of the Golgi complex are derived from one concentric layer of cisternae, a morphologic origin more akin to that observed in cells of the anterior pituitary. The origin of multivesicular bodies, and their differentiation and enzyme staining patterns, are similar to those in cells of the anterior pituitary and mammary glands. Dense-body-type lysosomes vary in number from cell to cell of the epithelium, their occurrence increasing as estrogen treatment is continued. (FIGURE 16). During treatment with estrogen only, limited numbers of dense-body-type lysosomes are seen in endothelial cells. They are infrequent in cells of the stroma.

Chlormadinone acetate, a halogenated derivative of 17-acetoxyprogesterone, is regarded as considerably more potent than endogenous progesterone and as having no estrogenic or androgenic properties. In our experiments (Smith & Henzl, 1969), doses of 25 μg/kg body weight of chlormadinone acetate (FIG-

URE 45) administered with estrogen, increased the size and enzyme staining capacity of the Golgi complex beyond that which could be obtained by simply extending the period of estrogen treatment. In the tall, columnar cells of the surface and of the glandular epithelial lining, the Golgi complex is elongated. AcPase reaction product appears as a deposit within the inner flattened layers of cisternae and along the membranes of the outer layers of distended cisternae (FIGURE 31). In these cells, there is also an increase in the number of enzyme staining Golgi vesicles, of multivesicular bodies and of dense-body-type lysosomes. The effect of chlormadinone acetate administration on the Golgi of endothelial cells is much the same; however, only one elongated, flattened layer of cisternae continues to contain enzyme reaction product and to produce vesicles (FIGURE 32). The administration of chlormadinone in combination with estrogen for three days brings about a distinct increase in size and staining of the Golgi elements in stromal cells; exogenous estrogen alone was not capable of doing so. Consequently, the origin and appearance of multivesicular bodies and dense bodies in stromal cells of the endometrium is an affirmation of progesterone activity.

The most dramatic changes in enzyme staining occur during the period of 24 hours to 4 days after both hormones have been withdrawn (FIGURE 45, group 3). We observed a striking increase in AcPase staining due to a progressive increase in number and size of lysosomal structures. These enzyme-staining structures appeared first in the apical cytoplasm of surface and glandular epithelial cells and, subsequently, at the base of the epithelial cells and in cells of the stroma (Smith & Henzl, 1969). They are membrane-limited, and the larger ones are clearly definable as autophagic bodies by virtue of their content, e.g., ribosomes, E.R., mitochondria and smooth membranes (FIGURES 37 and 38). Thus, once again, our findings can be teleologically interpreted with reference to lysosomal structure. While the endometrium undergoes proliferation and differentiation, the tissue programs-in a destructive potential that will eventually trigger and set into motion a chain of reactions leading to tissue regression.

Endometrial regression need not lead to menstruation, although regression by virtue of ischemia would accompany and follow menstrual bleeding. Consequently, our most recent observations of the effects of hormone withdrawal on the small arterioles and venules of the rabbit endometrium are of interest. Although the rabbit has no menses, its small arterioles respond to hormone withdrawal by hypertrophy and cytoplasmic rarefaction of the endothelial cells (Bruns & Palade, 1968a; 1968b; Friederici, 1967). Forty-eight hours after withdrawal of the hormone, the arteriole lumen has often become occluded by the endothelial enlargement (FIGURE 33). These morphologic alterations are concurrent with a progressive increase in AcPase staining and changes in sites of reaction-product localization. From the earliest stages of estrogen and chlormadinone acetate withdrawal, a shift begins in the staining pattern from Golgi cisternae and vesicles to lysosomes and cell membrane. A salient finding was the intense deposition of reaction product in the interspaces between opposed endothelial cell membranes. By 48 hours after withdrawal of the hormone, such localization was evident to some degree in almost every arteriole observed, while the incidence of reactive Golgi complexes in endothelial cells was infrequent. Of greatest interest, however, is the localization of AcPase reaction product in pinocytic vesicles and of that which is clearly on the cell membrane (FIGURES 34 through 36). The number of pinocytic vesicles reactive for AcPase was not so high as when ATP was used for substrate at pH 7.0. However, what makes

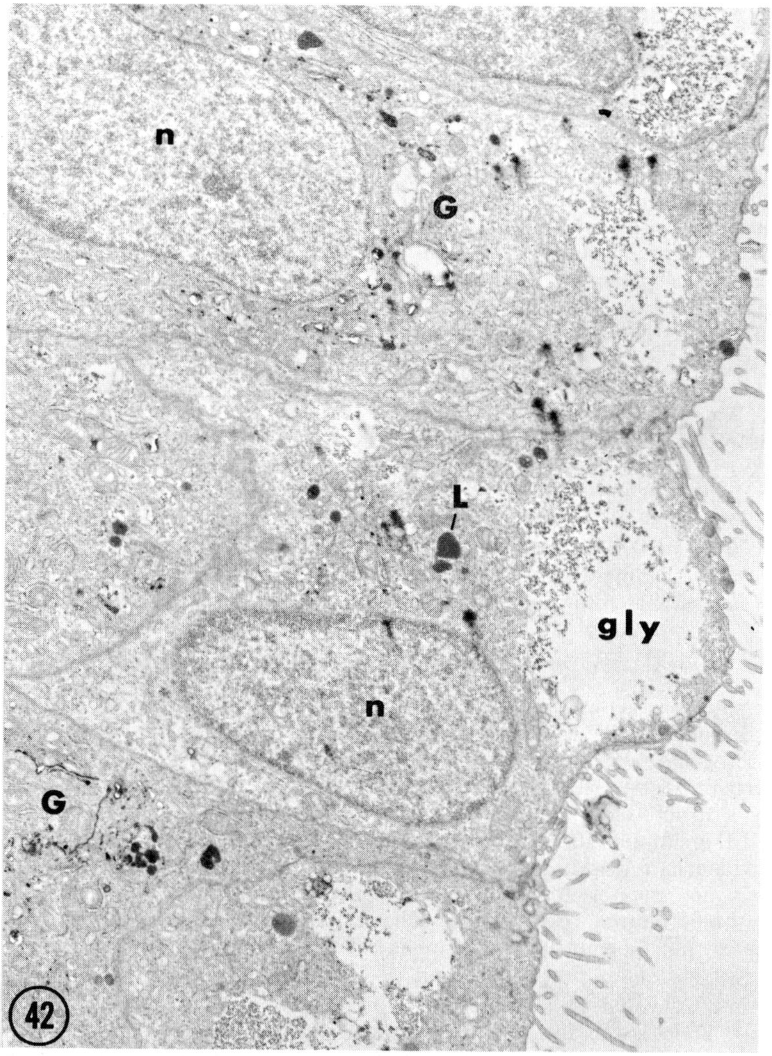

FIGURE 42. Normal human secretory endometrium stained for AcPase. Golgi complex (G) and lysosome (L) localization of reaction product. Note large areas of glycogen (gly) deposition. (×8,000)

the localization of AcPase reaction product so significant is that it has been observed only after both hormones have been withdrawn for at least 24 hours. No such changes have thus far been observed in the venules. Even four days after withdrawal of the hormone, the appearance and localization of reaction product in the endothelial cells of venules is much the same as it is during combined hormone administration. What physiologic significance can be attached to the endothelial localization of an acid hydrolase (Ancla *et al.*, 1967; Hall, 1968) is the subject of our continued efforts with both rabbit and human cytochemical preparations. Our belief, subject to more complete evidence, is that, in arterioles of the endometrium, these enzymorphologic events are related to interruptions of the vascular pattern, resulting in menstruation in primates. (Hisaw *et al.*, 1967; Wienke *et al.*, 1968).

A few remarks regarding our cytochemical studies of the human endometrium would seem in order. The principal reason for these studies was to determine whether or not we could identify any significant subcellular changes within the endometrium that could be associated with a continuing daily administration of 0.5 mg of chlormadinone acetate (Henzl, Smith & Tyler, 1968). Routine light microscopic preparations of human endometrium failed to reveal any major alterations in specimens taken during the proliferative phase of the cycle where hormone had been given, as compared with a specimen taken during the same phase where there was no treatment. Our electron microscopic studies have shown that the effects of chlormadinone acetate are apparent during the proliferative phase and can be evaluated as a premature occurrence of early secretory signs. Among other subcellular differences, lysosomes are more numerous than in the regular proliferative phase. A striking feature is the increase of AcPase staining in the stroma, which we have found to be more expressed than in the normal early secretory phase. The influence of chlormadinone acetate was even more accentuated during the secretory phase, AcPase reaction product being found in locations where, normally, no activity was detected, e.g., on epithelial and stromal cell membranes (FIGURES 42 and 43). These cell membrane localizations suggest that chlormadinone acetate has a labilizing effect (Weissman, 1965).

Speculations on the Relation of Hydrolytic Enzymes to Structure

Very little is actually known about the internal organization of the lysosome. The simplest model proposed was similar to a sac, with the enzymes present in a diffusible form enclosed in a semipermeable membrane (de Duve, 1963). Nevertheless, de Duve made it clear that "the picture of a bag does not necessarily imply a structureless interior." The bag model was suggested because it represented the simplest form compatible with experimental data of the time. As all the evidence is drawn together—morphologic, cytochemical and biochemical—there is more support for the proposition that dense-body-type lysosomes have at least some internal organization. The evidence arising from our own work indicates that the internal structure is a complex of membranes.

In order to defend a concept that the dense-body lysosome is a membranous structure, it would first be necessary to involve a multivesicular body in its genesis. There seems little doubt that some multivesicular bodies transform into dense bodies. As previously mentioned, situations analogous to those we observed have been reported in a variety of cells where there is a display of spheroid structures in forms varying between multivesicular bodies and dense bodies (Smith & Farquhar, 1966: FIGURES 10 through 12). However, the assumption that all multivesicular bodies are similar in origin and function is probably too general (Locke & Collins, 1968). Our premise of origin, therefore, may require amendment to acknowledge that not all multivesicular bodies have a kinship to dense bodies, but that dense bodies have a lineage through certain multivesicular bodies. Such a relationship depends upon whether or not the membranes of each have specific biochemical components in common (de Duve & Wattiaux, 1966; Revel *et al.* 1958).

Holtzman and coworkers (Holtzman & Dominitz, 1968; Holtzman & Petersen,

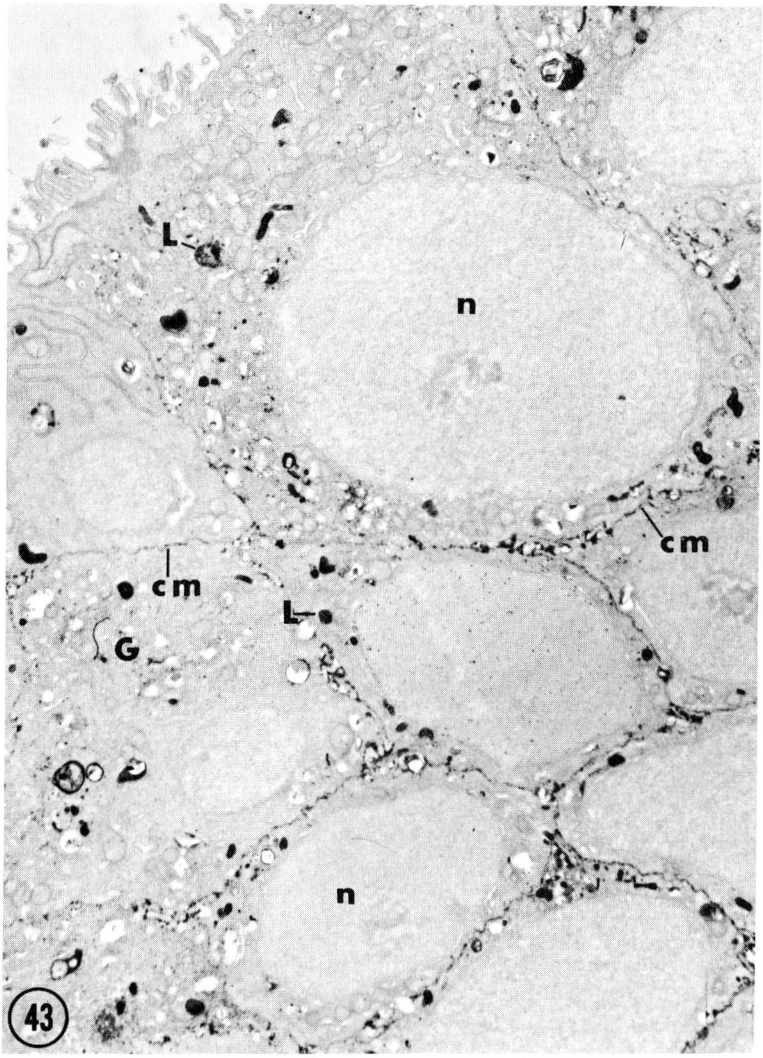

FIGURE 43. Secretory endometrium of a woman given 0.5 mg chlormadinone acetate each day throughout the cycle. Note increase in total AcPase activity from FIGURE 42. Golgi complex (G), lysosomes (L), and localization of reaction product along cell membranes not seen in FIGURE 42. (×8,000)

1968) have observed structures they define as "cuplike" and identify as precursors of multivesicular bodies. The fact that these cuplike structures contain peroxidase reaction product and are regularly seen near the cell surface strongly supports Holtzman's implication that they are derived from the cell membrane. The identification of phagocytized particles (Gordon *et al.*, 1965) and proteins (Maunsbach, 1966; Miller, 1960; Miller & Palade, 1964; Smith & Farquhar, 1966) within the matrix of multivesicular bodies has become common, and the fact that these structures stain for AcPase defines them as lysosomes (Gordon *et al.*, 1965; Holtzman & Petersen, 1968; Smith & Farquhar, 1966). In view of these and other findings (de Duve & Wattiaux, 1966, page 465), it seems conclusive that cell membrane is one source of multivesicular body-limiting membrane. Furthermore, the evidence grows ever stronger in support of the presumption that dense bodies are structures in a sequence between multivesicular bodies and bodies composed of residual lipoprotein in membranous form (Robbins *et al.*, 1964; Stoecknius, 1959).

Our observations support evidence that the classic dense-body lysosome has an internal organization. At low magnifications, the electron-dense matrix material usually appears structurally homogeneous throughout the body. However, Maunsbach (1966) noted that at high magnifications (X 250,000), such material in dense bodies often had regions with a layered appearance. In our view, a layered appearance could result from the internal coalescence of vesicles, principally of Golgi-cisternal origin, which, because of physical forces, eventually assume a concentric membrane arrangement (FIGURES 39 through 41), generally parallel to the limiting membrane of the structure. An internal organization may frequently not be recognized because of the compactness of the structure and the fixation and staining properties of its elements. FIGURE 46 is a diagrammatic illustration of the possible successive steps in the formation and organization of the dense-body lysosome. Essentially, the limiting membrane would be derived from the cell membrane as one vacuole (step 1) or through the fusion of vesicles (step 2) to form a cup-like structure. Anywhere within the cell, enzyme-containing vesicles–proto-lysosomes (Gordon *et al.*, 1965)–would enter the structure (FIGURES 7 through 9) with the formation of a multivesicular body (steps 3c and 4). As the number of vesicles continued to increase and coalesce, a more solid structure would be formed–a dense body. Material to be degraded may be present within the forming structure from the outset, or it may be taken in at any point, even after the structure could be defined as a dense body.

In the past two years, there has been increasing evidence that at least some of the lysosomal enzymes are membrane-bound (Brightwell & Tappel, 1968; Emmelot *et al.*, 1968; Furin & Allen, 1968; McDonald *et al.*, 1968; Mahadevan & Tappel, 1968; Nelson, 1966; Shibko & Tappel, 1964; Verity & Brown, 1968). It is possible that all may be bound, with some more easily released than others (Beck & Tappel, 1968). Moreover, other investigators have expressed the view that hydrolases may be properties of structural protein (Fishman *et al.*, 1967; Ide & Fishman, 1967). Certainly, the synthesis of lysosomal enzymes appears to be functionally linked with the formation of new protein. In FIGURE 47, a simple illustration of enzyme-to-membrane binding, the membrane structure is depicted as being in two general parts. Enzymes make up the graphic-structural layer, lipoprotein, the clear layer. Following enzyme action and digestion in such an arrangement, only lipoprotein would remain, taking membranous forms frequently identified as myelin figures. If this is so, it would be necessary to think of residual bodies as being composed not only of indigestible foreign material, but also of residue of lysosomal structure. The possibility is consistent with the opinion of Goldstone and Koenig (1968) that acid hydrolases are cationic glycoproteins ionically linked to lipoproteins. Furthermore, it is consistent with our observations that the more membranous a lysosome becomes, the less intense is its staining for AcPase, specifically over the membrane arrays themselves.

Consideration must now be given to the question of whether enzymorphologic

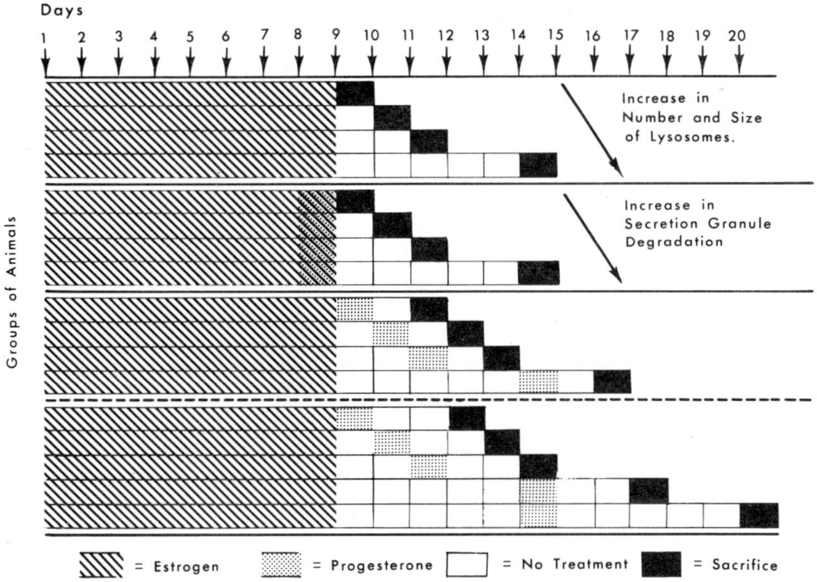

FIGURE 44. Effects of estrogen-progesterone withdrawal on AcPase activity in degradation of hormone, and regression of MT cells in the anterior pituitary of the ovariectomized rat.

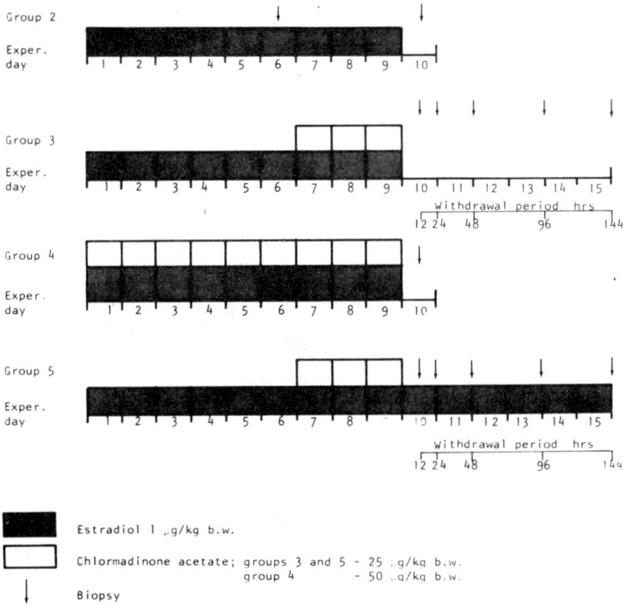

FIGURE 45. Hormonal treatment of ovariectomized rabbits.

information supports the biochemist's view of enzyme-to-membrane binding. We continue to think of acid phosphatase as being found within Golgi cisternae and vesicles because this is where lead salt reaction product is localized. In reality, the enzyme may be membrane-bound, but because of factors (e.g., technique) causing diffusion of enzyme or diffusion of reaction product, it appears as content. From our own studies, it is clear that the innermost Golgi-cisternal membrane that delimits secretion granules of anterior pituitary cells is the same membrane that forms AcPase-staining Golgi vesicles. Presently, there is no biochemical or cytochemical evidence to suggest that acid phosphatase mixes with exportable protein in secretion granule formation, as might be expected if both enzyme and hormone were contents of the same Golgi cisterna. Rather, there is strong cytochemical evidence that acid phosphatase is associated with the membrane in secretion-granule formation (FIGURES 1, 4 and 6). Furthermore, when progesterone, a membrane labilizer (Weissman, 1965), or chlormadinone acetate, a progesterone compound, is given to animals, the number of sites where enzyme is localized on the membrane increases. This increase would seem to strengthen the implication of enzyme-to-membrane binding.

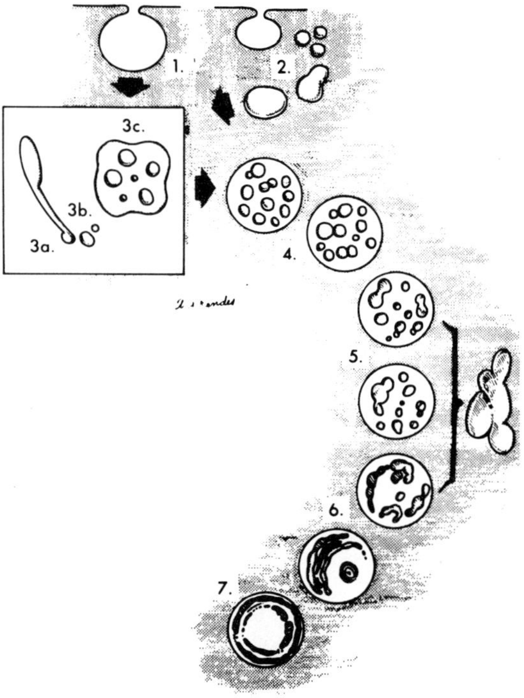

FIGURE 46. Diagrammatic sketch to illustrate possible successive steps in the formation of dense-body-type lysosomes from multivesicular bodies. The limiting membrane could be derived from the cell membrane as one vacuole (Step 1), by the fusion of vesicles (Step 2), or from a Golgi vacuole (not depicted). Enzyme-containing vesicles, principally of Golgi cisternal origin (Steps 3a and 3b), would enter the structure (Step 3c) with the formation of a multivesicular body (Step 4). As a number of vesicles coalesce, a more solid-appearing structure would be formed (Steps 5–7). Structures containing or composed of membranes (see FIGURES 39–41) suggest the formation of a residual body from a dense-body-type lysosome after enzyme action (see also Arstila & Trump, 1968).

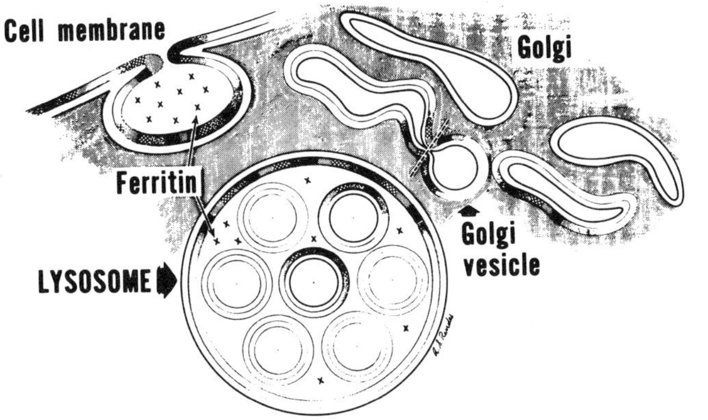

FIGURE 47. Diagrammatic sketch to illustrate the view of enzymes binding to membranes within the formation of a multivesicular body. The structure of the membrane is depicted in two general parts. Enzymes make up the graphic-structural part and lipoprotein makes up the clear component. Diffusion of enzymes would be to the matrix of the multivesicular body. The diagram implies that some of the enzymes are not contained within the Golgi vesicles, but rather that they are at one point a part of their membrane.

If the origin of the membrane that delimits secretion granules is the same as the origin of that which forms Golgi vesicles, and Golgi vesicles are constituents of multivesicular bodies, it may be fair to assume that enzymes of multivesicular bodies are, at one point, membrane-bound. Enzymorphologic evidence favors this assumption. Multivesicular bodies may contain reaction product to a limit that does not obstruct observation of the internal structure of the body. The reaction product localizes on the membrane of the vesicles, or is diffuse in the matrix, rather than localizing within the vesicles (FIGURE 11; see also Smith & Farquhar, 1966; FIGURE 28). In addition, we have observed less diffusion and more intense localization of reaction product around vesicles within multivesicular bodies if distilled, rather than commercial, glutaraldehyde is used as fixative, if sections are nonfrozen rather than frozen, and if sections are not placed in acid substrate media for prolonged periods of time.

The point at which there is physiologic diffusion of an enzyme is probably determined by changes in membrane properties. These changes are, in turn, related to the time at which a multivesicular body or dense body ingests material or at which conditions of "cell stress" occur. Unfortunately, with present methods of cytochemical staining, we are usually unable to differentiate between diffusion of enzyme related to physiologic causes and diffusion imposed by the necessities of our technique. Herein lies the limitation of subcellular enzymorphology—the difficulty of determining what, within the structure of the organelle, is genuine enzyme localization and what is artifact.

Acknowledgments

The author wishes to thank Dr. Robert Hill for his consultation and use of the animal facilities at Syntex Research, Palo Alto, Calif., in studies of the uterus; Mr. Albert Rendes for illustrative assistance; and Mrs. Irma Daehne and Mrs. Marla Hoag for technical support.

References

ABOLINS, L. & A. ABOLINS. 1949. Different kinds of acid phosphatase in various cytological structures of the anterior pituitary of the guinea pig. Nature (London) **164:** 455–456.

ANCLA, M., J. DE BRUX & P. SIMON. 1967. Aneurysmal microthrombosis associated with intrauterine devices in the human endometrium. Lab. Invest. **17:** 61–70.

ARSTILA, A. U. & B. F. TRUMP. 1968. Studies on cellular autophagocytosis. The formation of autophagic vacuoles in the liver after glucagon administration. Amer. J. Pathol. **53:** 687–733.

BAINTON, D. F. & M. G. FARQUHAR. 1966. Origin of granules in polymorphonuclear leukocytes. Two types derived from opposite faces of the Golgi complex in developing granulocytes. J. Cell Biol. **28:** 277–301.

BARRNETT, R. J., W. D. ROTH & J. SALZER. 1961. The histochemical demonstration of the sites of luteotropic hormone in the rat pituitary gland. Endocrinology **69:** 1047–1059.

BEAMS, H. W. & R. G. KESSEL. 1968. The Golgi apparatus: structure and function. *In* International Rev. of Cytology. G. H. Bourne & J. F. Danielli, Eds. **23:** 209–276. Academic Press, Inc., New York, N. Y.

BECK, C. & A. L. TAPPEL. 1968. Rat-liver lysosomal β-glucosidase: a membrane enzyme. Biochim. Biophys. Acta **151:** 159–164.

BEHNKE, O. & H. MOE. 1964. An electron microscope study of mature and differentiating Paneth cells in the rat, especially of their endoplasmic reticulum and lysosomes. J. Cell Biol. **22:** 633–652.

BRANDES, D. 1966. The fine structure and histochemistry of prostatic glands in relation to sex hormones. *In* International Rev. of Cytology. G. H. Bourne & J. F. Danielli, Eds. **20:** 207–276. Academic Press, Inc., New York, N. Y.

BRANDES, D., D. E. BUETOW, F. BERTINI & D. B. MALKOFF. 1964. Role of lysosomes in cellular lytic processes. I. Effect of carbon starvation in *euglena gracilis.* Exp. Molec. Path. **3:** 583–609.

BRIGHTWELL, R. & A. L. TAPPEL. 1968. Lysosomal acid pyrophosphatase and acid phosphatase. Arch. Biochem. **124:** 333–343.

BRUNS, R. R. & G. E. PALADE. 1968a. Studies on blood capillaries. I. General organization of blood capillaries in muscle. J. Cell Biol. **37:** 244–276.

BRUNS, R. R. & G. E. PALADE. 1968b. Studies on blood capillaries. II. Transport of ferritin molecules across the wall of muscle capillaries. J. Cell Biol. **37:** 277–299.

DAEMS, W. T. 1962. Mouse liver lysosomes and storage. Amorphological and histochemical study. Thesis. University of Leiden, The Netherlands.

DE DUVE, C. 1963. The lysosome concept. *In* Ciba Foundation Symposium on Lysosomes. A. V. S. de Reuck & M. P. Cameron, Eds. : 1–31. Little, Brown & Co., Boston, Mass.

DE DUVE, C. & R. WATTIAUX. 1966. Functions of lysosomes. Ann. Rev. Physiol. **28:** 435–492.

ELLIOTT, A. M. 1965. Primary lysosomes in Tetrahymena pyriformis. Science **149:** 640–641.

EMMELOT, P., A. VISSER & E. L. BENEDETTI. 1968. Studies on plasma membranes. VII. A leucyl-β-naphthylamidase-containing repeating unit on the surface of isolated liver and hepatoma plasma membranes. Biochim. Biophys. Acta **150:** 364–375.

ESSNER, E. & A. B. NOVIKOFF. 1961. Localization of acid phosphatase activity in hepatic lysosomes by means of electron microscopy. J. Biophys. Biochem. Cytol. **9:** 773–784.

FISHMAN, W. H., S. GOLDMAN & R. DELELLIS. 1967. Dual localization of beta-glucuronidase in endoplasmic reticulum and in lysosomes. Nature **213:** 457–460.

FRIEDERICI, H. H. R. 1967. The early response of uterine capillaries to estrogen stimulation. Lab. Invest. **17:** 322–333.

FRIEND, D. S. & M. G. FARQUHAR. 1967. Functions of coated vesicles during protein absorption in the rat *vas deferens.* J. Cell Biol. **35:** 357–376.

FURIN, B. & J. M. ALLEN. 1968. Relationship of soluble and bound lysosomal acid phosphatase in regenerating and control rat liver. J. Histochem. Cytochem. **16:** 512.

GOLDFISCHER, S., N. CARASSO & P. FARARD. 1963. The demonstration of acid phosphatase activity by electron microscopy in the ergastoplasm of the ciliate Campanella Umbellaria L. J. de Micros. **2:** 621.

GOLDSTONE, A. & H. KOENIG. 1968. Acid hydrolases and structural lipoproteins of kidney lysosomes. J. Histochem. Cytochem. **16:** 511–512.

GORDON, G. B., L. R. MILLER & K. G. BENSCH. 1965. Studies on the intracellular digestive process in mammalian tissue culture cells. J. Cell Biol. **25:** 41–55.

GREENBAUM, A. L., T. F. SLATER & D. Y. WANG. 1965. Lysosomal enzyme changes in enforced mammary-gland involution. Biochem. J. **97:** 518–522.

GREEP, R. O. 1961. Physiology of the anterior hypophysis in relation to reproduction. *In* Sex and Internal Secretions. W. C. Young, Ed., The Williams & Wilkins Co., Baltimore, Md.

HALL, K. 1968. Disappearance of histochemically-demonstrable adenosine triphosphatase and of PAS-reactive basement membranes in blood vessels in the decidua during ovum implantation in mice. J. Endocr. **41:** 53–59.

HARPEL, P. C., F. HOMBURGER & A. TREGER. 1968. Mouse uterine fluid plasminogen activator, acid phosphatase, and contraceptive hormones. Amer. J. Physiol. **215:** 928–931.

HENZL, M. R., R. E. SMITH, R. E. MAGOUN & R. HILL. 1968. The influence of estrogens on rabbit endometrium. An ultrastructural-cytochemical and biochemical study. Fertil. Steril. **19:** 914–935.

HENZL, M. R., R. E. SMITH & E. T. TYLER. 1968. Subcellular action of chlormadinone acetate on the rabbit and human endometrium. Part II. Acid phosphatase activity of the human endometrium during continuous administration of 0.5 mg chlormadinone acetate with special reference to the mechanism of break-through bleeding. Report submitted to Food & Drug Administration for Syntex Research, Palo Alto, Calif.

HISAW, F. L., F. L. HISAW, JR. & A. B. DAWSON. 1967. Effects of relaxin on the endothelium of endometrial blood vessels in monkeys (macaca mulatta). Endocrinology **81:** 375–385.

HOLLMANN, K. H. 1968. A morphometric study of subcellular organization in mouse mammary cancers and normal lactating tissue. Z. Zellforsch. **87:** 266–277.

HOLT, S. J. & R. M. HICKS. 1961. The localization of acid phosphatase in rat liver cells as revealed by combined cytochemical staining and electron microscopy. J. Biophys. Biochem. Cytol. **11:** 47–66.

HOLTZMAN, E. & R. DOMINITZ. 1968. Cytochemical studies of lysosomes, Golgi apparatus and endoplasmic reticulum in secretion and protein uptake by adrenal medulla cells of the rat. J. Histochem. Cytochem. **16:** 320–336.

HOLTZMAN, E. & E. PETERSEN. 1968. Cytochemical studies of protein uptake, lysosomes and GERL in neurons. J. Histochem. Cytochem. **16:** 502.

HOPKINS, C. R. & B. I. BAKER. 1968. The fine structural localization of acid phosphatase in the prolactin cell of the eel pituitary. J. Cell Sci. **3:** 357–364.

IDE, H. & W. H. FISHMAN. 1967. *De novo* synthesis of endoplasmic reticulum glycoprotein; androgen-stimulated mouse renal beta glucuronidase. J. Cell Biol. **35:** 60A.

JONES, F. W. 1924. Cytoclesis. A phenomenon explaining the course of embryonal development. Lancet **1:** 684–685.

KUROSUMI, K., Y. KOBAYASHI & N. BABA. 1968. The fine structure of mammary glands of lactating rats, with special reference to the apocrine secretion. Exp. Cell Res. **50:** 177–192.

LANE, N. J. 1968. Distribution of phosphatases in the Golgi region and associated structures cf the thoracic ganglionic neurons in the grasshopper, *Melanoplus differentialis*. J. Cell Biol. **37:** 89–104.

LOCKE, M. & J. V. COLLINS. 1968. Protein uptake into multivesicular bodies and storage granules in the fat body of an insect. J. Cell Biol. **36:** 453–483.

MCDONALD, J. K., I. J. REILLY, B. B. ZEITMAN *et al.* 1968. Dipeptidyl arylamidase II of the pituitary. Properties of lysylalanyl-beta-naphthylamide hydrolysis: inhibition of cations, distribution in tissues, and subcellular localization. J. Biol. Chem. **243:** 2028–2037.

MAHADEVAN, S. & A. L. TAPPEL. 1968. Lysosomal lipases of rat liver and kidney. J. Biol. Chem. **243:** 2849–2854.

MAUNSBACH, A. B. 1966. Observations on the ultrastructure and acid phosphatase activity of the cytoplasmic bodies in rat kidney proximal tubule cells. J. Ultrastruct. Res. **16:** 1–42.

MAUNSBACH, A. B. 1966. Absorption of I^{125}-labelled homologous albumin by rat kidney proximal tubule cells. J. Ultrastruct. Res. **15:** 197–241.

MILLER, F. 1960. Hemoglobin absorption by the cells of the proximal convoluted tubule in mouse kidney. J. Biophys. Biochem. Cytol. **8:** 689–718.

MILLER, F. & G. E. PALADE. 1964. Lytic activities in renal protein absorption droplets. An electron microscopical study. J. Cell Biol. **23:** 519–552.

NELSON, B. D. 1966. Rat liver acid phosphatase: differences in lysosomal and cytoplasmic forms. Proc. Soc. Exp. Biol. Med. **121:** 998–1001.

NOVIKOFF, A. B. 1967. Lysosomes in nerve cells. *In* The Neuron. H. Hyden, Ed. : 319. American Elsevier Publishing Co., Inc., New York, N. Y.

NOVIKOFF, A. B. 1964. GERL its form and function in neurons of rat spiral ganglia. Biol. Bull. **127:** 358.

NOVIKOFF, A. B. 1963. Lysosomes in the physiology and pathology of cells: contributions of staining methods. *In* Ciba Foundation Symposium on Lysosomes. P. 36. A. V. S. de Reuck & M. P. Cameron, Eds. : 36. Little, Brown & Co., Boston, Mass.

NOVIKOFF, A. B. 1961. Lysosomes and related particles. *In* The Cell. J. Brachet & A. E. Mirsky, Eds. **2:** 423–488. Academic Press, Inc., New York, N. Y.

NOVIKOFF, A. B. & E. ESSNER. 1962. Pathological changes in cytoplasmic organelles. Fed. Proc. **21:** 1130–1142.

NOVIKOFF, A. B., E. ESSNER & N. QUINTANA. 1964. Golgi apparatus and lysosomes. Fed. Proc. **23:** 1010–1022.

OSINCHAK, J. 1964. Electron microscopic localization of acid phosphatase and thiamine pyrophosphatase activity in hypothalamic neurosecretory cells of the rat. J. Cell Biol. **21:** 35.

PERDUE, J. F. & W. H. MCSHAN. 1962. Isolation and biochemical study of secretory granules from rat pituitary glands. J. Cell Biol. **15:** 159–172.

REVEL, J. P., S. ITO & D. W. FAWCETT. 1958. Electron micrographs of myelin figures of phospholipide simulating intracellular membranes. J. Biophys. Biochem. Cytol. **4:** 495–498.

ROBBINS, E., P. I. MARCUS & N. K. GONATAS. 1964. Dynamics of acridine orange-cell interaction. II. Dye-induced ultrastructural changes in multivesicular bodies (acridine orange particles). J. Cell Biol. **21:** 49–62.

SAMORAJSKI, T. & G. R. FITZ. 1960. Histochemical analysis of phosphomonoesterase in the hypothalamus and pituitary gland of the rat. Lab. Invest. **9:** 517–534.

SCHREIBER, V. & Z. LOJDA. 1967. Enzymes of the hypothalamo-hypophyseal system (review). Endocrinologia Experimentalis **1:** 237–259.

SEKHRI, K. K., D. R. PITELKA & K. B. DEOME. 1967a. Studies of mouse mammary glands. I. Cytomorphology of the normal mammary gland. J. Nat. Cancer Inst. **39:** 459–490.

SEKHRI, K. K., D. R. PITELKA & K. B. DEOME. 1967b. Studies of mouse mammary glands. II. Cytomorphology of mammary transplants in inguinal fat pads, nipple-excised host glands, and whole mammary gland transplants. J. Nat. Cancer Inst. **39:** 491–527.

SELIGMAN, A. M., M. J. KARNOVSKY, H. L. WASSERKRUG & J. S. HANKER. 1968. Nondroplet ultrastructural demonstration of cytochrome oxidase activity with a polymerizing osmiophilic reagent, diaminobenzidine (DAB). J. Cell Biol. **38:** 1–14.

SHIBKO, S. & A. L. TAPPEL. 1964. Distribution of esterases in rat liver. Arch. Biochem. **106:** 259–266.

SHIMIZU, H. & Y. OKAZAKI. 1967. The effects of administration of chlormadinone acetate on the body weight of female rats. Tohoku J. Agric. Res. **18:** 167–184.

SMITH, R. E. 1967. Effects of hormone replacement and withdrawal on acid phosphatase activity in anterior pituitary mammotrophic cells of ovariectomized rats. J. Cell Biol. **35:** 127A.

SMITH, R. E. 1963. Acid phosphatase activity of rat adenohypophysis during secretion. J. Cell Biol. **19:** 159.

SMITH, R. E. & M. G. FARQUHAR. 1966. Lysosome function in the regulation of the secretory process in cells of the anterior pituitary gland. J. Cell Biol. **31:** 319–347.

SMITH, R. E. & W. H. FISHMAN. 1969. *p*-(Acetoxymercuric) aniline diazotate; a reagent for visualizing the naphthol AS-BI product of acid hydrolase action at the level of the light and electron microscope. J. Histochem. Cytochem. **17:** 1–22.

SMITH, R. E. & M. R. HENZL. 1969. The role of mucopolysaccharides and lysosomal hydrolases in endometrial regression following withdrawal of estradiol and chlormadinone acetate. Endocrinology. (In press.)

SMITH, R. E., D. R. PITELKA & K. B. DEOME. 1969. Subcellular localization of acid hydrolytic enzymes in hyperplastic alveolar nodules of the mouse mammary gland. (In preparation.)

SOBEL, H. J. 1961a. The localization of acid phosphatase activity in the rat pituitary and thyroid glands, and its relation to secretory activity. Endocrinology **68:** 801–808.

SOBEL, H. J. 1961b. The relation of acid phosphatase activity of pituitary gonadotrophs and acidophils to secretory activity in the rat. Endocrinology **69:** 1108–1110.

STOECKENIUS, W. 1959. An electron microscope study of myelin figures. J. Biophys. Biochem. Cytol. **5:** 491–500.

STRAUS, W. 1967. Lysosomes, phagosomes and related particles. *In* Enzyme Cytology. D. B. Roodyn, Ed. : 239–319. Academic Press, Inc., New York, N. Y.

VERITY, M. A. & W. J. BROWN. 1968. Structure-linked activity of lysosomal enzymes in the developing mouse brain. J. Neurochem. **15:** 69–80.

WEISSMAN, G. 1965. Studies of lysosomes. VI. The effect of neutral steroids and bile acids on lysosomes *in vitro*. Biochem. Pharmacol. **14:** 525–535.

WELLINGS, S. R. & K. B. DEOME. 1963. Electron microscopy of milk secretion in the mammary gland of the C3H/CRGL mouse. III. Cytomorphology of the involuting gland. J. Nat Cancer Inst. **30:** 241–267.

WELLINGS, S. R., K. B. DEOME & D. R. PITELKA. 1960. Electron microscopy of milk secretion in the mammary gland of the C3H/CRGL mouse. I. Cytomorphology of the prelactating and the lactating gland. J. Nat. Cancer Inst. **25:** 393–421.

WIENKE, E. C., JR., F. CAVAZOS, D. G. HALL & F. V. LUCAS. 1968. Ultrastructure of the human endometrial stroma during the menstrual cycle. Amer. J. Obstet. Gynec. **102:** 65–77.

Discussion of the Paper

DR. RULCH (*Belgium*): Dr. Smith, you said a few times that you made a distinction between one or more cisterna of the Golgi being stained in different cells. Now do you feel this depends on the incubation time or on the concentration of lead in the medium, because I've seen this. You can, in the same cell, stain one cisterna when you incubate for a short time and stain five cisternae when you incubate a long time or when you increase the lead concentration. My second question is, are the details of the new procedure with the naphthyl AS-B1 substrates to be published soon? I would be interested in that. Could you comment on that?

DR. SMITH: In regards to the staining of the cisternae, we've stained cells of the anterior pituitary from 15 minutes up to two hours and, generally, there is no increase in localization of any of the cisternae beyond the innermost cisternae, regardless of the time; whereas 15 minutes' staining in the case of the uterus will show more than one cisterna frequently labeled, depending on whether exogenous hormones were given. So far as the naphthyl procedure is concerned, the paper is in press for the January issue of the Journal of Histochemistry and Cytochemistry.

C. DE DUVE: In one of your pictures, Dr. Smith, you showed a cluster of granules surrounded by acid phosphatase reaction product, and expressed the opinion that it was unlikely this was an image of autophagy owing to the absence of a membrane around this structure. Can you rule out the possibility of a disruption of such a membrane by fixation or some other artifact? It seemed to me that the preservation of the material was rather poor.

DR. SMITH: I was afraid I didn't make that quite clear. What I meant is that in our early studies on the lactating and postlactating animals we felt that the principle pathway of secretion granule degradation was simply by the incorporation of secretion granules into dense body lysosomes or occasionally into autophagic bodies that were not only sequestering cell organelles, but that also could take up secretion granules and degrade them. In this case, where there has been such a tremendous surge of synthesis induced by exogenous hormone, which are then withdrawn very quickly so that the gland gets back to its previous state, events of massive granule degradation occur. In this case, acid phosphatase has an entity, possibly with the granule itself, which may self-destruct. The structure demonstrated there was probably a group of secretion granules whose acid phosphatase activity was related to their limiting membrane as well as to membrane that came probably, from the endoplasmic reticulum. These, then, formed an autophagic structure, and there was just this delimiting membrane of the granule mass. There was no need for the incorporation of a dense body or Golgi vesicles into that structure. This is a strict morphological observation and certainly is open to a certain degree of criticism.

DR. DE DUVE: It certainly creates some misgivings in a biochemist, because the term self-destruction implies that such a granule must contain, presumably in some kind of latent form, a rather complicated apparatus, capable of bringing about an extensive breakdown of proteins. Is it not more likely that this enzyme system was provided by a lysosome and that what you showed was simply a large, badly preserved, autophagic vacuole, containing a number of secretion granules together with lysosomal hydrolases? Remember that the acid phosphatase reaction product was deposited outside the granules. But perhaps this interpretation will not be acceptable to you on morphological grounds.

DR. SMITH: Well, certainly I would be very much aware of your stated opinions there because they represent the general trend of thinking and the most acceptable one, but I think there is reason to keep an open mind about the existence of enzymes within the membrane itself.

5′-NUCLEOTIDASE OF PLASMA MEMBRANES OF THE RAT LIVER: STUDIES ON SUBCELLULAR DISTRIBUTION

Chull S. Song and Attallah Kappas
The Rockefeller University, New York, N. Y.

Oscar Bodansky
The Sloan-Kettering Institute for Cancer Research, New York, N. Y.

Introduction

5′-Nucleotidase (5′-ribonucleotide phosphohydrolase, EC 3.1.3.5) is a specific phosphohydrolase that selectively catalyzes the hydrolysis of 5′-monophosphates of nucleosides.[1] It is widely distributed in nature, particularly in mammalian tissues, including those of man. In a purified form, 5′-nucleotidase is highly specific for nucleoside 5′-monophosphates in its hydrolytic action.[2–4] Thus, it catalyzes the hydrolytic removal of phosphoryl groups from various nucleotides such as AMP, CMP, UMP, etc., and their 5′-deoxy analogues. The enzyme may act, at a reduced rate, on certain phosphomonoesters that are structurally similar to 5′-nucleotides, e.g., nicotinamide mononucleotide[2,3] and ribose-5-phosphate.[5] However, it does not act on such unrelated phosphomonoesters as glucose-6-phosphate, glycerophosphate, phenylphosphate, fructose-6-phosphate, etc.

There has recently been a considerable interest among biochemists and cytologists for 5′-nucleotidase of the liver,[6–9] primarily because of earlier histochemical evidence[10–12] for concentration of this enzyme in plasma membrane of the liver parenchymal cells and the possibility, therefore, of using its activity as a marker for hepatic plasma membranes during cell fractionation. In this paper, we report the results of our studies on subcellular distribution of 5′-nucleotidase in the rat liver based on isolation of individual structural components of the liver cell.

Materials and Methods

We used female Sprague-Dawley rats (Charles River Laboratories) weighing 150 to 250 grams and following a period of overnight fasting (12 to 18 hours). For the preparation of plasma membrane fraction, rats weighing 150 to 200 grams were used. The sources of chemicals employed in the present investigation have been indicated in previous publications.[9,13]

The activities of the following enzymes were used as specific markers for components of the parenchymal cells of the rat liver: glucose-6-phosphatase for microsomal fraction deriving from the endoplasmic reticulum,[14,15] assayed at pH 6.5 with 0.015 M glucose-6-phosphate as substrate;[16] acid phosphatase for lysosomes,[17] assayed at pH 5.0 with 0.025 M β-glycerophosphate as substrate;[18] glutamate dehydrogenase for mitochondria,[19] determined by oxidation of NADH with 0.01 M α-ketoglutarate and 0.05 M NH_4Cl as substrates;[20] and NAD pyrophosphorylase (ATP:NMN adenylyl-transferase, EC 2.7.7.1.) for nuclei.[21] The assay for the latter enzyme was based on the rate of NAD produced from 0.003 M NMN and 0.004 M ATP in the presence of 0.015 M Ni^{++}.[9] 5′-Nucleotidase was assayed at pH 7.5 with 0.005 M AMP as substrate in the presence of 0.01 M Mg^{++}.[22] The activity of all the marker enzymes as well as 5′-nucleotidase remained relatively stable during various procedures for isolation of cell components. The loss of enzyme activity in all cases was less than 10%, and most of the small losses were due partly to problems inherent in transfering from one vessel to another and partly to slight inactivations.

Nuclei were isolated from the rat liver by the method originally reported by Chauveau *et al.*[23] with subsequent modifications by Maggio *et al.*[24] and Conover and Siebert.[25] This method consists essentially of subjecting the crude nuclear fraction (600 *g* pellet) of the homogenate to differential flotation in 2.2 M solution of sucrose containing $CaCl_2$ to obtain a relatively pure pellet of nuclei, N-1. N-1 was then further purified by pelleting it through 2.2 M solution of sucrose again to obtain the final preparation, N-2. A cell fraction containing both mitochondria and lysosomes, but relatively free from other cytoplasmic components, was prepared according to the method of Schneider.[26] During washing procedures, we retained the light, fluffy upper layer of the mitochondrial pellets. The method of Palade and Siekevitz[27] was used to isolate the microsomal fraction. Plasma membranes were isolated according to the procedure reported by Neville.[28] This procedure consists of rupturing the liver cells by Dounce homogenizer (Blaessig Glass Specialties) and repeatedly washing the resulting homogenate in a hypotonic medium to obtain a crude preparation of plasma membranes, M-1. M-1 was then further purified by flotation through 1.76 M solution of sucrose, which yields the final preparation, M-2.

A plasma membrane fraction rich in intact bile canaliculi was prepared according to the following procedure,[13] which is a modification of the method of Neville[28] and of Emmelot *et al.*[29] Minced rat livers were homogenized in large Dounce homogenizers with loose-fitting pestles, then diluted and centrifuged essentially as reported previously.[28] The pellets were pooled and suspended by gentle shaking in 0.001 M $NaHCO_3$ (pH 7.5) to the final volume (ml) corresponding to the original weight of the liver (g). To this suspension of crude plasma membrane preparations, exactly 5.5 volumes of sucrose solution of density 1.26 (70.74%, w/v) were added, and the mixture was gently homogenized in a Dounce homogenizer until the membranes became evenly dispersed (2 to 10 strokes). Ten-ml aliquots of this suspension were placed in cellulose nitrate tubes (Beckman, No. 302237) and overlaid successively with 7 and 5 ml of sucrose solutions of densities 1.18 (48.45%, w/v) and 1.16 (42.9%, w/v), respectively. The tubes were then placed in a Spinco No. 30 rotor and centrifuged for 60 min at 66,000 *g*. The white sheet of tissue fraction collected at the upper interface of sucrose solutions in the tube was collected by means of a syringe, diluted with 4–5 volumes of 0.001 M $NaHCO_3$ buffer and centrifuged for 10 min at 1,500 *g*. The pellet was washed once in the same buffer and used for morphological and enzymatic studies.

The microsomal fraction was separated into two subfractions, one containing primarily smooth membrane vesicles and the other containing largely rough membrane vesicles with attached ribosomes, according to the method reported by Dallner *et al.*[30] The final centrifugation was for 45 min at 134,000 *g* in a Spinco Type 50 Titanium Rotor. This method depends on the difference in the buoyant density of the two microsomal subfractions for separation in discontinuous gradient of sucrose solution. Free ribosomes contained in the microsomal fraction were separated in continuous density-gradient solution of sucrose as reported by Henshaw *et al.*[31]

Tissue fractions were fixed in glutaraldehyde with or without osmium tetroxide, dehydrated in graded concentrations of ethanol and propylene oxide. Thin sections were stained with lead hydroxide or lead citrate. All specimens were examined in a Siemens Elmiskop 1A or a Philips EM-200 electron microscope.

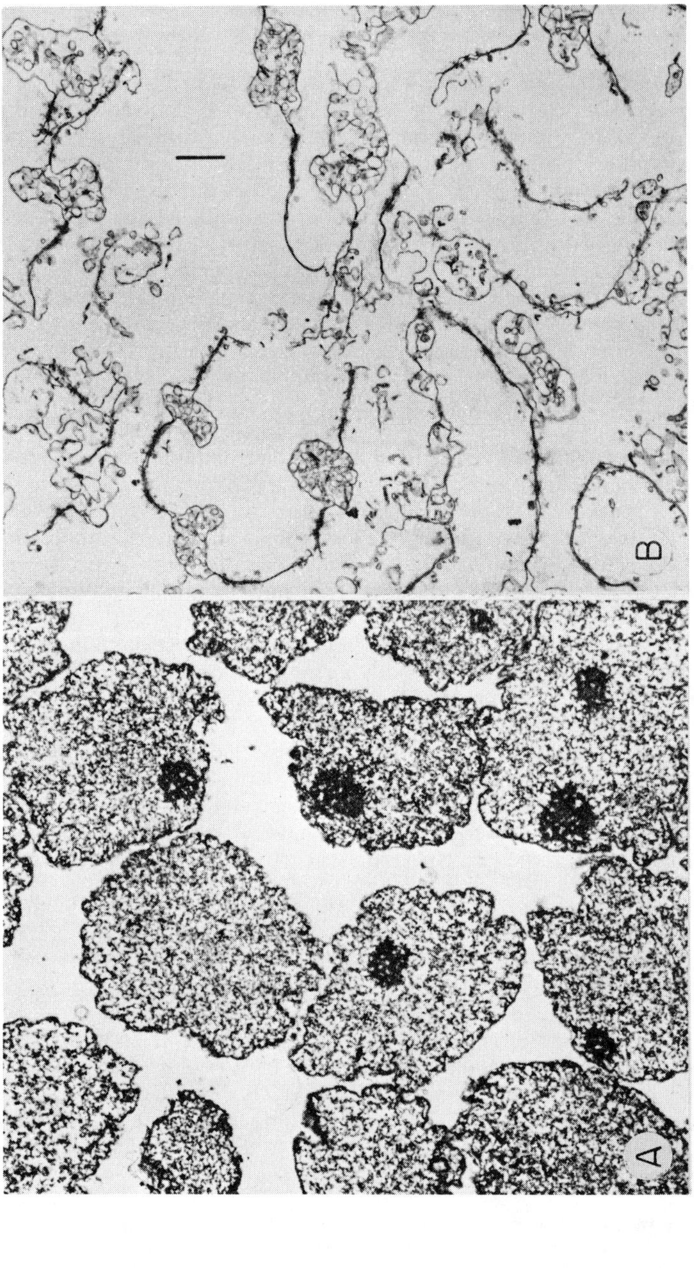

FIGURE 1. Electron micrographs of nuclei (A) and plasma membrane fraction containing bile canaliculi (B) isolated from the rat liver. Magnifications: (A), ×4,800; (B), ×6,000.

Results

The final preparation of nuclei, N-2, when examined in the electron microscope, consisted of nuclei of parenchymal cells with double-layered nuclear membrane (FIGURE 1 A). Although many nuclei appeared slightly crenated, most of the nuclear membranes were intact. Very few membrane fragments or vesicles of cytoplasmic origin were noted in the preparation of nuclei.

The recovery of nuclei at each preparatory step was followed by assaying for DNA and NAD pyrophosphorylase (TABLE 1). In terms of DNA, the final preparation (N-2) yielded about 30% of the total liver cell nuclei. The recovery of nuclear marker enzyme, NAD pyrophosphorylase, although somewhat less in each fraction due to slight inactivation, roughly paralleled the DNA recovery. The specific activity for NAD pyrophosphorylase in N-2 was 16 times as high as that in the initial homogenate. The recovery and specific activity of glucose-6-phosphatase, an enzyme used as a marker for fragments of endoplasmic reticulum (or microsomal membranes), showed a marked decrease with the purification of nuclei in N-1 and N-2. The recovery of this enzyme in N-2 was practically negligible. 5′-Nucleotidase behaved in a similar fashion during isolation of the nuclei, so that N-2 contained less than 0.2% of the activity present in the original homogenate.

A cell fraction containing primarily mitochondria and lysosomes yielded about 40% of the mitochondrial marker, glutamate dehydrogenase, and about 20% of the lysosomal marker, acid phosphatase. Again, practically no glucose-6-phosphatase or 5′-nucleotidase was detectable in the final preparations, indicating little contamination of the mitochondria-lysosomal fraction with microsomal components and the absence of 5′-nucleotidase in mitochondrial or lysosomal fractions of the rat liver.

The final yields of glucose-6-phosphatase and 5′-nucleotidase in microsomal fraction ranged from 23 to 27%, with an approximately twofold increase in their specific activities (TABLE 2). The microsomal fractions contained a small amount of lysosomes as shown by approximately 7.5% recovery of the total acid phosphatase activity in this fraction. The specific activity for this enzyme, however, was lower in the microsomal fraction than in the original homogenate.

The microsomal fraction of the liver was separated into free ribosomes and the membrane-containing fraction by centrifugation through a density-gradient solution of sucrose (FIGURE 2). In studies in which the overall recovery of 5′-

TABLE 1

RECOVERY OF DNA, PROTEIN, 5′-NUCLEOTIDASE, GLUCOSE-6-PHOSPHATASE AND NAD PYROPHOSPHORYLASE DURING ISOLATION OF RAT LIVER NUCLEI*

Fraction	Total DNA Phosphorus	Total Protein	Enzymes Recovered: Glucose-6-Phosphatase	Enzymes Recovered: 5′-Nucleotidase	Enzymes Recovered: NAD pyrophosphorylase
	(μg)	(mg)	(μg P/min/ml)	(μg P/min/ml)	(μmole NAD/min)
Homogenate	1370	1150	437	308	0.644
600 *g* Pellet	1110	290	62	72	0.510
N–1	398	18	0.8	1.2	0.163
N–2	417	16	0.4	0.4	0.142

* A rat liver weighing 8 g was used to obtain a preparation of nuclei according to the method described in the text. The units of glucose-6-phosphatase and 5′-nucleotidase activities are expressed as μg phosphorus released/min/ml reaction mixture. The unit of NAD pyrophosphorylase activity is expressed as μmole NAD formed/min.

TABLE 2

RECOVERY OF PROTEIN, 5′-NUCLEOTIDASE, GLUCOSE-6-PHOSPHATASE AND ACID PHOSPHATASE IN ISOLATED MICROSOMAL FRACTION OF RAT LIVER*

Fraction	Total Protein	Enzymes Recovered: Glucose-6-phosphatase	Enzymes Recovered: 5′-Nucleotidase	Enzymes Recovered: Acid Phosphatase
	(mg)	(μg P/min/ml)	(μg P/min/ml)	(μg P/min/ml)
Homogenate	1120	367	353	174
Microsomes	130	99	79	13

* A rat liver weighing 6.3 g was used to prepare the microsomal fraction. The units of enzyme activity in all cases are defined as μg phosphorus released/min/ml reaction mixture.

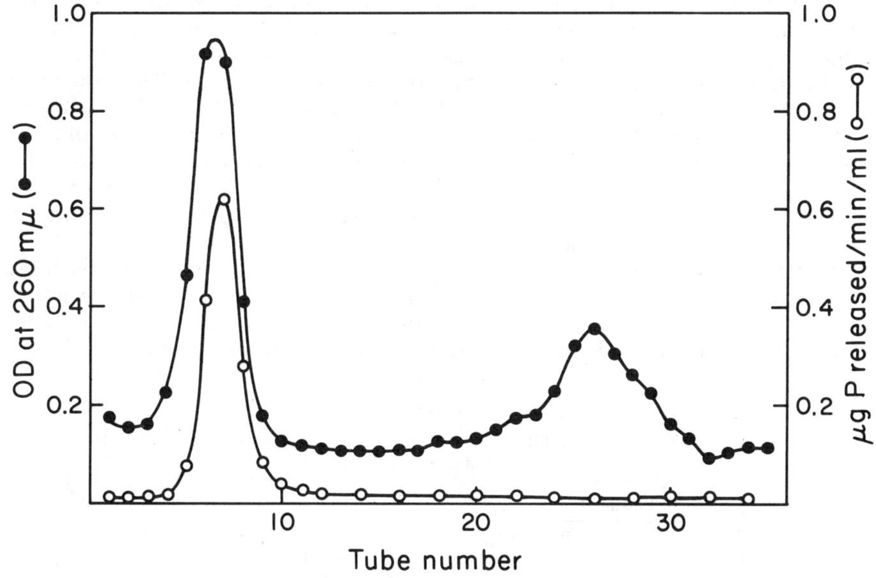

FIGURE 2. Centrifugation of the microsomal fraction of the rat liver through density-gradient solution of sucrose. Microsomal pellet was suspended in a medium containing 0.05 M Tris (pH 7.8), 0.1 mM $MgCl_2$, and 0.05 M KCl. One ml of this suspension was layered over 20 ml of sucrose solution in a linear gradient from 5 to 20% (w/v). Each tube, in addition, contained a 5-ml cushion of 50% (w/v) sucrose solution at the bottom. All sucrose solutions were prepared in the same medium. The tubes were centrifuged for 150 min at 20,000 rpm in a Spinco SW25.1 rotor. Fractions were collected from the bottom of each tube and analyzed for absorbance at 260 mμ (●——●) and 5′-nucleotidase activity (○——○). The fractions are numbered from the bottom of the gradient.

nucleotidase in the effluent fractions was essentially complete, more than 90% of the enzyme activity was associated with the membrane-containing fraction of the microsomes. No 5′-nucleotidase activity was detectable in effluent fractions corresponding to the free ribosomes sedimenting at the rate of 83 S. When microsomal membranes were solubilized in 0.5% solution of sodium deoxycholate, a large proportion of microsomal 5′-nucleotidase was released from the membrane component that remained in the supernatant following centrifugation at 105,000 *g* for two hours.

The specific activities of glucose-6-phosphatase and 5′-nucleotidase in microsomal subfractions, viz. the lighter fraction consisting chiefly of smooth membrane vesicles and the heavier fraction mainly of rough membrane vesicles with attached ribosomes,[30] are given in TABLE 3. Some divergence in concentration of these phosphohydrolases was noted. Glucose-6-phosphatase was concentrated more in the heavier microsomal membranes, while 5′-nucleotidase was more active in the lighter membranes. The heavier fraction, presumably consisting primarily of rough membrane vesicles and thus membranes deriving from the endoplasmic reticulum, contained a considerable amount of 5′-nucleotidase activity. The difference in specific activity of 5′-nucleotidase between the lighter and heavier fractions amounted to only about 22%. Since the heavier fraction contained proteins of free and attached ribosomes, the actual difference in specific activity would be less than this value.

A marked increase in the specific activity for 5′-nucleotidase was noted during the isolation of plasma membranes (TABLE 4). The specific activity in N-2, the final preparation, was about 12 times as high as in the starting homogenate. It should be noted, however, that the total recovery of 5′-nucleotidase in the final preparation was no more than 1.4% of the activity present in the homogenate. An enrichment of 5′-nucleotidase of comparable magnitude[13] was obtained in plasma membrane fractions containing a high concentration of intact bile canaliculi (FIGURE 1 B). The total recovery of 5′-nucleotidase in the final preparations was approximately 3%. Trace activity of glucose-6-phosphatase was detectable in all preparations of plasma membranes.

Repeated washings of the plasma membrane preparations in various buffer solutions or in an isotonic solution of NaCl did not release 5′-nucleotidase activity from the membranes. Prolonged sonic oscillation of microsomal suspension[32] only partially released 5′-nucleotidase into the suspending medium, with con-

TABLE 3

SPECIFIC ACTIVITIES OF GLUCOSE-6-PHOSPHATASE AND 5′-NUCLEOTIDASE IN MICROSOMAL SUBFRACTIONS*

Glucose-6-Phosphatase		5′-Nucleotidase	
(Top)	(Bottom)	(Top)	(Bottom)
0.91	1.42	0.50	0.39

* Microsomal fraction of the rat liver was separated into a heavier fraction (bottom) containing rough membrane vesicles, and a lighter fraction (top) containing smooth membrane vesicles. The heavier fraction also contained free ribosomes. The units of enzyme activity are defined as μg phosphorus released/min/ml reaction mixture. Specific activity is defined as Units/mg protein.

TABLE 4

RECOVERY OF PROTEIN AND ENZYME ACTIVITIES DURING ISOLATION OF RAT LIVER PLASMA MEMBRANES*

Fraction	Total Protein	Glucose-6-Phosphatase Total Activity	Glucose-6-Phosphatase Specific Activity	5′-Nucleotidase Total Activity	5′-Nucleotidase Specific Activity
	(mg)	(μg P/min/ml)	(U/mg protein)	(μg P/min/ml)	(U/mg protein)
Homogenate	1680	956	0.57	705	0.42
N–1	13.0	1.69	0.13	22.4	1.72
N–2	2.0	0.14	0.07	9.8	4.89

* Pooled rat livers weighing 10 g were used to obtain a preparation of plasma membranes. The units of enzyme activity are defined as μg phosphorus released/min/ml reaction mixture. Specific activity is defined as Units/mg protein.

comitant dissociation into subunits of antigenic materials of the microsomal membranes. The enzyme activity was readily solubilized, however, in solutions of sodium deoxycholate.[9]

Discussion

Our studies indicate that 5′-nucleotidase of the rat liver is located solely in the microsomal membranes. When the liver nuclei are isolated in a state virtually free from cytoplasmic membranes, they exhibit no more than a trace of 5′-nucleotidase activity. Thus, a substantial recovery of this enzyme in the crude nuclear fraction[33,34] must be attributable to contamination of this fraction with microsomal membranes.

It is now well known that microsomal membranes are of heterogeneous origin and, although they derive mostly from fragments of endoplasmic reticulum, other minor cell components such as Golgi apparatus and plasma membranes make contributions.[27] Our studies show that a high concentration of 5′-nucleotidase activity is present in the plasma membranes and the bile canaliculi of the rat liver.

Comparison of specific activities suggests that a large proportion of the 5′-nucleotidase of the microsomal membranes may actually derive from plasma membrane fragments. However, because of the low yield of plasma membranes prepared according to the existing methods (1.4% to 3% of the original 5′-nucleotidase activity), it is not possible to estimate quantitatively the fraction of microsomal 5′nucleotidase activity that can be assigned to the plasma membrane fragments.

The distribution of 5′-nucleotidase between the heavier and lighter subfractions of the microsomal preparations suggest that a substantial proportion of total microsomal 5′-nucleotidase may be present in the heavier fraction, i.e., in those membranes with attached ribosomes (rough membranes) and therefore deriving primarily from the endoplasmic reticulum rather than the plasma membrane. These findings also have to be interpreted with caution because of difficulties with existing methods for a clean, total separation of smooth from rough membrane vesicles making up the microsomal fraction.[30,35]

A better separation of microsomal subfractions, together with quantitative counting of smooth and rough vesicles, when coupled with direct enzymatic assay, may clarify these problems. Further development in the use of a high-speed zonal centrifuge[6,36] may prove to be of considerable use. Until such studies are available, 5′-nucleotidase should be used with caution as a quantitative marker for hepatic plasma membranes.

References

1. HEPPEL, L. A. 1961. "5-Nucleotidase." *In* The Enzymes. Ed. by P. D. Boyer, H. Lardy & K. Myrbäck, Eds. **5**: 49. Academic Press, Inc., New York, N. Y.
2. HEPPEL, L. A. & R. J. HILMOE. 1951. J. Biol. Chem. **188**: 665.
3. SONG, C. S. & O. BODANSKY. 1966. Biochem. J. **101**: 5c.
4. LEVIN, S. J. & O. BODANSKY. 1966. J. Biol. Chem. **241**: 51.
5. SCHWARTZ, M. N. & N. O. KAPLAN. 1956. Science **123**: 50.
6. EL-AASER, A. A., E. REID, E. KLUCIS, P. ALEXANDER, J. T. LETT & J. SMITH. 1966. Nat. Cancer Inst. Monogr. **21**: 323.
7. REID, E. 1967. *In* Enzyme Cytology. D. B. Roodyn. : 321. Academic Press, Inc., New York, N. Y.
8. COLEMAN, R., R. M. MICHELL & J. B. FINEAN. 1967. Biochem. J. **105**: 5.
9. SONG, C. S. & O. BODANSKY. 1967. J. Biol. Chem. **242**: 694.
10. WACHSTEIN, M. & E. MEISEL. 1957. Amer. J. Clin. Path. **27**: 13.

11. WACHSTEIN, M. & E. MEISEL. 1959. J. Histochem. Cytochem. 7: 189.
12. ESSNER, E., A. B. NOVIKOFF & B. MASEK. 1958. J. Biophys. Biochem. Cytol. 4: 711.
13. SONG, C. S., W. RUBIN, A. B. RIFKIND & A. KAPPAS. 1969. J. Cell Biol. 41: 124.
14. DE DUVE, C., B. C. PRESSMAN, R. GIANETTO, R. WATTIAUX & F. APPLEMANS. 1955. Biochem. J. 60: 604.
15. TICE, L. W. & R. J. BARNETT. 1962. J. Histochem. Cytochem. 10: 754.
16. SCHWARTZ, M. K. & O. BODANSKY. 1961. Meth. Med. Res. 9: 5.
17. BEAUFAY, H., D. S. BENDALL, P. BAUDHUIN, R. WATTIAUX & C. DE DUVE. 1959. Biochem. J. 73: 628.
18. APPLEMANS, F., R. WATTIAUX & C. DE DUVE. 1955. Biochem. J. 59: 438.
19. BEAUFAY, H., D. S. BENDALL, P. BAUDHUIN & C. DE DUVE. 1959. Biochem. J. 73: 623.
20. HOGEBOOM, G. H. & W. C. SCHNEIDER. 1953. J. Biol. Chem. 204: 233.
21. HOGEBOOM, G. H. & W. C. SCHNEIDER. 1952. J. Biol. Chem. 197: 611.
22. BODANSKY, O. & M. K. SCHWARTZ. 1963. J. Biol. Chem. 238: 3420.
23. CHAUVEAU, J., Y. MOULÉ & C. ROUILLER. 1956. Exp. Cell Res. 11: 317.
24. MAGGIO, R., P. SIEKEVITZ & G. E. PALADE. 1963. J. Cell Biol. 18: 267.
25. CONOVER, T. E. & G. SIEBERT. 1965. Biochim. Biophys. Acta 99: 1.
26. SCHNEIDER, W. C. 1948. J. Biol. Chem. 176: 259.
27. PALADE, G. E. & P. SIEKEVITZ. 1956. J. Biophys. Biochem. Cytol. 2: 171.
28. NEVILLE, D. M. 1960. J. Biophys. Biochem. Cytol. 8: 413.
29. EMMELOT, P., C. J. BOS, E. L. BENEDETTI & P. RÜMKE. 1964. Biochim. Biophys. Acta 90: 126.
30. DALLNER, G., S. ORRENIUS & A. BERGSTRAND. 1963. J. Cell Biol. 16: 426.
31. HENSHAW, E. C., T. B. BOJARSKI & H. H. HIATT. 1963. J. Molec. Biol. 7: 122.
32. SONG, C. S., J. S. NISSELBAUM, B. TANDLER & O. BODANSKY. 1967. Biochim. Biophys. Acta 150: 300.
33. NOVIKOFF, A. B., E. PODBER & J. RYAN. 1950. Fed. Proc. 9: 210.
34. DE LAMIRANDE, G., C. ALLARD & A. CANTERO. 1958. J. Biophys. Biochem. Cytol. 4: 373.
35. FOUTS, J. R. 1961. Biochem. Biophys. Res. Comm. 6: 378.
36. ANDERSON, N. G. 1966. Science 154: 103.

Acknowledgments

Thanks are due to Dr. Walter Rubin and Mr. Robert Erlandson for help in preparing the electron micrographs used in the present investigation. The capable technical assistance of Miss Linda Almazon in some of the present studies is gratefully acknowledged.

Discussion of the Paper

R. C. NORDLIE: I wonder whether the biphasic pH activity curve that you described was observed with all concentrations of magnesium you used or whether it was somewhat dependent upon the particular concentration of magnesium. In other words, could you type the polyphasic effect right away if you were to raise magnesium from the levels that you used?

DR. SONG: This has been extensively studied by Doctors Levin and Bodansky,[4] and there is some concentration effect. At 0.005 M, one begins to observe the biphasic effects.

DR. NORDLIE: Well, we saw something quite similar to this effect with inorganic pyrophosphatase, and in this case we could type right away completely the biphasic curve by increasing magnesium. We attributed this to a very complex phenomenon in which magnesium binds to pyrophosphate. pH affects not only the affinity of the substrate for the enzyme but the affinity of pyrophosphate for magnesium. We presume that this is the complex. I was wondering whether there might be a similarity here, although I realize that the compound you're using doesn't bind the metal to anywhere near the extent that pyrophosphate does.

Dr. Song: Yes, that is very interesting. The kinetic studies of Drs. Levin and Bodansky[4] have shown some evidence that there is indeed a magnesium binding site also on the enzyme.

F. Roels (*Ames Research Laboratory, Elkhart, Ind.*): I have two questions and one comment. There have been numerous papers published by Leon Heppel and Harold Nieu from Columbia. In their studies, they have shown about three-fold higher activation by cobalt as against that by magnesium. Did you find, or did you try, cobalt for activation?

Dr. Song: Yes, cobalt is a slight activator of nucleotidase from mammalian sources. However, it does not activate the enzyme at alkaline pH to the extent that magnesium does, so we do not observe a double pH profile with cobalt.

Dr. Madre: Also in their studies on selective release by osmotic shock, they showed that there was an inhibitor present in spheroplast if you use simply the frequency methods.

Dr. Song: We have on numerous occasions attempted to demonstrate possible inhibitors. We haven't been able to detect any such inhibitor activity, at least in the rat liver homogenate.

C. de Duve: Concerning the relationship between plasma membranes and lysosomes, I might mention briefly some recent results obtained in Louvain by Drs. J. Berthet, H. Beaufay and their coworkers. Using isopycnic density gradient centrifugation in sucrose gradients, they have found that the 5′-nucleotidase activity of microsomal fractions equilibrates at a distinctly lower density than do many other microsomal constituents, except cholesterol, which follows exactly the distribution of 5′-nucleotidase. Their tentative interpretation is that these two constituents are associated with membrane fragments originating from, or related to, the plasma membrane, and not with the endoplasmic reticulum itself. There is a difficulty, however, in the interpretation of all results obtained on purified plasma membranes. So far, enzymes typically attached to the plasma membrane, such as 5′-nucleotidase, have been purified no more than 30 to 50-fold in such preparations, suggesting that the total amount of protein associated with the plasma membrane may be as much as 2 to 3% of the total cell content. This is a very high amount for what is believed to be only a surface film. Possibly, the plasma membrane may be highly convoluted, or many of the vesicles seen in the cytoplasm may be surrounded by a membrane of plasma membrane type. Such could, of course, be the case for endocytic vesicles and also for secondary lysosomes derived from them

Dr. Song: Thank you, Dr. de Duve. We've noticed in most of the preparations of plasma membranes that there is a weak but detectable amount of glucose-6-phosphatase activity, and it is probable that these preparations are not really completely pure in the sense that they derive exclusively from the surrounding membranes of the cells. At least by histochemistry, glucose-6-phosphatase does not localize on the surface membrane. We have tried using the Anderson zonal rotor[36] for the type of a separation Dr. de Duve has just mentioned. We did notice a larger proportion of 5′-nucleotidase on the light fraction; however, some was always associated with the heavier fraction, presumably containing microsomal membranes, which had a lot of glucose-6-phosphatase activity; so we haven't been able to reach a firm conclusion in this regard.

Dr. de Duve: The separations I mentioned were based on density equilibration, not on zonal differential sedimentation through a gradient.

SOLUBLE AND MEMBRANE-ASSOCIATED FORMS OF ACID PHOSPHATASE ASSOCIATED WITH THE LYSOSOMAL FRACTION OF RAT LIVER

Barbara Furin Sloat* and John M. Allen

Department of Zoology
The University of Michigan
Ann Arbor, Mich.

Introduction

As initially formulated (de Duve, 1959), the lysosome concept held that the hydrolytic enzymes associated with lysosomes are contained within the particles and that constraint from hydrolytic action is provided by the particle membrane, which acts as a barrier to enzyme-substrate interaction. Rupture of the lysosomal membrane, within this context, should result in the simultaneous release of all internal enzymes in a soluble and fully active form, rendering them accessible to substrates of the cytoplasm. A disparity between the total acid phosphatase activity of the intact lysosomal fraction and the unsedimentable activity of the released enzyme was noted, however, as early as 1951 (Berthet *et al.*, 1951). This discrepancy was accounted for on the basis of secondary adsorption of enzyme to lysosomal structure (Berthet *et al.*, 1951; Appelmans & de Duve, 1958; de Duve, 1959).

Recently, morphological and biochemical data have become available suggesting that this view of the association between the lysosomal hydrolases and lysosomal structure may have to be revised. Electron microscopic observations show that the lysosome may possess a complex internal structure (Novikoff *et al.*, 1956; Van Lancker & Sempoux, 1958; Daems & Van Rijssel, 1961; Koenig, 1962), and biochemical determinations suggest that lysosomes may possess structure-bound enzymes that are not released by simple physical disruption. An inability to release all acid phosphatase from rat liver lysosomes by physical disruption was reported by Shibko and Tappel (1963). Similarly, Allen and Gockerman (1964) were unable to effect total release of acid phosphatase from rat liver lysosomes by physical disruption, but did achieve total solubilization in the presence of Triton X-100. These authors further demonstrated the presnce of two electrophoretically distinct acid phosphatases in their mitochondrial-lysosomal fraction. These forms exhibited differential release properties, one being released by physical disruption of the particles and the other only after treatment of the fraction with Triton X-100. In addition to these instances, other lysosomal enzymes reported to be bound in part to lysosomal structure include aryl sulfatase A (Ugazio & Pani, 1963), an esterase (Shibko & Tappel, 1964), β-acetyl glucosaminidase (Weissman *et al.*, 1967), and β-glucosidase (Beck & Tappel, 1968).

This paper deals with a more definitive localization of a bound form of acid phosphatase to the lysosomal fraction of rat liver, with some physical and biochemical properties of the bound and soluble acid phosphatase of this fraction, and with the behavior of these enzymes in the lysosomes of regenerating rat liver.

* Portions of this work were submitted in partial fulfillment of the requirements for the Ph.D. degree. The work was supported by funds from an NIH training grant in the Department of Zoology, The University of Michigan, (NIH 5T 01GM00989).

Materials and Methods

Preparation of Liver Homogenates

Normal tissue. Normal tissue used in quantitative and electrophoretic studies was obtained from 300 to 400-gram albino male rats. Animals were fed a diet of Purina Lab Chow and water *ad libitum.* After a starvation period of 12 to 18 hours, animals were sacrificed by cervical dislocation. The liver was removed immediately, weighed, and an initial 20% (w/v) homogenate prepared by bringing 20 g of tissue to a final volume of 100 ml with 0.25 M sucrose (Merck, reagent grade). Tissue was homogenized at O°C in a smooth glass homogenizer with a Teflon pestle using 5 to 8 up-down strokes at 1200 rev/min.

Regenerated tissue. Animals were partially hepatectomized under Nembutal anesthesia (Merck, 20 mg/kg body weight) according to the method of Higgins and Anderson (1931). At the time of partial hepatectomy, the median and left lateral lobes were ligated and removed. This tissue was homogenized as above and utilized as control tissue. During the first 24 hours after the operation, animals were provided with 20% dextrose (Mallinckrodt analytical) *ad libitum.* After this period, food and water were given as usual. After the required regeneration period, animals were sacrificed and homogenates prepared as previously described.

Differential Centrifugation

Normal and regenerated whole tissue homogenates were subjected to differential centrifugation at 4° C according to one of the following schemes. Centrifugation times and *g* values are designated exclusive of acceleration and deceleration times and are based on average r-values.

Scheme 1:

Nuclear fraction. Whole homogenates were centrifuged at 480 × *g* for 10 minutes followed by two washes (5 up-down strokes each), resuspensions, and recentrifugations at 270 × *g* for 10 minutes each. The washed pellet was resuspended to starting volume in 0.25 M sucrose to yield a final 20% fraction. All other pellets were resuspended to starting volume in the same manner.

Mitochondrial-lysosomal fraction. The combined supernatants from the nuclear step were centrifuged at 22,000 × *g* for 30 minutes to sediment mitochondria and lysosomes.

Microsomal-soluble fraction. The supernatant remaining after the mitochondrial-lysosomal centrifugation was designated the microsomal-soluble fraction. All centrifugations were carried out in a Servall RC 2 refrigerated centrifuge equipped with an SS-34 rotor.

Scheme 2:

Nuclear fraction. Whole homogenates were centrifuged at 270 × *g* for 10 minutes. Two resuspensions (homogenized with 8 up-down strokes at 1,200 rev/min) and recentrifugations followed at the same speed and time. The washed pellet was brought to starting volume with 0.25 M sucrose.

Mitochondrial fraction. The combined supernatants from the nuclear sedimentation were centrifuged at 2,500 × *g* for 10 minutes. The pellet was resuspended, homogenized by hand, and recentrifuged at the same speed and time to yield the final mitochondrial pellet. Resuspension to starting volume with 0.25 M sucrose followed.

Lysosomal fraction. Mitochondrial supernatants were combined and centrifuged at 8,700 × *g* for 20 minutes. The lysosomal pellet was brought to starting volume in 0.25 M sucrose as described. All steps to this point were carried out using a Servall refrigerated centrifuge (RC 2) equipped with an SS-34 rotor. Subsequent fractions were obtained using a Spinco Ti50 rotor in a Spinco L2-50 centrifuge.

Microsomal fraction. The lysosomal supernatant was centrifuged at 165,000 × *g* for 60 minutes to yield a microsomal pellet that was resuspended to starting volume in 0.25 M sucrose.

Soluble fraction. The supernatant from the microsomal centrifugation constituted the soluble fraction.

Recoveries of enzymatic activity, calculated as percent of whole homogenate activity present in summed fractions, averaged 98% for acid phosphatase; 98% for glucose-6-phosphatase; and 100% for succinic dehydrogenase.

Density Gradient Centrifugations

Gradients were made and fractions collected using a Buchler density gradient device following the method of Martin and Ames (1961). Linearity of the gradients was confirmed by spectrophotometric measurement of dichlorophenolindophenol (DCIP) incorporated into gradients during preparation. Three types of gradients were utilized:

1. Density equilibrium centrifugation was carried out at 4° C according to Beaufay *et al.*, (1964), using a Spinco SW 39 rotor in a Spinco Model L2-50 centrifuge. Sucrose gradients of density 1.12 to 1.26 were prepared and stored 12 to 18 hours at 4° C before use. Four hundred μl samples of 20% homogenates from which nuclei had been removed were layered on 4.6 ml gradients to yield a final tube volume of 5.0 ml. Centrifugation at 124,000 × *g* was carried out at 4° C for 2.5 hours.

2. *Sedimentation* behavior of released soluble and bound forms of acid phosphatase was examined employing 5 to 20% sucrose: water gradients (density 1.017 to 1.074) according to the method of Martin and Ames (1961). One hundred μl of a 20% sample were layered on gradients prepared 12 to 18 hours before use and stored at 4° C. Final tube volume was 4.7 ml. Centrifugation was carried out at 4° C for 4 and 8 hours at 124,000 × *g* using a Spinco L 2–50 centrifuge equipped with a Spinco SW 39 rotor.

3. *Velocity density gradient centrifugation* experiments were carried out using 0.25 M to 0.7 M sucrose: water gradients (density based on sucrose concentration, 1.032 to 1.090. Gradients were made 1.0 M with KCl (Baker reagent grade) and prepared at 4° C just prior to use. A 200 μl cushion of 2.0 M sucrose was utilized to facilitate collection of sedimented material. Prior to layering, homogenates were made 0.2 M with respect to sucrose and 1.0 M with KCl. Two hundred μl of a 4% homogenate from which the nuclei had been removed were layered on gradients to yield a tube volume of 5.0 ml. Centrifugation was carried out at 4° C for 20 minutes at 4,000, 8,000, and 124,000 × *g* using a Spinco L2-50 centrifuge equipped with a Spinco SW 39 rotor.

Data are presented as relative activities, calculated as the enzyme activity present in each fraction divided by the calculated mean enzyme activity per fraction. Sedimentation behavior of particles as determined by marker enzyme positions in the gradients is described in terms of median density position in centimeters from the axis of rotation (Hogeboom & Kuff, 1954).

Enzyme Assays

Biochemical determination of enzyme activity was made according to the following methods. For all assays, substrate was not limiting. Reaction rates were linear with time and enzyme concentration.

Acid phosphatase activity was determined using (a) α-naphthyl acid phosphate (Sigma), (b) *p*-nitrophenyl phosphate (Sigma), and (c) sodium β-glycerophosphate (Sigma) as substrates.

(a) α-naphthol liberated enzymatically from sodium α-naphthyl acid phosphate at pH 5.0 was determined according to the method of Allen and Gockerman (1964).

(b) *p*-nitrophenol liberated enzymatically at pH 5.0 from *p*-nitrophenyl phosphate was determined according to Sigma Technical Bulletin 104 (1963).

(c) Measurement of phosphate produced by enzymatic hydrolysis of β-glycerophosphate at pH 5.0 was accomplished by a modification of the method of Shinowara *et al.* (1942) and Dryer *et al.* (1957). The reaction mixture contained sodium acetate-acetic acid buffer, pH 5.0, 45 mM and sodium β-glycerophosphate, 34 mM. After incubation at 37° C, the reaction was stopped by adding 30% trichloroacetic acid (Baker), two parts to ten parts of reaction mixture. Precipitated protein was removed by centrifugation. Samples of TCA-supernatant were assayed for inorganic phosphate using the following proportions of reactants: ammonium molybdate (Baker), 0.04 M, 1 part; TCA-supernatant, 3 parts; *N*-phenyl-*p*-phenylenediamine monohydrochloride (Eastman), 0.05 M in 1% sodium bisulfite (Mallinckrodt), 6 parts. Color was developed at room temperature for 10 minutes. Optical density was measured at 700 mμ with a Coleman Model 6A spectrophotometer.

Glucose-6-phosphatase activity was determined by measuring inorganic phosphate enzymatically released from glucose-6-phosphate at pH 6.5 according to Swanson (1955). The inorganic phosphate produced was determined as above.

Succinic dehydrogenase activity was measured by the enzymatic reduction of 2,6 dichlorophenolindophenol as described by Allen and Beard (1965).

Enzyme Activity in Supernatants and Sediments

Supernatant portions of lysosomal fractions were obtained by subjecting fractions to blending for 5 minutes at 4° C (Eberbach microattachment, Waring Blendor, 2 cm blade, 15,000 rev/min), followed by centrifugation at 4° C in a Spinco Model L centrifuge at 100,000 $\times$ *g* for 60 minutes. The acid phosphatase activity associated with this supernatant was termed soluble acid phosphatase. Sediments derived after centrifugation were resuspended to starting volume with 0.25 M sucrose. Acid phosphatase activity associated with the sediment was termed bound acid phosphatase. Bound enzyme was released into the soluble phase and rendered electrophoretically mobile in the presence of a 5% final concentration of Triton X-100 (Rohm and Haas). When biochemical or electrophoretic studies required bound enzyme free of soluble enzyme contamination, pellets were subjected to four cycles of washing with 0.25 M sucrose or water, resuspension, and centrifugation at 100,000 $\times$ *g* for 20 minutes before final resuspension to starting volume. Summed supernatant and sediment activities approached 100% of the activity of whole unseparated fractions. Physically solubilized enzyme accounted for 58% of the acid phosphatase activity of the lysosomal fraction, while 38% of the total activity was associated with the sediment.

Electrophoretic Separation of Enzymes

Acrylamide electrophoresis. Electrophoretic separation of bound and soluble acid phosphatase in acrylamide gels was accomplished according to the method of Allen and Gockerman (1964). Localization of acid phosphatase in gels was achieved by incubating gels in a reaction mixture containing 0.005 M sodium a-naphthyl acid phosphate and o-aminoazotoluene (Diazo Garnet GBC, Dajac), as described by Allen and Gockerman (1964). Gels were incubated at 25° C. The reaction was stopped by replacement of the reaction mixture with 7.5% acetic acid. Densitometric measurement of dye deposited in the gels was accomplished with a scanning device attached to a Beckman DU spectrophotometer (Johnson & Starkweather, 1962). Gels were scanned in 7.5% acetic acid. Optical density was measured at 545 mμ using a Beckman potentiometric recorder. Deposition of enzymatically produced reaction product was linear with incubation time and enzyme concentration within the limits used for assay.

Small-scale preparative electrophoresis. A small-scale preparative electrophoretic system was constructed according to the specifications of Racusen and Calvanico (1964). Gel stocks and buffers were prepared exactly as for routine acrylamide electrophoresis (Allen & Gockerman, 1964). Three ml (1 cm height) of lower gel solution was added to the separating chamber (1.8 cm I.D.). After polymerization, 6 ml of a sample:sample gel mixture (1:2) was layered onto the separating gel. Polymerization was effected for 20 minutes with an ultraviolet light source. Eluates were collected from a plastic eluting chamber fitted with an inlet and outlet of polyethylene tubing (Intramedic, I.D. .062′ × O.D. .082′). Height of the eluting chamber was ⅛ in., yielding a volume of 0.8 cm^3. Electrophoresis was carried out for four hours at 300 v starting potential. Fractions were collected for 5 minutes at a flow rate of 0.6 ml eluate per minute using a Beckman Model 746 Solution Metering Pump and an automatic fraction collector. The fractions were assayed for acid phosphatase using a-naphthyl acid phosphate as substrate.

RESULTS

Acrylamide Electrophoresis of Mitochondrial-Lysosomal Fractions

The appearance of two electrophoretically distinguishable forms of acid phosphatase in mitochondrial-lysosomal fractions of rat liver (Allen & Gockerman, 1964) was confirmed. When 20% fractions obtained by Scheme 1 were made 5% with Triton X-100 prior to electrophoresis, two bands of enzyme activity were detected, a fast-migrating component and a slow-migrating one. The slow-migrating component was detectable only after Triton treatment; the fast band was evident in untreated preparations. When mitochondrial-lysosomal fractions were blended, centrifuged for 30 minutes at 100,000 × *g*, and the supernatant made 5% with Triton X-100 prior to electrophoresis, only the fast-migrating band was evident. When the sediment was washed and made 5% with Triton X-100 prior to electrophoresis, only the slow-migrating component was visualized. The fast-migrating component was taken to represent soluble acid phosphatase released from mitochondrial-lysosomal fractions by physical disruption of particles. The slow-migrating component, appearing only after Triton treatment, was taken to represent the bound form of acid phosphatase.

Separation of Two Forms of Acid Phosphatase Using Small-Scale Preparative Electrophoresis in Acrylamide Gels

That two electrophoretically distinct forms of acid phosphatase are present in the mitochondrial-lysosomal fraction of rat liver was further demonstrated

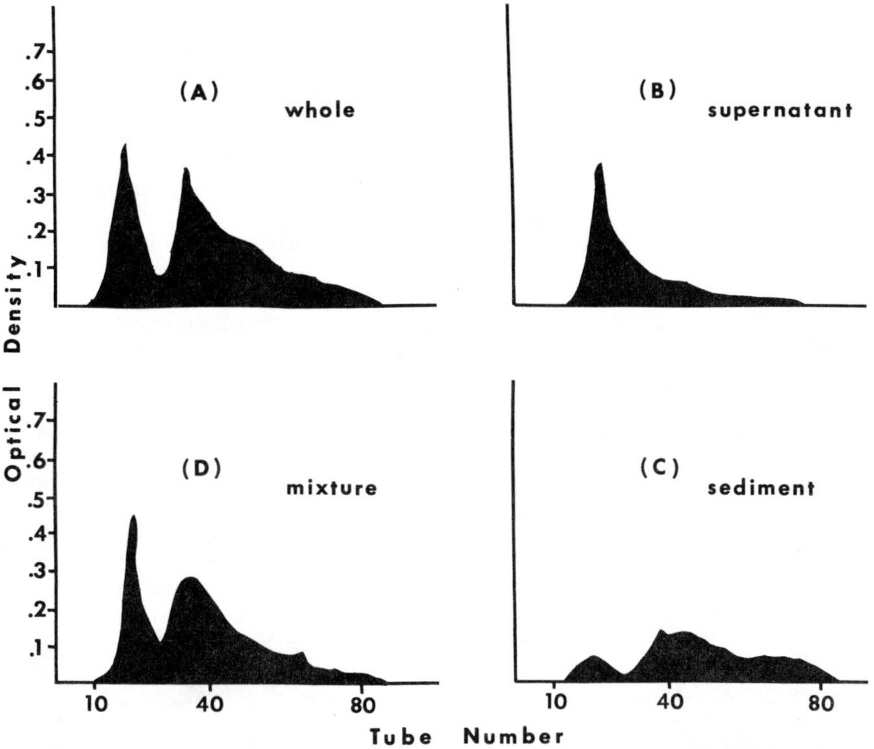

FIGURE 1. Preparative electrophoretic separation of soluble and bound acid phosphatase in 10% acrylamide gels. Mitochondrial-lysosomal fractions were derived according to differential centrifugation Scheme 1. Electrophoresis was accomplished as described in the text. Eluates were assayed using sodium α-naphthyl acid phosphate as substrate. Two hundred μl of eluate were assayed routinely, and incubation was for 30 minutes at 37° C. (A) Whole fractions were made 5% with Triton X-100 and subjected to electrophoresis. Two elution peaks of activity were present. (B) Fractions were subjected to blending and centrifugation at 100,000 × *g* for 30 minutes. Supernatants were made 5% with Triton X-100 before electrophoresis. One fast-migrating peak was evident. (C) Fraction sediments from (B) were resuspended and made 5% with Triton X-100. Electrophoresis followed, and one, slow-migrating, diffuse area of activity was detected. (D) Separated supernatants and sediments (B and C) were mixed prior to electrophoresis.

using small-scale preparative electrophoresis in acrylamide gels. Cell preparations were made 5% with Triton X-100. When mitochondrial-lysosomal fractions were subjected to electrophoresis, two elution peaks of acid phosphatase activity were detected (FIGURE 1, A). Soluble and bound fractions, when subjected to electrophoresis, resolved into one peak each, a fast-migrating one when soluble preparations were utilized (FIGURE 1, B), and a more slowly migrating, diffuse one (FIGURE 1, C) when preparations containing the bound form were subjected to electrophoresis. The elution peaks of separated supernatant and sediment portions of the mitochondrial-lysosomal fraction coincided in position with those of the whole fraction. The integrity of the separated forms was maintained when they were subjected to electrophoresis as a mixture (FIGURE 1, D). When sodium β-glycerophosphate was employed as substrate, Triton X-100 interfered with the formation of phosphomolybdenum blue. *N-N′*-methylenebisacrylamide tetramethylethylene diamine (TEMED, Rohm and Haas) also interefered with the visualization process in the assay. Recovery of total enzyme activity, loaded onto gels before electrophoresis, was low; 30% when total eluate activity was compared to the activity of the starting sample.

Biochemical and Physical Characterization of Separated Forms

Sedimentation behavior. Ten percent mitochondrial-lysosomal fractions were made 5% with Triton X-100 to render all acid phosphatase soluble. These preparations were subjected to density gradient centrifugation in 5 to 20% sucrose-water gradients. After centrifugation, acid phosphatase activity was present as a single peak with a median position at a density of 1.032. When soluble acid phosphatase was osmotically released from the mitochondrial-lysosomal fraction by resuspension in distilled water and subjected to centrifugation as above, a single peak was found at a median position of density 1.031. Repeated experiments with whole, soluble, bound and mixed preparations yielded the same, single peak of enzyme activity. The presence of both electrophoretic forms in peak activity gradient fractions derived from intact mitochondrial-lysosomal material, and of only the fast-migrating form in peak activity gradient fractions derived from soluble material, was confirmed by subjecting these fractions to acrylamide electrophoresis. Since no differences in the sedimentation behavior of the two forms were found, it is probable that the slower electrophoretic mobility of the bound form is not due to association of the enzyme with membranous components. When centrifugation time was extended to eight hours, similar preparations also yielded a single acid phosphatase activity peak.

pH. Whole, supernatant, and sediment preparations showed identical activity profiles in the range of pH 3.0 to 6.5 when assayed in the presence of sodium α-naphthyl acid phosphate, *p*-nitrophenyl phosphate or sodium β-glycerophosphate, although the forms of the profiles varied somewhat between substrates (FIGURE 2).

Inhibition studies. No differences in response to 2.5 to 20 mM sodium tartrate, 2.5 to 20 mM sodium fluoride, 0.1 to 1.3 M formaldehyde, or 0.01 to 0.2 M alloxan were noted among supernatant, sediment, and whole mitochondrial-lysosomal preparations when assayed in the presence of sodium α-naphthyl acid phosphate, *p*-nitrophenyl phosphate, or sodium β-glycerophosphate. Activity could not be measured with sodium α-naphthyl acid phosphate as substrate in the presence of alloxan due to its interference with color formation.

Heat inactivation. When whole, supernatant and sediment preparations, resuspended in 0.25 M sucrose, were subjected to treatment at 50° C for 10, 20, 40, and 80 minutes before enzyme assay, a striking difference in behavior was found between soluble and membrane-associated forms (FIGURE 3). Utilizing sodium α-naphthyl acid phosphate (FIGURE 3, A), *p*-nitrophenyl phosphate (FIGURE 3, B), and sodium β-glycerophosphate (FIGURE 3, C) as substrates, the membrane-associated form showed no loss in activity after treatment at 50° C for 80 minutes, while 60% of the acid phosphatase activity of the soluble preparation was inhibited. Whole mitochondrial-lysosomal preparations showed an inactivation curve intermediate between soluble and bound curves. Identical results were obtained with or without Triton X-100 treatment of preparations, indicating that the heat stability of the bound form was not conferred by association of the enzyme with membraneous material.

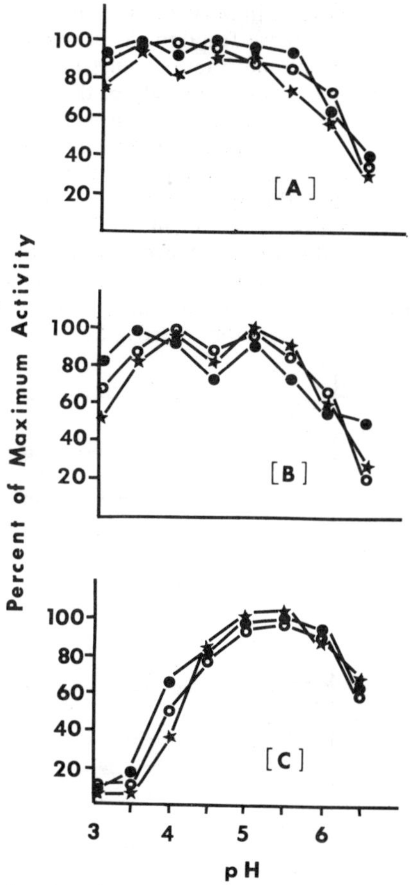

FIGURE 2. The pH optima for whole, supernatant, and sediment portions of mitochondrial-lysosomal fractions prepared according to differential centrifugation Scheme 1 and assayed in the presence of (A) *p*-nitrophenyl phosphate, (B) sodium β-glycerophosphate, and (C) sodium α-naphthyl acid phosphate. Fractions (○) were blended and centrifuged at 100,000 $\times$ *g* for 30 minutes at 4° C. Supernatants (*) were used for soluble activity. Sediments (●) were washed four times with water before final resuspension and use for bound enzyme activity. Activity is expressed as percent of activity at optimal pH.

Lysosomal Localization of Soluble and Bound Forms of Acid Phosphatase

Differential centrifugation. Differential centrifugation distribution patterns (Scheme 2) for lysosomes, mitochondria, and microsomes were obtained using acid phosphatase, succinic dehydrogenase, and glucose-6-phosphatase, respectively, as marker enzymes (FIGURE 4). When calculated as percent of whole homogenate activity present in each fraction, 40 to 50% of the total acid phosphatase activity was recovered in the lysosomal fraction, with approximately 10% of the enzyme appearing in the soluble fraction. Sixty percent of the succinic dehydrogenase activity was recovered in the mitochondrial fraction; 60% of the glucose-6-phosphatase activity, in the microsomal fraction.

The distribution pattern for bound acid phosphatase alone (FIGURE 5, bottom), was obtained by subjecting differential centrifugation fractions (Scheme 2), made

5% in TX-100, to electrophoresis in acrylamide gels. The electrophoretic forms of acid phosphatase present in these fractions are shown in FIGURE 5 (top). No activity was detectable in the soluble fraction. Distribution of the bound enzyme was established by measuring the optical density of the slow-migrating band in the gels. A comparison of the bound enzyme pattern with that of the lysosomal and microsomal patterns of FIGURE 4 shows that the distribution of the bound enzyme follows that of the lysosomal population and not that of the microsomal one. It was noted, however, that while the major portion of bound enzyme appeared to reside in the lysosomal fraction, the enzyme did not follow exactly the lysosomal pattern obtained by differential centrifugation alone. A larger-than-expected amount of the bound form appeared to be associated with the microsomal fraction. Percent of total activity found in each fraction after differential centrifugation, and for bound enzyme after electrophoresis, is shown in TABLE 1.

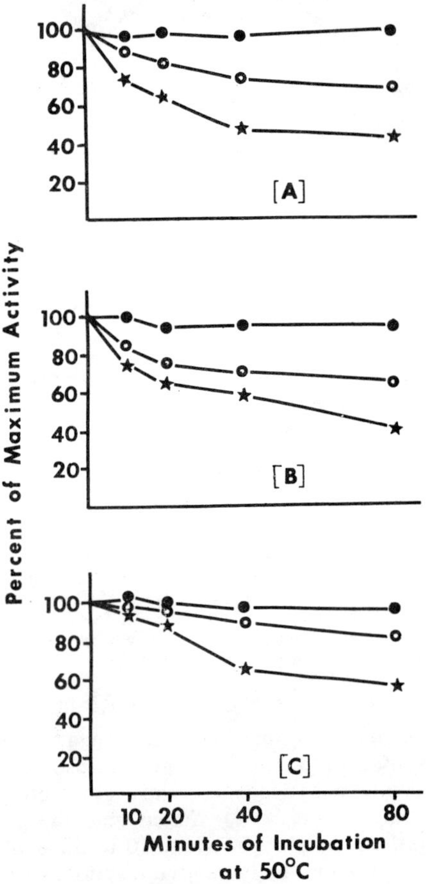

FIGURE 3. Heat inactivation of whole, soluble, and bound forms of acid phosphatase at 50° C. Whole (○), supernatant (★), and sediment (●) portions of mitochondrial-lysosomal fractions were prepared as in FIGURE 2. Incubation at 50° C was for 10, 20, 40, and 80 minutes prior to assay using (A) sodium α-naphthyl acid phosphate, (B) *p*-nitrophenyl phosphate, and (C) sodium β-glycerophosphate. Activity is expressed as percent of control, untreated activity.

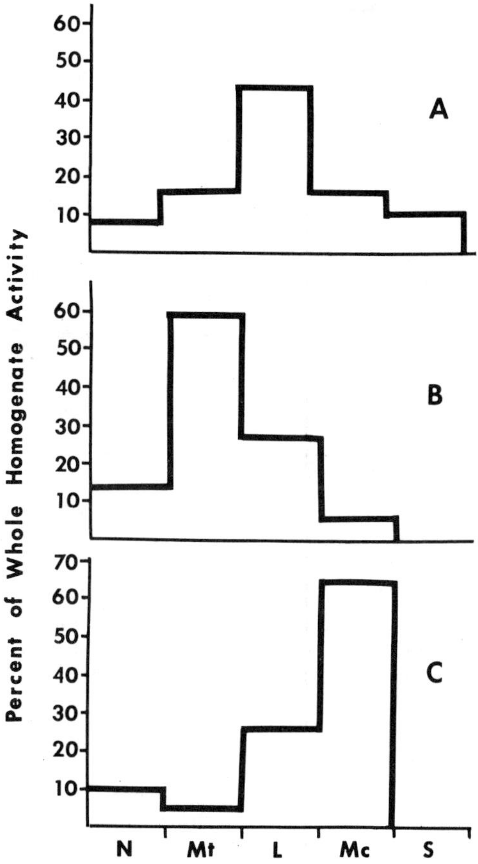

FIGURE 4. Distribution of (A) acid phosphatase, using sodium α-naphthyl acid phosphate as substrate; (B) succinic dehydrogenase; and (C) glucose-6-phosphatase after differential centrifugation (Scheme 2). N = nuclear; Mt = mitochondrial; L = lysosomal; Mc = microsomal; S = soluble.

Fourteen percent of the total acid phosphatase activity after differential centrifugation was attributed to the microsomal fraction, with 48% of the activity in the lysosomal fraction. However, 24% of the total bound enzyme activity was present in the microsomal fraction, with 41% localized in the lysosomal fraction.

Density gradient centrifugation. Density equilibrium centrifugation further established the lysosomal localization of both electrophoretic forms of acid phosphatase, and indicated a proportionately greater association of bound enzyme with "light" material. FIGURE 6 illustrates the distinctly different distribution patterns for total acid phosphatase and for glucose-6-phosphatase when homogenates from which the nuclei had been removed were subjected to centrifugation. Median particle density for the lysosomal population was 1.200; for the microsomal population, 1.166. Distribution patterns for soluble and bound enzymes alone were obtained after electrophoresis of gradient fractions and subsequent photometric assay (FIGURE 7). Both enzyme forms clearly followed the lysosomal distribution as compared to the microsomal one. Proportionately larger

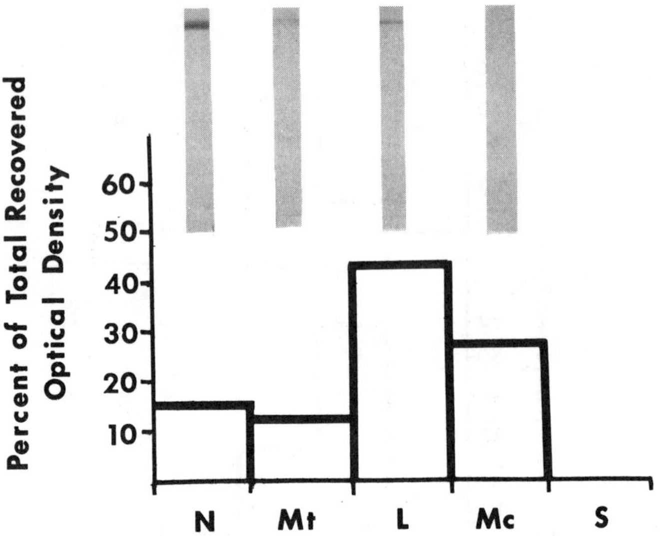

FIGURE 5. Distribution pattern (bottom of figure) of acid phosphatase in 10% acrylamide gels after electrophoresis of fractions obtained by differential centrifugation. Electrophoretic forms are shown at top of figure: 200 μl of sample:sample gel (1 part 20% fraction made 5% with Triton X-100:1 part sample gel) was layered on lower gel; Incubation in a sodium α-naphthyl acid phosphate-Diazo Garnet GBC reaction mixture was at 25° C for 4 minutes. No activity was detected in the soluble fraction. Migration is toward the anode (bottom of figure). N = nuclear; Mt = mitochondrial; L = lysosomal; Mc = microsomal; S = soluble. Optical density of the slow-migrating component was measured by scanning gels with a modification of a Beckman DU spectrophotometer (Johnson & Starkweather, 1962).

TABLE 1

PERCENT OF TOTAL ACTIVITY IN FRACTIONS (SCHEME 2) CALCULATED FOR TOTAL ACID PHOSPHATASE AND BOUND ACID PHOSPHATASE

Fractions	Total Acid Phosphatase (Biochemical Assay) % Total Activity	Bound Acid Phosphatase (Photometric Scanning) % Total Activity
Nuclear	15	24
Mitochondrial	14	12
Lysosomal	48	41
Microsomal	14	24
Soluble	9	—

amounts of the bound form in less dense regions of the gradient, however, suggested that a larger proportion of this form is associated with light components. That these components are lysosomal and not microsomal, is suggested by the close similarity of the bound enzyme pattern to that of the total lysosomal one, and its dissimilarity to the microsomal pattern.

A further distinction between the lysosomal and microsomal populations was established using velocity density gradient centrifugation in sucrose-water gradients. When homogenates were layered on these gradients, aggregation of particulate material occurred, with subsequent pelleting during centrifugation. This problem was circumvented by making gradients and homogenates 1.0 M in KCl prior to centrifugation. When gradients were centrifuged for 20 minutes at 4,000, 8,000, and 16,000 × *g*, two distinct distribution patterns were obtained for acid phosphatase and glucose-6-phosphatase (FIGURE 8). Acid phosphatase-associated particles were observed to move further into the gradient with increasing gravitational forces. At 4,000 × *g*., the median position occupied by the lysosomal population was at a distance of 6.64 cm from the axis of rotation. At 8,000 × *g*, the position was 7.15 cm from the axis; at 16,000 × *g* 8.18 cm from the axis of rotation. At 16,000 × *g*, some lysosomes pelleted in the 2.0 M sucrose cushion. Microsomes, on the other hand, remained at the top of the gradient under the same gravitational forces. At 4,000 × *g*, 8,000 × *g*, and 16,000 × *g*, the median position of the microsomal population was, respectively, 6.42, 6.62 and 6.64 cm from the axis of rotation. Thus, the distinction between the position of the lysosomal and microsomal populations was maintained to the extent that little overlap between the populations was found.

A determination of altered acid phosphatase distribution due to release of soluble enzyme in gradients containing 1.0 M KCl was made by pelleting all particulate material present in a lysosomal preparation made 1.0 M with KCl (FIGURE 9). Centrifugation was at 124,000 × *g* for 10 minutes. Material in the top fraction was designated solubilized acid phosphatase (unshaded), and accounted for 10% of the total acid phosphatase of the fraction. This value compared with that observed for solubilization in 0.25 M sucrose without KCl.

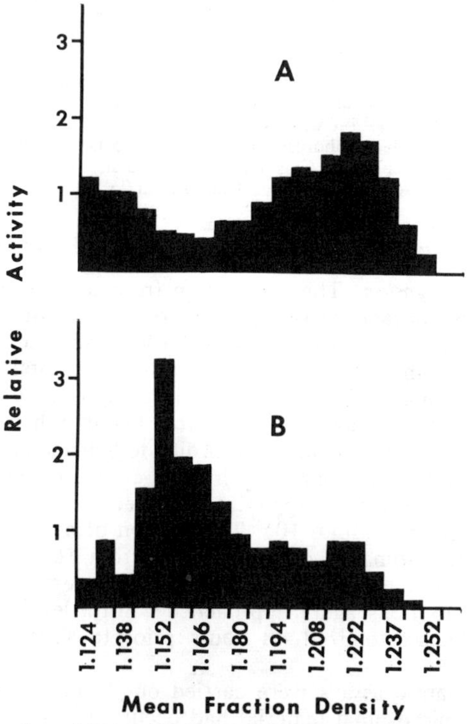

FIGURE 6. Distribution of (A) acid phosphatase, assayed using α-naphthyl acid phosphate as substrate; and (B) glucose-6-phosphatase after density gradient equilibrium centrifugation. Nuclei were removed from 20% homogenates by centrifugation at 480 × *g* for 10 minutes prior to layering on gradients. For the gradient illustrated, median position of acid phosphatase was at a density of 1.205. Glucose-6-phosphatase median density was 1.168.

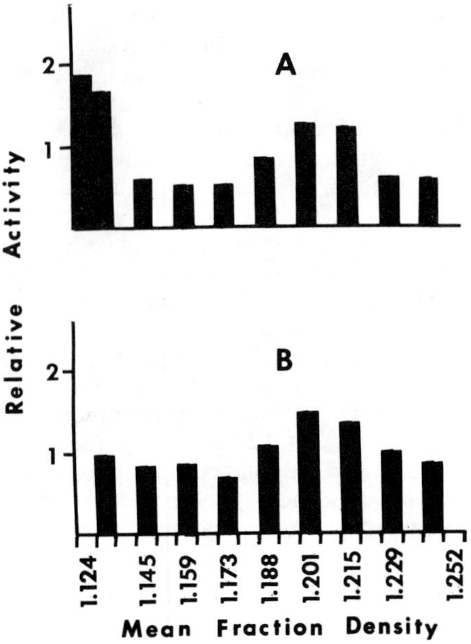

FIGURE 7. Distribution of (A) Soluble (fast-migrating band) and (B) Bound (slow-migrating band) acid phosphatase after density equilibrium centrifugation and electrophoresis in 10% acrylamide gels. Preparation was as in FIGURE 6. Gradient fractions were made 5% with Triton X-100 prior to electrophoresis. Density of enzyme-produced dye deposited was determined by photometric scanning. Gels were incubated in sodium α-naphthyl acid phosphate:Diazo Garnet GBC reaction mixture for 4 minutes at 25° C.

Distribution of Acid phosphatase in Regenerating Liver

Differential centrifugation. The suggestion from previous data that a higher proportion of the membrane-associated form of acid phosphatase is associated with slowly sedimenting lysosomes rather than with nonlysosomal material was further investigated using regenerating liver as experimental tissue. Tissue was examined at 24, 48, and 72 hours after partial hepatectomy. Liver removed at the time of the operation was used as control tissue. When such tissues were subjected to differential centrifugation according to Scheme 2, an altered distribution of acid phosphatase in regenerated liver as compared to control tissue was noted. This was manifested as an apparent increased proportion of the enzyme in the microsomal fraction (FIGURE 10). The portion of acid phosphatase activity recovered in the microsomal fraction increased from 16% in control tissue to 36% in 24 and 48-hour experimental tissue. At 72 hours after partial hepatectomy, fraction distributions again approached control levels. Liver tissue from animals partially hepatectomized 48 hours prior to sacrifice was chosen for further work.

Glucose-6-phosphatase assays were carried out to determine if alteration in the distribution of microsomal material had occurred in regenerating liver. Results of such analyses showed no differences in the distribution of microsomes between regenerating and control tissue (FIGURE 11). In both control and experimental tissue, 50% of the glucose-6-phosphatase activity was recovered in the microsomal fraction, and approximately 20% in the lysosomal fraction.

These results suggested that the distributional shift of acid phosphatase in experimental animals was probably not related to an association of the enzyme with the endoplasmic reticulum, but to an altered character of the lysosomal population.

Velocity density gradient studies. To confirm an altered character of the lysosomal population, typified by more slowly sedimenting acid phosphatase-associated particles in regenerating liver, velocity density gradient analysis was undertaken. At 4,000 $\times$ *g*, a difference between the distribution profiles of particles in control and regenerated tissue was noted (FIGURE 12, A). Regenerating liver contained a greater proportion of slowly sedimenting lysosomes than did control liver. The median position occupied by the lysosomal population in control tissue was at a distance of 6.64 cm from the axis of rotation; in regenera-

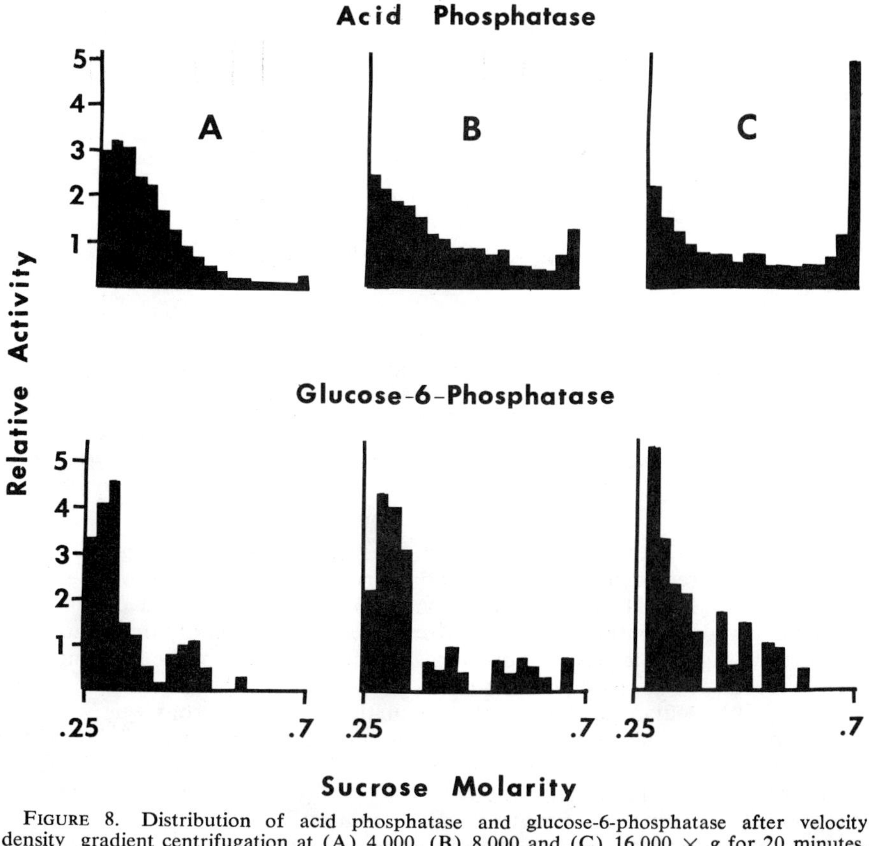

FIGURE 8. Distribution of acid phosphatase and glucose-6-phosphatase after velocity density gradient centrifugation at (A) 4,000, (B) 8,000 and (C) 16,000 $\times$ *g* for 20 minutes. Nuclei were removed from 20% homogenates by centrifugation at 270 $\times$ *g* for 10 minutes followed by two resuspensions and recentrifugations at the same speed and time. Homogenates were made 0.2 M with respect to sucrose and 1.0 M with KCl before layering. Acid phosphatase was assayed using sodium α-naphthyl acid phosphate as substrate. The median position occupied by acid phosphatase at 4,000, 8,000 and 16,000 $\times$ *g* for 20 minutes was 6.60, 7.09 and 8.19 cm from the axis of rotation for the experiment shown. For glucose-6-phosphatase under these conditions, median position occupied by the population was at a distance of 6.42, 6.62 and 6.64 cm from the axis of rotation.

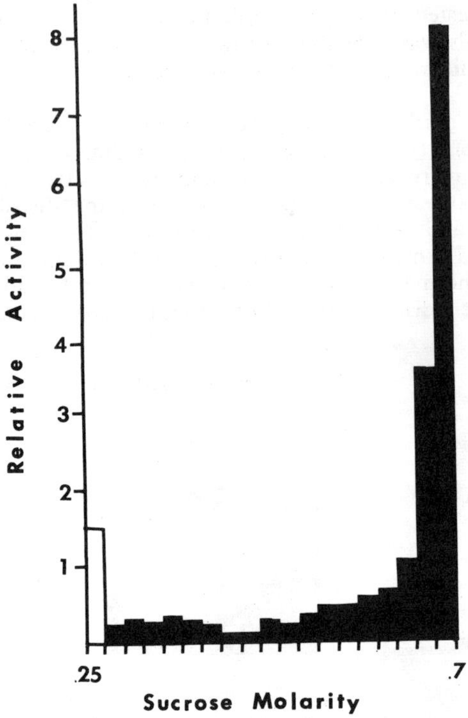

FIGURE 9. Separation of particulate and soluble acid phosphatase after velocity density gradient centrifugation at 124,000 × *g* for 10 minutes. A lysosomal fraction was obtained from a 20% homogenate by differential centrifugation Scheme 2. The fraction was made 4%, 0.2 M with respect to sucrose, and 1.0 M with KCl prior to layering on gradients. Pelleted material was collected in a 2.0 M sucrose cushion. Acid phosphatase was assayed using sodium α-naphthyl acid phosphate as substrate.

ted tissue, the median distance was 6.48 cm from the axis. When gravitational forces were increased to 8,000 × *g*, the distributional differences were emphasized (FIGURE 12, B). Under these conditions, particles associated with acid phosphatase from control tissue were distributed more generally throughout the gradient. In regenerated tissue, however, a larger proportion of the acid phosphatase associated with particles remained in the lower density portions of the gradient. The median position of the population in the control tissue was 7.15 cm from the axis of rotation, while in regenerated tissue, the median position of the population was 6.68 cm from the axis. When control and experimental tissue was subjected to centrifugation at 124,000 × *g* for 20 minutes to determine enzyme solubilization, particulate material from both experimental and control tissue pelleted (FIGURE 12, C). Solubilization in both tissues was comparable in all experiments, and ranged from 7 to 20% of the total acid phosphatase activity.

Concomitant acid phosphatase and glucose-6-phosphatase assays were carried out on regenerated liver after centrifugation for 20 minutes at 4,000, 8,000 and 16,000 × *g* (FIGURE 13). Such experiments confirmed a difference in the distribution patterns between the lysosomal and microsomal populations as defined

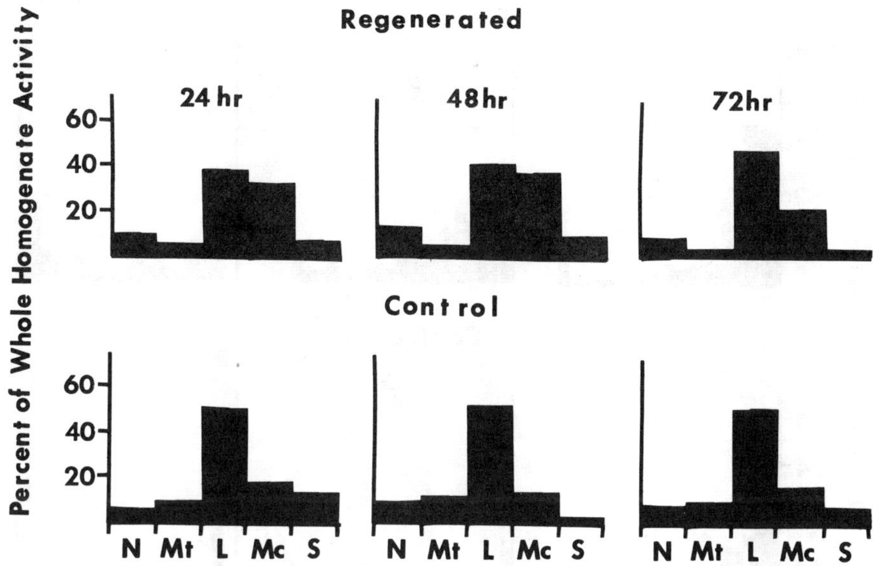

FIGURE 10. Distribution of acid phosphatase after differential centrifugation of control and regenerated liver at 24, 48 and 72 hours after partial hepatectomy. Differential centrifugation was carried out according to Scheme 2, N = nuclear; Mt = mitochondrial; L = lysosomal; Mc = microsomal; S = soluble. Acid phosphatase was assayed using sodium α-naphthyl acid phosphate as substrate.

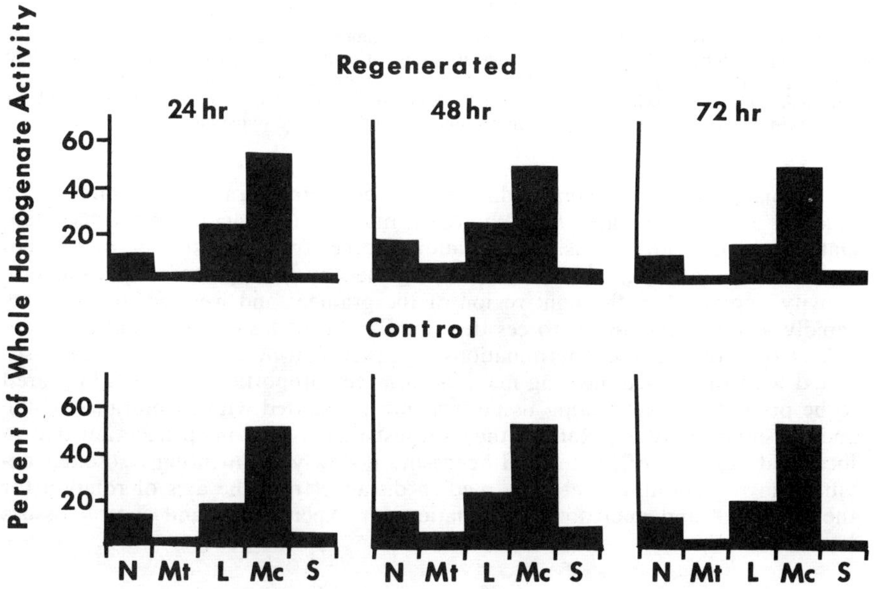

FIGURE 11. Distribution of glucose-6-phosphatase after differential centrifugation of control and regenerated liver at 24, 48 and 72 hours after partial hepatectomy. Differential centrifugation was carried out according to Scheme 2. N = nuclear; Mt = mitochondrial; L = lysosomal; Mc = microsomal; S = soluble.

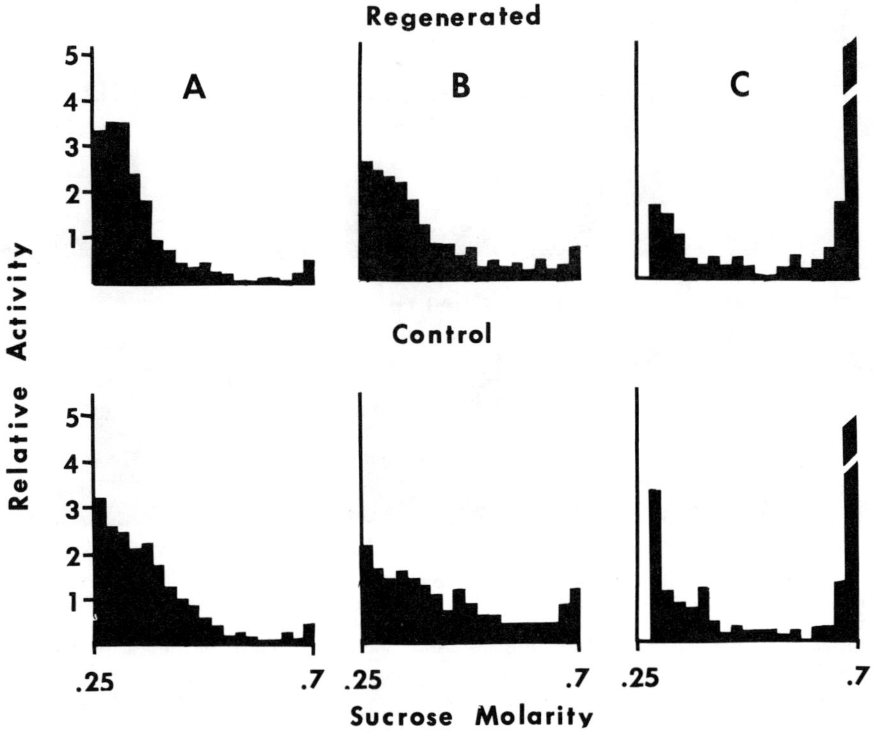

FIGURE 12. Distribution of acid phosphatase in regenerated and control liver 48 hours after partial hepatectomy following velocity density gradient centrifugation at (A) 4,000, (B) 8,000 and (C) 124,000 × *g* for 20 minutes. Nuclei were removed as in FIGURE 8. Homogenates were made 4%, 0.2 M with respect to sucrose, and 1.0 M with KCl. Gradients contained 1.0 M KCl. Acid phosphatase was assayed using sodium α-naphthyl acid phosphate as substrate.

by the marker enzymes. Similar differences were demonstrated for control tissue (FIGURE 10). Regenerated liver showed a movement of acid phosphatase-associated particles with increasing gravitational forces from 6.48 to 6.68 to 7.94 cm from the axis of rotation. Microsomes, indexed by their glucose-6-phosphatase activity, remained in the light region of the gradient and were sedimented less rapidly at the gravitational forces described (6.20 to 6.39 to 6.64 cm from the axis of rotation). These determinations suggested that the acid phosphatase associated with slowly sedimenting material, a larger proportion of which appeared to be present in regenerating tissue, was not associated with membranes of the endoplasmic reticulum. Rather, they suggest that a shift in distribution due to increased numbers of lighter and hence more slowly sedimenting lysosomes occurred in regenerating liver. The median distance from the axis of rotation for the lysosomal and microsomal populations of experimental and control tissues is summarized in TABLE 2.

Ratio of Soluble to Bound Acid Phosphatase in Control and Regenerating Tissue

Supernatant-sediment analysis. Lysosomal and microsomal fractions derived from control and regenerated liver 48 hours after partial hepatectomy were

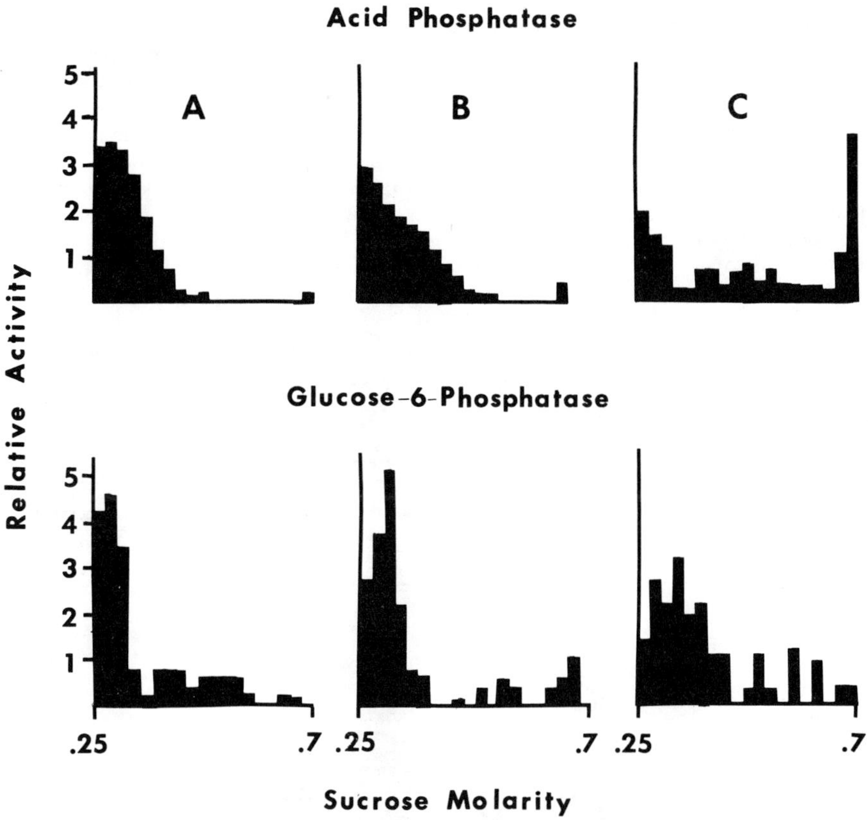

FIGURE 13. Distribution of acid phosphatase and glucose-6-phosphatase in liver 48 hours after partial hepatectomy following velocity density gradient centrifugation at (A) 4,000 × *g* for 20 minutes, (B) 8,000 × *g* for 20 minutes and (C) 16,000 × *g* for 20 minutes. Nuclei were removed as in FIGURE 8. Homogenates were made 4%, 0.2 M with respect to sucrose, and 1.0 M with KCl. Gradients contained 1.0 M KCl. Acid phosphatase was assayed using sodium α-naphthyl acid phosphate as substrate. For the gradient illustrated, the median position occupied by acid phosphatase after centrifugation at 4,000, 8,000 and 16,000 × *g* for 20 minutes was at a distance of 6.40, 6.62 and 7.94 cm from the axis of rotation, respectively. Glucose-6-phosphatase under the same conditions was at a median distance of 6.20, 6.39 and 6.64 cm, respectively, from the axis of rotation.

TABLE 2

MEDIAN DISTANCE FROM THE AXIS OF ROTATION OF ACID PHOSPHATASE AND GLUCOSE-6-PHOSPHATASE IN CONTROL AND REGENERATED LIVER 48 HOURS AFTER PARTIAL HEPATECTOMY

Assays	Median Position of Population in cm From the Axis of Rotation		
	4000 × *g* 20 Min	8000 × *g* 20 Min	16,000 × *g* 20 Min
Acid Phosphatase			
Control Tissue	6.64	7.15	8.18
Regenerated Tissue	6.48	6.68	7.94
Glucose-6-Phosphatase			
Control Tissue	6.42	6.62	6.64
Regenerated Tissue	6.20	6.39	6.64

blended and centrifuged to yield a supernatant containing the soluble enzyme and a sediment containing the membrane-associated form. When the two preparations were made 5% with Triton X-100 and assayed for acid phosphatase activity using sodium α-naphthyl acid phosphate as substrate, differences in the amount of acid phosphatase present in the supernatant and sediment portions of the fractions were found. Results were calculated as percent of the whole blended fraction recovered in the supernatant or sediment (TABLE 3). Analysis of microsomal fractions from control and regeneration tissue showed a higher proportion of bound enzyme in these fractions than in the lysosomal fraction from control tissue. However, the lysosomal fraction from regenerated tissue displayed a higher proportion of bound enzyme than did the control preparation for this

TABLE 3
DISTRIBUTION OF ACID PHOSPHATASE IN THE SUPERNATANT AND SEDIMENT PORTIONS OF LYSOSOMAL AND MICROSOMAL FRACTIONS (SCHEME 2) OF CONTROL AND REGENERATED LIVER 48 HOURS AFTER PARTIAL HEPATECTOMY

Analysis	Percent of Whole Blended Fraction			
	Lysosomal		Microsomal	
	Control	Regenerated	Control	Regenerated
Supernatant	58	52	41	41
Sediment	45	53	55	52

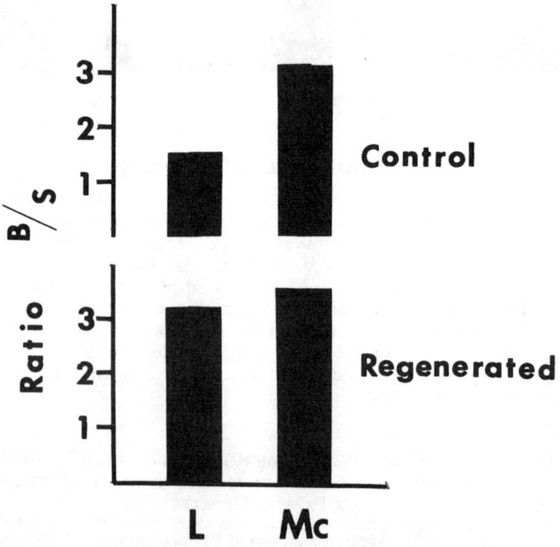

FIGURE 14. Ratio of bound (B) to soluble (S) acid phosphatase in lysosomal and microsomal fractions of control and regenerated liver after electrophoresis in 10% acrylamide gels. Lysosomal (L) and microsomal (Mc) fractions, obtained from animals partially hepatectomized 48 hours prior to sacrifice, and from control animals, were derived according to Scheme 2. Ten-percent fractions were made 5% with Triton X-100 and mixed with sample gel (1:1). Two hundred μl of this mixture were layered onto polymerized lower gels. Electrophoresis was carried out for 90 minutes at 4° C. Incubation at 25° C in sodium α-naphthyl acid phosphate-Diazo Garnet GBC reaction mixture followed for 5 minutes. Optical density was measured by scanning gels as for FIGURE 5. Activity is expressed as the ratio of bound to soluble enzyme activity based on optical density of the dye deposit formed per unit time.

fraction. Assuming, from previous data, that the acid phosphatase in both fractions is largely lysosomal, it appeared that slowly sedimenting lysosomes (microsomal fraction) showed a higher proportion of the membrane-associated form, and that the larger percentage of this form in the lysosomal fraction of regenerated liver was associated with new and more slowly sedimenting lysosomes in this fraction. Analysis of tissue from animals sacrificed 72 hours after partial hepatectomy gave similar results. At 24 hours after partial hepatectomy, an increase in the proportion of the membrane-associated enzyme in the microsomal fraction was noted, with no change in proportion apparent in the lysosomal fraction.

Electrophoresis. The above observations were extended using acrylamide electrophoresis of lysosomal and microsomal fractions. FIGURE 14 shows the relative proportions of bound to soluble enzyme in control and experimental tissue 48-hours after partial hepatectomy, as determined by densitometric measurement. A higher proportion of membrane-associated enzyme in the microsomal fraction was noted when compared to control tissue. After tissue regeneration for 48 hours, the proportion of membrane-associated to soluble enzyme in the lysosomal fraction increased from 1.5 to 3.3; in the microsomal fraction the change was from 3.0 in control to 3.7 in experimental tissue. Electrophoretic analysis of tissue obtained 24 hours after partial hepatectomy showed an increase in the proportion of the bound to soluble acid phosphatase in the lysosomal fraction from 1.5 in control tissue to 3.0 in experimental tissue. An increase from 3.0 to 4.5 was noted for the microsomal fraction. At 72 hours after partial hepatectomy, the proportion of bound to soluble acid phosphatase in both lysosomal and microsomal fractions increased, but the effect was complicated by a decreased detection of the soluble electrophoretic band.

The shift in proportion of bound to soluble enzyme between control and

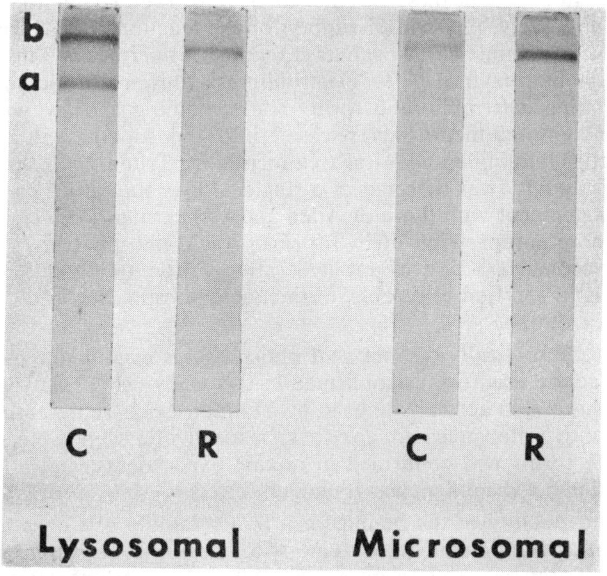

FIGURE 15. Distribution of acid phosphatase in 10% acrylamide matrices after electrophoresis of lysosomal and microsomal fractions of control (C) and regenerated (R) liver 48 hours following partial hepatectomy; (a) designates fast-migrating component (soluble enzyme), (b) slow-migrating component (bound enzyme). Preparations and electrophoresis as for FIGURE 14. Migration is toward the anode (bottom of figure).

experimental tissue, derived 48 hours after partial hepatectomy, was readily apparent after visual examination of gels (FIGURE 15). Control lysosomal fractions showed the typical qualitative pattern, with slow- and fast-migrating components evident. Little of either band was evident in the microsomal fraction. Lysosomal fractions from regenerated liver showed a decrease in activity for both bands, with an increased proportion of the bound form. An increase in the activity of the bound form was evident in the microsomal fraction of this tissue.

Discussion

The multiple nature of rat liver acid phosphatases has been recognized for many years. Roche, in 1950, distinguished multiple forms of the enzyme on the basis of pH data and response to Mg^{++} ions. Goodlad and Mills (1956; 1957) reported evidence for the existence of two or more forms of acid phosphatase in unfractionated rat liver, the forms exhibiting differential responses to Mg^{++} ions, acetate and veronal buffers, and possessing different pH optima. Further, they exhibited different mobilities after electrophoresis in a Tiselius apparatus. No intracellular localization was established.

Barka in 1961 (Barka, 1961a) effected the separation of acid phosphatases of rat liver on polyacrylamide gels. He demonstrated three bands of activity, but obtained no evidence for differential substrate specificities at acid pH. Chromatographically distinct acid phosphatases were separated by Moore and Angeletti (1961) and by Barka (1961b) from rat liver. Barka found four elution peaks of acid phosphatase activity, one of which was detectable only after treatment of homogenates with Triton X-100.

In this study, two electrophoretic forms of acid phosphatase were found in the lysosomal fraction. One of these was detectable only after Triton treatment. When assayed quantitatively, physical disruption of the fraction resulted in the release of only 60% of the total acid phosphatase activity of the fraction into the supernatant phase (soluble enzyme). After electrophoresis, this preparation displayed one rapidly migrating electrophoretic form. The remaining activity was associated with the fraction sediment, was released into the supernatant and rendered electrophoretically mobile only after treatment with Triton X-100. After electrophoresis, this activity was detected as a single, slowly migrating band. These results are in agreement with those of Allen and Gockerman (1964), who effected the electrophoretic separation of two forms of acid phosphatase from the mitochondrial-lysosomal fraction of rat liver after Triton treatment, and with the earlier finding of a Triton-releasable, distinct acid phosphatase in rat liver homogenates (Barka, 1961b).

That electrophoretically distinct acid phosphatases exist in the mitochondrial-lysosomal fraction was further confirmed in this study using small-scale preparative electrophoresis in acrylamide gels. Two elution peaks representing physically solubilized and Triton-released enzymes, respectively, were detected. The integrity of the forms was confirmed in mixing experiments, and no evidence of interconversion between them was found.

The slower mobility of the bound form in acrylamide gels does not appear to be due to an association of the enzyme with membraneous components. When soluble and Triton-released forms were subjected to sedimentation analysis in density gradients, no differences in sedimentation properties were noted between them. Had the bound form been associated with membrane material under these conditions, differences in sedimentation behavior would have been expected.

The biochemical properties of the bound and soluble enzymes are similar. No differences between the forms were noted in response to sodium fluoride and sodium tartrate, as were reported for the multiple forms of rat liver acid phosphatase by Shibko and Tappel (1963) and Nelson (1966), and for guinea pig liver acid phosphatases by Neil and Horner (1964). The latter investigators also reported differential responses of lysosomal and soluble acid phosphatases to alloxan and formaldehyde. Differential responses to these inhibitors were not found for the enzymes reported here.

No differences in pH optima between the soluble and bound forms of the enzyme were detected. However, the nature of the pH optima curves varied somewhat among substrates. This behavior is consistent with earlier reports, and may form the basis for the reported multiple forms of rat liver acid phosphatase of other workers (Roche, 1950; Goodlad & Mills, 1956; Nelson, 1966).

In 1966, Nelson implied the existence of both a heat-stable and a heat-labile form of acid phosphatase in rat liver lysosomal fractions. His report is consistent with the finding of this study that membrane-bound acid phosphatase, associated with the lysosomal fraction, is heat stable at 50° C, while physically solubilized acid phosphatase loses up to 60% of its activity under such conditions. Differences in heat stability have also been detected for the acid phosphatases of plants (Williams & Staples, 1964; Ikawa *et al.*, 1964; Staples *et al.*, 1965; Blum, 1965). It is unlikely that the heat stability of the bound form is conferred by an association of the enzyme with membranous components. Identical results were obtained whether or not the bound enzyme was heated while associated with the lysosomal sediment or after it was solubilized by Triton treatment. This difference in heat stability, coupled with the integrity exhibited by the electrophoretic forms after mixing experiments, suggests that the electrophoretic species are distinct enzymatic entities and are not artifacts of preparation or technique.

Quantitative studies of the distribution of acid phosphatase after differential centrifugation showed, as expected, a localization of the enzyme distinct from that of mitochondria and microsomes. Likewise, in a variety of density gradient sedimentations, the distribution of particles containing acid phosphatase was distinctly different from that of particles containing glucose-6-phosphatase. However, it was noted that an increased amount of acid phosphatase was associated with the microsomal fraction after differential centrifugation of liver homogenates from animals partially hepatectomized for 48 hours. Liver is a tissue in which synthesis of acid phosphatase (Walakinshaw & Van Lancker, 1964) and acid phosphatase-associated particles (Bernhard & Rouiller, 1956) occurs. However, this tissue did show a distribution of glucose-6-phosphatase identical to that found in control preparations. The identity of sedimentation behavior of particles containing glucose-6-phosphatase in both control and experimental tissues suggests that the increase in acid phosphatase in the microsomal fraction may not be due to an association between acid phosphatase and microsomes, but rather may represent an association of the enzyme with the newly developed, small, less dense lysosomes presumably present in regenerating tissue.

This point was further examined utilizing velocity density gradient centrifugation. Again it was found that the distribution profiles and the rate of sedimentation of particles containing acid phosphatase and those containing glucose-6-phosphatase were distinctly different in both control and experimental tissues. In addition, these studies confirmed that a greater proportion of acid phosphatase is associated with more slowly sedimenting particles in homogenates derived from regenerated liver.

Electrophoretic evidence confirmed the lysosomal localization of both forms of acid phosphatase by showing the major portion of each to be associated with the lysosomal fractions derived from both control and regenerated liver. It was found, however, that after electrophoresis of fractions obtained by differential centrifugation, the distribution of bound acid phosphatase differed from that of the soluble enzyme. A greater-than-expected proportion of the membrane-bound component was present in the microsomal fraction. This effect was particularly pronounced in preparations derived from regenerated liver. Comparison of the pattern of bound enzyme distribution with that of glucose-6-phosphatase, however, again suggested a lysosomal localization of the enzyme rather than an association with the endoplasmic reticulum, since, as noted above, the distribution of the latter enzyme was identical in control and experimental samples. Electrophoretic analysis of the distribution of the bound and soluble forms of acid phosphatase after density equilibrium centrifugation likewise suggested that both forms of the enzyme are associated with lysosomal rather than with microsomal material. This type of analysis again indicated that a proportionately greater amount of the bound enzyme was associated with particles occupying less dense regions of the gradients.

The above interpretation is based upon the assumption that acid phosphatase and glucose-6-phosphatase are valid markers reflecting the existence of two distinct subcellular populations. That the microsomal population reflects endoplasmic reticulum membranes vesiculated during fractionation procedures, was established by the biochemical and electron microscopic study of Palade and Siekevitz in 1956. Glucose-6-phosphatase is exclusively a microsomal enzyme (Swanson, 1955) and the one generally employed as marker enzyme for the population. In electron micrographic cytochemical studies, all sections of the endoplasmic reticulum are reported to contain the enzyme (Orrenhius & Ericsson, 1966). Acid phosphatase, on the other hand, is the classical marker for lysosomes, with little or no reaction product found associated with the endoplasmic reticulum (Novikoff *et al.,* 1964; Novikoff, 1961).

The localization of some acid phosphatase in the endoplasmic reticulum has been suggested for rat and mouse liver by Fishman, *et al.* (1967), and for rat liver, especially after regeneration, by Walkinshaw and Van Lancker (1964). The presence of acid phosphatase, or any enzyme, in the endoplasmic reticulum is consistent with the fact that most enzyme synthesis occurs there, and a transient localization of enzymes in the endoplasmic reticulum is implicit in the theory of zymogen granule formation and storage established by Caro and Palade (1964). Thus, while the lysosomal and microsomal populations are clearly distinct, at any one time both acid phosphatase and glucose-6-phosphatase may, in fact, be present simultaneously in particles where these populations overlap in sedimentation behavior, making total distinction between them impossible. In spite of this region of uncertainty, the above data suggest that the preponderance of bound acid phosphatase resides in the lysosomal population and not in the endoplasmic reticulum.

The prevalent theory of lysosome formation implicates the Golgi apparatus in the formation of primary lysosomes as Golgi vesicles (Novikoff *et al.*, 1964). As suggested by the theory of zymogen granule formation (Caro & Palade, 1964), acid hydrolases may travel through channels of the endoplasmic reticulum to the Golgi apparatus where they are subsequently packaged as vesicles. This theory is supported by the evidence of Bainton and Farquhar (1966) that granules of rabbit leukocytes are primary lysosomes (de Duve, 1963; Hirsch & Cohn,

1964), and that they form from the Golgi apparatus. The existence of membrane-bound lysosomal acid phosphatase is not readily accounted for by this theory, however, since the transport form of the enzyme would be expected to be soluble or at least not part of the membrane components of the particle.

If, as seems likely on the basis of the data presented here, the bound acid phosphatase of lysosomes is associated with lysosomal membranes, they are likely to be derived from either the membrane of the Golgi vesicles or from the membranes of the endoplasmic reticulum. The existence of bound acid phosphatase in these cellular membranes is consistent with the theory that such membranes may be a mosaic of functionally different patches (Korn, 1966) that have been simultaneously assembled from their component lipids, structural proteins and enzymatic proteins (Dallner, *et al.* 1966). Development of lysosomes directly from membranes of the endoplasmic reticulum has been suggested for protozoa (Elliott, 1965), rat kidney (Ericsson, 1964) and rat liver (Novikoff & Shin, 1964). Similarly autophagic vesicles appear to develop directly from endoplasmic reticulum sites (Van Lancker, 1964; Ashford & Porter, 1962; Ericsson, 1964; de Duve & Wattiaux, 1966 Deter & de Duve, 1967; Deter *et al.*, 1967). Thus, lysosomes may originate as small, membrane-bound vesicles with structural hydrolases composing an integral part of the membrane.

Whether small lysosomes containing more membrane-bound enzyme represent a developmental sequence from primary lysosomes to older, secondary particles cannot be unequivocally answered, although data derived from regenerating tissue support the suggestion. Deter and de Duve (1967) indicated such a possibility in their report of the existence of a population of small dense bodies after glucagon treatment and their implication of an enlargement of the particles with the development of autophagic vacuoles. Such a sequence also seems consistent with the general evolutionary sequence suggested by de Duve and Wattiaux (1966), in which lysosomes in early cells were represented by vacuolar sections of the endoplasmic reticulum, which contained hydrolases.

The nature of the binding of acid phosphatase to the lysosomal membrane is unknown. That it is very firm is indicated by the failure of strenuous physical treatment to remove it. Extraction with acetone and carbon tetrachloride effected no solubilization of the component (Allen & Gockerman, 1964). It was, however, readily extracted by them with digitonin, Triton X-100, and to some extent with butanol, treatments which disperse lipoprotein complexes (Morton, 1955). That such complexes may occur at the lysosomal membrane or within the particles, has been suggested by Koenig (1962). According to his theory, release may involve cleavage of glycoprotein, enzyme bonds, making enzyme accessible to substrate. Sawant *et al.* (1964a) implicated electron binding as a factor in the attachment of acid phosphatase, β-glucuronidase, cathepsin and aryl sulfatase to lysosomal membranes. Bound acid phosphatase has been reported by Shibko and Tappel (1963) and Sawant *et al.* (1964b). These workers reported that 30% or more of the acid phosphatase remains in the sedimentable phase after physical treatments. Shibko and Tappel (1963) found a membrane-bound esterase; Ugazio and Pani (1963), aryl sulfatase a; Beck and Tappel (1968), β-glucosidase; and Weissman *et al.* (1967), β-acetylglyucosaminidase, all in rat lysosome fractions. In terms of lysosomal function, such enzymes may be implicated in a postulated two-stage release of hydrolases (Shibko *et al.*, 1964; Beck & Tappel, 1968), in one step of which enzyme becomes accessible to substrate, but remains sedimentable, and in the next step becoming soluble and unsedimentable. The mechanism of release of bound acid phosphatase from membranes to an actively hydrolytic role as a soluble enzyme is open to question.

Summary

Two varieties of acid phosphatase associated with lysosomal fractions derived from rat liver have been identified after electrophoresis in acrylamide gels. One form is a rapidly migrating enzyme released after physical disruption of lysosomal fractions. The other form is electrophoretically mobile only after treatment of lysosomal fractions with 5% Triton X-100. This enzyme appears to be associated with lysosomal membranes and accounts for approximately 40% of the total acid phosphatase of the lysosomal fraction.

The membrane-associated and soluble forms identified electrophoretically have been individually isolated by a preparative electrophoretic technique. The integrity of these forms is maintained when they are subjected to reelectrophoresis singly or as mixtures. The soluble enzyme and Triton-solublized bound enzyme show identical activity profiles when subjected to density equilibrium centrifugation in sucrose : water gradients, suggesting that the bound form is no longer associated with membraneous components. Biochemical assays of fractions derived by differential and density gradient centrifugation combined with photometric assay after electrophoresis indicated that both soluble and membrane-bound forms are associated with the lysosomal population.

Lysosomal fractions, disrupted by blending, were centrifuged to yield a supernatant fraction containing the soluble enzymes and a sediment containing the membrane-associated form. Biochemical studies of these preparations indicated that the membrane-associated acid phosphatase is heat stable (50° C for 80 minutes) in contrast to the soluble enzyme, which lost 70% of its activity under these conditions. Bound and soluble enzymes possess a similar pH optimum and respond to inhibition by L-tartrate, fluoride, alloxan and formaldehyde in the same manner.

Studies of regenerating and control liver were undertaken at 24, 48 and 72 hours after partial hepatectomy. A distributional shift of acid phosphatase toward an association with lighter particles was noted after differential and density gradient centrifugation. Such a shift appears to be related to a change in the characteristics of the lysosomal population rather than to any association with the elements of the endoplasmic reticulum. Biochemical and electrophoretic data indicated that lysosomal fractions derived from regenerating liver contain a larger proportion of bound to soluble enzyme than fractions from control animals. Such data suggest that a proportionately larger amount of bound enzyme may be associated with a more slowly sedimenting and presumably smaller population of lysosomes.

References

Allen, J. M. & M. E. Beard. 1965. L-Hydroxy acid oxidase: Localization in renal microbodies. Science **149:** 1507–1509.

Allen, J. M. & J. Gockerman. 1964. Electrophoretic separation of multiple forms of particle associated acid phosphatase. Ann. N. Y. Acad. Sci. **121:** 616–633.

Appelmans, F. & C. deDuve. 1958. Tissue fractionation studies. 3. Further observations on the binding of acid phosphatase by rat-liver particles. Biochem. J. **59:** 426–433.

Ashford, T. P. & K. R. Porter. 1962. Cytoplasmic components in hepatic cell lysosomes. J. Cell Biol. **12:** 198–202.

Bainton, D. F. & M. G. Farquhar. 1966. Origin of granules in polymorphonuclear leukocytes. Two types derived from opposite faces of the Golgi complex in developing granulocytes. J. Cell Biol. **28:** 277–301.

BARKA, T. 1961a. Studies of acid phosphatase. I. Electrophoretic separation of acid phosphatases of rat liver on polyacrylamide gels. J. Histochem. Cytochem. **9:** 542–547.
BARKA, T. 1961b. Studies of acid phosphatase. II. Chromatographic separation of acid phosphatases of rat liver. J. Histochem. Cytochem. **9:** 564–571.
BEAUFAY, H., P. JACQUES, P. BAUDHUIN, O. SELLINGER, J. BERTHET & C. DEDUVE. 1964. Resolution of mitochondrial fractions from rat liver into three distinct populations of cytoplasmic particles by means of density equilibration in various gradients. Biochem. J. **92:** 184–205.
BECK, C. & A. L. TAPPEL. 1968. Rat liver lysosomal B-glucosidase; a membrane enzyme. Biochim. Biophys. Acta **151:** 159–164.
BERNHARD, W. & C. ROUILLER. 1956. Close topographical relationship between mitochondria and ergastoplasm of liver cells in a definite phase of cellular activity. J. Biophys. Biochem. Cytol. Suppl. to **2:** 73–77.
BERTHET, J., L. BERTHET, F. APPELMANS & C. DEDUVE. 1951. Tissue fractionation studies. 2. The nature of the linkage between acid phosphatase and mitochondria in rat liver tissue. Biochem. J. **50:** 182–189.
BLUM, J. J. 1965. Observations of acid phosphatases of *Euglena gracilis.* J. Cell Biol. **24:** 223–234.
CARO, L. G. & G. E. PALADE. 1964. Protein synthesis, storage, and discharge in the pancreatic exocrine cell. J. Cell Biol. **20:** 473–495.
DAEMS, W. T. & T. G. VAN RIJSSEL. 1961. The fine structure of the peribiliary dense bodies in mouse liver tissue. J. Ultrastruct. Res. **5:** 263–290.
DALLNER, G., P. SIEKEVITZ & G. PALADE. 1966. Biogenesis of ER membranes. II. Synthesis of constitutive microsomal enzymes in developing rat hepatocytes. J. Cell Biol. **30:** 97–117.
DE DUVE, C. 1959. Lysosomes, a new group of cytoplasmic particles. *In* Subcellular Particles. T. Hayashi, Ed. : 128–159. Ronald Press, N. Y.
DE DUVE, C. 1963. The lysosome concept. *In* Ciba Foundation Symposium on Lysosomes. A. V. S. Reuck & M. P. Cameron, Eds. : 1–31. Little, Brown & Co., Boston, Mass.
DE DUVE, C. & R. WATTIAUX. 1966. Functions of lysosomes. Ann. Rev. Physiol. **28:** 435–492.
DETER, R. L., P. BAUDHUIN & C. DE DUVE. 1967. Participation of lysosomes in cellular autophagy induced in rat liver by glucagon. J. Cell Biol. **35:** C11–C16.
DETER, R. L. & C. DE DUVE. 1967. Influence of glucagon, an inducer of cellular autophagy, on some physical properties of rat liver lysosomes. J. Cell Biol. **33:** 437–449.
DRYER, R. L., A. R. TAMMES & J. I. ROUTH. 1957. The determination of phosphorus and phosphatase with N-phenyl-p-phenylenediamine. J. Biol. Chem. **225:** 177–183.
ELLIOTT, A. M. 1965. Primary lysosomes in *Tetrahymena pyriformis,* Science **149:** 640–641.
ERICSSON, J. L. E. 1964. Absorption and decomposition of homologous hemoglobins in renal proximal tubular cells. Acta Path. Microbiol. Scand. Suppl. to **168:** 1–121.
FISHMAN, W. H., S. S. GOLDMAN & D. DELELLIS. 1967. Dual localization of β-glucurodinase in endoplasmic reticulum and in lysosomes. Nature (London) **213:** 457–460.
GOODLAD, G. A. J. & G. T. MILLS. 1956. The multiple nature of rat liver acid phosphatase activity. Biochem. J. **63:** 14.
GOODLAD, G. A. J. & G. T. MILLS. 1957. The acid phosphatases of rat liver. Biochem. J. **66:** 346–354.
HIGGINS, G. M. & R. M. ANDERSON. 1931. Experimental pathology of the liver. I. Restoration of the liver of the white rat following partial surgical removal. Arch. Path. (Chicago) **12:** 186–202.
HIRSCH, J. G. & Z. A. COHN. 1964. Digestive and autolytic function of lysosomes in phagocytic cells. Fed. Proc. **23:** 1023–1025.
HOGEBOOM, G. H. & E. L. KUFF. 1954. Sedimentation behavior of protein and other materials in a horizontal preparative rotor. J. Biol. Chem. **210:** 733–751.
IKAWA, T., K. NISIZAWA & M. TOMOE. 1964. Specificities of several acid phosphatases from plant sources. Nature (London) **203:** 939–940.
JOHNSON, J. D. & W. STARKWEATHER. 1962. A simple, improved microdensitometric recording method for slide mounted electrophoretic systems. Proceedings of the Tenth Annual Detroit Conference, Assoc. Anal. Chemists (Paper No. 15).
KOENIG, H. 1962. Histological distribution of brain gangliosides; lysosomes as glycolipoprotein granules. Nature (London) **195:** 782–784.
KORN, E. D. 1966. Structure of biological membranes. Science (London) **153:** 1491–1498.
MARTIN, R. G. & B. N. AMES. 1961. A method for determining the sedimentation behavior of enzymes: application to protein mixtures. J. Biol. Chem. **236:** 1372–1379.
MOORE, B. W. & P. U. ANGELETTI. 1961. Chromatographic heterogeneity of some enzymes in normal tissues and tumors. Ann. N. Y. Acad. Sci. **94:** 659–667.

MORTON, R. K. 1955. Methods of extraction of enzymes from animal tissues. *In* Methods in Enzymology. S. Colowick & N. Kaplan, Eds., **I**: 25–51. Academic Press, Inc., New York, N. Y.

NEIL, M. W. & M. W. HORNER. 1964. Studies on acid hydrolases in adult and foetal tissues. Acid phosphatase p-nitrophenyl-phosphate phosphehydrolases of adult Guinea-pig liver. Biochem. J. **92**: 217–224.

NELSON, B. D. 1966. Rat liver acid phosphatase: differences in lysosomal and cytoplasmic forms. Proc. Soc. Exp. Biol. Med. **121**: 998–1001.

NOVIKOFF, A. B. 1961. *In* The Cell. J. Brachet & A. E. Mirsky, Eds., **II**: 423–488. Academic Press, Inc., New York, N. Y.

NOVIKOFF, A. B., BEAUFAY, H. & C. DE DUVE. 1956. Lysosome rich fractions from rat liver. J. Biophys. Biochem. Cytol. **2**: 179–184.

NOVIKOFF, A. B., ESSNER, E. & N. QUINTANA. 1964. Golgi apparatus and lysosomes. Fed. Proc. **23**: 1010–1022.

NOVIKOFF, A. B. & W. Y. SHIN. 1964. The endoplasmic reticulum in the Golgi zone and its relations to microbodies, Golgi apparatus, and autophagic vacuoles in rat liver cells. J. Mikroskopie **3**: 187–206.

ORRENHIUS, S. & J. L. E. ERICSSON. 1966. On the relationship of liver glucose-6-phosphatase to the proliferation of endoplasmic reticulum in phenobarbital induction. J. Cell Biol. **31**: 243–256.

PALADE, G. E. & P. SIEKEVITZ. 1956. Liver microsomes. An integrated morphological and biochemical study. J. Biophys. Biochem. Cytol. **2**: 171–200.

RACUSEN, D. & N. CALVANICO. 1964. Preparative electrophoresis on polyacrylamide gel. Anal. Biochem. **7**: 62–66.

ROCHE, J. 1950. *In* The Enzymes. J. B. Sumner & K. Myrback, Eds., **I**: 473–510. Academic Press, Inc., New York, N. Y.

SAWANT, P. L., I. D. DESAI & A. L. TAPPEL. 1964a. Factors affecting the lysosomal membrane and availability of enzymes. Arch. Biochem. **105**: 247–253.

SAWANT, P. L., S. SHIBKO, U. S. KUMTA & A. L. TAPPEL. 1964b. Isolation of rat liver lysosomes and their general properties. Biochim. Biophys. Acta **85**: 82–92.

SHIBKO, S. & A. L. TAPPEL. 1963. Acid phosphatases of the lysosomal and soluble fractions of rat liver. Biochim. Biophys. Acta **73**: 76–86.

SHIBKO, S. & A. L. TAPPEL. 1964. Distribution of esterases in rat liver. Arch. Biochem. **106**: 259–266.

SHINOWARA, G., L. JONES & H. REINHART. 1942. The estimation of serum inorganic phosphate and acid and alkaline phosphatase activity. J. Biol. Chem. **142**: 921–933.

SIGMA CHEMICAL COMPANY. 1963. Sigma Technical Bulletin No. 104. St. Louis, Mo.

STAPELS, R. C., W. J. MCCARTHY & M. A. STAHMANN. 1965. Heat stabilities of acid phosphatases from Pinto bean leaves. Science **149**: 1248–1249.

SWANSON, M. 1955. *In* Methods in Enzymology. Vol. II. S. P. Colowick & N. O. Kaplan, Eds., **II**: 541–546. Academic Press, Inc., New York, N. Y.

UGAZIO, G. & P. PANI. 1963. Differential release of bound hydrolases from rat liver lysosomes treated by a non-ionic surface active substance. Exp. Cell Res. **31**: 424–427.

VAN LANCKER, J. L. 1964. Fed. Proc. **23**: 1050–1052.

VAN LANCKER, J. L. & D. G. SEMPOUX. 1958. Regeneration of various cellular components in rat livers after subtotal hepatectomy. Arch. Biochem. **77**: 129–137.

WALKINSHAW, C. H. & J. L. VAN LANCKER. 1964. Molecular mechanisms of liver regeneration. II. Intracellular distribution of biochemical markers in normal and regenerating liver. Lab. Invest. **13**: 513–523.

WEISSMANN, B., G. ROWIN, J. MARSHALL & D. FRIEDERICI. 1967. Mammalian a-acetylglucosaminidase. Enzymic properties, tissue distribution, and intracellular localization. Biochemistry (Wash.) **6**: 207–214.

WILLIAMS, P. H. & R. C. STAPLES. 1964. Acid phosphatases from healthy and rust infected Pinto bean leaves. Contrib. Boyce Thompson Inst. **22**: 269–282.

DISCUSSION OF THE PAPER

C. DE DUVE: Dr. Allen, have you explored the possibility of a precursor-product relationship between the two acid phosphatases? Partial proteolysis, a process believed to take place within lysosomes, could be responsible for the physical changes you have described. Have you studied the effect of autolysis on the ratio of the two activities?

Dr. Allen: We've not studied the effect of autolysis on the ratios. We have looked at autolysis in terms of electrophoretic phenomenon and, unfortunately, we cannot detect in these experiments any conversion of bound-to-soluble enzyme. This is a very intriguing point, and we would like to understand it. We simply can't.

Dr. Aminoff (*University of Michigan, Ann Arbor, Mich.*): Might I suggest that, rather than proteolytic release, you could be adding a sugar, making it soluble.

Dr. Allen: Adding a sugar and thereby solublizing it. Well, these are of course, possibilities that have occurred to us in terms of the electrophoretic studies. It would take only a very minor difference in charge—the association of enzyme with substrate, perhaps—to give rise to these differences. However, I would point out that the binding between this bound phosphatase in membrane is very tight indeed. You simply cannot shake it off by any physical treatment we have that does not completely destroy the enzyme.

SUMMATION OF THE SESSION ON INTRACELLULAR LOCALIZATION

Christian de Duve

The Rockefeller University, New York, N. Y.

Few enzymes have attracted as much attention as have the phosphatases, whether in biochemistry, enzymology, clinical chemistry or cytochemistry. It is certainly remarkable, and to some extent frustrating, that such an enormous amount of work has yielded so little definitive information concerning the function of these ubiquitous enzymes. There are a number of exceptions, of course, but on the whole I think it is fair to state that we are still very ignorant of the role played by many phosphatases in cellular economy.

Some phosphatases have a relatively narrow specificity, and this property has helped us to identify their functions and to fit them in some known metabolic sequence. For instance, the role of glucose 6-phosphatase in glucose production, that of hexose-diphosphatase in gluconeogenesis, and that of phosphatidic acid phosphatase in the synthesis of phospholipids have all been clearly established on such a basis.

Unfortunately, most phosphatases have a rather broad specificity, and their function is not immediately apparent from the nature of their substrates. In a few instances, the consequences of genetic loss have provided useful indications. The clearest such case is that, already discussed, of the bacterial alkaline phosphatase, the function of which is obviously related to the ability of the bacteria to grow on organic phosphates as sole source of inorganic phosphate. Again, the lack of glucose 6-phosphatase in one form of glycogen storage disease has given additional support to our belief that this enzyme plays an essential role in the production of glucose.

A third approach to the function of phosphatases is the one that was covered in the previous session. It involves investigating the intracellular localization of the enzymes, and has been fostered by the availability of excellent biochemical and cytochemical techniques. Indeed, considerable factual information has been gained in this manner, but it has, in itself, been depressingly unilluminating. Take, for example, alkaline phosphatase, which has been studied by countless histochemists and cytochemists. We know a great deal about its localization in certain structures. However, we are still completely ignorant of its true function. It has been credited with roles in protein synthesis, in DNA synthesis, in RNA synthesis, in the absorption of sugars by the kidney and the intestine, in bone calcification, and in many other processes. But so far, there is no clear evidence supporting any of these hypotheses. Nor have we any satisfactory explanation for the high amounts of alkaline phosphatase that are found, for instance, in the brush borders of kidney and intestine, or in osteoblasts.

Again, the very nice work presented earlier by Dr. Song, while clearly establishing the localization of 5′-nucleotidase in the plasma membrane, nevertheless leaves us guessing as to what the function of this enzyme may be.

Even acid phosphatase, of which much has been heard here, has not truly betrayed its function by revealing its intracellular localization. I doubt that the nice pictures shown by Dr. Smith, or any of the others that have been obtained by the numerous users of the Gomori method, could be interpreted, were we not aware from biochemical work that acid phosphatase is usually associated with numerous other acid hydrolases – at least 30 such enzymes are now known in liver lysosomes – acting on proteins, nucleic acids, polysaccharides and lipids. This information tells us that acid phosphatase is but a small part of a complex digestive system. Presumably, its function in the lysosome is to hydrolyze the phosphate esters arising, for instance, from the digestion of nucleic acids and phospholipids. Armed with this information, we may now attempt to interpret these cytochemical pictures as revealing either the sites of digestive foci in the cell, or stages in the synthesis, transport and storage of the digestive enzymes.

In this respect, Dr. Smith's work, and the previous investigations he carried out in collaboration with Dr. Farquhar, have been particularly valuable in that they have brought to light a new form of lysosomal digestion. It has been known for some time that lysosomes are involved in the intracellular digestion of exogenous material taken in by endocytosis and of endogenous constituents segregated by autophagy. The phenomenon discovered by Smith and Farquhar, which I like to call crinophagy, concerns the digestion of excess secretory products stored in glandular cells. It is different from autophagy in that it involves direct fusion between a secretion granule and a lysosome. Some of the pictures shown by Dr. Smith were not illustrative of crinophagy. Whether they represent massive autophagy of secretion granules, or some other phenomenon, is not entirely clear. The possibility, raised by Novikoff several years ago, that lysosomes may sometimes be involved in a more specific type of processing of secretory material, certainly deserves to be kept in mind.

Several biochemists working on lysosomes have been puzzled by the fact that some lysosomal enzymes readily go into solution after disruption of the particles, whereas others tend to remain attached to their insoluble stroma or membrane. The possibility that adsorption artifacts may be involved has been raised repeatedly, but the careful work described by Dr. Allen makes this explanation rather unlikely so far as the acid phosphatases are concerned, since the soluble and insoluble forms clearly have distinct physical properties. At present, the functional significance of the membrane-bound acid hydrolases in the lysosomes is unclear.

To conclude this brief survey of the phosphatases, I should mention an additional possibility that has been considered by numerous authors, namely that these enzymes may act not as hydrolases, but as transferases in the living cell. Certainly, we cannot discard such a possibility concerning enzymes that are strongly attached to a membrane component and could perform their function in a relatively hydrophobic medium. There are good indications, for example, that the mitochondrial ATPase may fall within this category, and that its normal function is to act as a phosphoryl transferase in oxidative phosphorylation. However, for the phosphatases that are readily accessible to water in the living cell, I doubt that conditions that would allow them to act efficiently as transferases could be realized *in vivo*. This point will come up again when Dr. Nordlie discusses the possible transferase functions of glucose 6-phosphatase. The enzyme is membrane-bound and, therefore, could conceivably be shielded to some extent from the surrounding aqueous environment. On the other hand, there is definite evidence that it can and does act as a hydrolase.

Obviously, we are not through yet with the phosphatases. This conference has been timely in allowing us to assess our present knowledge or lack of knowledge. It will certainly spur all of us to new efforts. In the meantime, we must thank the phosphatases for having provided us with particularly intriguing objects of study, as well as with valuable markers, both in cytochemistry and in clinical medicine, even though they have been so coy in keeping their true function hidden from us.

PART IV. BIOCHEMISTRY

PURIFICATION AND MOLECULAR PROPERTIES OF PLACENTAL AND INTESTINAL ALKALINE PHOSPHATASES

Nimai K. Ghosh*

Department of Medicine, Roger Williams General Hospital
Division of Bio-Medical Sciences, Brown University, Providence, R. I.
and Institut du Cancer de Montréal, Laboratoires de Recherche, Hôpital Notre Dame
Montréal, Quebec

INTRODUCTION

During the last 20 years, extensive efforts have been made by many workers to purify and crystallize alkaline phosphatase (orthophosphoric monoester phosphohydrolase, EC. 3.1.3.1) from bacterial, animal and human sources. Notable success has been achieved in this area by a number of investigators.[1–23] In 1964, Malamy and Horecker[24] made a major breakthrough in this field by crystallizing alkaline phosphatase for the first time from *E. Coli* (FIGURE 1). Human placenta and intestine have long been known to possess alkaline phosphatase activity. Moss and his coworkers[25–27] used human intestinal tissue to purify alkaline phosphatase. The earliest report in which human placenta was shown to exhibit alkaline phosphatase activity appeared about three decades ago[28] and was reconfirmed later.[29] In recent years, a revived interest has been centered around human placenta, especially in the attempt to elucidate the mechanism of elevation of serum alkaline phosphatase level in pregnancy. In 1957, Anagnostopoulos and Matsudaira[4] recognized placenta as a very rich source of alkaline phosphatase and initiated studies on the partial purification of the enzyme. In 1960, Ahmed and King[30] made considerable advances in purification and were successful in obtaining reasonably pure alkaline phosphatase from this tissue. In the present work, methods of purifying human placental alkaline phosphatase have been reinvestigated. Attention has been focused on the existence of multiplicity in the molecular forms of human placental alkaline phosphatase on the basis of their molecular weights. Current studies, therefore, relate to the preparation of placental alkaline phosphatase variant at a very high state of purity and in homogeneous condition, to properties of the purified molecular weight variants, to comparison of the biochemical behaviors of placental and intestinal enzymes, to the mechanism of L-phenylalanine inhibition of the two isoenzymes and to characterization of the "placental type" alkaline phosphatase in human pregnancy sera as well as in neoplastic pleural effusion. Finally, purified preparation of human placental alkaline phosphatase, a sialoglycoenzyme, is proven to exhibit viral hemagglutination inhibitory potency.

MATERIALS AND METHODS

Specimens of human placental alkaline phosphatase used in the present study were purified as outlined below. Rat intestinal alkaline phosphatase was made by the method of Portmann and his associates.[12,13] Butanol extracts of the homogenates of human intestinal mucosa were employed. Alkaline phosphatase of human neoplastic pleural effusion of a cancer patient was prepared by exposure to heat, ammonium sulfate fractionation and continuous curtain electrophoresis in Beckman Spinco Model CP unit with Model CPF fraction collector.

Unless mentioned otherwise, alkaline phosphatase activity was measured with 72 mM disodium phenylphosphate in 50 mM Na_2CO_3-$NaHCO_3$ buffer, pH 10.7

* Mailing Address: 825 Chalkstone Avenue, Providence, R. I.

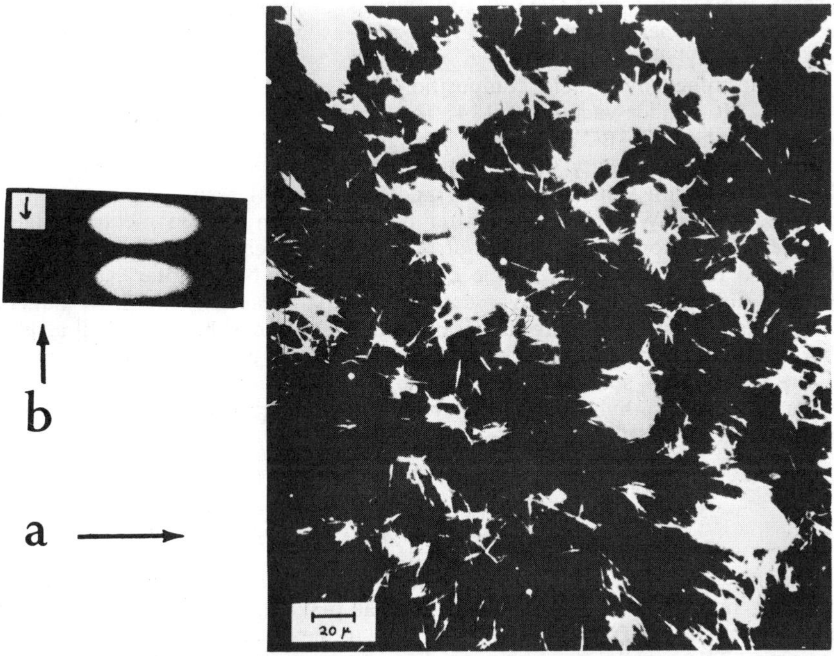

FIGURE 1. *E. coli* alkaline phosphatase crystals (a) prepared by Malamy and Horecker. The crystalline material showed three electrophoretic variants (b). Thanks are due to Dr. M. H. Malamy for supplying the photomicrograph from his Ph.D. thesis.

and 10 mM $MgCl_2$. Enzyme solution (0.1 ml) was added to the preheated (5 minutes) digest to initiate the reaction. The amount of phenol liberated in 15 minutes at 37° was determined by the diazocoupling technique with Fast Red B salt.

Protein determination was done by the method of Lowry *et al.*[31] and also by Microkjeldahl's method, whenever necessary. Starch gel electrophoresis was carried out in a Buchler apparatus with 12% starch in discontinuous tris-citrate-borate buffer system for 16 hours at 6 v/cm at 4 to 6°. Horizontal slices of the gel were stained for protein with 0.5% Nigrosin. Alkaline phosphatase was located in the gel by incubating with alpha-naphthyl phosphate and then either exposing the gel to ultraviolet light or diazocoupling the liberated alpha-naphthol with Fast Blue RR.

Sucrose density gradient centrifugation of the different enzyme specimens and of standard marker proteins was done with a 5 to 20% linear gradient of sucrose. The centrifugation was carried out in a Beckman Spinco Model L Ultracentrifuge at 4° for 17 hours at 25,000 rpm with SW 25.1 rotor.

Radioactivity of ^{14}C-RNA was measured in Nuclear-Chicago Mark I Liquid-Scintillation Counter. Uutracentrifugal analysis was carried out in a Beckman Spinco Model E. Analytical Ultracentrifuge. Ouchterlony double-diffusion tests for imunochemical study of the enzyme were performed in 1% agarose gel made in 0.05 M Veronal-HCl buffer at pH 8.6 for 40 hours at room temperature. L-phenylalanine inhibition of alkaline phosphatase was computed by the relation:

percent inhibition = D-L/D × 100, where D was the enzyme activity in presence of D-phenylalanine and L, the activity with an equivalent concentration of L-phenylalanine in the digest.

To determine amino acid composition, the enzyme protein was hydrolyzed with 6 N HCl under vacuum at 114° for 20 hours, and the protein hydrolysate analyzed in the JLC-3BC amino acid analyzer.

Neuraminidase activity was measured by assaying sialic acid liberated from N-acetyl neuramin lactose at pH 5.5 and 37°. The released sialic acid was determined by the Warren method after oxidation with sodium metaperiodate.[32]

Paper chromatographic analysis of the enzyme specimens was carried out by putting 10 to 40 μl of the sample onto a Whatman No. 1 filter paper (20 × 40 cm) and subjecting it to ascending chromatography with 25% aqueous acetone as solvent. The chromatogram was run for five hours. Alkaline phosphatase was visualized as violet zones after drying the paper chromatogram with cold air and then spraying 0.2% diazo dye, Fast Blue RR containing 1% sodium alpha-naphthyl acid phosphate in 0.1 M carbonate-bicarbonate buffer adjusted to a pH of 10.6.

Results

Isolation and Properties of Molecular Weight Variants of Human Placental Alkaline Phosphatase

Alkaline phosphatase of human placenta was purified by a procedure[33-35] involving homogenization with tris buffer at pH 8.6, extraction with butanol, ammonium sulfate fractionation, exposure to heat, ethanol fractionation, gel filtration, TEAE-cellulose anion exchange chromatography and continuous curtain electrophoresis in a Beckman Model CP unit (TABLE 1). Two major molecular weight variants, designated as A and B, were separated by molecular sieving with Sephadex G-200 (FIGURES 2 and 3), and variant A was purified 4,000-fold. Methods for both laboratory-scale and large-scale preparations[35] were devised. Enzyme specimens isolated at later stages of purification exhibited no acid phosphatase and beta-glucuronidase activities that were demonstrable in materials obtained at earlier steps (TABLE 2). Variant B, which came off the Sephadex G-200 column before variant A, was an electrophoretically slower moving species on starch gel and stayed closer to the origin, whereas variant A was the faster moving component. Two variants differed in their rates of gel filtration and were separable by molecular sieving with Sephadex G-200. They could not be separated from each other by alcohol fractionation (FIGURE 4). Slow moving variants were noted to be predominant in concentration in 0 to 30% ammonium sulfate fraction, while a 30 to 60% sample contained both variants A and B. Variant A needed a higher concentration of amonium sulfate for precipitation, due possibly to its lower molecular weight, *vide infra*. Paper chromatographic analysis showed that acetone (25%) could fractionate the enzyme (60% alcohol fraction, laboratory method[35]) into three bands with R_f values 0, 0.7 and 0.82. Continuous electrophoresis on paper curtain (FIGURE 5) was an efficient means of removing nonenzymic contaminant (identified as albumin) of placental alkaline phosphatase. The separation of the variant A from placental albumin was also achieved by repeated TEAE-cellulose anion exchange chromatography. The final preparation of variant A was completely free from variant B and placental albumin. It was homogeneous on starch gel electrophoresis (FIGURE 6) and thin-layer Sephadex G-200 gel electrophoresis. It showed only one protein band. Ultracentrifugal analysis of variant A (FIG-

TABLE 1

PURIFICATION OF HUMAN PLACENTAL ALKALINE PHOSPHATASE VARIANTS A AND B

Purification Step:	Tris	Butanol	Ammonium Sulfate	Heat	Sephadex G-200		TEAE-Cellulose	Electrophoresis	
Variants:					A	B	A	A	B
Total Activity $\times 10^{-4}$:	223.0	193.0	7.2	6.4	2.6	0.86	0.6	0.03	0.02
Specific Activity (Activity/mg Protein):	0.28	2.6	7.7	16.3	100.7	38.0	250.0	1171.0	212.0
Purification Fold:	1.0	7.0	27.0	59.0	395.0	134.0	892.0	4192.0	757.0

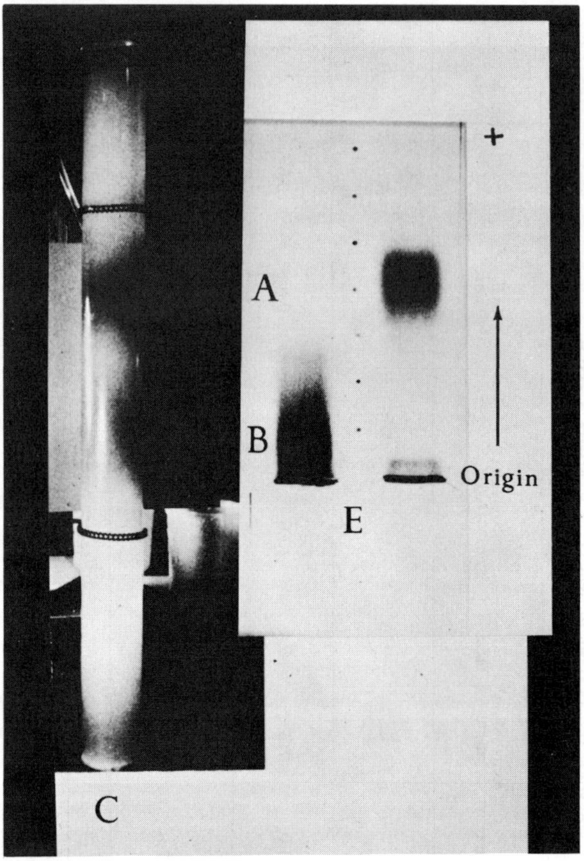

FIGURE 2. Sephadex G-200 column showing two zones (C) of human placental alkaline phosphatase with their starch gel electrophoretic patterns (E). The two major variants are designated as A and B.

URE 7) in Beckman Model E Analytical Ultracentrifuge also exhibited essentially one protein species. Svedberg sedimentation coefficient ($S_{20,w}$) computed from the slopes of log x vs. t plots (FIGURE 8) were 4.1, 4.3 and 4.2 S at protein concentrations 3.8, 3.9 and 1.5 mg/ml, respectively. The final preparation of variant A exhibited one precipitin line on immunodiffusion, indicating immunologic homogeneity (FIGURE 9). The ultraviolet absorption spectrum of purified enzyme sample revealed the presence of a peak at 278 mμ, and the ratio of the absorbance at 278 mμ vs. 255 mμ was 0.65.

When purified variant A, or a mixture of variants A and B, were precipitated with 60% alcohol, dissolved in water and subjected to the process of equilibrium dialysis with a system in which the pH of the enzyme solution was gradually changed during dialysis from 7 to 5.6,[35] crystalline material was obtained. On starch gel, crystals exhibited a broad, slow-moving alkaline phosphatase band comparable to that of variant B and showed only one enzyme spot of $R_f = 0$ on the paper chromatogram, as it did not move at all. The highest specific activity

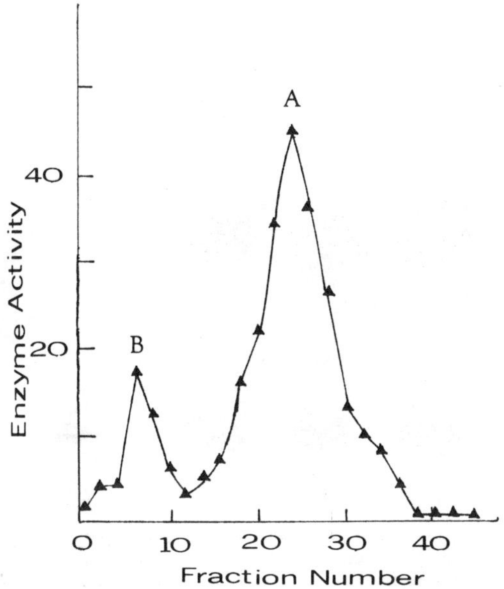

FIGURE 3. Molecular sieve chromatogram of human placental alkaline phosphatase (large-scale method) in Sephadex G-200 column. Elution of the two major variants, **A** and **B**, is shown.

TABLE 2

ACID PHOSPHATASE AND BETA-GLUCURONIDASE CONTENTS IN DIFFERENT ENZYME FRACTIONS OBTAINED DURING PURIFICATION OF PLACENTAL ALKALINE PHOSPHATASE[35]

Steps	Acid Phosphatase* (μmoles phenol/ml/hr)	Beta-Glucuronidase† (μmoles phenolphthalein/ ml/hr) $\times 10^3$
Centrifuged tris-homogenate	5.3	356
Butanol supernatant	3.2	362
First ammonium sulfate precipitate from butanol supernatant	4.3	1656
Supernatant from heat-denatured material	0.0	0
50-60% Ammonium sulfate fraction	0.0	0
65% Alcohol fraction	0.0	0
Sephadex gel filtrate	0.0	0

* Acid phosphatase was assayed by measuring phenol liberated from 3 mM phenylphosphate at pH 4.9 (citrate buffer, 100 mM).

† Beta-glucuronidase activity was measured by determining the amount of phenolphthalein liberated from 1 μmole/ml phenolphthalein glucuronide in 100 mM acetate buffer, pH 4.5.

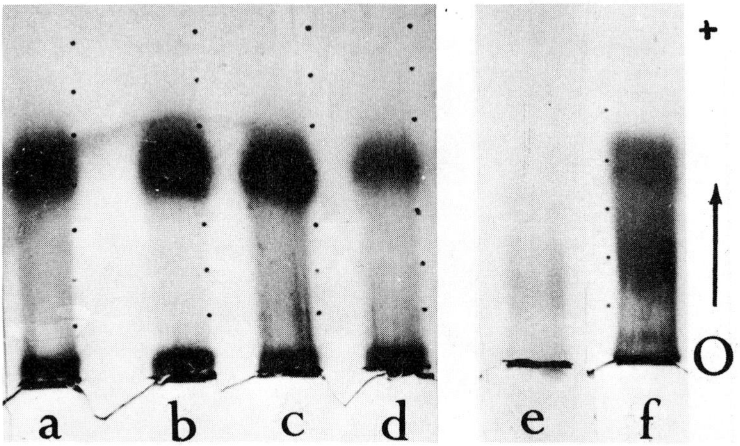

FIGURE 4. Starch gel enzymogram of different alcohol and ammonium sulfate fractions of human placental alkaline phosphatase. Columns a, b, c and d are enzyme specimens obtained (from best ammonium sulfate fraction, a mixture of variants A and B) with 40%, 50%, 60% and 70% alcohol, respectively. Columns e and f are 0–30% and 30–60% ammonium sulfate fractions from butanol extracts of placenta. O is the origin, and the arrow shows the direction of migration toward anode.

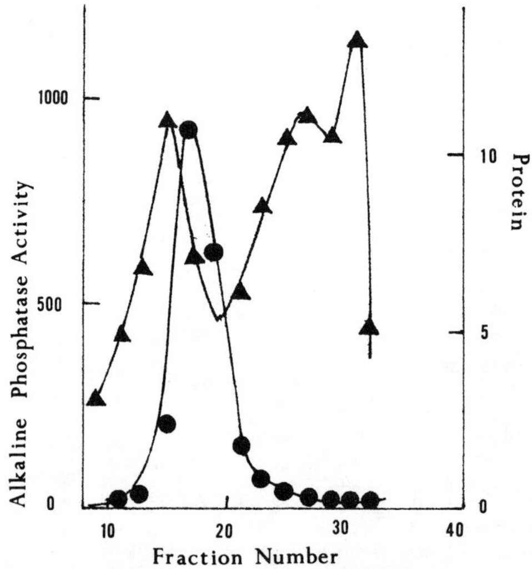

FIGURE 5. Typical continuous curtain electrophoretic profile of variant A. The fractions 25 and 32 were identified as placental albumin by starch gel electrophoresis. Enzyme activity is represented by closed circles and protein, by closed triangles.

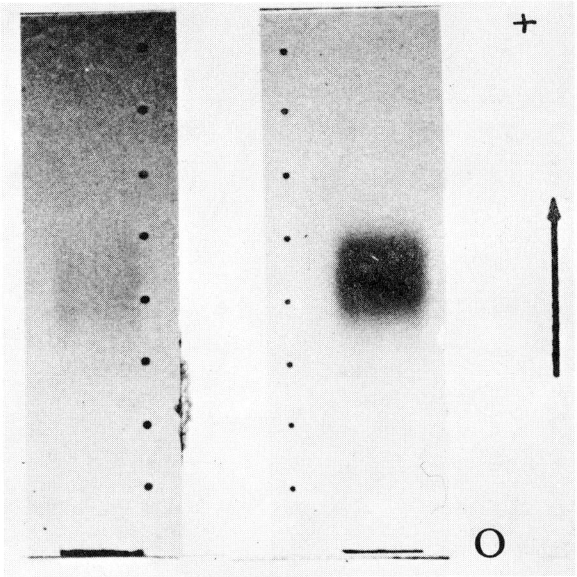

FIGURE 6. Homogeneity of variant A by starch gel electrophoresis. A single protein band (left) corresponds in location with a single enzyme band (right). The application slot was at 0. and the arrow indicates the migration toward anode.

shown by the crystalline product (FIGURE 10) was 400 units/mg protein. The specific activity was much lower than the highest activity achieved for variant A (TABLE 1). However, a similar difference in the specific activity of the variants of an enzyme present in a single tissue was observed in other systems such as carbonic anhydrase,[36,37] hexokinase[38] and arginine kinase.[39] The method of equilibrium dialysis employed to obtain hexagonal prism-shaped crystalline variant B appeared to involve association of enzyme proteins of low molecular weight to high molecular species. Crystals, insoluble in water and sparingly soluble in buffer, underwent gradual disaggregation, yielding the lighter variant A as shown by ultracentrifugal and electrophoretic studies (FIGURE 11). Crystalline product might also be obtained with 60% ammonium sulfate, but the needle-shaped crystals did not exhibit expected specific activity. Its low specific activity was possibly due to the ability of ammonium sulfate to coordinate with Z_n^{++} present in the active center of the enzyme, as pointed out by Vallee and Simpson.[40] Very recently, Harkness[41] reported the preparation of needle-shaped crystals with ammonium sulfate as the crystallizing agent.

Sucrose density gradient centrifugation profiles of the isozymes were compared with each other in FIGURE 12. The rate of sedimentation of variant B is faster than that of A, indicating higher molecular weight of the B form. Higher electrophoretic mobility of A on starch is compatible with its lower rate of sedimentation in the sucrose gradient and slower rate of filtration on Sephadex gels. The rates of sedimentation of the variants were compared with those of three standard molecular weight markers such as crystalline bovine serum albumin, crystalline bovine liver catalase and 4 S, 16 S, 23 S ^{14}C-RNA. The molecular weight of variant A, as determined from the sedimentation data, was 69,000, the same as that of crystalline bovine serum albumin. Variant B was a

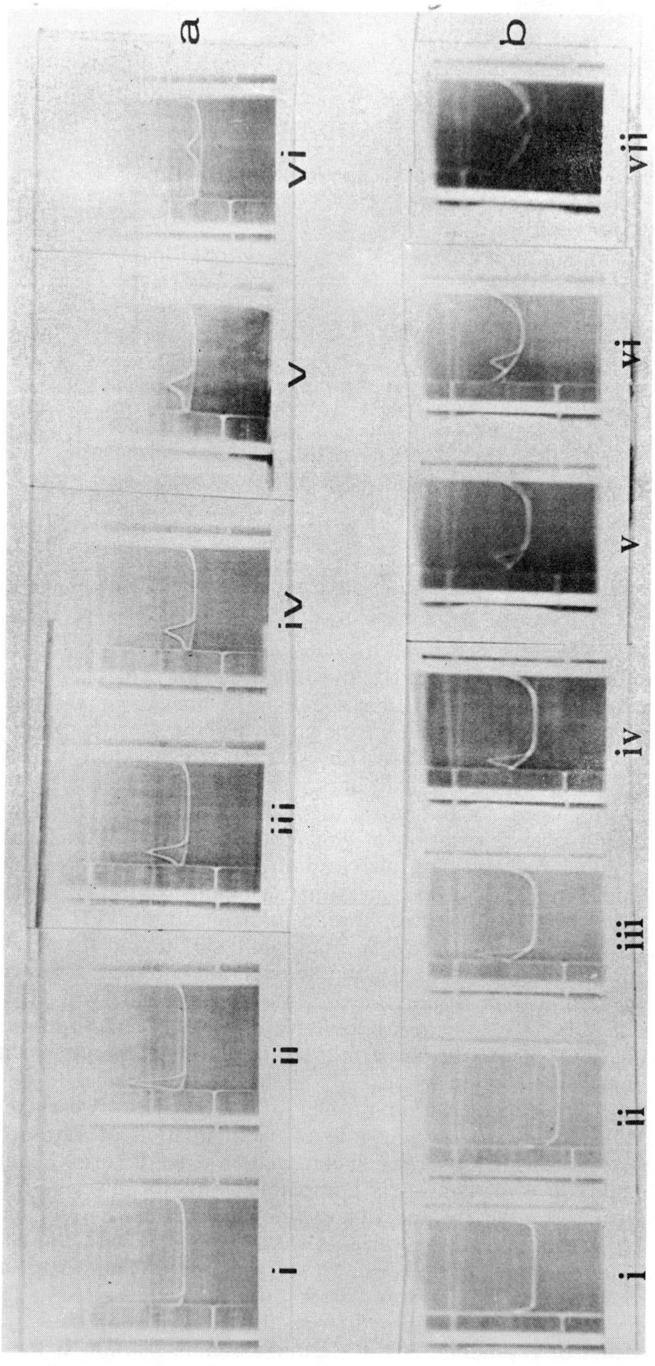

FIGURE 7. Ultracentrifugal pattern of variant A. The photographs of the protein boundaries of the purified variant A in Tris-HCl buffer, pH 8.6 (a) were snapped sequentially after 8 (i), 16 (ii), 32 (iii), 48 (iv), 64 (v) and 128 (vi) minutes with 70° diaphragm angle for the first snap and 60° for the rest, with the exposure time of 2 seconds in each case. Ultracentrifugation was repeated with veronal-HCl buffer, pH 8.6 (b), and the pictures were taken at 0 (i), 9 (ii), 17 (iii), 25 (iv), 41 (v), 57 (vi and 121 ((vii) minutes after the attainment of the maximum speed of 59,780 rpm) with the bar angles of 70° for i), 55° for (ii), (iii) and (iv), and 50° for the rest.

Thanks are due to Dr. R. H. Haschemeyer for his help in carrying out the ultracentrifugal analysis.

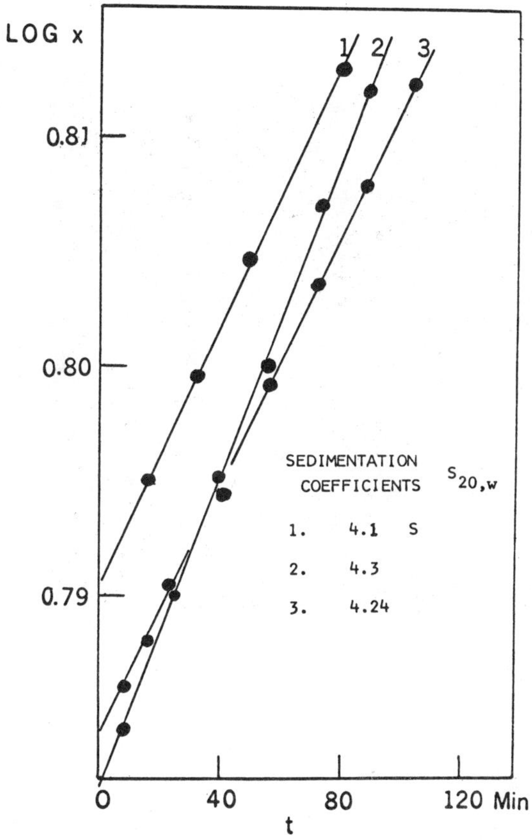

FIGURE 8. Log x vs. t plots for determining Svedberg sedimentation constants of variant A, x being the distance of the protein boundary from the axis of rotation of the rotor in the ultracentrifuge and t the time of centrifugation (min).

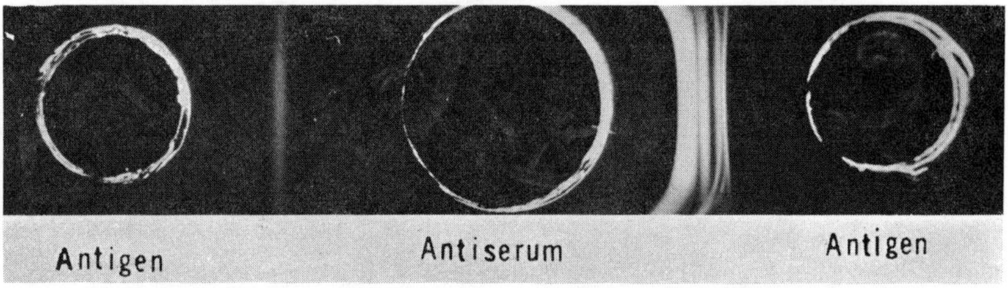

FIGURE 9. Ouchterlony immunodiffusion patterns of placental alkaline phosphatase preparations. The antigen number 2 (right) was the best ammonium sulfate fraction after exposure to heat and dialysis, and antigen number 5 (left), the best specimen of variant A obtained by continuous curtain electrophoresis and Sephadex G–200 gel filtration of number 2. In the central well is the antiserum against antigen number 2. Grateful thanks are due to Dr. Arnold Reif for his directions and help in preparing the antienzyme.

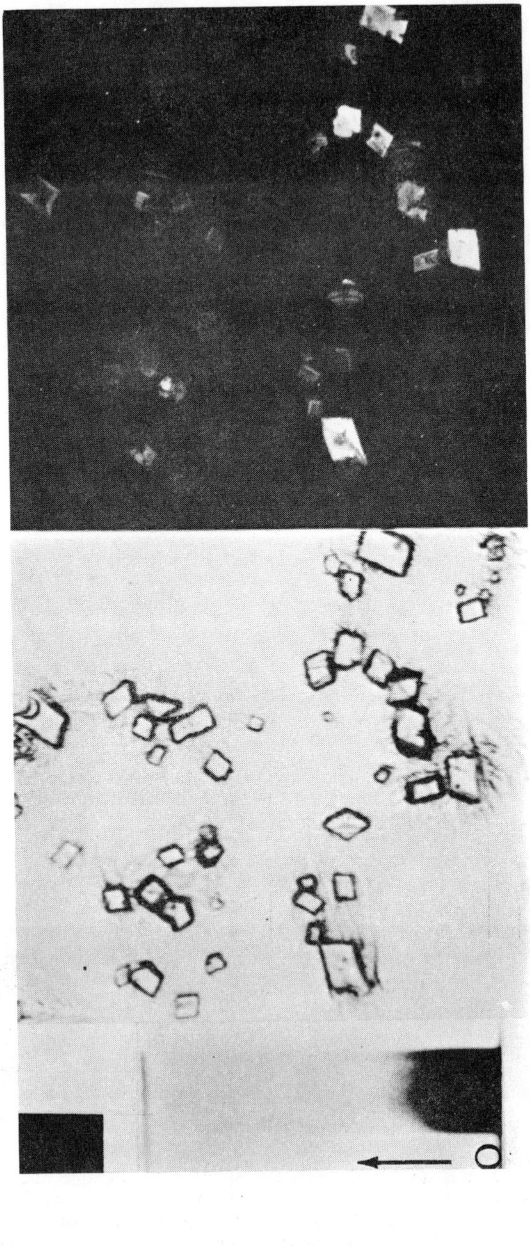

FIGURE 10. Crystalline human placental alkaline phosphatase (variant B) obtained by the method of equilibrium dialysis in bright light (left) and in polarized light (right). Magnification $\times 450$. The starch gel enzymogram of the material exhibiting only slow-moving band is shown at far left. Origin on the starch gel is indicated by 0, and the direction of migration toward anode, by the arrow.

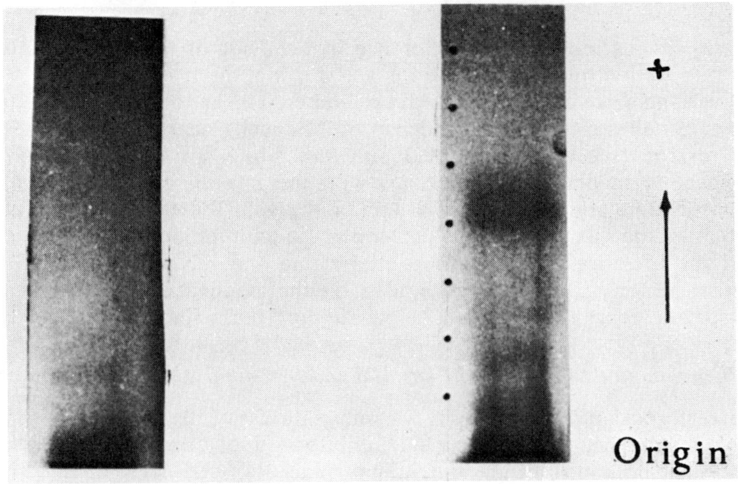

FIGURE 11. Crystalline variant B before (left) and after (right) storage. The crystalline material was kept in 0.05 M carbonate-bicarbonate buffer at pH 9.2 for four months in the cold room (4–6°). Aging produced fast-moving variant A from crystalline variant B. The arrow indicates the direction of anodal migration.

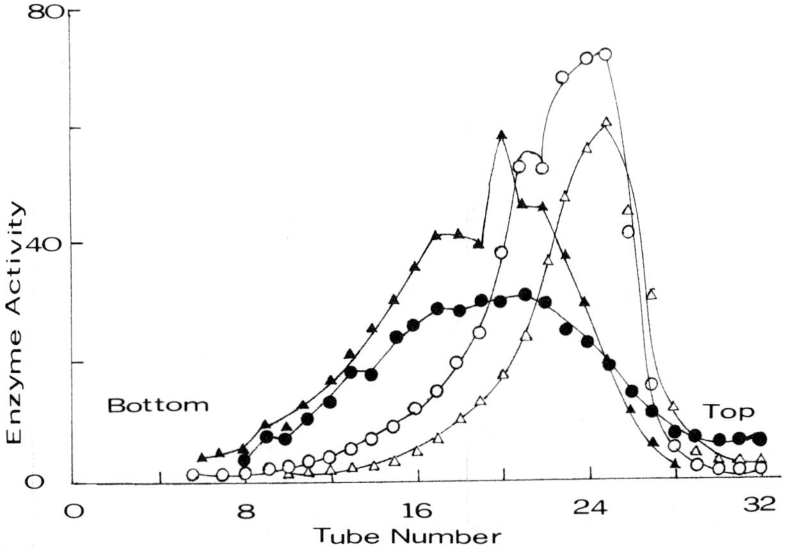

FIGURE 12. Sucrose density gradient centrifugation profiles of variant A (△), variant B (▲), crystalline variant B (●) and variant A contaminated with variant B (○).

heterogeneous mixture of several high molecular species (FIGURE 12) of the enzyme.

Kinetic studies indicated no difference in behavior of the two variants. The linear rate of hydrolysis of substrate and pH optimum of the two molecular weight variants were comparable with each other. The Dixon plot for pK_m vs. pH (FIGURE 13) illustrates the dependence of Michaelis constant on pH. The pK values for the free enzyme are 9.3 and 9.9, which are changed to 9.7 and 10.3 when phenylphosphate combines with the enzyme to form intermediate enzyme-substrate complex. This pK data, along with those of intestinal alkaline phosphatase, the Dixon plot of which showed discontinuities at pH 8.6 and 9.6, suggest the presence of thiol group of cysteine and ϵ-NH_2 group of lysine in the active center of the enzyme. Studies on the inactivation of the enzyme by group-specific reagents described below support these findings.

L-Phenylalanine Inhibition of Placental and Intestinal Alkaline Phosphatases

The reciprocal plots of velocity vs. substrate concentrations in the presence of L-phenylalanine, the sterospecific inhibitor[42–51] of alkaline phosphatases of rat intestine, human intestine and human placenta, were straight lines parallel to those obtained in the presence of noninhibitory D-phenylalanine. The nature of these curves with human placental alkaline phosphatase was identical to those of rat and human intestinal alkaline phosphatases, both of which evidenced "uncompetitive" inhibition by L-phenylalanine (FIGURE 14). The extent of L-phenylalanine inhibition of the variants A and B was dependent on pH and substrate concentrations. Results presented in TABLE 3 showed that Michaelis constant, maximal velocity and the first-order rate constant for the decomposition of the enzyme-substrate complex into products (k_3) of rat intestinal alkaline phosphatase were reduced by L-phenylalanine, while the energy of activation

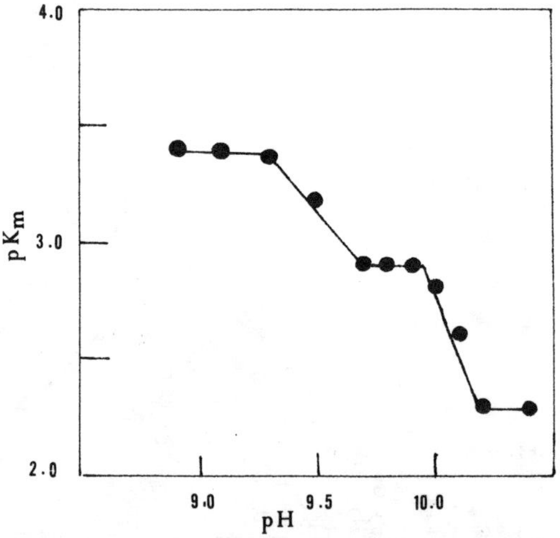

FIGURE 13. Profile showing pK_m ($-Log_{10}K_m$) vs. pH plot of placental alkaline phosphatase. The enzyme used in making this profile was purified by the procedure outlined above, except that steps involving treatment and fractionation with ammonium sulfate were omitted. Ammonium sulfate treatment during purification could change the pK_m-pH profile, as it might act as an inhibitor of the enzyme.[4]

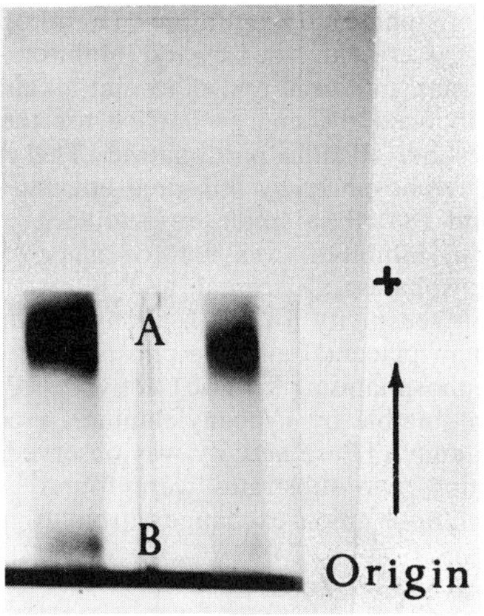

FIGURE 14. Starch gel enzymogram of placental alkaline phosphatase containing both variants A and B, developed with 5 mM D-phenylalanine (left) and 5 mM L-phenylalanine (right). The arrow has the same significance as in FIGURE 11.

TABLE 3

KINETIC AND THERMODYNAMIC PARAMETERS* FOR THE BINDING REACTION OF INTESTINAL ALKALINE PHOSPHATASE† WITH L-PHENYLALANINE

Parameters	Without Inhibitor	With Inhibitor
Activation Energy	6,000	18,000
k_3 at pH 9.2	3.0×10^{-3}	1.05×10^{-3}
K_m at pH 9.2	1.8×10^{-4}	0.9×10^{-4}
V_{max}	1.9×10^{-3}	0.8×10^{-3}
Optimum pH for Beta-Glycerophosphate	8.8	9.3
Phenylphosphate	9.8	10.2
Optimum Temperature for Maximal Velocity, V_{max}	38°	45°
Δ H(kcal/mole)	—	−5.52
K_i (mM)	—	2.1
Δ F(kcal/mole)	—	−3.5
Δ S(cal/mole/degree)	—	−6.4

* At 37° C.

† Activity of rat intestinal alkaline phosphatase, the detailed data on which are presented in this table, was measured with 18 mM phenylphosphate in 0.05 M carbonate-bicarbonate buffer, pH 9.8. Human intestinal alkaline phosphatase exhibited an optimum pH of 9.8 with alpha-naphthyl phosphate as the substrate. L-phenylalanine changed the pH optimum to 10.1. The pH optimum for human placental alkaline phosphatase with 18 mM phenylphosphate as substrate were 10.6 and 11.1 with and without the inhibitor, respectively.

for the cleavage of phenylphosphate, optimum pH and optimum temperature for maximal velocity, V_{max}, were enhanced by the inhibitor. A similar situation was also observed with human intestinal and placental alkaline phosphatases.

L-Phenylalanine enhanced the energy barrier for the hydrolysis of phenylphosphate by rat intestinal alkaline phosphatase. The energy of activation for the hydrolysis of phenylphosphate by intestinal enzyme with D- and L-phenylalanine were 6,000 and 18,000 cal/mole, respectively.

The optimum pH of inhibition was 9.6 for placental enzyme and 9.2 for intestinal alkaline phosphatase. Placental and intestinal isoenzymes behaved similarly so far as their sensitivity toward L-phenylalanine was concerned. Purified specimens of human placental alkaline phosphatase exhibited pyrophosphatase and adenosine triphosphatase (ATPase) activities. Pyrophosphatase activity of the enzyme was inhibitable by L-phenylalanine. A concomitant purification of phenylphosphatase and ATPase activity was observed, and the peaks for the enzyme activities against two substrates were found[52] to coincide with each other in the TEAE-cellulose anion exchange chromatogram. The release of in-

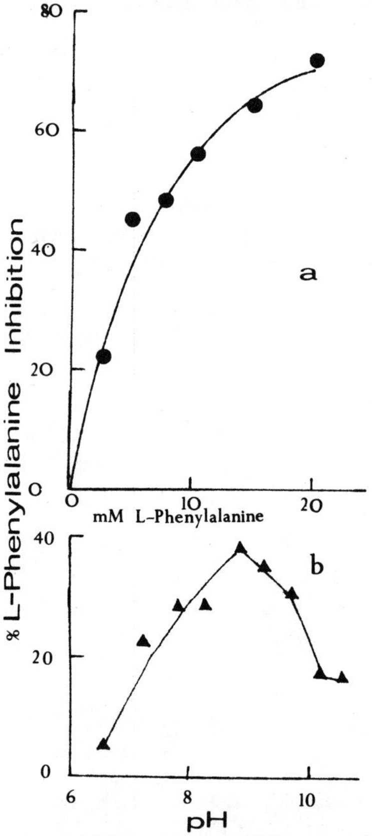

FIGURE 15. L-phenylalanine inhibition (%) of ATPase activity of purified placental alkaline phosphatase as a function of inhibitor concentration at pH 8.4 (a) and pH (b). The inhibitor concentration of the curve b was 5 mM. D-Phenylalanine (5 mM) was used in the control experiments.

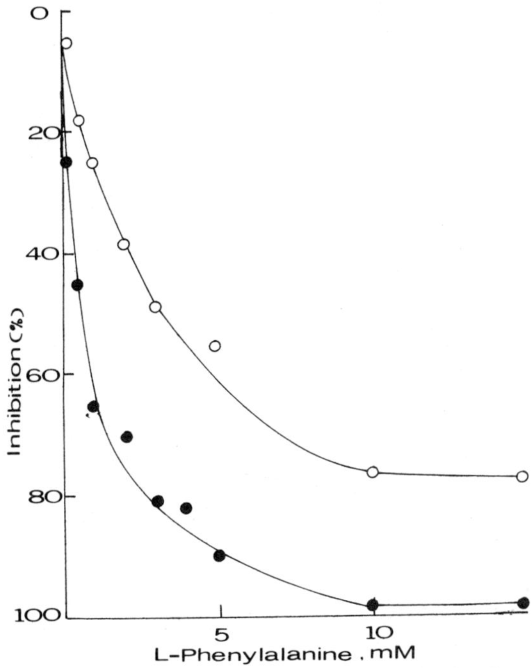

FIGURE 16. L-phenylalanine inhibition of rat intestinal alkaline phosphatase as a function of inhibitor concentration at 0° (●) and 45° (○).

organic phosphorus from ATP was a function of pH with an optimum pH of 9.1. ATPase activity of the purified enzyme was inhibited up to 40% by 5 mM L-phenylalanine (FIGURE 15b) at pH 8.4, the optimum pH for inhibition. The L-phenylalanine inhibition was a function of inhibitor concentration and, hence, could be enhanced up to 75% with 20 mM inhibitor (FIGURE 15a).

Papain digestion, heat denaturation and treatment with urea and diethylstilbestrol, which altered tertiary structure of the enzyme protein, did not lower the extent of L-phenylalanine inhibition of the enzyme, although a loss in enzyme activity was noted in each case. The number (n) of L-phenylalanine molecules that combined with one molecule of the enzyme was computed to be unity. The change of enthalpy during inhibition was −5.52 kcal, while the changes in free energy ranged from −3.6 to −3.3 kcal/mole in the temperature range of 0 to 45°. The change of entropy, Δ S for inhibition was −6.7 entropy units/mole. The inhibitor constant K_i was evaluated at four different temperatures, 0, 23.5, 37 and 45°. K_i values were directly proportional with temperature. Thermodynamic parameters, especially the low entropy change and the figure of unity for n, suggested that L-phenylalanine inhibition of intestinal alkaline phosphatase was not of the allosteric type. The nonallosteric nature of the inhibition was also corroborated by the nonsigmoid, hyperbolic curves obtained by plotting the extent of inhibition against either inhibitor (FIGURE 16) or substrate concentration. L-Phenylalanine inhibition decreased with an increase of temperature, and the optimum temperature for the maximal velocity was enhanced by the inhibitor. Inhibition of alkaline phosphatase by L-phenylalanine may thus be classified under the category of McElroy's homosteric transition in which the modifier conceivably combines at or near the active center of the enzyme and not at a distant site, as encountered in allosteric interactions.

The ϵ-NH_2 group of lysine, thiol group of cysteine and metal site are implicated in the mechanism of catalysis by alkaline phosphatase. Intestinal alkaline phosphatase could be inactivated by metal-binding agents such as EDTA, 8-hydroxyquinoline, pyridine-2, 6-dicarboxylic acid, alpha-alpha′-dipyridyl, *o*-phenanthroline and sodium cyanide; sulfhydryl reagents like *p*-hydroxymercuribenzoate, iodoacetamide and iodine (TABLE 4). The enzyme also lost activity on being reacted with amino-group-blocking reagents such as formaldehyde-acetamide and *o*-methylisourea, a reagent specific for ϵ-amino group of lysine. The diminution of enzyme activity was proportional to the concentration of the amino-group-modifying reagents, acetic anhydride, nitrous acid, succinic anhydride, formaldehyde and formaldehyde-acetamide. Treatment with acetic anhydride, succinic anhydride and formaldehyde-acetamide produced enzymes with electrophoretic migration greater than that of the untreated sample (FIGURE 17). The *o*-methylisourea-treated enzyme however, did not show increase in mobility, probably because the guanidino side chain introduced into the protein did not alter its negative charge. Chemical modification of the amino groups of alkaline phosphatase did not change the optimum pH but increased the K_m value, indicating reduced substrate affinity of the modified enzyme. The enzyme could be protected from inactivation by thiol-group reagents by pretreatment with substrate, and the inhibition was reversed by treatment with cysteine. Acetylated intestinal alkaline phosphatases showed "cooperative" activation by D-phenylalanine. The data on the order of stability constants of metal-binding agents compared with the order of effectiveness as inactivators of intestinal enzyme indicated the presence of Zn in the active center. Metal-binding agents not only altered enzyme activity but also reduced the extent of L-phenylalanine inhibition. This could be interpreted to suggest the probable role of metal, both in the

TABLE 4

INHIBITORS OF INTESTINAL ALKALINE PHOSPHATASE*

Metal-Binding Agents	Concentration (mM)	% Inhibition
EDTA (0.4)	1.0	89.1
8-Hydroxyquinoline (0.4)	1.0	92.0
Pyridine-2:6-Dicarboxylic Acid (0.4)	1.0	71.5
Sodium Cyanide (0.4)	10.0	82.0
Amino Group Reagents		
Acetic Anhydride (0.16)	91.0	94.0
Nitrous Acid (30)	200.0	47.0
Succinic Anhydride (48)	500.0	82.0
Formaldehyde (0.5)	4500.0	87.0
Formaldehyde-Acetamide (24)	2500.0	82.0
O-Methyl Isourea (114)	175.0	68.0
Thiol Group Reagents		
PHMB (1)	10.0	62.0
Iodoacetamide (16)	45.0	95.0
Iodine (1)	0.08	90.0

* The figures in parentheses after the name of each reagent refer to the time of reaction in hours. The enzyme used was purified from rat intestine.

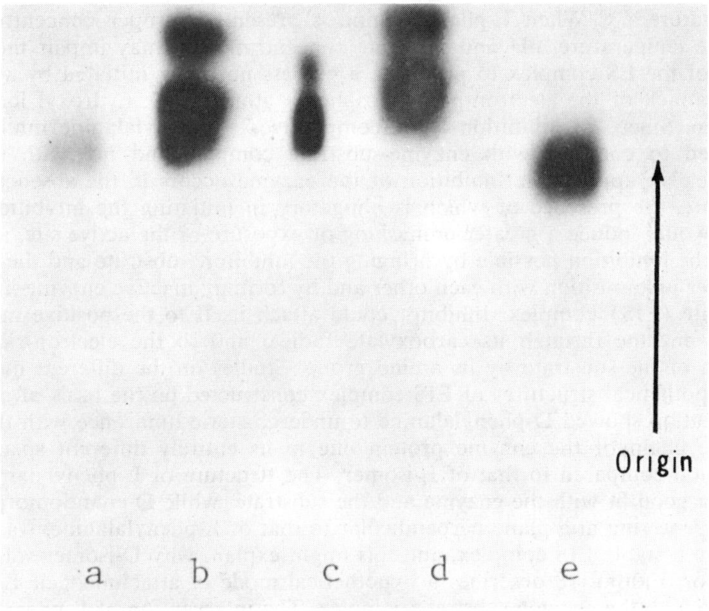

FIGURE 17. Starch gel enzymogram of purified rat intestinal alkaline phosphatase: a is untreated; b, acetylated; c, formaldehyde-acetamide treated; d, succinylated; and e, *o*-methylisourea-treated enzyme specimens. The arrow indicates the direction of migration toward anode.

binding of the substrate during catalysis and in the attachment of L-phenylalanine during inhibition.

As in other enzyme-catalyzed reactions, hydrolysis of phenylphosphate (S) or other phosphate esters by alkaline phosphatase (E), proceeds through the formation of an intermediate enzyme-substrate (ES) complex in the Michaelis-Menten scheme:

$$\begin{array}{c} E + S \underset{k_2}{\overset{k_1}{\rightleftharpoons}} ES \xrightarrow{k_3} E + \text{Products} \\ \quad\;\; \downarrow I \\ \quad\;\; EIS \end{array}$$

In the phosphoryl group of the substrate, the double-bonded oxygen may acquire a partial negative charge due to its greater electrophilicity than phosphorus (FIGURE 18). The electron-rich oxygen may be hydrogen-bonded with the thiol group during attachment of the substrate with the enzyme. One of the ionic oxygen atoms and the bridge oxygen can be pictured to coordinate with positively charged metal site of the enzyme. The other electron-rich ionic oxygen of the substrate may donate its electrons to the positively charge $\epsilon{-}NH_3^+$ group of lysine side chain, the presence of which at the active center was indicated by the studies with lysine-specific reagent, *o*-methylisourea. The enzyme-substrate complex is thus formed as diagrammatically depicted in FIGURE 18. The influence of electron attraction or repulsion by the substituents in the benzene ring of the substituted phenylphosphates, and of other factors, on the rate of formation of ES complex and its hydrolysis to products and enzyme back has been reported in literature.[53–59] When L-phenylalanine is present in proper concentration at suitable temperature, pH and substrate concentration, it may impair the breakdown of the ES complex to products, a process normally initiated by a nucleophilic attack of the electron-poor phosphorus atom by the hydroxyl ion of the medium. Since the inhibition is "uncompetitive," L-phenylalanine inhibition is expected to combine with enzyme-substrate complex and not with the free enzyme. No appreciable inhibition of the enzyme occurs in the absence of the substrate, the presence of which is obligatory in initiating the inhibition. Substrate would induce a greater unmasking or exposure of the active site, and thus make the inhibition possible by bringing the inhibitor, substrate and the enzyme in closer juxtaposition with each other and by forming inactive enzyme-inhibitor-substrate (EIS) complex. Inhibitor could attach itself to the positive metal site of the enzyme through its carboxylate radical and to the electron-rich ionic oxygen of the substrate by its amino group. Studies on the different models of the hypothetical structures of EIS complex constructed on the basis of available information showed D-phenylalanine to undergo steric hindrance with the polypeptide chain of the enzyme protein due to its entirely different spatial configuration compared to that of L-isomer. The structure of L-phenylalanine provided a good fit with the enzyme and the substrate, while D-enantiomorph, with its benzene ring at a plane perpendicular to that of L-phenylalanine, was unable to form a stable EIS complex, and this might explain why D-isomer was not an inhibitor. FIGURE 18 describes a hypothetical mode of attachment of L-phenylalanine with the enzyme-substrate complex. The intervention of L-phenylalanine at the active center of the enzyme to impede the cleavage of the ES complex into products is consistent with the "uncompetitive" homosteric mechanism of inhibition.

Distinctions Between Placental and Intestinal Isoenzymes of Alkaline Phosphatase

Human placental and intestinal alkaline phosphatases were inhibited to the same extent (80%) by 5 mM L-phenylalanine. Hence, treatment of L-phenylalanine could not be employed to identify and measure placental alkaline phosphatase in the presence of intestinal isoenzymes, although L-phenylalanine in-

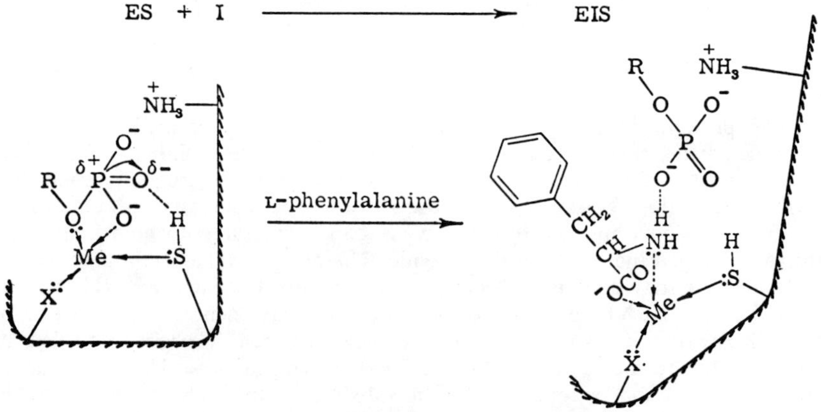

FIGURE 18. Hypothetical mode of attachment of L-phenylalanine with the enzyme-substrate (ES) complex to form enzyme-inhibitor-substrate (EIS) complex.

TABLE 5

DISTINCTIONS BETWEEN PLACENTAL AND INTESTINAL ISOENZYMES OF ALKALINE PHOSPHATASE

Parameters		Tissue Source	
		Human Placenta	Human Intestine
10.7/9.8 R*	2.0 mM	1.10	0.11
	10.0 mM	1.50	0.49
K_m			
	pH 9.2	0.31	0.06
	pH 9.4	0.45	0.20
	pH 9.8	2.3	0.66
Optimum pH (18 mM Phenylphosphate)		10.6	9.8
Susceptibility to Neuraminidase:		Neuraminidase-sensitive	Neuraminidase-resistant

* Ratio of enzyme activity at pH 10.7 versus that at pH 9.8.

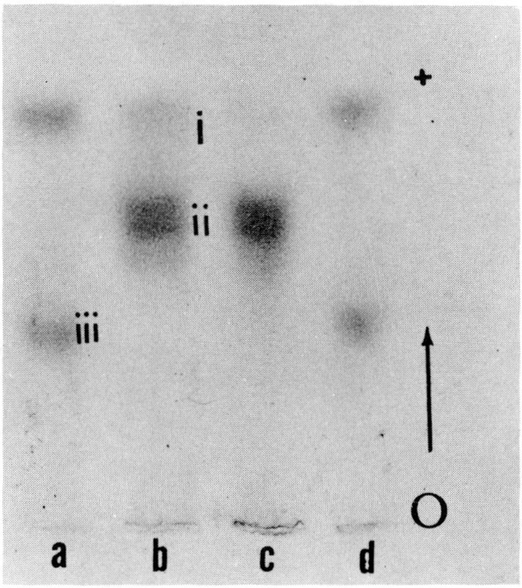

FIGURE 19. Thin layer Sephadex G-200 gel electrophoresis of serum alkaline phosphatase: i designates fast-moving nonplacental band in a, b, c and d; ii designates placental isoenzyme of alkaline phosphatase in pregnancy sera (b and c), *vide infra,* and iii designates slow-moving intestinal isoenzyme in cirrhotic serum (a and d). Origin was at O, and the arrow shows the anodal migration.

hibition provided a convenient means of distinguishing them from liver, bone and other nonintestinal alkaline phosphatases. However, various biochemical parameters (TABLE 5) such as optimum pH, neuraminidase sensitivity, Michaelis constant and the ratio of activity of pH 10.7 vs. 9.8 could be utilized to distinguish the two isoenzymes.[60] The relative proportions of these two isoenzymes in pregnancy sera (*vide infra*) may be determined by studying these parameters of the serum enzyme. Besides, the electrophoretic mobilities of placental and intestinal isoenzymes of serum alkaline phosphatase are different from each other. A remarkably good separation of the two isoenzymes present in pregnancy sera was achieved with a newly developed technique[61] of thin-layer Sephadex G-200 gel electrophoresis (FIGURE 19). While rat and human placental alkaline phosphatases were found sensitive to neuraminidase, intestinal isoenzymes were resistant to it and, hence, did not show any reduction of electrophoretic mobility by treatment with neuraminidase (FIGURE 20), an enzyme specific for cleaving sialic acid residues.

Intestinal Neuraminidase in Relation to Slow-Moving Isoenzyme of Serum Alkaline Phosphatase

Slow-moving L-phenylalanine-sensitive intestinal isoenzyme of alkaline phosphatase[51] was present in considerable amount in human sera of blood group O and B subjects, especially those who are secretors of ABH blood group sub-

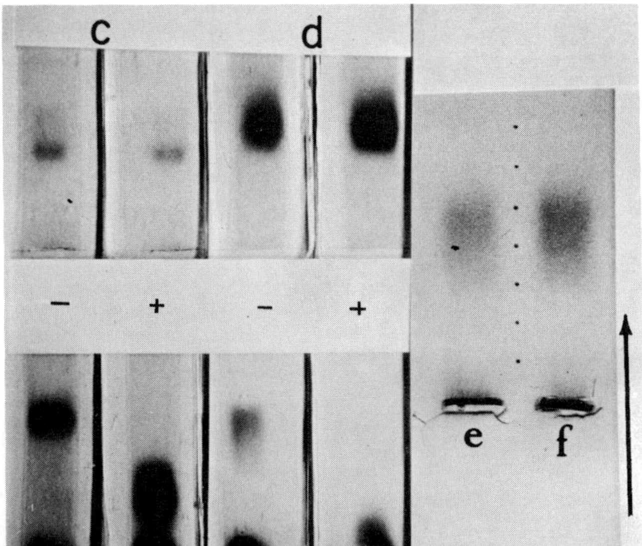

FIGURE 20. Starch gel electrophoresis of alkaline phosphatase in human placenta (a), rat placenta (b), human intestine (c), rat intestine (d), and human ileostomy drainage before (e) and after (f) treatment with neuraminidase. The plus sign in a, b, c and d indicates the pattern after being treated with neuraminidase, and the minus sign shows the same before neuraminidase treatment.

TABLE 6

NEURAMINIDASE ACTIVITIES* IN DIFFERENT HUMAN TISSUES

Tissue Source†	Neuraminidase Activities (Sample No.)					
	1	2	3	4	5	6
Liver	0	3690	0	0	0	0
Bone	0	1844	0	0	0	0
Kidney	0	1890	0	0	0	0
Intestine	631	5145	970	485	970	2910
Spleen	0	ND‡	0	0	0	0
Lung	0	ND‡	0	0	0	0
Placenta	0	0	0	0	0	0
Vibrio cholerae§	6165	6165	5340	5825	5825	6165

* Expressed as mμmoles sialic acid liberated by 1 ml of 10% homogenate in 1 hr from N-acetylneuramin lactose in acetate buffer, pH 5.5 at 37°.[59] While samples no. 1, 3, 4, 5 and 6 were normal tissues, the possibility of viral infection of different tissue specimens in sample no. 2 could not be excluded.

† Different postmortem tissue specimens, except placenta, in a particular sample were obtained from the same subject.

‡ Not determined.

§ Purified *Vibrio cholerae* neuraminidase (Calbiochem, 500 units/ml) was used to compare its activity with those of human tissue homogenates.

stances in saliva. Intestinal component of serum alkaline phosphatase is neuraminidase-resistant, the electrophoretic mobility of the enzyme not being reduced by pretreatment with sialidase. Moss and his associates reported that alkaline phosphatases prepared from human liver and kidney exhibited reduced electrophoretic migration on starch gel after incubation with neuraminidase.[51] Human placental alkaline phosphatase is also neuraminidase-sensitive,[32,51] and the enzyme is a sialoprotein, *vide infra.* Neuraminidase action helped greatly in the genetic studies of Robson and Harris[62] on placental alkaline phosphatase polymorphism. The mobility of alkaline phosphatase in gastric juice, and in duodenal and intestinal secretions, as well as in ileostomy drainage, are not affected by neuraminidase. A question may be posed as to whether the neuraminidase insensitivity of human intestinal and other related alkaline phosphatases is due to the presence of endogenous neuraminidase.[63] Activities of neuraminidase in different human tissues presented in TABLE 6 show that the intestinal mucosa is by far the richest source of neuraminidase compared to other organs such as liver, bone, kidney, spleen, lung and placenta. The nonintestinal tissues had none or comparatively small amounts of neuraminidase. Intestinal and duodenal secretions, gastric juice and ileostomy drainage also contained demonstrable amounts of neuraminidase. Alkaline phosphatases in the tissues of the gastrointestinal tract were neuraminidase-resistant, probably because endogenous neuraminidase present in comparatively high level in these tissues induced *in vivo* cleavage of the sialic acid residues of the enzyme. Any further treatment with purified neuraminidase *in vitro* did not lead to any more reduction in the electrophoretic migration of the enzyme, as its neuraminidase sensitivity had already been impaired *in vivo.* Unlike that of liver, bone and other tissues, the pH of intestinal and gastric secretions was close to 5.6, the optimum pH for neuraminidase activity, and this might be another contributing factor for the removal of sialic acid from intestinal alkaline phosphatase. Partially purified human intestinal neuraminidase could split off sialic acid from N-acetyl neuramin lactose and human placental alkaline phosphatase.[63]

Characterization of the Isoenzyme of Placental Alkaline Phosphatase in Human Pregnancy Serum

The level of serum alkaline phosphatase was enhanced in pregnancy,[47,64,65] the elevation being a function of the period of gestation (FIGURE 21 a). L-phenylalanine inhibition of serum alkaline phosphatase increased (FIGURE 21 b) concomitantly with the rise of serum enzyme level. The extent of heat (55°, 16 minutes) inactivation of serum alkaline phosphatase diminished with the progress of pregnancy and became minimum at parturition. It returned back to normal (FIGURE 22 b) several weeks after the delivery.

The ratio of serum alkaline phosphatase activity at pH 10.7 vs. 9.8 (10.7/9.8 R) was found to be 1.1 for placenta and around 0.11 for intestine, liver, bone and lung. The ratio (10.7/9.8 R) increased from 0.2 to 0.8 and from 0.4 to 1.0 with unheated and heated pregnancy sera, respectively (FIGURE 22 a). After the puerperium, the ratio was gradually reduced and returned back to 0.15 14 weeks after parturition. A new band (p) of alkaline phosphatase isoenzyme appeared (FIGURE 23) and increased in intensity as the pregnancy advanced. The bands p and B (variants B of placenta) disappeared about four weeks after the birth of the infant. When placenta was no longer a source of alkaline phosphatase in the postpartum weeks, intestine started to contribute at a larger concentration, and a distinct slow-moving intestinal band (i) appeared (FIGURE 23) in the sera of the patient (a blood group B subject). Starch gel patterns of alkaline phospha-

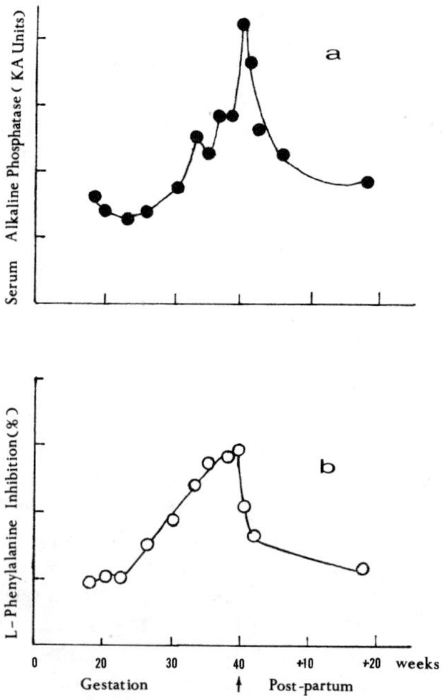

FIGURE 21. Serum alkaline phosphatase activity (a) and L-phenylalanine inhibition (b) as a function of the period of gestation in pre- and postnatal stages of pregnancy. The arrow indicates the time of puerperium. Blood samples used in experiments, the results of which are presented in these plots and in FIGURES 22, 23 and 24, were collected from the same subject (B.G.). I am thankful to my wife for volunteering herself to be the subject of this investigation, despite great apprehension at the beginning.

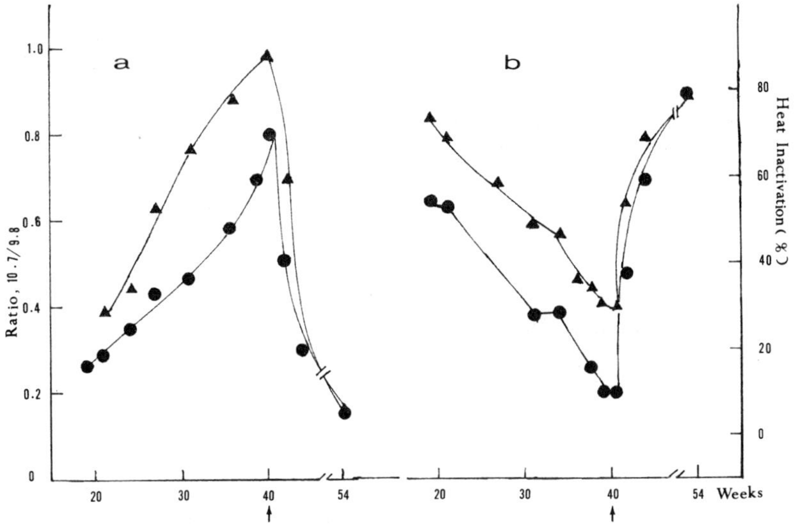

FIGURE 22. Change in the ratio of serum alkaline phosphatase activity at pH 10.7 vs. 9.8 (a) and heat inactivation of serum alkaline phosphatase (b) during pregnancy. The numbers in the abscissae refer to pregnancy weeks of gestation. The arrow has the same significance as in FIGURE 21. The triangles and the circles in (a) represent heated and unheated sera respectively. The heat stabilities of L-phenylalanine sensitive (●) and insensitive (○) moities of serum alkaline phosphatase are obtainable from (b).

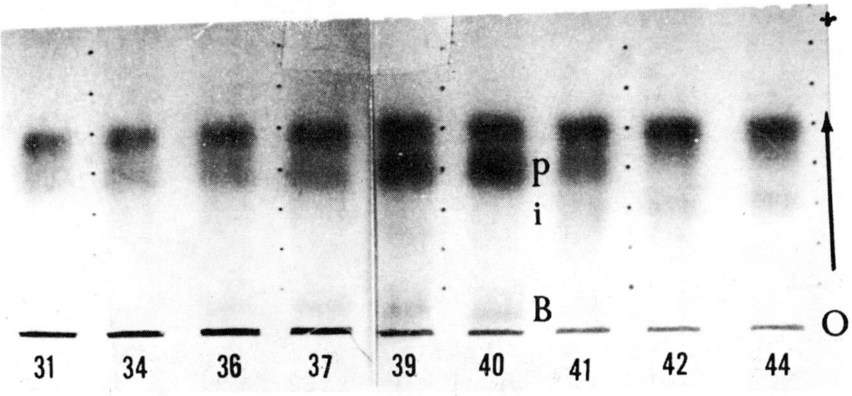

FIGURE 23. Starch gel electrophoretic patterns of serum alkaline phosphatase at different periods of pregnancy. Weeks of gestation are indicated by the numbers, origin by O, and the anodal direction by the arrow.

tase in neuraminidase-treated and untreated control serum sample were compared with the corresponding patterns of purified placental alkaline phosphatase variant A. The electrophoretic migration of the heat-stable serum isoenzyme was similar to those of placental isoenzyme (FIGURE 24). The biochemical parameters (TABLE 7), including electrophoretic behavior and neuraminidase sensitivity of heat-stable alkaline phosphatase in pregnancy sera at term were comparable to those of purified placental alkaline phosphatase but different from the values for alkaline phosphatase in cord serum of the newborn infant. The values for 10.7/9.8 R of the pregnancy sera of women in their third trimesters were higher than those of sera from normal, nonpregnant women. The difference was found to be statistically significant at 1% level. On the basis of these observations, the enhanced level of pregnancy serum alkaline phosphatase seemed to be due to the enrichment of the circulation with an isoenzyme of placental origin.

Characterization of "Placental Type" Alkaline Phosphatase in Human Neoplastic Pleural Effusion

Alkaline phosphatase isoenzyme of "placental type" was found in certain neoplastic cells and malignant tissues.[66-71] Placental-type alkaline phosphatase was characterized in human neoplastic pleural effusion of a cancer patient. Biochemical parameters of placental alkaline phosphatase were similar to those of alkaline phosphatase isolated from neoplastic pleural effusion (TABLE 8, FIGURES 25 and 26).

Human Placental Alkaline Phosphatase; a Sialoprotein

Human placental alkaline phosphatase is a substrate for bacterial and viral neuraminidases. *Vibrio cholerae* neuraminidase exhibited greater potency than influenza virus neuraminidase in releasing sialic acid from placental enzyme preparation. As pointed out earlier, the enzyme is also a substrate for human intestinal neuraminidase. Warren-thiobarbiturate chromogen of the compound released from the enzyme by 0.1 N sulfuric acid or by neuraminidase showed an absorption maximum at 550 mμ, as did pure N-acetyl neuraminic acid. *Vibrio*

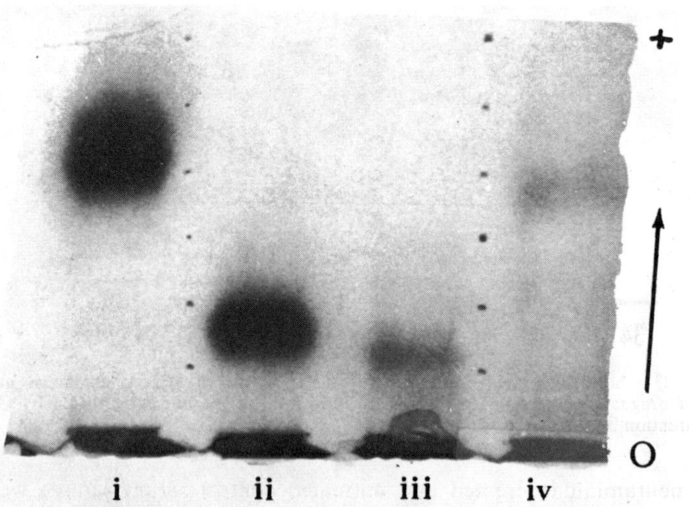

FIGURE 24. Starch gel enzymograms of the purified placental alkaline phosphatase variant A isolated from the placental tissue of the same subject whose blood specimens have been investigated (FIGURES 21, 22 and 23) before (i) and after (ii) treatment with neuraminidase. The gel patterns of placental alkaline phosphatase isoenzyme were compared with the corresponding enzymograms (iii, with neuraminidase; iv, without neuraminidase) of alkaline phosphatase present in heated (55°, 60 min) term serum. See FIGURE 23 for the significance of O and the arrow.

TABLE 7

PROPERTIES OF ALKALINE PHOSPHATASE IN MATERNAL TERM SERUM, CORD SERUM AND PLACENTA

Properties	Maternal Term Serum Unheated	Maternal Term Serum Heated	Cord Serum	Placenta* (Purified Variant A)
Inhibition (%) by 5 mM L-Phenylalanine at pH 9.6	56.4	71.3	20.7	75.0
Heat Stability (%) at 55°, 16 min	69.4	—	7.3	99.0
10.7/9.8 R†	0.9	1.0	0.3	1.1

* Variant A of placental alkaline phosphatase purified by butanol extraction, ammonium sulfate fractionation, exposure to heat and molecular sieve chromatography with Sephadex G-200.

† The ratio of enzyme activity at pH 10.7 to that at 9.8 with 2 mM disodium phenylphosphate as the substrate.

TABLE 8

COMPARISON OF SOME BIOCHEMICAL PARAMETERS* OF ALKALINE PHOSPHATASE IN HUMAN PLACENTA AND NEOPLASTIC PLEURAL EFFUSION

Parameters	Placenta	Neoplasm
K_m	0.51	0.55
Optimum pH (18 mM Phenylphosphate)	10.6	10.6
10.7/9.8 R (4.5 mM Phenylphosphate)	1.37	1.80
L-Phenylalanine (10 mM) inhibition (%)	87.5	89.5
n	0.82	0.70
Electrophoretic Migration		
Variant A	0.64	0.57
Variant B		
1st Component	0.28	0.36
2nd Component	0.03	0.03
Heat Stability (55°, 120 min)	100.0	100.0
K_i (M), EDTA	1.4×10^{-5}	1.4×10^{-5}
DTNB	5.6×10^{-3}	5.4×10^{-3}
HCHO-Acetamide	2.57	1.66

* Thanks are due to Mr. Everett Schaner for his skillful technical assistance in collecting the data presented in this table.

cholerae neuraminidase could liberate up to 80% of the total sialic acid of alkaline phosphatase under optimal conditions of hydrolysis. Specific activity and the extent of L-phenylalanine inhibition of placental alkaline phosphatase did not change by treatment with sialidase. The pH optimum for alkaline phosphatase-neuraminidase interaction was around 5.3. The presence of N-glycosidic bond in the enzyme was suggested by an extra peak at 385 mμ in its ultraviolet spectrum.[32] These results indicate that the enzyme is a sialoprotein.

Amino Acid and Carbohydrate Residues of Placental Alkaline Phosphatase

TABLE 9 shows the amino acid composition and carbohydrate residues of the purified enzyme. Lysine, serine and cysteine, which are implicated in the mechanism of catalysis by the enzyme were present in the protein-hydrolysate along with other amino acids. Sialic acid, glucosamine and galactosamine were believed to be the integral parts of the enzyme molecule. In a recent study[72] undertaken in conjunction with Professor R. J. Winzler, State University of New York

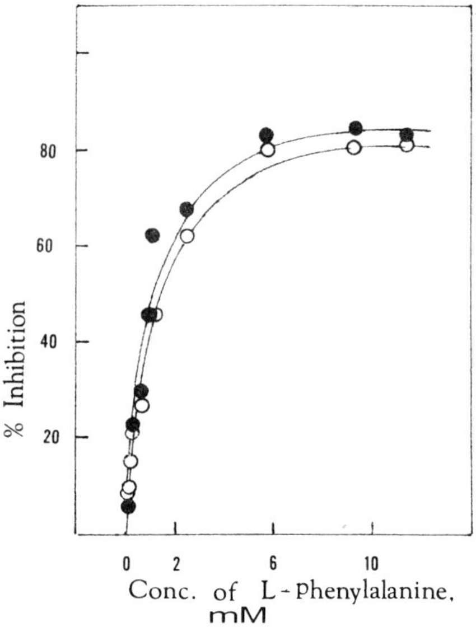

FIGURE 25. L-phenylalanine inhibition of alkaline phosphatase isolated from placenta (○) and neoplastic pleural effusion (●) as a function of inhibitor concentration.

at Buffalo, a number of neutral carbohydrate residues, such as fucose, mannose, galactose and glucose, were identified in purified placental alkaline phosphatase preparations.

Viral Hemagglutination Inhibitory Potency of Human Placental Alkaline Phosphatase Preparations

Many well-documented reports suggested that sialoglycoproteins might act as inhibitors of myxoviruses. The viral hemagglutination inhibitory property of different preparations of human placental alkaline phosphatase, a sialoglycoenzyme, has been discovered very recently. In this study, I have collaborated with Dr. Magdalena Usategui-Gomez and Dr. Helene Wallace Toolan of the Putnam Memorial Hospital Institute for Medical Research, Bennington, Vt. H-1 virus used in this work was isolated by Dr. Toolan from a transplantable human malignant tumor and is known as Toolan's virus. If this small DNA virus is treated with human placental alkaline phosphatase *in vitro,* it loses the ability to agglutinate red blood cells. All the enzyme-rich fractions at different stages of purification exhibited the capacity to inhibit agglutination of red blood cells by Toolan's H-1 virus.[73] The best TEAE-cellulose anion exchange fraction with more than a 1,000-fold increase in purity evidenced hemagglutination inhibitory potency of 51,000/mg of protein.[74,75] In TEAE-cellulose chromatogram (FIGURE 27), the enzyme activity peak coincided with the corresponding peak for hemagglutination inhibitory potency. Thus, it is quite probable that the hemagglutination inhibitory factor and the alkaline phosphatase present in the placental tissue are the same glycoprotein. Lyophilization, contamination with bacteria and, especially, treatment with neuraminidase removed the hemagglutination inhibitory potency of the enzyme. While the active center of the enzyme is in the polypeptide chain, the hemagglutination inhibitory site is perhaps located in its carbohydrate moiety.

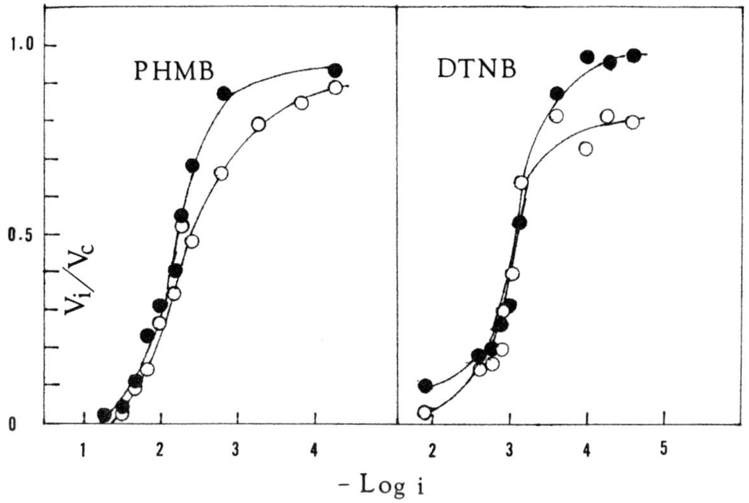

FIGURE 26. The plots of Vi/Vc vs. —Log i for *p*-hydroxymercuribenzoate (PHMB) and 5:5′-dithio-bis-2-nitro-benzoic acid (DTNB) with alkaline phosphatase purified from placental tissue (○) and neoplastic pleural effusion (●), Vi and Vc are enzyme activities with and without inhibitor (molar conc. = i), respectively.

TABLE 9

AMINO ACID AND CARBOHYDRATE RESIDUES OF PLACENTAL ALKALINE PHOSPHATASE VARIANT A

Residues	Moles per 70,000 g of Protein
Lysine	18
Histidine	8
Ammonia	92
Arginine	12
Aspartic acid	37
Threonine	20
Serine	23
Glutamic acid	43
Proline	17
Glycine	25
Alanine	32
Half Cystine	20
Valine	23
Methionine	7
Isoleucine	12
Leucine	36
Tyrosine	12
Phenylalanine	17
Tryptophan	4
Hexosamine	4
Sialic acid	7
Fucose*	1
Mannose*	4
Galactose*	6
Glucose*	1

* Determined by gas liquid chromatography and expressed in moles per 70,000 g of dry weight of a mixture of variants A and B. I am grateful to Professor R. J. Winzler for his cooperation in collecting these data. A detailed investigation on the carbohydrate contents of alkaline phosphatase variants is being pursued in collaboration with him.

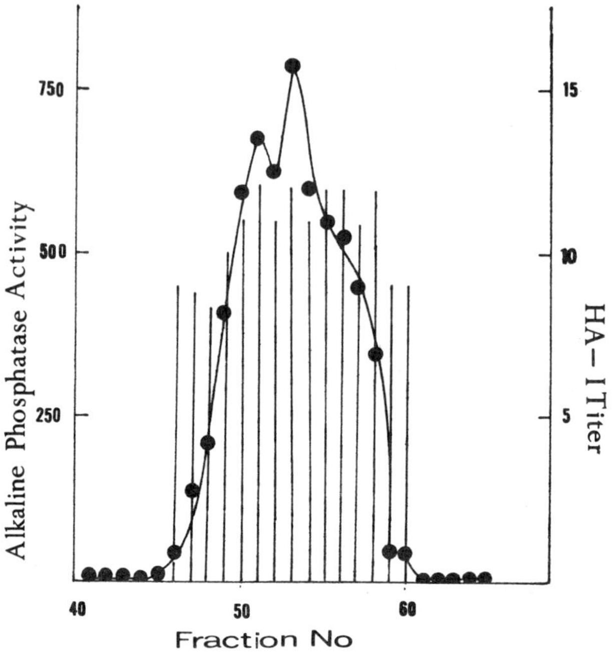

FIGURE 27. Enzyme activity (●) and hemagglutination inhibitory (HA–I) potency (vertical lines) of TEAE-cellulose anion exchange fractions obtained by stepwise elutions of placental alkaline phosphatase. The HA–I titers are expressed in arbitarary units comparable to the highest dilution of the enzyme specimen that completely inhibits agglutination of red blood cells by H–1 virus.

DISCUSSION

Placental alkaline phosphatase exists in at least two major forms, A and B, which have identical reaction kinetics but differ from one another in their molecular weights, although other differences cannot be discounted at this time. Variant A has a molecular weight comparable to that of bovine serum albumin, while the B form is a mixture of several heavy molecular species, which may probably be designated as B_1, B_2, B_3, etc. Molecular weight variants of the enzyme not separable by alcohol fractionation were isolated by Sephadex G-200 gel filtration. Placental albumin, the tenacious contaminant of variant A could be removed by TEAE-cellulose anion exchange chromatography and continuous curtain electrophoresis. The final preparation of A was homogeneous. The crystalline product, prepared by equilibrium dialysis, had properties similar to those of variant B and was sparingly soluble in aqueous buffered solutions. The crystalline variant B might be made soluble in water by precipitation with alcohol, which, however, was found to be deleterious to the enzyme activity of the crystals. The lower specific activity of variant B compared to that of A was not unusual Störmer[76] recently noted low solubility and reduced specific activity of his crystalline enzyme. As in the present study, pure crystalline amino acid oxidase,[77] *E. coli* alkaline phosphatase,[24,78] hexokinase[79] and other enzymes were found to contain more than one component and, hence, crystallinity is no longer a criterion of absolute homogeneity. Characteristic molecular properties of purified placental alkaline phosphatase were utilized to study the abundance of placental isoenzyme of alkaline phosphatase in pregnancy sera and in the neoplastic pleural effusion.

The existence of multiple molecular forms of enzymes within a single tissue may be due to a variety of reasons such as polypeptide synthetic machinery itself, enzymatic alteration, nonenzymic processes such as folding, aggregation, dissociation, chemical modification (FIGURE 17), catabolic changes and artifacts of isolation. According to "one gene-one enzyme" theory, the variants may be explained as the products of several genes or the result of hybrid molecules formed from different polypeptide chains. Molecular weight variants of placental alkaline phosphatase characterized in this work appeared to be due to aggregation and dissociation. The genetic variants of placental alkaline phosphatase have also been reported in the literature.[62–80] It was observed that, in stages of acute infection, many patients' sera showed frequent presence of heavy molecular aggregates[81] of alkaline phosphatase, whereas in normal subjects they could be found only very rarely. However, the physiologic advantage derived by the patients through aggregation of alkaline phosphatases was far from known. Fennely and his associates[82] recently reported similar phenomenon demonstrating the occurrence of heavy molecular weight species of alkaline phosphatase in pathological sera. This isoenzyme disappeared from the circulation when the patients recovered after long-term chemotherapy or other treatments. It may be mentioned in this connection that the heavy molecular variant B of placental alkaline phosphatase appeared to have greater antigenicity than A. I am thus tempted to make an open conjecture that variant B, observed in neoplastic pleural effusion, might have some role to play in coping with the challenge of infection.

Tomkins and his coworkers[79] showed the existence of multiple molecular forms of *E. coli* beta-galactosidase. The isoenzymes differed in their molecular weights and could be separated by Sephadex gel filtration and sucrose density gradient centrifugation. Moreland and Watts[39] identified and separated molecular weight isoenzymes of arginine kinase with Sephadex G-100. I guess that perhaps on careful scrutiny, molecular weight variants of alkaline phosphatase will be found also in other human tissues (heavy molecular species being present in infected organs) besides the placenta, and such findings may help in the clarification of the present perplexing picture of human alkaline phosphatase isoenzymes in pathological sera and infected tissues.

In recent years, human intestine has been considered as a possible contributor of normal adult serum alkaline phosphatase. Intestinal alkaline phosphatase, which is absorbed by lymph gland, may be conceived to be transported to the liver through the portal circulation. Intestinal enzyme may acquire sialic acid from endogenous donors during its transport to, or storage in, the liver. The attachment of sialic acid, which may lead to the formation of neuraminidase-sensitive fast-moving isoenzyme, may be mediated through hitherto unidentified sialic acid-transferring enzyme systems. It is known that a large amount of slow-moving, unmodified L-phenylalanine-sensitive intestinal component is present in relatively large amounts in cirrhotic sera, particularly of blood group O and B subjects. Perhaps degenerated liver cells produced by cirrhosis lose sialyl transferase[83] enzyme systems and can no longer function properly in handling alkaline phosphatase of intestinal origin. Hence, the unmodified intestinal isoenzyme, with its L-phenylalanine sensitivity and neuraminidase resistance intact, appears in substantial amounts (sometimes up to 99%) in the peripheral circulation.

Neuraminidase resistance of intestinal alkaline phosphatase may be due to the presence of neuraminidase in the intestinal tissue itself. This postulation offers an explanation of the slower electrophoretic migration of intestinal isoenzyme and throws some light on the origin of the slow-moving component of serum alkaline phosphatase.

Specimens of placental alkaline phosphatase isolated by different routes of purification have been found to contain essentially similar amounts of neutral carbohydrates,[72] and the enzyme is thus believed to be a glycoprotein. Besides, placental alkaline phosphatase activity was observed to be associated[75,84] with human placental inhibitor (proven to be a glycoprotein) to hemagglutination by H-1 virus. The combination of myxovirus with the cellular receptors are known to be mediated through terminal sialic acid residues of glycoproteins. The impairment of hemagglutinating potency of H-1 virus by pretreatment with placental alkaline phosphatase may be due to blocking or damage of the agglutination-specific sites at the surface structure of the virus by the enzyme itself or by its sialic acid.

Summary

Human placental alkaline phosphatase was purified by procedures involving butanol treatment, precipitation and extraction with ammonium sulfate, exposure to heat, alcohol fractionation, molecular sieving with Sephadex G-200, TEAE-cellulose anion exchange chromatography, continuous curtain electrophoresis and equilibrium dialysis. The enzyme exists in more than one interconvertible molecular form separable by Sephadex gel filtration. One of the variants with higher electrophoretic mobility and lower molecular weight attained 4,000-fold purity and was isolated in a homogeneous condition as judged by starch and Sephadex gel electrophoreses, ultracentrifugation and immunodiffusion. The heavy molecular form, which was obtained in crystalline condition, was electrophoretically slow-moving. Purified molecular weight variants exhibited similar kinetic properties.

Unlike alkaline phosphatases of other tissues, the isoenzymes of intestine and placenta undergo "uncompetitive" homosteric inhibition by L-phenylalanine. Intestinal and placental isoenzymes were inactivated by reagents reacting with metal, amino and sulfhydryl groups. Purified placental enzyme possessed L-phenylalanine-sensitive ATPase activity. Characteristic molecular properties of placental alkaline phosphatases were utilized to identify the placental isoenzyme in human pregnancy sera and in neoplastic pleural effusion. The amino acid composition of placental alkaline phosphatase was determined. Placental alkaline phosphatase, a substrate for bacterial, viral and human intestinal neuraminidases, was found to be a glycoprotein, and this sialoglycoenzyme exhibited the ability to inhibit hemagglutination of red blood cells by H-1 virus.

Acknowledgment

I am deeply indebted to Professor William H. Fishman, Tufts New England Medical Center, Boston, Mass. for his support, inestimable help and constant encouragement.

References

1. Schmidt, G. & S. J. Thannhauser. 1943. Intestinal phosphatase. J. Biol. Chem. **149:** 369.
2. Thoai, Nguyen-Van, J. Roche & L. Sartori. 1944. Isolement et cristallisation de la phosphatase alcaline du rein (phosphomonoeste'rase). C. R. Soc. Biol. (Paris) **138:** 47.
3. King, E. J., M. A. M. Abdul-Fadl, Nguyen-Van Thoai & J. Roche. 1949. Purification of alkaline phosphatase. Biochem. J. **44:** 428.

4. ANAGNOSTOPOULOS, C. & H. MATSUDAIRA. 1957. Purification and kinetic studies of the alkaline phosphatase of human placenta. Proc. Intern. Symp. Enzyme Chem., Tokyo-Kyoto, K. Ichihara, Ed. : 166.
5. MORTON, R. K. 1954. The purification of alkaline phosphatase of animal tissues. Biochem. J. **57**: 595.
6. MORTON, R. K. 1957. The kinetics of hydrolysis of phenylphosphate by alkaline phosphatases. Biochem. J. **65**: 674.
7. MATHIES, J. C. 1958. Preparation and properties of highly purified alkaline phosphatase from swine kidneys. J. Biol. Chem. **233**: 1121.
8. GAREN, A. & C. LEVINTHAL. 1960. A fine-structure genetic and chemical study of the enzyme, alkaline phosphatase of *E. Coli*. Biochim. Biophys. Acta **38**: 470.
9. ENGSTROM, L. 1961. Studies on calf intestinal alkaline phosphatase I. Chromatographic purification, microheterogeneity and some other properties of the purified enzyme. Biochim. Biophys. Acta **52**: 36.
10. ENGSTROM, L. 1964. Studies on bovine-liver alkaline phosphatase, purification, phosphate incorporation. Biochim. Biophys. Acta **92**: 71.
11. MOOG, F., H. R. VIRE & R. D. GREY. 1966. The multiple forms of alkaline phosphatase in the intestine of the young mouse. Biochim. Biophys. Acta **113**: 336.
12. PORTMANN, P. 1957. Zur Kenntis der alkalischen darmphosphatase. Z. Fiz. Khim. **309**: 87.
13. PORTMANN, P., R. ROSSIER & H. CHARDENNERS. 1960. Zur Kenntis der alkalischen darm phosphatase II. Untersuchungen uber die Homogenitat und den chemieschen Aufban der reiner alkalischen Phosphomonoesterase. Helv. Physiol. Pharmacol. Acta **18**: 414.
14. SCHALES, O. & K. ARAI. 1959. Preparation and properties of highly purified alkaline kidney phosphatase. Arch. Biochem. Biophys. **83**: 152.
15. PLOCKE, D. J., C. LEVINTHAL & B. L. VALLEE. 1962. Alkaline phosphatase of *Escherichia Coli*. A zinc metalloenzyme. Biochemistry **1**: 373.
16. BINKLEY, F. 1961. Purification and partial characterization of alkaline phosphatase of swine kidney. J. Biol. Chem. **236**: 735.
17. SARASWATHI, S. & B. K. BACHHAWAT. 1966. Heterogeneity of alkaline phosphatase in sheep brain. J. Neurochem. **13**: 237.
18. SARASWATHI, S. & B. K. BACHHAWAT. 1963. Phosphatases from human brain. I. Purification and properties of pyridoxal phosphate phosphatase. J. Neurochem. **10**: 127.
19. SUSSMAN, H. H., P. A. SMALL & E. COTLOVE. 1968. Human alkaline phosphatase. Immunochemical identification of organ-specific isoenzymes. J. Biol. Chem. **243**: 160.
20. COX, R. P., P. GILBERT, JR. & M. J. GRIFFIN. 1967. Alkaline inorganic pyrophosphatase activity of mammalian-cell alkaline phosphatase. Biochem. J. **105**: 155.
21. NISSELBAUM, J. S., M. SCHLAMOWITZ & O. BODANSKY. 1961. Immunochemical studies of functionally similar enzymes. Ann. N. Y. Acad. Sci. **94**: 970.
22. COX, R. P. & M. J. GRIFFIN. 1968. Alkaline phosphatase I. Comparison of the physical and chemical properties of enzyme preparation from mammalian cell culture, various animal tissues and *Escherichia Coli*. Arch. Biochem. Biophys. **122**: 552.
23. SCHLESINGER, M. J. & L. ANDERSON. 1968. Multiple molecular forms of the alkaline phosphatase of *Escherichia Coli*. Ann. N. Y. Acad. Sci. **151**: 159.
24. MALAMY, M. H. & B. L. HORECKER. 1964. Purification and crystallization of the alkaline phosphatase of *Escherichia Coli*. Biochemistry **3**: 1893.
25. MOSS, D. W., D. M. CAMPBELL, E. ANAGNOSTOU-KAKARAS & E. J. KING. 1961. Characterization of tissue alkaline phosphatases and their partial purification by starch gel electrophoresis. Biochem. J. **81**: 441.
26. MOSS, D. W. 1969. Biochemical studies on phosphohydrolase isoenzymes. Ann. N. Y. Acad. Sci. (This monograph.)
27. MOSS, D. W. 1967. Association of inorganic-pyrophosphatase activity with human alkaline phosphatase preparations. Biochem. J. **102**: 53.
28. REIS, J. 1937. Uber du aktivitat der 5-nukleotidase in der tierischen und menschlichen geweben. Enzymologia **2**: 183.
29. SEELICH, F. & H. EHRLICH-GOMOLKA. 1951. Uber du "Saure" und "alkalische" phosphatase in placenta and fruchtwasser. Enzymologia **15**: 96.
30. AHMED, Z. & E. J. KING. 1960. Purification of placental alkaline phosphatase. Biochim. Biophys. Acta **40**: 320.
31. LOWRY, O. H., N. J. ROSEBROUGH, A. L. FARR & R. J. RANDALL. 1951. Protein measurement with the Folin phenol reagent. J. Biol. Chem. **193**: 265.
32. GHOSH, N. K., S. S. GOLDMAN & W. H. FISHMAN. 1967. Human placental alkaline phosphatase; a sialoprotein. Enzymologia **33**: 113.

33. GHOSH, N. K. & W. H. FISHMAN. 1967. Characterization of human placental alkaline phosphatase isoenzymes. Fed. Proc. **26:** 558.
34. GHOSH, N. K., N. I. INGLIS & W. H. FISHMAN. 1966. Properties of purified and crystalline human placental alkaline phosphatase. Abstract of the 152nd National Meeting of the American Chemical Society, New York City, pg. 281C.
35. GHOSH, N. K. & W. H. FISHMAN. 1968. Purification and properties of the molecular weight variants of human placental alkaline phosphatase. Biochem. J. **108:** 779.
36. RICKLI, E. E. & J. T. EDSALL. 1962. Zinc binding and sulfhydryl group of human carbonic anhydrase. J. Biol. Chem. **237:** PC258.
37. EDSALL, J. T. 1968. Multiple molecular forms of carbonic anhydrase in erythrocytes. Ann. N. Y. Acad. Sci. **151:** 31.
38. GAZITH, J., R. H. GODDING, I. T. SCHULZE, F. C. WOMACK & S. P. COLOWICK. 1968. Multiple forms and subunits of yeast hexokinase. Ann. N. Y. Acad. Sci. **151:** 307.
39. MORELAND, B. & D. C. WATTS. 1967. Molecular weight isoenzymes of arginine kinase in the mollusca and their association with muscle function. Nature (London) **215:** 1092.
40. VALLEE, B. L. & R. R. SIMPSON. 1969. Zinc and cobalt alkaline phosphatases. Ann. N. Y. Acad. Sci. (This monograph.)
41. HARKNESS, D. R. 1968. Studies on human placental alkaline phosphatase I. Purification and crystallization. Arch. Biochem. Biophys. **126:** 503.
42. FISHMAN, W. H., S. GREEN & N. I. INGLIS. 1962. Organ-specific behavior exhibited by rat intestine and liver alkaline phosphatase. Biochim. Biophys. Acta **62:** 363.
43. FISHMAN, W. H., S. GREEN & N. I. INGLIS. 1963. An organ-specific, stereospecific inhibitor of human intestinal alkaline phosphatase. Nature (London) **198:** 685.
44. FISHMAN, W. H. & J. H. KREISHER. 1963. Stereospecific, organ-specific inhibition of intestinal alkaline phosphatase. Ann. N. Y. Acad. Sci. **103:** 951.
45. GHOSH, N. K. & W. H. FISHMAN. 1966. On the mechanism of inhibition of intestinal alkaline phosphatase by L-phenylalanine I. Kinetic studies. J. Biol. Chem. **241:** 2516.
46. FISHMAN, W. H., N. I. INGLIS, F. SARKE & N. K. GHOSH. 1966. Distinguishing characteristics of serum alkaline phosphatase isoenzymes. Fed. Proc. **25:** 748.
47. GHOSH, N. K. & W. H. FISHMAN. 1969. Characterization of placental isoenzyme of alkaline phosphatase in human pregnancy serum. Canad. J. Biochem. **47:** 147.
48. GHOSH, N. K. & W. H. FISHMAN. 1968. L-Phenylalanine inhibition of rat intestinal alkaline phosphatase; a homosteric phenomenon. Arch. Biochem. Biophys. **126:** 700.
49. GHOSH, N. K. & L. KOTOWITZ. 1969. On the intracellular distribution of alkaline phosphatase in human liver and intestine. Enzymologia **36:** 54.
50. FISHMAN. W. H. & N. K. GHOSH. 1967. Influence of reagents reacting with metal, thiol and amino sites on catalytic activity and L-phenylalanine inhibition of rat intestinal alkaline phosphatase. Biochem. J. **105:** 1163.
51. FISHMAN, W. H. & N. K. GHOSH. 1967. Isoenzymes of human alkaline phosphatase. *In* Advances in Clinical Chemistry. O. Bodansky & C. P. Stewart, Eds. **10:** 255.
52. GHOSH, N. K. (Unpublished observations.)
53. NATH, R. L. & N. K. GHOSH. 1963. Studies on serum phosphatases. Effect of dilution on acid and alkaline phosphatases of human serum. Enzymologia **25:** 182.
54. NATH, R. L. & N. K. GHOSH. 1963. Studies on serum phosphatases II. Increase in active site of serum alkaline phosphatase on dilution. Enzymologia **25:** 350.
55. NATH, R. L. & N. K. GHOSH. 1963. Studies on serum phosphatases III. Influence of structure on the hydrolysis of substituted phenylphosphates by serum alkaline phosphatase. Enzymologia **26:** 141.
56. NATH, R. L. & N. K. GHOSH. 1963. Studies on serum phosphatases IV. Energy changes during complex formation between substituted phenylphosphates and serum alkaline phosphatase. Enzymologia **26:** 297.
57. GHOSH, N. K. 1963. Studies on serum phosphatases. Ph.D. Thesis, Calcutta University, Calcutta, India.
58. NATH, R. L. & N. K. GHOSH. 1964. Use of 16-β-methyl-9-α-fluoro-prednisolone (betamethasone) phosphate as a substrate for the estimation of human serum alkaline phosphatase. Bull. Calcutta School Trop. Med. **12:** 111.
59. NATH, R. L. & N. K. GHOSH. 1967. Studies on serum phosphatases V. Nonspecific human alkaline phosphatase and FDPase in normal and pathological conditions. Enzymologia **32:** 378.
60. FISHMAN, W. H., N. I. INGLIS & N. K. GHOSH. 1968. Distinctions between intestinal and placental isoenzymes of alkaline phosphatase. Clin. Chim. Acta **19:** 71.
61. INGLIS, N. R., N. K. GHOSH & W. H. FISHMAN. 1968. Sephadex G-200 gel electrophoresis of human serum phosphatase. Anal. Biochem. **22:** 382.

62. Robson, E. B. & H. Harris. 1966. Further studies on the genetics of placental alkaline phosphatase. Ann. Hum. Genet. **30:** 219.
63. Ghosh, N. K., L. Kotowitz & W. H. Fishman. 1968. Neuraminidase in human intestinal mucosa. Biochim. Biophys. Acta **167:** 201.
64. Neale, F. C., J. S. Clubb, D. Hotchkis & S. Posen. 1965. Heat stability of human placental alkaline phosphatase. J. Clin. Path. **18:** 359.
65. McMaster, Y., R. Tennant, J. Clubb, F. C. Neale & S. Posen. 1964. The mechanism of the elevation of serum alkaline phosphatase in pregnancy. J. Obstet. Gynaec. Brit. Comm. **71:** 735.
66. Fishman, W. H., N. R. Inglis, M. J. Krant & L. L. Stolbach. 1968. A serum alkaline phosphatase isoenzyme of neoplastic tissue origin. Cancer Res. **28:** 150.
67. Inglis, N. I. & N. K. Ghosh. 1967. L-Phenylalanine sensitive alkaline phosphatase (LPSAP) of intestine, placenta and neoplastic tissue. Abstract of the VIIth International Congress of Biochemistry, Tokyo, I-62, p. 928.
68. Fishman, W. H., E. Schaner, N. K. Ghosh, S. Green & N. R. Inglis. 1968. Biochemical and immunologic evaluation of the Regan isoenzyme of alkaline phosphatase in cancer patients. Abstract of the 156th Annual Meeting of the American Chemical Society, Atlantic City (September 8–13), pg. 265.
69. Fishman, W. H., N. R. Inglis, S. Green, C. L. Anstiss, N. K. Ghosh, A. E. Reif, R. Rustigian, M. Krant & L. L. Stolbach. 1968. Immunology and biochemistry of Regan Isoenzyme of alkaline phosphatase in human cancer. Nature (London) **219:** 697.
70. Fishman, W. H. 1969. Immunologic and biochemical approaches to alkaline phosphatase isoenzyme analysis: The Regan Isoenzyme. Ann. N. Y. Acad. Sci. This Monograph.
71. Stolbach, L. 1969. Clinical application of alkaline phosphatase isoenzyme analysis. Ann. N. Y. Acad. Sci. This Monograph.
72. Ghosh, N. K. & R. J. Winzler. (Unpublished work.)
73. Toolan, H. W. 1968. The Picodna Viruses; H, Rv and AAV. Int. Rev. Exp. Path. **6:** 135.
74. Ghosh, N. K. & M. Usategui-Gomez. 1969. Viral haemagglutination inhibitory potency of human placental alkaline phosphatase. Biochim. Biophys. Acta **177:** 565.
75. Usategui-Gomez, M., N. K. Ghosh & H. W. Toolan. 1969. Association of placental alkaline phosphatase activity with preparations of the human placental inhibitor to haemagglutination by H-1 virus. Proc. Soc. Exp. Biol. Med. **130:** 1128.
76. Störmer, F. C. 1967. Isolation of crystalline pH 6 acetoacetate-forming enzyme from *Aerobacter aerogenes*. J. Biol. Chem. **242:** 1756.
77. Wellner, D. & M. B. Hayes. 1968. Multiple molecular forms of L-amino acid oxidase. Ann. N. Y. Acad. Sci. **151:** 118.
78. Malamy, M. H. 1963. The alkaline phosphomonoesterase of *Escherichia Coli.* Its localization and physiological function. Ph.D. Thesis, New York University, New York, N. Y.
79. Alpers, D. H., E. Steers, Jr., S. Shifrin & G. Tomkins. 1968. Isoenzymes of the lactose operon of *Escherichia Coli.* Ann. N. Y. Acad. Sci. **151:** 545.
80. Beckman, L., B. Björling & C. Christodoulou. 1966. Pregnancy enzymes and placental polymorphism II. Leucine aminopeptidase. Acta Genet (Basel) **16:** 122.
81. Ghosh, N. K. (Unpublished observations.)
82. Fennely, J. J., J. Dunne, K. McGeeney, L. Chung & M. Fitzgerald. 1969. The importance of varying molecular size, differential heat and urea inactivation of phosphatase in the identification of disease patterns. Ann. N. Y. Acad. Sci. (This monograph.)
83. Kaufman, B., S. Basu & S. Roseman. 1968. Enzymatic synthesis of disialogangliosides from monosialogangliosides by sialyltransferases from embryonic chicken brain. J. Biol. Chem. **243:** 5804.
84. Ghosh, N. K. & M. Usategui-Gomez. (Unpublished data.)

Discussion of the Paper

M. Etzler: I should like to ask Dr. Ghosh what was the blood type of the donor of tissue used in the characterization of the enzyme carbohydrate? Do you know this?

Dr. Ghosh: No. This was pooled placentae. To prepare a large amount of enzyme, one has to start with a large number of placenta. The tissue used was a mixture of more than one placenta.

DR. ETZLER: You made no attempt to determine the blood group. I mean, this may have come from people with the same blood group. You have no information on this?

DR. GHOSH: We have not done that yet. No.

L. BECKMAN: There are a few points that may add to your study, that is, the genetic variation of placental alkaline phosphatase, which has been studied in many laboratories–above all, in the Galton Laboratory in London. It struck me that you're speaking of the enzyme as *the* enzyme, although there are frequent variants. May I show a few slides?

DR. HORECKER: Yes, very briefly please.

DR. BECKMAN: There are three main variants that occur rather frequently (FIGURE 1). In Caucasians, the F variant is rather frequent. In a Nigerian population, you would have, almost exclusively, the variant you have shown us, that is, S. So, since you are dealing with these three main types, F the heterozygous type FS, and S, it puzzles me that you get one zone if you're dealing with pooled material, since the FS type is very frequent there and you're bound to get it. The slow-moving band at the bottom is what you refer to as B. We have observed that the B bands do not separate on polyacrylamide, paper and agarose. They only separate on starch gel. If you run two-dimensional electrophoresis on acrylamide and starch gel in the second dimension, you will find that each B variant has exactly the same mobility as its main A variant. In sucrose density centrifugation, we and several other people have found that there's practically no difference

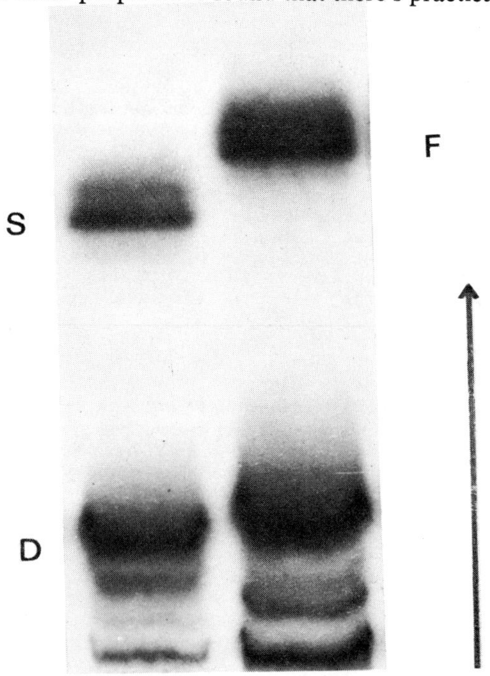

FIGURE 1. Starch gel electrophoresis at pH 8.2 showing isozymes of alkaline phosphatase in two individual placentas. F and S are two common genetic variants. The D variants are rare and are separable on starch gel, but not on paper, polyacrylamide and agarose. (Reproduced, with permission, from Beckman, L. & G. Beckman. 1969. A genetic variant of placental alkaline phosphatase with unusual electrophoretic properties. Acta Genet. (In press.)

at all between A and B, and that the fast-moving enzyme A has a molecular weight of about 120,000, and that the slow-moving component B is possibly a little bit larger. Would you please comment on this?

DR. GHOSH: Yes. I remember yesterday your electrophoretic migration of the placental alkaline phosphatase was much faster than liver and bone. We didn't observe this phenomenon in our laboratories. Secondly, as I've stated in response to Dr. Etzler's question, we did not restrict ourselves to a particular population or a particular genetic background of the individual. The starting material was pooled placentae. Many of the chemical reagents like persulfates, used to polymerize acnylamide during preparation of the gel are found to be inhibitors of alkaline phosphatase. . . . I think the starch gel should be used to separate these isoenzymes. . . as it does not involve the use of reagents with deleterious effects on enzyme activities.

DR. BECKMAN: No, it's not a matter of inhibition. You can show it does not separate.

DR. GHOSH: What was the material you used in this study?

DR. BECKMAN: This was the extract of the enzyme.

DR. GHOSH: How did you prepare this extract?

DR. BECKMAN: It was prepared by homogenization only.

DR. GHOSH: Did you take the whole homogenate or the center piece, or what was it?

DR. BECKMAN: It was water-extracted placentas without . . .

DR. GHOSH: With all the particles in it or the supernatant of the homogenate?

DR. BECKMAN: The supernatant.

DR. GHOSH: It has usually been found that the major amount of variant B, the heavier molecular weight species is present in particulate fractions (mitochondria, microsomes, etc.), not in the supernatant fractions, and one would have to release this B variant by butanol treatment.

DR. BECKMAN: No, you don't have to. You can do this with water extraction. This strong component called Δ only separates on starch gel electrophoresis at pH 8.2, and this separation can be completely abolished by adding EDTA.

DR. GHOSH: The lower band, which you're showing–is that your variant of variant B, or what?

DR. BECKMAN: This is a genetic variant that behaves the same way as B; it's well separated, but this happens only on starch gel.

DR. GHOSH: Yes, that's what I mean. Starch gel would have to be used.

H. H. SUSSMAN: We did comparable studies with a purified placental alkaline phosphatase that we made in two batches a couple of years apart, and our findings have always been that in purified form it's essentially a molecule of molecular weight 116,000 that can be dissociated into two monomers, each of which have a molecular weight of 58,000. However, when we dialyze the molecule to equilibrium above pH 10.5, then we get a reversible multimer-monomer system in which, at high pH, the multimer form is favored and constitutes approximately 90 to 95% of the material in the centrifuge cell. The rest of the material is essentially a tetramer of about 240,000, and this system is reversible by simple titration.

DR. GHOSH: I'd like to comment on that. I remember that you have obtained a molecular weight of 125,000, and I believe that your enzyme is a dimer. I think that in your isolation technique the pH was maintained at 6.5. This might be the reason why, finally, you get the dimeric species at 125,000 because, as you know, this transformation of one form to the other is pH dependent, and if one takes the precipitate forming at a lower acidic pH, one may expect to get the heavier molecular species.

D. AMINOFF (*University of Michigan, Ann Arbor, Mich.*): I believe you showed that there were some seven molecules of sialic acid in the alkaline phosphatases. Is that right?

DR. GHOSH: Yes, that's right.

DR. AMINOFF: You would expect, then, I suppose, to get the number of variants with mild or short treatments with sialidase. Have you done that at all?

DR. GHOSH: Well, this was done in Dr. Harris's laboratory, and they found that if one treats the enzyme with a gradient concentration of neuraminidase, one gets about seven different bands, which can be observed in the electrophoretic field.

DR. AMINOFF: Well, there shouldn't be more bands than the number of sialic acid molecules you have there.

DR. GHOSH: No. It is not over seven. We have found this to be five to six.

BIOCHEMICAL STUDIES ON PHOSPHOHYDROLASE ISOENZYMES

D. W. Moss*

Department of Clinical Chemistry, University of Edinburgh
The Royal Infirmary, Edinburgh, U.K.

The widespread occurrence in animal tissues of enzymes that *in vitro,* hydrolyse phosphate esters at alkaline pH has been recognized for many years, and the results of numerous biochemical studies on these alkaline phosphatases have been reported. In spite of these investigations, several features of the biochemistry of the alkaline phosphatases have remained in doubt, notably the precise limits of their substrate specificity, the identity or dissimilarity of alkaline phosphatases from the several tissues of a species, and the number of such phosphatases to be found within a given tissue. Although active extracts of phosphatase-containing tissues can readily be obtained, preparation of highly purified alkaline phosphatases from human sources has proved more difficult, and at least some of the uncertainties concerning these enzymes can be attributed to the use of enzyme preparations of a low degree of purity. One human alkaline phosphatase–that from the placenta–has now been crystallized,[1] however, and the present paper describes studies on the phosphatases of human liver, bone and small intestine after purification of the order of 1000- to 2000-fold.[2,3] The results of these investigations are considered from the viewpoint of enzyme specificity and inter- and intra-tissue heterogeneity.

Substrate Specificity

For some years, the consensus was that alkaline phosphatases acted only on orthophosphate monoesters and did not hydrolyze inorganic or organic pyrophosphates. In 1965, Russell[4] suggested that the excess of pyrophosphate in the urine of patients suffering from hypophosphatasia represented a failure to break down this substance due to alkaline phosphatase deficiency, a characteristic of this condition. Cox and Griffin[5] subsequently reported that inorganic pyrophosphatase activity is associated with several human and other animal alkaline phosphatases, and in view of these reports, the pyrophosphatase activity of the human liver, bone and intestinal enzymes was investigated during purification.

The purification stages included extraction of the tissues with *n*-butanol followed by acetone and ammonium sulphate precipitation, filtration through Sephadex G-200 gel, anion-exchange chromatography on DEAE-cellulose and finally, for the phosphatases of liver and intestine, recycling gel filtration. At all stages, fractions possessing alkaline orthophosphatase activity (substrate, *p*-nitrophenyl phosphate at pH 10) also liberated inorganic phosphate from sodium pyrophosphate (at pH 8.5); while at the chromatographic and gel-filtration stages the peaks of orthophosphatase and pyrophosphatase activity were exactly coincident. The ratios of ortho- to pyrophosphatase activity did not vary significantly during purification and were of the order of 15 to 1 for liver and bone phosphatases and 3 to 1 for the intestinal enzyme.[3,6] (The slight variations noted in these ratios may have resulted from alterations in the content of metal ions, which have a differential action on the two activities.).

Inorganic pyrophosphatase activity was confirmed as a property of the purified alkaline phosphatases by the following additional criteria: coincident zones for

* Present address: Postgraduate Medical School of London (University of London) Ducane Road, Shepherd's Bush, London, W. 12.

both activities on starch gel electrophoresis, the zones remaining coincident after treatment with neuraminidase, which reduces the electrophoretic mobility of bone and liver phosphatases; parallel decline of the two activities during inactivation by heat and concentrated urea solutions; and nonadditive ortho- and pyrophosphatase velocities in mixed substrate experiments with a similar response to inhibitors.[6,7] In addition, ortho- and pyrophosphatase activities were found to be strongly correlated in blood samples from patients with a raised alkaline phosphatase activity due to liver or bone diseases.[8]

The alkaline phosphatases also release inorganic phosphate from organic pyrophosphates such as adenosine diphosphate (ADP) and adenosine triphosphate (ATP).[9] The relative activities of the bone and liver phosphatases toward these and other substrates are rather similar when referred, in each case, to activity toward the reference substrate *p*-nitrophenyl phosphate, but intestinal phosphatase is relatively more effective in its action on ADP and ATP. Addition of magnesium ions further alters the specificity patterns, markedly depressing the action of intestinal phosphatase on pyrophosphates (FIGURE 1).

Magnesium ions also inhibit hydrolysis of inorganic pyrophosphate by the enzymes, and this contrasts with the well-known activating effect of these ions on orthophosphatase action. Zinc ions also have a differential action on the two activities, inhibiting orthophosphatase powerfully and noncompetitively, pyro-

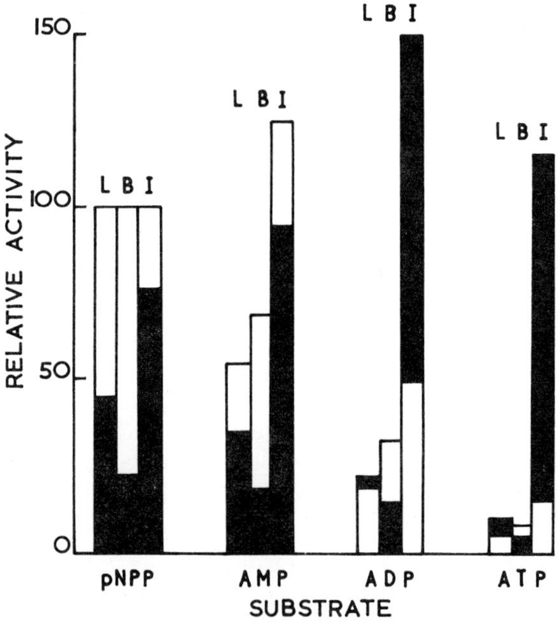

FIGURE 1. Relative release rates of inorganic phosphate from ortho- and pyrophosphate substrates by purified alkaline phosphatases of human liver (L), bone (B) and small intestine (I). Activity toward each substrate was measured at optimum pH for that substrate at 2 mM concentration. Solid bars represent activity without the addition of magnesium ions; open bars, activity with 10 mM magnesium present. For each enzyme, the activity toward all substrates has been expressed in terms of hydrolysis of 2 mM *p*-nitrophenyl phosphate (pNPP) plus 10 mM magnesium as 100. Substrates are adenosine monophosphate (AMP); adenosine diphosphate (ADP); and adenosine triphosphate (ATP).

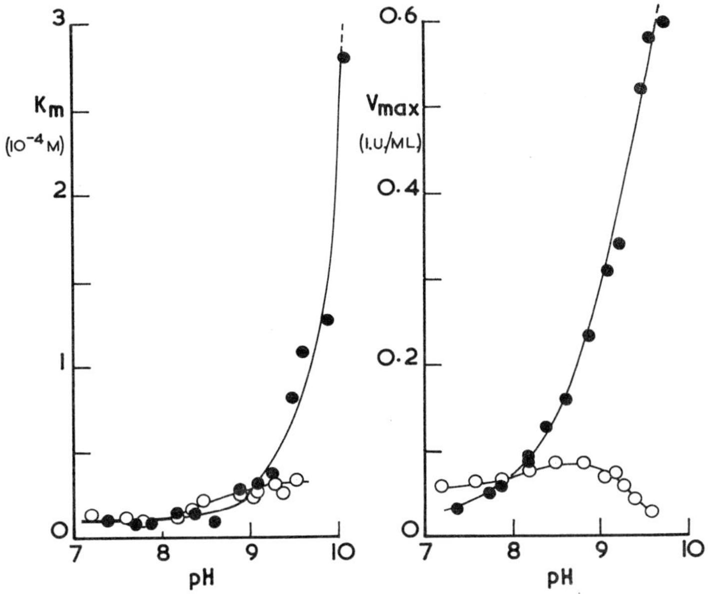

FIGURE 2. Variation of Michaelis constant (K_m) and maximum velocity (V_{max}) for the action of purified human bone alkaline phosphatase on *p*-nitrophenyl phosphate (●) and inorganic pyrophosphate (○). (Data from Eaton & Moss.[10])

phosphatase less strongly and competitively. It is apparent that these differences are due to interaction of metal ions with pyrophosphate rather than to the existence of separate enzymes; for example, zinc ions appear to form a complex with inorganic pyrophosphate, which is a competitive inhibitor of hydrolysis of both classes of substrate.

At the alkaline pH values usually chosen for *in vitro* measurements, the orthophosphatase activity of these enzymes is several times greater than their inorganic pyrophosphatase action, particularly in the case of liver and bone phosphatases. However, when measurements are extended toward pH 7, the maximum velocities for the hydrolysis of inorganic pyrophosphate and *p*-nitrophenyl phosphate approach each other;[10] similarly, values of Michaelis constant for the two substrates are of the same order in the range of pH 7 to 8.5 (FIGURE 2). Thus, under conditions that may be more closely approximate to those *in vivo,* the alkaline phosphatases appear to be as effective inorganic pyrophosphatases as orthophosphatases, an observation that may lend support to hypotheses regarding their physiological roles, e.g., the suggested pyrophosphatase function of the bone enzyme in calcification.[4]

Distinctions Between Alkaline Phosphatases From Different Human Tissues

One of the main objectives of the present work was to define differences in properties between the phosphatases from the three tissues and, if possible, to account for such differences on a molecular basis. One of the first tissue-specific characteristics of alkaline phosphatases to be discovered was Bodansky's observation that intestinal phosphatase resists inhibition by bile acids,[11] and this approach has been further extended by Fishman and his colleagues, who have demonstrated the selective inhibition of intestinal phosphatase by L-phenylalanine.[12] Other evidence has been accumulated that clearly differentiates intestinal alkaline phosphatase from the enzymes of other tissues; in fact, intestinal phosphatases from different species resemble each other more closely than phosphatases from other tissues of the same species. Similar evidence also identifies placental alkaline phosphatase as being in a separate category. Thus, at least three tissue-specific forms of these enzymes exist: (1) placental, (2) intestinal, and (3) nonplacental, nonintestinal phosphatases (TABLE 1).

Of the evidence that supports this classification in the present study, the differences in substrate specificity between human intestinal phosphatase, on the one hand, and the liver and bone enzymes on the other, have already been mentioned. The comparatively greater resistance to denaturation by heat, urea solutions and acid pH on the part of intestinal phosphatase was also noted, as was the lack of effect of incubation with neuraminidase on the electrophoretic mobility of this enzyme.[13]

Within the nonplacental, nonintestinal group of phosphatases, however, differences between the enzymes are much less clear-cut, and this is particularly true of the liver and bone phosphatases. There are small differences in the mobilities of the main bone and liver enzyme zones on starch gel electrophoresis, but both are retarded by treatment with neuraminidase. The substrate specificities of the two phosphatases are similar without being completely identical, and there are reproducible differences also in Michaelis constants.[14] Liver phosphatase is more resistant to inactivation by heat, urea and acid pH than bone phosphatase,[3] and these differences are maintained in mixtures of the two enzymes. The sum of biochemical evidence, therefore, suggests that tissue-specific variations exist within the nonplacental, nonintestinal group of phosphatases, and this conclusion is reinforced by the recent demonstration of an immunochemical distinction between liver and bone phosphatases.[15]

Although there are basic similarities between alkaline phosphatases from different tissues – for example, they are probably all enzymes with an active serine residue – the differences between placental phosphatase, intestinal phosphatase and those in the nonplacental, nonintestinal group are such that at least three separate structural genes seem to be involved, one controlling each of the three groups. In the case of placental alkaline phosphatase, an inherited polymorphism has been observed that further indicates a separate genetic control for this enzyme.[16,17] However, the evidence is not conclusive enough to determine whether the phosphatases within the nonplacental, nonintestinal group are genetically heterogeneous, or whether the differences observed can be attributed to cytoplasmic factors operating in each tissue on a fundamentally similar enzyme molecule. Analyses of primary structures will eventually determine whether genetically distinct alkaline phosphatases exist within each tissue and – for those phosphatases that are almost certainly the products of distinct genes (i.e., placental and intestinal phosphatases) – whether the differences have arisen by modification of a common prototype or by convergent evolution from separate precursors.

The Heterogeneity of Alkaline Phosphatases Within a Single Tissue

As with many other enzymes, the availability of separation methods of high resolving power – notably gel electrophoresis – has stimulated an investigation

TABLE 1

DIFFERENCES BETWEEN THREE MAIN CATEGORIES OF HUMAN ALKALINE PHOSPHATASES

Properties	Placental Phosphatase	Intestinal Phosphatase	Nonplacental, Nonintestinal (Liver, Bone, etc.) Phosphatases	References
Catalytic Properties				
1. Substrate specificity	Hydrolyzes β-glycerophosphate and phenyl phosphate at similar rates (others more active on phenyl phosphate).	Hydrolyzes AMP and PP_1 faster with respect to *p*-nitrophenyl phosphate than nonintestinal enzymes.	Similar relative rates of hydrolysis of various substrates by enzymes within this group.	3, 6, 9, 24
2. Inhibition				
(a) By Bile Acids	—	Not Inhibited	Inhibited	11
(b) By L-Phenylalanine	Inhibited	Inhibited	Not Inhibited	12
Molecular Properties				
1. Resistance to denaturation (a) Time for Half-Inactivation at 55° C	Completely Stable	60 Min	Varies slightly for different phosphatases (bone 5–10, liver 30–40 min).	3, 18, 25
(b) Urea Concentration for Irreversible Inactivation	8 M	6–7 M	Varies with source of enzyme (liver 3 M, bone and kidney < 3 M).	3, 26, 27
(c) Exposure to Low pH	—	More Stable Than Non-Intestinal enzymes.	Liver phosphatase more stable than bone phosphatase.	3, 28
2. Effect of Neuraminidase on Electrophoretic Mobility	Retarded	Not Retarded	Retarded	3, 13, 21, 29
3. Immunochemical	Antigenically distinct (partial cross-reaction with intestinal enzymes.)	Antigenically distinct (partial cross-reaction with placental enzymes.)	Antigenically distinct from placental and intestinal enzymes. Antiserum to liver phosphatase does not cross-react with bone and kidney phosphatases.	15, 30, 31

into the molecular variations of alkaline phosphatase within a single tissue. When phosphatase-containing extracts of human tissues are submitted to starch gel electrophoresis at pH 8.6, the main zones of activity show various degrees of heterogeneity, ranging from a fairly compact band in liver extracts to a very diffuse region in extracts of kidney. Additional, slowly-migrating, minor zones are present in all extracts.

Earlier investigations of the properties of these zones after recovery from starch gels – e.g., their Michaelis constants and stabilities to heating – indicated that, within a single tissue, the properties of the main enzyme zone are reflected in the minor bands, and that, within the more diffuse main zones such as those of intestinal and kidney phosphatases, there is apparently no variation in properties.[18,19] These observations suggest that there is only a single alkaline phosphatase within each tissue, and that the observed heterogeneity is a consequence of modification of this single enzyme in some way.

A more detailed examination of the heterogeneity of liver and intestinal phosphatases was made during the present study. The starch gel electrophoresis appearances of these enzymes at different stages of purification are represented diagrammatically in FIGURES 3 and 4.

In the case of the liver enzyme (FIGURE 3), the compact, slow-moving zone

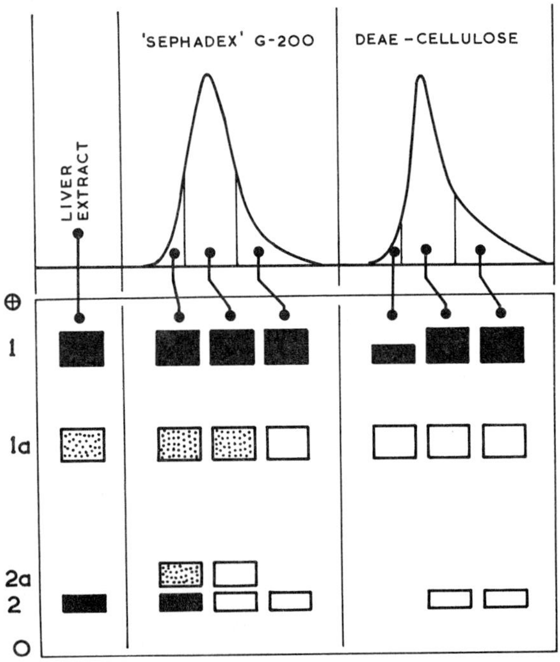

FIGURE 3. Diagram showing appearance on starch gel electrophoresis of active zones of human liver alkaline phosphatase in a butanol-extract of the tissue and in fractions taken from Sephadex G-200 gel filtration and DEAE-cellulose chromatography. The gel filtration and chromatography peaks are represented in the upper part of the figure with the corresponding electrophoresis patterns (at pH 8.6) in lower part. The direction of migration is upward. The shading indicates relative intensities of active zones; open rectangles are faint zones and solid rectangles, strong zones, with dotted areas corresponding to zones of intermediate activity. (Data from Smith *et al.*[2])

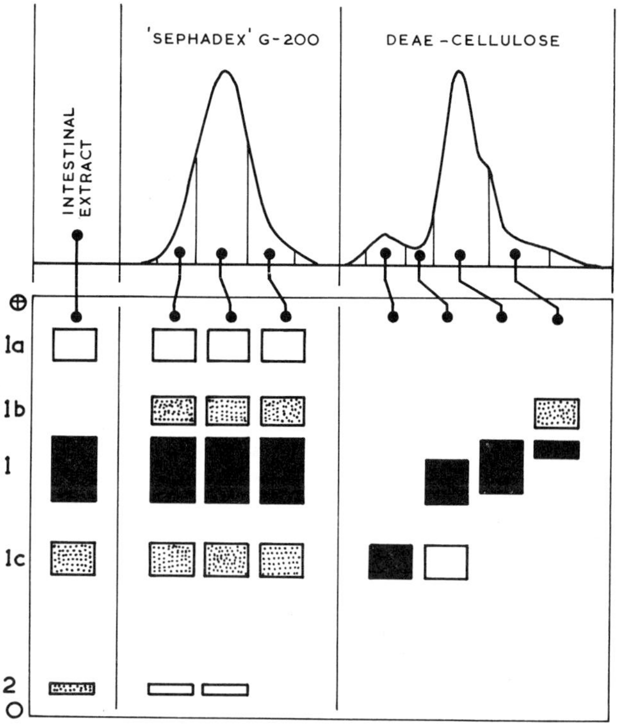

FIGURE 4. Starch gel electrophoresis appearance of human intestinal alkaline phosphatase fractions during extraction and purification. Representation as in FIGURE 3.

(2) is enriched in the early fractions from gel-filtration, suggesting that this zone may represent an aggregate of the enzyme, either with itself or with nonenzymic proteins such as lipoprotein. The fainter intermediate zone (2a) is also enriched in the same fractions, and thus may be due to a partial degradation of zone 2. The major enzyme zone (1) is not resolved on gel-filtration, but is heterogeneous on anion-exchange chromatography. The intermediate band (1a) is present in variable amount during purification and may represent a product of partial degradation of zone 1. The status of these minor zones (1a and 2a) as possible degradation products is reinforced by the observation that their appearance is governed to some extent by the method used to prepare the tissue extract.[20]

The pattern of zones of intestinal phosphatase is broadly similar (FIGURE 4), except that the degree of heterogeneity within the main active region is much greater. This heterogeneity is apparently due to a variation in net charge. The intensity of the subsidiary zones (1a, 1b and 1c) is again variable throughout purification and from one preparation to another, and these zones may represent degradation products; the stability to urea of zone 1c is much lower than that of the other fractions.

Some of the heterogeneity of the main alkaline phosphatase zones may be due to a variable content of sialic acid residues, at least in certain tissues such as kidney or liver, since preincubation with neuraminidase reduces the mobility of the enzyme zones and also the degree of heterogeneity.[21] However, intestinal phosphatase does not appear to contain sialic acid, at least not in a combination accessible to the action of neuraminidase. It is interesting that treatment with neuraminidase also reduces the mobility of zone 2 of liver extract, providing additional support for the view that the several zones have a common origin.

The extreme heterogeneity of the alkaline phosphatases presents several problems of interpretation. While attachment of varying numbers of sialic acid residues to the enzyme protein may provide part of the explanation, variation in the protein core of the enzyme cannot be ruled out, and the apparent absence of sialic acid from intestinal phosphatase makes such an explanation untenable regarding that enzyme. Alkaline phosphatases are fairly large enzyme molecules, gel-filtration indicating molecular weights of about 200,000 and it may be possible for considerable alteration in the structure of the enzyme molecule to take place without serious modification of its catalytic properties. Since these are enzymes of very low specificity, the structural requirements for enzyme activity are presumably less strict than would be the case for an enzyme of absolute specificity.

It is also relevant to consider to what extent the properties of the alkaline phosphatases observed *in vitro* reflect the situation as it exists in the living cell. Alkaline phosphatases apparently do not exist free in solution in the cytoplasm but are associated with subcellular structures such as microsomes, and purification processes involve the disruption of this association by autolysis or extraction with butanol. To this degree, therefore, studies carried out *in vitro* are performed on unphysiological or degraded enzyme, and it may be that this dissociation process is responsible for the great degree of heterogeneity observed on electrophoresis and chromatography. Thus, the compact, slowly migrating phosphatase zones present in extracts of most tissues may represent a closer approach to the condition of these enzymes in the living state.

As with other enzymes, the answers to the unsolved problems presented by the alkaline phosphatases must come ultimately from investigations into their primary, secondary and tertiary structural levels. These, in turn, depend on the availability of pure enzymes in some quantity, and while solutions may not be imminent, there are promising developments to be recorded. The recent crystallization of human placental alkaline phosphatase[1] is such a development, while limited amino acid sequence studies by means of labeling with radioactive phosphate[22,23] show promise as a way of attacking the primary structure of the phosphatases.

Discussion of the Paper

S. Posen: Would Dr. Moss care to speculate on the reason for the pH optimum differences between orthophosphatase or the phosphatase activity toward orthodox substrates and pyrophosphatase activity.

Dr. Moss: I think that, possibly, part of that explanation may be that at lower pH, binding the ionized phosphate groups may be responsible for combination with the enzyme, and this is perhaps what's necessary for activity, but when you get to higher pH's, there may be binding sites coming into play that are able to attach to the nonphosphate part of orthophosphate substrates and these may have an effect on the reaction rates and the binding of the substrate, but they're just not seen when the substrate is entirely a phosphate, for example, a pyrophosphate molecule.

Dr. Naughety (*Ohio State University, Columbus, Ohio*): You mentioned that the variants seen could be breakdown products. Dr. Ghosh mentioned a few moments ago that intestine contains quite a bit of neuraminidase, and I'm wondering if you have an opinion as to whether or not the lack of sialic acid in the preparation of intestinal alkaline phosphatase might be due to an attack of neuraminidase during the preparation of the enzyme.

DR. MOSS: I believe this suggestion has been made by Dr. Fishman, that he thought this might be a reasonable explanation. I think it might. I don't know really about the relative positions of these two enzymes in intestinal mucosa, whether such a thing would be possible, but this explanation has occurred to Dr. Fishman. It does seem reasonable, certainly.

J. NAVIA (*Massachusetts Institute of Technology, Cambridge, Mass.*): I wonder if you have investigated the effect of bone or intestinal alkaline phosphatase on other substrates, such as phosphoproteins, say, something like casein or vitellin.

DR. MOSS: We haven't done this. I don't know whether this is all part of the difficulty of deciding what these enzymes are, in fact, doing *in vivo*. It may be that they are phosphoprotein phosphatases, but I think we've got to regard them as much more widely active than we believed them to be a few years ago, and it may be that this is a possibility. All sorts of substrates are now possible.

N. K. GHOSH: With regard to the earlier question about neuraminidase, we have reported that in all tissues, of the intestinal or gastrointestinal tract, which contains the neuraminidase-resistant alkaline phosphatase–that is, alkaline phosphatase whose electrophoretic mobility could not be reduced by treatment–contain a considerable amount of neuriminidase.

DR. ALCOCK: (*Sloan Kettering Institute, New York, N. Y.*): I wondered if you had looked into the effect of calcium, especially on inorganic pyrophosphatase activity.

DR. MOSS: No, this we haven't tried, and calcium I think is usually a mild activator of phosphatase activity. With pyrophosphate I would expect that it would have a similar effect to that which it has on all the phosphatases, provided that the relative concentrations of the pyrophosphate and calcium was such that there was free substrate present.

DR. ALCOCK: I would like to make a comment on inorganic pyrophosphatase, which I've been studying in rat costal cartilage. This tissue begins to calcify when the rat is about 35 to 40 grams in weight, and, associated with the initiation of calcification, there is a marked increase in inorganic pyrophosphatase activity. There appears to be no correlation between this activity and alkaline phosphatase in the tissue. The optimum pH is between 6.8 and 7.0, and the effect of magnesium ions is different from that which you've described. Maximum activity is with 10 mM of magnesium concentration, and the activity remains the same between 10 and 18 mM magnesium, but the enzyme is totally inhibited in the presence of magnesium by very low concentrations of calcium. So this does seem to be a case where, perhaps, inorganic pyrophosphatase associated with calcification is at least not also an alkaline phosphatase.

DR. MOSS: The human alkaline phosphatase seems not only to be different from that enzyme, but also different from the red cell inorganic pyrophosphatase, which has been described in which you get maximum activity in the presence of excess magnesium. In other words, the relative ratio of the magnesium to the substrate must be greater than 1, I think, or are optimal at about 3.8, I seem to remember. With these enzymes you don't get activity unless you've got excess pyrophosphate present. In other words, it seems to be free pyrophosphate that's the substrate, not the metal complex. These are difficulties that you mentioned for the calcification theory. I think that what we're trying to do is to find a role for alkaline phosphatase in bone calcification to explain the fact that in hypophosphatasia, the really important, and in fact the only, pathological sign is deficient calcification, and the corresponding chemical finding is low alkaline phosphatase activity. So the relation is no stronger than that. It's just an attempt to relate two events that may, in fact, be unrelated.

F. Moog: I would like to raise an objection to the idea that the variants that are shown by electrophoresis, for example, may be degradation products. As we tried to show with the mouse, the variants that we've been able to identify by electrophoresis, and in other ways, are differentially distributed on the villus. I would like to suggest that if you were to find some stable and reliable means of characterizing the enzyme in the homogenate so that you could then identify it with your different variants, you might be able to say whether or not these were really a result of the preparative processes. It seems to me it's quite important to know whether these variants are real, and whether they exist in the tissue, and whether they have specific distribution there.

Dr. Moss: Yes, I agree it is important, and there's no real evidence for suggesting that these are not real enzymes or enzyme variants. The only observations we've made on this point are that, first of all, there's no variation in the actual pattern, the gross pattern, in the human intestine by going up and down the intestine, that is, taking segments near to the stomach and then down to the distal parts.

Dr. Moog: Well, that's not what I'm speaking of.

Dr. Moss: No, I agree. The second point is that there is apparently no relative difference in extractability. If you take a piece of human intestine and set it to antolyze for various periods and electrophorese the extracts, you see the whole pattern at once. You see it faintly at first, and then it grows progressively stronger throughout. In other words, there is no more easily extractable part, but I agree that this doesn't necessarily provide an answer to your comment.

Dr. Moog: Yes, certainly we have no evidence of our variants in any way differing in extractability, but they are real in distribution.

R. C. Nordlie: I find your observations on pyrophosphatase activity of alkaline phosphatase quite interesting, but I think a false impression in some ways could be created here by attributing too much significance to the enzyme relative to this activity. For instance, in liver, at least in rat and guinea pig and other smaller animals, there is an extremely potent inorganic pyrophosphatase very specifically stimulated by magnesium, which I would speculate would be at least a hundred times, perhaps several hundred times, more active than alkaline phosphatase of any sort in liver. In heart and in aorta, we've demonstrated pyrophosphatase activity that is extremely sensitive to calcium, and have suggested that this may be involved in the calcification process or in the prevention of calcification, so that I believe we would have to think in terms of these pyrophosphatases, or specific pyrophosphatases, with respect to this particular function, since so many of these very active enzymes have been found in various tissues of the body.

Dr. Moss: I think this is the difficulty throughout with alkaline phosphatase. When Robison described the bone enzyme in 1923, it was much easier to assign its function. As time has gone on, more and more specific phosphatases have been described for every substrate that's been suggested for alkaline phosphatase; a specific enzyme acting on that substrate has been found. The observation that you made about inorganic pyrophosphatase represents to us just another step in this. All the time, alkaline phosphatase has been pushed further and further into the background by the finding of specialized and specific enzymes that act on the various substrates that have been suggested for it.

References

1. GHOSH, N. K. & W. H. FISHMAN. 1968. Purification and properties of molecular-weight variants of human placental alkaline phosphatase. Biochem. J. **108:** 779–792.
2. SMITH, J. K., R. H. EATON, L. G. WHITBY & D. W. MOSS. 1968. Large-scale gel-filtration in the purification of human liver and small intestine alkaline phosphatases. Anal. Biochem. **23:** 84–96.
3. EATON, R. H. & D. W. MOSS. 1968. Partial purification and some properties of human bone alkaline phosphatase. Enzymologia **35:** 31–39.
4. RUSSELL, R. G. G. 1965. Excretion of inorganic pyrophosphate in hypophosphatasia. Lancet **ii:** 461–464.
5. COX, R. P. & M. J. GRIFFIN. 1965. Pyrophosphatase activity of mammalian alkaline phosphatase. Lancet **ii:** 1018–1019.
6. MOSS, D. W., R. H. EATON, J. K. SMITH & L. G. WHITBY. 1967. Association of inorganic-pyrophosphatase activity with human alkaline-phosphatase preparations. Biochem. J. **102:** 53–57.
7. EATON, R. H. & D. W. MOSS. 1967. Inhibition of the orthophosphatase and pyrophosphatase activities of human alkaline-phosphatase preparations. Biochem. J. **102:** 917–921.
8. EATON, R. H. & D. W. MOSS. 1967. Alkaline orthophosphatase and inorganic pyrophosphatase activities in human serum. Nature (London) **214:** 842–843.
9. EATON, R. H. & D. W. MOSS. 1967. Organic pyrophosphates as substrates for human alkaline phosphatases. Biochem. J. **105:** 1307–1312.
10. EATON, R. H. & D. W. MOSS. 1968. Kinetic studies on the orthophosphatase and inorganic pyrophosphatase activities of human alkaline phosphatases. Enzymologia **35:** 168–178.
11. BODANSY, O. 1937. Are the phosphatases of bone, kidney, intestine and serum identical? The use of bile acids in their differentiation. J. Biol. Chem. **118:** 341–362.
12. FISHMAN, W. H., S. GREEN & N. I. INGLIS. 1962. Organ-specific behaviour exhibited by rat intestine and liver alkaline phosphatase. Biochim. Biophys. Acta **62:** 363–375.
13. MOSS, D. W., R. H. EATON, J. K. SMITH & L. G. WHITBY. 1966. Alteration in the electrophoretic mobility of alkaline phosphatase after treatment with neuraminidase. Biochem. J. **98:** 32–33C.
14. MOSS, D. W., D. M. CAMPBELL, E. ANAGOSTOU-KAKARAS & E. J. KING. 1961. Characterization of tissue alkaline phosphatases and their partial purification by starch-gel electrophoresis. Biochem. J. **81:** 441–447.
15. SUSSMAN, H. H., P. A. SMALL & E. COTLOVE. 1968. Human alkaline phosphatase. Immunochemical identification of organ-specific isoenzymes. J. Biol. Chem. **243:** 160–166.
16. BOYER, S. H. 1961. Alkaline phosphatase in human sera and placentae. Science **134:** 1002–1004.
17. ROBSON, E. B. & H. HARRIS. 1965. Genetics of the alkaline phosphatase polymorphism of the human placenta. Nature (London) **207:** 1257–1259.
18. MOSS, D. W. & E. J. KING. 1962. Properties of alkaline-phosphatase fractions separated by starch-gel electrophoresis. Biochem. J. **84:** 192–195.
19. MOSS, D. W. 1965. Properties of alkaline-phosphatase fractions in extracts of human small intestine. Biochem. J. **94:** 458–462.
20. MOSS, D. W. 1962. Isoenzymes of alkaline phosphatase in autolysed and butanol-extracted liver preparations. Nature (London) **193:** 981–982.
21. BUTTERWORTH, P. J. & D. W. MOSS. 1965. Action of neuraminidase on human kidney alkaline phosphatase. Nature (London) **209:** 805–806.
22. MILSTEIN, C. 1964. The amino acid sequence around the reactive serine residue in alkaline phosphatase from *Escherichia coli.* Biochem. J. **92:** 410–422.
23. ENGSTROM, L. 1964. The amino acid sequence around the reactive serine in calf-intestinal alkaline phosphatase. Biochem. Biophys. Acta **92:** 79–84.
24. AHMED, Z. & E. J. KING. 1960. Kinetics of placental alkaline phosphatase. Biochim. Biophys. Acta **45:** 581–592.
25. NEALE, F. C., J. S. CLUBB, D. HOTCHKIS & S. POSEN. 1965. Heat stability of human placental alkaline phosphatase. J. Clin. Path. **18:** 359–363.

26. Birkett, D. J., R. A. J. Conyers, F. C. Neale, S. Posen & J. Brudenell-Woods. 1967. Action of urea on human alkaline phosphatases: with a description of some automated techniques for the study of enzyme kinetics. Arch. Biochem. **121:** 470–479.
27. Butterworth, P. J. & D. W. Moss. 1967. The effect of urea on human alkaline-phosphatase preparations. Enzymologia **32:** 269–277.
28. Scutt, P. B. & D. W. Moss. 1968. Reversible inactivation of alkaline phosphatase in acid solution. Enzymologia **35:** 157–167.
29. Ghosh, N. K., S. S. Goldman & W. H. Fishman. 1967. Human placental alkaline phosphatase; a sialoprotein. Enzymologia **33:** 113–124.
30. Schlamowitz, M. & O. Bodansky. 1959. Tissue sources of human serum alkaline phosphatase, as determined by immunochemical procedures. J. Biol. Chem. **234:** 1433–1437.
31. Boyer, S. H. 1963. Human organ alkaline phosphatases: discrimination by several means including starch-gel electrophoresis of antienzyme-enzyme supernatant fluids. Ann. N. Y. Acad. Sci. **103:** 938–950.

INFLUENCE OF STRUCTURE OF SUBSTRATE ON THE HYDROLYSIS OF ALKYL AND ARYL PHOSPHATES BY PHOSPHOHYDROLASES : MECHANISM OF ACID AND ALKALINE PHOSPHATASES*

R. L. Nath

Calcutta School of Tropical Medicine, Calcutta, India

The influence of the structure of a reactant on the rate of a chemical reaction is well known. Hammett,[1] in his method of approaching this problem regarding the reaction at the side chain of the benzene ring, gave quantitative values to the electron displacement powers of substituents in the benzene ring and called them substituent constants (σ). If, in a series of the same side chain reaction of differently substituted phenyl compounds, the logarithms of the rate constants are plotted against the σ-values of the substituents in the benzene ring, then a straight line plot is obtained. A positive slope of this straight line meant that the reaction is facilitated by electron attraction of substituents, while a negative slope meant facilitation by electron release. The method was first used successfully in an enzyme-catalyzed reaction by Nath and Rydon[2] in their study of the hydrolytic action of emulsin on a series of substituted phenyl- β-D-glucosides. These workers determined the equilibrium constant for the reversible formation of the intermediate enzyme-substrate complex as envisaged by Michaelis and Menten[3] and the velocity constant for its irreversible hydrolysis into the products. Correlating these rate constants with substituent constants after Hammett, they arrived at an electronic mechanism for the hydrolysis of phenyl β-D-glucosides by emulsin.

The present study on acid and alkaline phosphatases was started with the same idea of using Hammett's approach and, if possible, of developing an electronic mechanism for the phosphohydrolase activity of these enzymes. This paper aims at coordinating all the published work on this subject from the author's laboratory and comparing the mechanism of action of the two phosphatases.

Methods

Acid phosphatase was obtained from leaves of *Phaseolus vulgaris*, L. and *Dolichos lablab*; alkaline phosphatase, from human serum. Pooled human serum was obtained from the blood of various donors. One portion was used as native serum, another was precipitated with ethanol to get the alcohol precipitate, while a third portion was precipitated with acetone. The native serum, as well as the alcohol and acetone precipitates, had considerably high alkaline phosphatase activity.[4] To get active preparations of acid phosphatase, petiole-free leaves, collected fresh, were homogenized in the Waring blendor and washed chlorophyll-free with acetone. Dry powdered material passing through a 30-mesh sieve was finally kept as acetone powder. Another partially purified preparation was obtained by extracting this powder with water and precipitating the extract with ethanol. Details are given by Nath and Pradhan[5] and by Nath and Das.[6,7]

These enzyme preparations were kept at $-20°C$ and used throughout the whole of the work.

* The author expresses his thanks to the Council of Scientific and Industrial Research of the Government of India and to the School of Tropical Medicine, Calcutta, India, for the facilities and funds provided by them for this study.

The substrates consisted of disodium phenylphosphate and barium salts of *o*-methyl, *m*-methyl, *p*-methyl and *m*-methoxy phenylphosphates. Besides these, barium salts of alkyl phosphates containing *n*-propyl, *iso*-propyl, *n*-butyl, *iso*-butyl, *sec.*-butyl, *tert.*-butyl, *n*-amyl, *iso*-amyl and *tert.*-amyl groups, were also used for acid phosphatase. Disodium phenylphosphate was obtained from the British Drug Houses Ltd. Other compounds were prepared by a modification[4,8,9] of the method of King and Nicholson,[10] in which phosphorus oxychloride was condensed with appropriate phenol or alcohol in pyridine solution. The final product was isolated as barium salt, and the purity determined by analysis of barium. In performing the hydrolytic experiments, freshly prepared solutions of the sodium salt were directly prepared, while the barium salts were first dissolved in cold dilute HCl, the barium precipitated with a requisite amount of 0.25 M K_2SO_4 solution, then filtered, and the volume of the filtrate made up with washings to get the desired concentration.

Acetate buffer prepared according to Green[11] was used for acid phosphatase, and carbonate-bicarbonate buffer after Colowick and Kaplan[12] was used for alkaline phosphatase in doing the hydrolytic experiments. The degree of hydrolysis of any substrate was found by estimating the liberated inorganic orthophosphate during a particular interval under well defined experimental conditions. The phosphate was analyzed by a modification of the method of Lowry and Lopez,[13] using KH_2PO_4 as the standard. With acid phosphatase, the final blue color stabilized after five minutes, but with alkaline phosphatase, in which a trichloracetic acid filtrate of the reaction mixture was used, the final color increased continuously; this necessitated taking readings at definite intervals, obtaining the value for zero minute by extrapolation, and using that value for the calculation.[14]

In all experiments, the reaction mixture was analyzed at definite intervals, and the first-order velocity constant, k_o for the overall reaction, was calculated from the slope of the straight line obtained by plotting the decadic logarithm

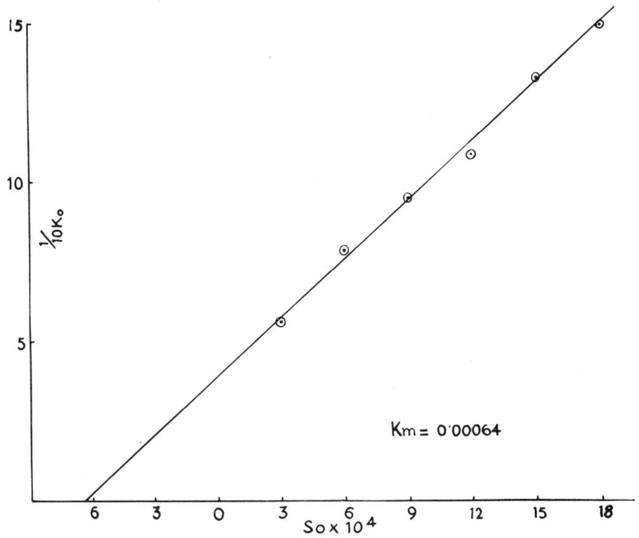

FIGURE 1. Determination of K_m-value for alkaline phosphatase using native serum at 35° C. (phenyl phosphate as substrate).

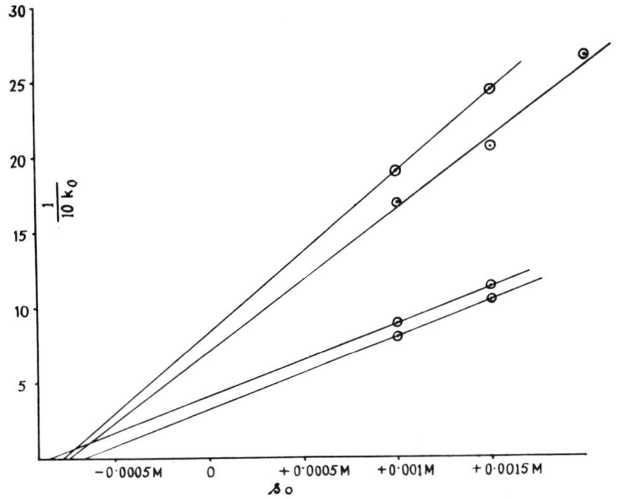

FIGURE 2. Determination of K_m-value for acid phosphatase using acetone powder at 40° C. (phenyl phosphate as substrate). Mean K_m = 0.00075. (Reproduced by permission of Enzymologia.)

of the molar concentration of unhydrolyzed substrate against time in minutes. The activity of an enzyme was expressed by the initial velocity of the reaction as determined by the product of the velocity constant and the initial molar concentration of the substrate. A Klett-Summerson photoelectric colorimeter was used in the work, and the thermostat maintained at an accuracy of ± 0.1° C.

For the determination of the Michaelis constant K_m, the velocity constant k_o was obtained experimentally at different substrate concentrations (s_o), and the plot of $1/k_o$ against s_o gave a straight line with its intercept on the X-axis equal to $-K_m$ (cf. Veibel[15]; Veibel & Lillelund[16]; Nath & Rydon[2]). The reciprocal of this was the equilibrium constant (termed affinity constant K_a in this paper) for the formation of the enzyme-substrate complex. The first-order velocity constant k_3' for the hydrolysis of the complex into the products was calculated by:

$$k_3 = \frac{(K_m + s_o)\, k_o}{e_o}$$

(in which e_o' was the weight/volume concentration of the enzyme preparation). Although it was not possible to obtain the absolute molar concentration of the enzyme, the above method, as used by Nath and Rydon,[2] allowed comparison of the results from a set of experiments using the same enzyme preparation retaining the same activity. The rate of formation of the complex was considered very much higher than that of its decomposition into products. The latter, therefore, determined the overall reaction rate.

Determination of the Michaelis constant for alkaline phosphatase against disodium phenyl phosphate using native serum is shown in FIGURE 1. A single concentration of the enzyme is used here because any other concentration would have required dilution of the serum, involving an increase in enzyme activity, as shown by Nath and Ghosh.[14] However, more than one concentration could be used with alcohol and acetone precipitate. FIGURE 2 illustrates determination of the Michaelis constant for acid phosphatase against the same substrate using acetone-dry powder from *Dolichos lablab* leaves as the enzyme source. More than one concentration of the enzyme is used here, with all straight lines tending to meet at the same point, thus increasing the accuracy. TABLE 1 shows the system for determination of rate constants in the hydrolytic experiments, using the data for a particular experiment of alkaline phosphatase.[4]

RESULTS

Ortho-methyl phenyl phosphate was resistant to the action of both acid and alkaline phosphatases.[7,17] Alkaline phosphatase was studied against substituted phenyl phosphates only, but acid phosphatase was studied against both phenyl phosphates and alkyl phosphates. The results were as follows.

TABLE 1

SYSTEM FOR DETERMINATION OF RATE CONSTANTS, USING DATA FOR A PARTICULAR EXPERIMENT OF ALKALINE PHOSPHATASE (AQUEOUS EXTRACT OF ACETONE PRECIPITATE OF SERUM) CARRIED OUT AT pH 9.8

e'_o	s_o	t	$X .10^4$	$1/k_o .10^{-1}$	K_m	K_a	$k'_3 .10^6$
1	0.0006	20	0.60				
		40	1.15				
		60	1.76	17.40			11.1
	0.0012	20	0.96				
		40	1.85				
		60	2.90	21.86			11.6
	0.0018	20	1.25				
		40	2.42				
		60	3.60	26.95	0.00141		11.7
2	0.0006	20	1.20				
		40	2.30				
		60	3.50	6.94			14.0
	0.0012	20	1.90				
		40	3.65				
		60	5.60	9.63			13.1
	0.0018	20	2.43				
		40	4.78				
		60	7.05	12.09	0.00129	740.8	13.0
					Mean — 0.00135		Mean — 12.4
					S.E. — ± 0.00006		S.E. — ± 0.46

Buffer: 0.05 M carbonate-bicarbonate; Substrate: disodium phenyl phosphate; Unit of enzyme concentration: 1 ml. of the preparation taken as 1 unit arbitrarily.

k_o = First-order velocity constant for overall reaction, min.$^{-1}$
K_m = Michaelis constant.
K_a = Affinity constant (Equilibrium constant for the formation of the enzyme-substrate complex) l./mole.
k'_3 = First-order velocity constant for the hydrolysis of complex, min.$^{-1}$
e'_o = Units of enzyme concentration.
s_o = Initial molar concentration of the substrate in the reaction mixture.
t = Time in minutes.
X = Molar concentration of the substrate decomposed.

TABLE 2

CORRELATION OF RATE CONSTANTS WITH ELECTRONIC EFFECTS OF SUBSTITUENTS IN THE REACTION OF ALKALINE PHOSPHATASE WITH ARYL PHOSPHATES

Enzyme Preparation	Substituent	σ-Value	K_a-Value	Log_{10} K_a	10^6. k'_3-Value	Log_{10} k'_3
Native Serum	*p*–CH_3	−0.170	1047	3.0200	15.6	−4.8069
	m–CH_3	−0.069	1307	3.1162	18.0	−4.7447
	H	0.000	1550	3.1903	17.8	−4.7496
	m–OCH_3	+0.115	2703	3.4319	3.7	−5.4318
Acetone Precipitated Proteins (Aqueous Extract)	*p*–CH_3	−0.170	1818	3.2596	7.5	−5.1249
	m–CH_3	−0.069	1250	3.0969	10.9	−4.9626
	H	0.000	740.8	2.8697	12.4	−4.9066
	m–OCH_3	+0.115	333.4	2.5229	4.7	−5.3279
Alcohol Precipitated Proteins (Aqueous Extract)	*p*–CH_3	−0.170	668.9	2.8254	19.4	−4.7212
	m–CH_3	−0.069	1450	3.1614	16.1	−4.7932
	H	0.000	1923	3.2840	13.0	−4.8861
	m–OCH_3	+0.115	4348	3.6383	2.7	−5.5686

K_a and k'_3 as in TABLE 1.
σ = Hammett's substituent constant.

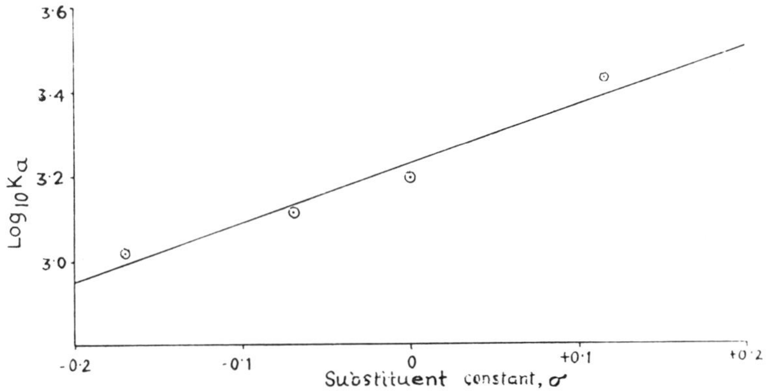

FIGURE 3. Correlation of K_a with substituent constant for alkaline phosphatase using native serum. (Reproduced by permission of Enzymologia.)

A. Alkaline Phosphatase Studied Against Substituted Phenyl Phosphates[18]

The values of the rate constants were obtained at 35° for each substrate at its own optimum pH, which ranged from 9.8 to 10.0. TABLE 2 shows the results.[4]

The plots of $\log_{10} K_a$ against substituent constant are shown in FIGURES 3, 4 and 5.

In all these three cases, the plot is a straight line. With native serum and its alcohol precipitate (FIGURES 3 and 5), the reaction appears to be facilitated by electron attraction by substituents, while with acetone precipitate (FIGURE 4), it is facilitated by electron release.

The plots of $\log_{10}k_3'$ had no such correlation with substituent constants,[4] as demonstrated in FIGURE 6.

The above facts are explained by the following mechanism presented in FIGURE 7. The enzyme is considered to possess hydrogen donating centers q_1H, q_2H, q_3H and q_4H and electron-rich center p_1. The electron attraction by the substituents, the inductive effect toward the oxygen, and the opening of one of the bonds of P = 0 make the phosphorus atom acquire a positive charge. The possibility of the ionic oxygen atoms supplying electrons to phosphorus to counteract the latter's electron loss is minimized by their participation in the formation of hydrogen bonds with q_1H and q_2H of the enzyme. The phosphorus atom, therefore, may form a strong bond with the center p_1 of the enzyme. Further hydrogen bonding is postulated for the other two oxygen atoms with q_3H and q_4H.

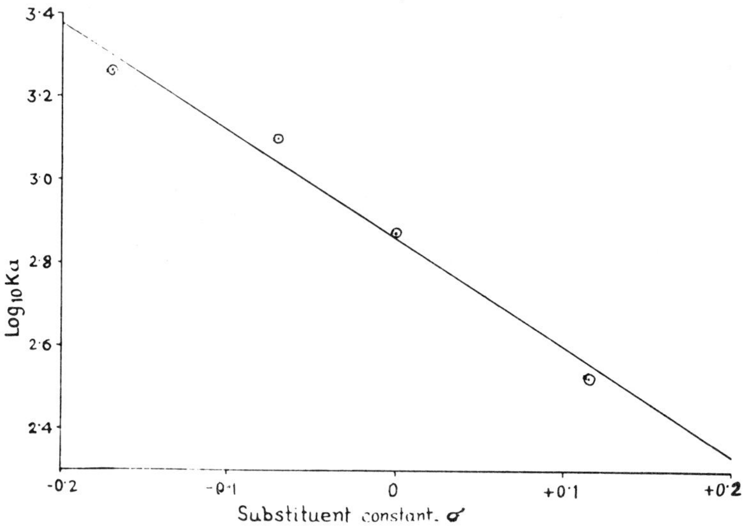

FIGURE 4. Correlation of K_a with substituent constant for alkaline phosphatase using acetone-precipitate. (Reproduced by permission of Enzymologia.)

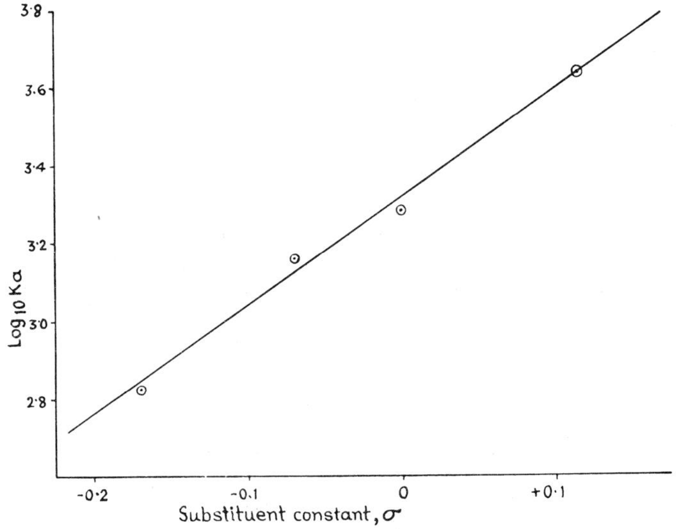

FIGURE 5. Correlation of K_a with substituent constant for alkaline phosphatase using alcohol precipitate. (Reproduced by permission of Enzymologia.)

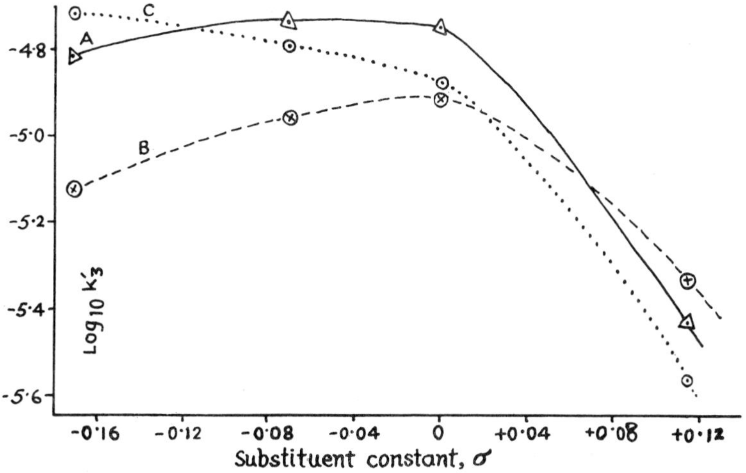

FIGURE 6. Plot of $\log_{10}k'_3$ against substituent constant. A indicates native serum; B, acetone precipitate; C, alcohol precipitate. (Reproduced by permission of Enzymologia.)

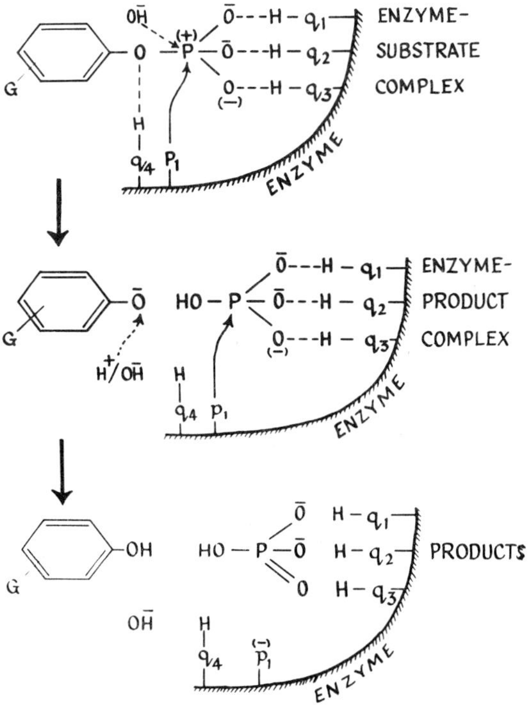

FIGURE 7. Mechanism of action of serum alkaline phosphatase upon aryl phosphates.

On treatment with acetone, the center p_1 may be wholly or partially inactivated; the hydrogen bonds predominate, and the reaction is facilitated by electron release.

Alcohol precipitation may wholly or partially inactivate the hydrogen donating sites of the enzyme, and the phosphorus-enzyme bond predominates. The reaction is then facilitated by electron attraction.

With native serum, although the two opposing processes of bond formation may be working simultaneously, the resultant effect is the facilitation of the reaction by electron attraction, indicating thereby that the attachment of the phosphorus to the enzyme is much stronger than the hydrogen bonds.

The thermodynamic parameters, namely, Δ H, Δ F, and Δ S, for the complex formation between the different substrates and alkaline phosphatase using native serum, were also obtained as usual by determining K_a-values at 25°, 30° and 35° and then plotting $\log_{10}K_a$ against 1/T (T = absolute temperature), and calculating the Δ H-values from the slope of the straight line plot. Δ S-values were obtained from the relation :

$$\log_{10}K_a = \frac{\Delta S}{2.303\,R} - \frac{\Delta H}{2.303\,R} \cdot 1/T$$

(R = gas constant). The Δ F-values at 30° C were calculated from the relation:

$$\Delta F = \Delta H - T\Delta S$$

All these values are presented in TABLE 3. Details have been given by Nath and Ghosh.[19]

The change in free energy is negative in all cases, agreeing with the usual observation in spontaneously occurring chemical reactions. It is also decreased proportionately with increasing value of the substituent constant as expected in this reaction, which is facilitated by electron attraction by the substituents. But the heat of reaction and entropy change are both positive, and roughly increase in a similar way with σ-values. The positive ΔS-values, changing from substrate to substrate, are contrary to the observation in chemical reactions in which they are not effected by the nature of the substituent (cf. Laidler[20]; Zawidzki, Papee and Laidler[21]). Laidler and Hoare,[22] as well as Casey and Laidler,[23] attribute this positive entropy change in an enzymatic reaction to a configurational change in the enzyme molecule during the reaction. Accepting this view, it is postulated in the present case that the molecule of alkaline phosphatase undergoes a configurational change when it forms a complex with the substrates. This change is somewhat influenced by the electron displacement by the substituent in the

TABLE 3

THERMODYNAMIC PARAMETERS FOR THE ENZYME-SUBSTRATE COMPLEX FORMATION USING NATIVE SERUM AS SOURCE OF ALKALINE PHOSPHATASE

Substrate	σ-Value	Δ H	Δ F at 30°	Δ S
p-Methyl Phenyl Phosphate	−0.170	+ 4.296	−4.146	+27.86
m-Methyl Phenyl Phosphate	−0.069	+ 3.878	−4.276	+26.91
Phenyl Phosphate	0.000	+ 5.276	−4.347	+31.76
m-Methoxy Phenyl Phosphate	+0.115	+14.499	−4.484	+62.65

σ = Hammett's substituent constant.
Δ H = Heat of complex formation, kcal/mole.
Δ F = Change in free energy during complex formation at 30°, kcal/mole.
Δ S = Change in entropy during complex formation, cal/mole/degree.

TABLE 4

CORRELATION OF RATE CONSTANTS WITH ELECTRONIC EFFECTS OF SUBSTITUENTS IN THE REACTION OF ACID PHOSPHATASE WITH ARYL PHOSPHATES

Enzyme Preparation	Substituent	σ-Value	K_a-Value	$Log_{10} K_a$	$10^6 . k'_3$-Value	$Log_{10} (10^6 . k'_3)$
Acetone-Dry Powder	p-CH_3	−0.170	1370	3.1367	9.20	0.9368
(Temp. 35°)	m-CH_3	−0.069	1449	3.1612	15.41	1.1878
	H	0.000	1538	3.1870	16.15	1.2082
	m-OCH_3	+0.115	3842	3.5845	4.80	0.6812
Partially Purified	p-CH_3	−0.170	4878	3.6882	9.552	0.9801
Enzyme	m-CH_3	−0.069	2000	3.3010	17.85	1.2516
(Temp. 37°)	H	0.000	909	2.9586	30.40	1.4777
	m-OCH_3	+0.115	1460	3.1644	9.854	0.9936

K_a and k'_3 as in TABLE 1.
σ as in TABLE 2.

substrate molecule. Such a hypothesis agrees with the "induced fit" theory of Koshland,[24] who thinks that when this substrate fits to the active site of the enzyme, a considerable change in the geometry of the enzyme may take place. Linderstrom-Lang and Schellman[25] also consider that appreciable dependence of slight changes of the structure of the substrate on the entropy of binding may indicate configurational changes in the enzyme molecule.

Although no correlation could be obtained by plotting $\log_{10} k'_3$ against the substituent constant, we have postulated a nucleophilic attack by a hydroxyl ion upon the phosphorus atom of the substrate as the mechanism for breakdown of the complex. This is similar to the postulation of Stein and Koshland[26] concerning the hydrolysis of phenylphosphate and of Cohn[27] for the hydrolysis of glucose-l-phosphate. The medium being alkaline, hydroxyl ions are freely available.

B. Acid Phosphatase Studied Against Substituted Phenyl Phosphates[28]

This study was first taken up by Nath and Pradhan using acetone powder from leaves of *Phaseolus vulgaris* L. against phenyl phosphate and *m*-methyl, *p*-methyl, *m*-methoxy–and *p*-nitro phenyl phosphates, the last compound being obtained as disodium salt from the California Corporation of Biochemical Research, Los Angeles, Calif. Their results showed that both the formation and the breakdown of the complex were facilitated roughly by electron attraction by substituents, although the *p*-nitro compound showed a sluggish reaction in both.[8] The work was repeated with further purification of the enzyme by acetone precipitation. This time, the electronic effect was reversed during complex formation, the *p*-nitro-compound retaining its anomaly and the *m*-methoxy compound occupying a more anomalous position by having a much higher rate of complex formation and a much slower rate of breakdown than expected from its electronic effect as measured by the substituent constant.[29] The work was then continued using acid phosphatase preparation from *Dolichos lablab,* and the same set of substrates, but with the exclusion of the *p*-nitro phenyl phosphate. Acetone-dry powder and the partially purified preparation were both used. Hydrolytic experiments were carried out at 37° and pH 5.0, which fell in the optimum range for all the substrates, and the values of K_a and k'_3 were determined and correlated with σ-values. The results[7] are presented in TABLE 4.

As shown in FIGURE 8, the complex formation is facilitated by electron attraction with acetone-dry powder and by electron release with partially purified

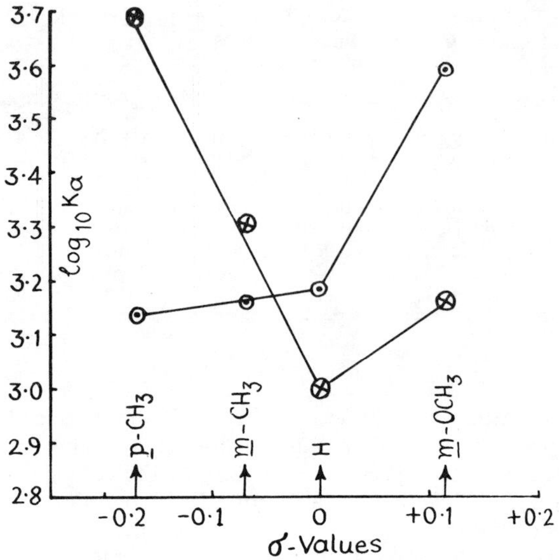

FIGURE 8. Correlation of K_a with substituent constant for acid phosphatase from *Dolichos lablab*. (⊙ is for acetone powder at 35° C.; ⊗, for partially purified enzyme at 37° C.)

enzyme. The *m*-methoxy compound shows unexpectedly higher values in both cases.

In FIGURE 9, the velocity constants for breakdown of the complex are correlated with structure. Electron attraction can be seen to facilitate the reaction with both preparations, the *m*-methoxy compound showing a slower rate than expected in both cases.

The following mechanism, presented in FIGURE 10, is proposed to explain the above facts regarding acid phosphatase action upon aryl phosphates: The hydrogen atoms of the substrate hydroxyl groups take part in hydrogen bonding with electron-rich centers p_1 and p_2 of the enzyme, an action facilitated by electron attraction of the substituents. The hydrogen-donating centers q_1H and q_2H of the enzyme attach themselves to the electron-rich oxygen atoms of the substrate through hydrogen bonds; this is facilitated through electron release by substituents. In the reaction with acetone-dry powder, the centers p_1 and p_2 are more active than the centers q_1H and q_2H, while with partially purified material, the reverse takes place. Another center, q_3H, in the enzyme molecule attaches itself through its hydrogen atom to the oxygen atom of the *m*-OCH_3 group when the corresponding substrate is used. This is an additional factor apart from the electronic effect as measured by the σ-value for this group. Thus, the *m*-methoxy compound shows an increased power of attachment with the enzyme and a reduced tendency to separate out.

Since the hydrolysis of the complex is facilitated by the substituents' electron attraction, the postulated mechanism subsumes an attack by a bound hydroxyl ion upon the carbon atom of the C-O-P bond. The medium being acidic, availability of free hydroxyl ion is very much reduced, and the attacking hydroxyl ion is thought to be formed by the attachment of a water molecule to a primary amino group of the enzyme. The enzyme-substrate complex may be so placed

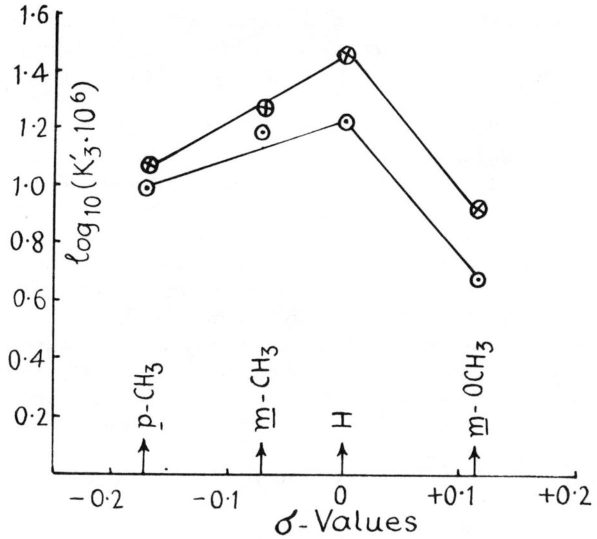

FIGURE 9. Correlation of k′$_3$ with substituent constant for acid phosphatase from *Dolichos lablab*. (⊙ stands for acetone powder at 35° C.; ⊗, for partially purified enzyme at 37° C.)

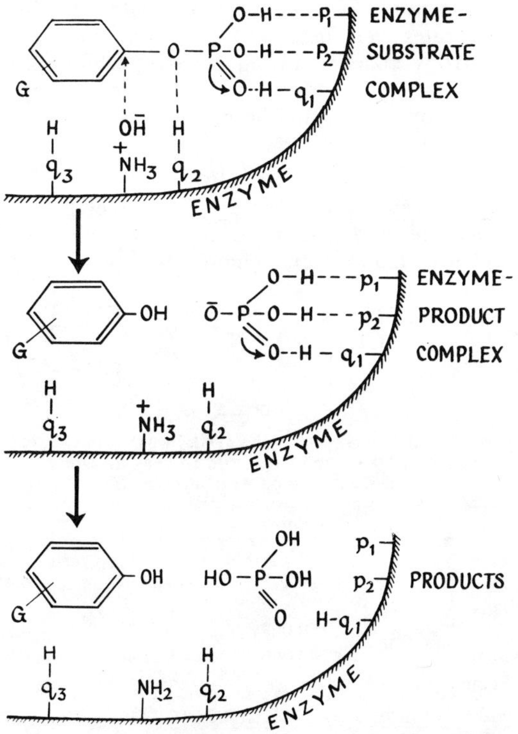

FIGURE 10. Mechanism of action of plant acid phosphatase upon aryl phosphates.

in space that this bound hydroxyl ion is nearest to the ring carbon forming the linkage. Electron withdrawal by substituents makes this carbon atom electron-deficient, and hence, a vulnerable site for the attack of the hydroxyl ion.

The thermodynamic functions ΔH, ΔF and ΔS were determined, as in the case of alkaline phosphatase, by working at 25°, 30°, 35° and 40° C. The ΔF-value was calculated at 30° C. The results[7] are given in TABLE 5.

Here also, the free energy change is negative, all substrates thus agreeing with the usual observations in spontaneously occurring chemical reactions. But the correlation with σ-values is not as satisfactory as in the case of alkaline phosphatase. Moreover, the heat of reaction, although negative for others, is positive for the *m*-methoxy compound, whose entropy change is also significantly positive; in other substrates, it is either negative or insignificantly positive. As in the case of alkaline phosphatase, the positive entropy change found with the *m*-methoxy compound is considered an indication that a configurational change takes place in the acid phosphatase molecule when it forms a complex with this substrate; perhaps the change facilitates a new attachment between the free electrons of the methoxy oxygen and some electron-poor site in the enzyme. This may explain both the especially high rate of complex formation and the low rate of its breakdown.

The significance of considerable negative entropy change appears to be an open question. Laidler[20] has explained the positive and negative entropy changes in enzyme-catalyzed reactions as being based on the nature of the substrates, i.e., on whether or not they are charged. He supports his conclusions with data on different enzymes acting upon different substrates, but in the present work, the same set of substrates were used with two different enzymes. With alkaline phosphatase, the entropy changes are all positive, while with acid phosphatase some are positive and some negative. Evidently, the sign of the entropy is dependent on the nature of the enzyme here.

C. Acid Phosphatase Studied Against Alkyl Phosphates[28]

It is known that saturated alkyl groups release electrons toward an electronegative atom at one end and that branching in the alkyl group produces this effect to a greater degree than a single chain[30] as shown below (x represents the electronegative atom):

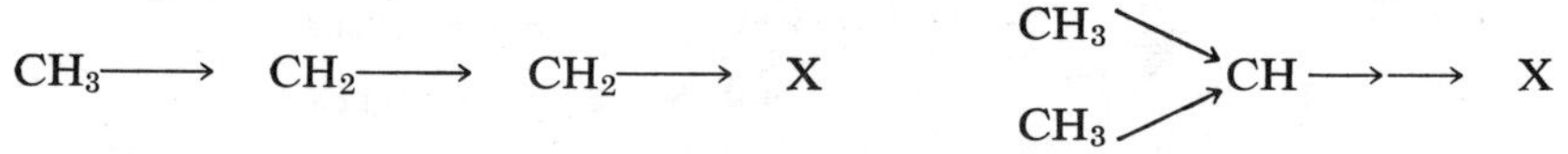

TABLE 5

THERMODYNAMIC PARAMETERS FOR THE ENZYME-SUBSTRATE COMPLEX FORMATION USING ACETONE-DRY POWDER OF THE LEAVES OF *Dolichos lablab* AS THE SOURCE OF ACID PHOSPHATASE

Substrate	σ-Value	Δ H	Δ F at 30° C	Δ S
p-Methyl Phenyl Phosphate	−0.170	−4.3792	−4.452	+ 0.241
m-Methyl Phenyl Phosphate	−0.069	−6.1732	−4.519	− 5.46
Phenyl Phosphate	0.000	−9.2046	−4.635	−15.08
m-Methoxy Phenyl Phosphate	+0.115	+5.520	−4.438	+32.68

Significance of σ-value, Δ H, Δ F and Δ S are as in TABLE 3.

TABLE 6

RATE CONSTANTS FOR THE REACTION BETWEEN ACID PHOSPHATASE AND DIFFERENT ALKYL PHOSPHATES

Name of Substrate	K_a-Values, L./Mole			k'_3-Values, Min^{-1}		
	20° C	25° C	30° C	20° C	25° C	30° C
n-Propyl Phosphate		4762	6061		5.63	5.65
iso-Propyl Phosphate	11111	13333	28571	2.92	3.21	4.50
n-Butyl Phosphate		4444	5714		3.42	4.73
sec.-Butyl Phosphate	5128	4444	4167	2.54	3.45	5.04
iso-Butyl Phosphate	10000	7692	6060	3.04	3.37	5.30
tert.-Butyl Phosphate	9302	8333	7843	4.23	4.94	6.85
n-Amyl Phosphate		4651	6451		3.78	3.77
iso-Amyl Phosphate	28571	15385	11111	1.34	2.75	3.68
tert.-Amyl Phosphate		9524	12500		3.89	5.57

The values have the same significance as in TABLE 1.

But unlike Hammett's σ-values[1] for the substituents in the benzene ring, there is no quantitative measure available for the electron displacement power of the alkyl groups along open chains, either single or branched. The first evidence of the special influence of branched chain alkyl group in the reaction of a phosphohydrolase was obtained by Nath and Pradhan,[5] who showed that a phosphodiesterase preparation from leaves of *Phaseolus vulgaris,* L., hydrolyzed di-*iso*-propyl phosphate much more rapidly than the corresponding normal propyl compound. A detailed study was made with acid phosphatase preparation from leaves of *Dolichos lablab,* using a series of alkyl phosphates having different propyl, butyl and amyl groups. Hydrolytic experiments were carried out with the acetone-dry powder at the optimum pH of each substrate, which varied from 4.6 to 5.0, the experimental method being the same as with aryl phosphates. K_a-values, and k'_3-values were determined[31] (TABLE 6).

As seen in this table, the affinity constants for the *iso*-amyl, *iso*-butyl and *iso*-propyl phosphates are higher than the corresponding normal compounds. The higher affinity of the former group may be due to the branched chain configuration because the higher inductive effect of a branched alkyl group, as compared to a normal group with the same number of carbon atoms, may produce greater electron density around the oxygen atom of the C-O-P bond, thereby increasing its capacity to form a hydrogen bond with a hydrogen-donating center of the enzyme, as proposed with aryl phosphates. But this alone does not explain all the results. For instance, *tert.*-butyl phosphate with three branches is expected to have a higher affinity, due to greater inductive effect, than the *iso*-compound, but although it agrees at 30°, it is narrowly so at 25° and quite the opposite at 20°. Similarly, *tert.*-amyl phosphate, having three branches, is expected to show greater affinity than the *iso*-compound, but it is narrowly so at 30° and quite the reverse at 25°. There appear to be additional superimposed factors, other than the inductive effect of the alkyl groups, that are influenced considerably by change in temperature. It is suggested that, at the appropriate temperature, a recess of suitable size may form in the acid phosphatase molecule into which the *iso*-propyl group nearest to the reactive bond may fit, thereby endowing the substrate containing this group with a greater capacity to form the complex with the enzyme. The attachment of the enzyme at other points in the phosphoryl group, as proposed with aryl phosphate, (FIGURE 9) and a similar mechanism for the hydrolysis of the complex, may also be working with alkyl phosphates. As indicated in FIGURE 11, the recess in the acid phosphatase molecule may have a spacing of 2.51 Å. We found no systematic relation of the velocity constant of the complex decomposition with the alkyl groups of substrates.

The thermodynamic parameters for the enzyme-substrate complex formation were determined, as in the case of aryl phosphates, and the values are shown in TABLE 7.[32]

Here also, as with aryl phosphates, the free energy change for all the substrates is negative but the change in the heat of reaction and the entropy are both positive and negative, the values being sometimes insignificant. No correlation could be found between these values and the structure of substrates.

In conclusion, a few lines of comparison may be drawn between the reactions of acid phosphatase and alkaline phosphatase with the common substrates used in this study. The two enzymes have not yet been differentiated by their substrate specificities, and the International Union of Biochemistry has given the same systematic name to both, their index numbers being EC. 3.1.3.2 and EC. 3.1.3.1, respectively. They act at different pH, their levels are altered in blood in entirely

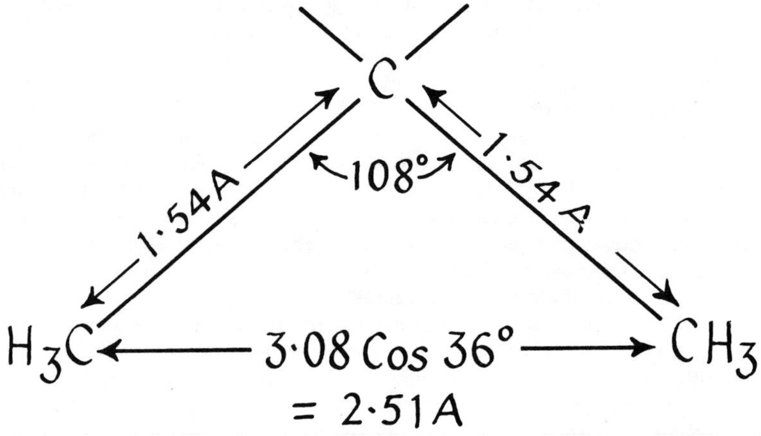

FIGURE 11. Spacing in the acid phosphatase molecule into which the *iso*-propyl group may fit. (Reproduced by permission of Enzymologia.)

TABLE 7

THERMODYNAMIC PARAMETERS FOR THE COMPLEX FORMATION BETWEEN ACID PHOSPHATASE AND ALKYL PHOSPHATES

Substrate	Δ H Kcal/Mole	Δ F Kcal/Mole	Δ S Cal/Mole/Degree
n-Propyl Phosphate	+10.16	−5.29	+51.0
iso-Propyl Phosphate	+14.56	−6.1	+68.2
n-Butyl Phosphate	+ 9.96	−5.24	+50.16
sec.-Butyl Phosphate	− 4.88	−5.02	+ 0.47
iso-Butyl Phosphate	− 8.86	−5.28	−11.8
tert.-Butyl Phosphate	− 6.06	−5.36	− 2.31
n-Amyl Phosphate	+10.59	−5.29	+52.4
iso-Amyl Phosphate	−19.40	−5.56	−45.7
tert.-Amyl Phosphate	+10.17	−5.71	+52.4

The values have same significance as in TABLE 3.

different clinical conditions, and their mode of combination with the substrate also appears to differ to some extent, as found in this study. Although both attach themselves by virtue of their electron-rich and electron-poor centers, combining with points of opposite nature in the phosphoryl group of the substrates, alkaline phosphatase may undergo structural change when combining with any of the substrates while acid phosphates does so only with the *m*-methoxy compound. The latter also combines with the oxygen atom of the methoxy group, which can thereby exert electronic influence apart from that envisaged by the Hammett's sigma value for this group. Alkaline phosphatase does not show any such special behavior with this substrate. Another factor that has not yet been studied with respect to alkaline phosphatase is that the acid phosphatase molecule appears to possess a recess into which an *iso*-propyl group of the substrate close to the C-O-P bond may fit.

Also, in applying Hammett's approach to enzyme-substrate combination, one should bear in mind that the substituents–and particularly those containing atoms with free electrons, such as *m*-OCH_3–may not act simply by electron displacement along the benzene ring, but that, in certain cases, there may be direct attachments of such atoms with the enzyme molecule. Failure to obtain a direct correlation between affinity constants and substituent constants may be due to such multi-point attachments, which may influence the rate while not necessarily being confined to the bond of cleavage or its neighborhood.

References

1. Hammett, L. P. 1940. Physical Organic Chemistry. : 184. McGraw-Hill. New York, N. Y.
2. Nath, R. L. & H. N. Rydon. 1954. Biochem. J. **57**: 1.
3. Michaelis, M. & M. L. Menten. 1913. Biochem. Z. **49**: 333.
4. Nath, R. L. & N. K. Ghosh. 1963. Enzymologia **26**: 141.
5. Nath, R. L. & T. K. Pradhan. 1962. Enzymologia **24**: 81.
6. Nath, R. L. & I. Das. 1963. Bull. Calcutta Sch. Trop. Med. **11**: 13.
7. Nath, R. L. & I. Das. 1963. Enzymologia **26**: 269.
8. Nath, R. L. & T. K. Pradhan. 1962. Enzymologia **24**: 184.
9. Nath, R. L. & I. Das. 1964. Bull. Calcutta Sch. Trop. Med. **12**: 59.
10. King, E. J. & T. F. Nicholson. 1939. Biochem. J. **33**: 1181.
11. Green, A. A. 1933. J. Amer. Chem. Soc. **55**: 2336.
12. Colowick, S. P. & N. O. Kaplan. 1955. Methods in Enzymology **1**: 146. Academic Press, New York, N. Y.
13. Lowry, O. H. & J. A. Lopez. 1946. J. Biol. Chem. **162**: 421.
14. Nath, R. L. & N. K. Ghosh. 1963. Enzymologia **25**: 182.
15. Veibel, S. 1936–37. Kgl. Danske Videnskab. Selskab. Meth-fys. Medd. **14**: 15.
16. Veibel, S. & H. Lillelund. 1940. Kgl. Danske Videnskab. Selskab. Meth-fys. Medd. **17**: 6.
17. Nath, R. L. (Unpublished.)
18. Ghosh, N. K. 1963. Ph.D. Thesis.. Calcutta University, Calcutta, India.
19. Nath, R. L. & N. K. Ghosh. 1963. Enzymologia **26**: 297.
20. Laidler, K. J. 1956. The Physical Chemistry of Enzymes. Discussions of the Faraday Society No. **20**: 83. Aberdeen University Press, Aberdeen, Scotland.
21. Zawidzki, T. W., H. M. Papee & K. J. Laidler. 1959. Trans. Farad. Soc. **55**: 1743.
22. Laidler, K. J. & J. P. Hoare. 1950. J. Amer. Chem. Soc. **72**: 2489.
23. Casey, E. J. & K. J. Laidler. 1950. J. Amer. Chem. Soc. **72**: 2159.
24. Koshland, D. E., Jr. 1959. *In* The Enzymes. **1**: 334. P. D. Boyer, H. Lardy & K. Myrback, Eds., Academic Press, New York, N. Y.
25. Linderstrom-Lang, K. U. & J. A. Schellman. 1959. *In* The Enzymes **1**: 443, 480. P. D. Boyer, H. Lardy & K. Myrback, Eds. Academic Press, New York, N. Y.
26. Stein, S. S. & D. E. Koshland. 1952. Arch. Biochem. **39**: 229.
27. Cohn, M. 1949. J. Biol. Chem. **180**: 771.
28. Das, I. 1965. Ph.D. Thesis. Calcutta University, Calcutta, India.
29. Nath, R. L. & T. K. Pradhan. 1962. Enzymologia **25**: 117.

30. FINAR, I. L. 1955. *In* Organic Chemistry. : 103. Longmans. London, England.
31. NATH, R. L. & I. DAS. 1964. Enzymologia **28:** 32.
32. NATH, R. L. & I. DAS. 1966. Enzymologia **31:** 163.

ACKNOWLEDGMENTS

The present study was made possible through the collaboration of Drs. T. K. Pradhan, N. K. Ghosh and I. Das. Drs. Pradhan and Das worked during the periods of 1959–1962 and 1962–1965, respectively, as Research fellows of the Council of Scientific and Industrial Research, Government of India, on studies relating to plant enzymes. Studies by Dr. Pradhan were entitled 'Studies on enzymes from some vegetable sources' while those by Dr. Das were entitled 'Studies on plant phosphatases'. Dr. Ghosh worked for the period 1960–1964 as Chemist of the School of Tropical Medicine, Calcutta. 'Studies on serum alkaline phosphatases' formed his most important research work.

DISCUSSION OF THE PAPER

B. L. HORECKER: I was a little confused by the distinction between binding and reaction velocity. In the case of the effective compounds, are you postulating that the electron-donating group in the serum phosphatase is involved in binding rather than in catalytic reaction? The one you showed was involved in electron-donating to the phosphorus atom.

DR. NATH: Just for the binding.

DR. HORECKER: Only for the binding. Because this is the group that you suggested was destroyed during acetone treatment and–

DR. NATH: The effect was altered.

C. DE DUVE: Your mechanism for the acid phosphatase reaction implies that if the reaction were run in O^{18} water, the oxygen would bind to the phenolic group rather than to the phosphate. Do you know of any evidence in the literature indicating that such is the case for acid phosphatase.

DR. NATH: The binding of the substrate with acid phosphatase takes place with the hydroxyl group of the phosphate as well as with the oxygen of the COP bond.

DR. DE DUVE: If I remember rightly, the diagram you showed indicated attack by a hydroxyl group on the carbon and not on the phosphorus. This would indicate that the 0^{18} would bind to the carbon of the phenyl group and not phosphate. Now, as far as I know, all phosphatases that have been investigated in this respect have attached the oxygen to the phosphate group. And I was wondering whether there was any evidence about acid phosphatase indicating that it was different.

DR. NATH: Yes, now I follow. We have also seen that the phosphorus has more binding capacity and is more positive. But in the case of the acid phosphatase, we had postulated the attack on C-O bond. Well, we do not really say that the C-O bond breaks; the O-P bond might, as well, but we have no proof to distinguish between the two. And we just put the positive charge on the carbon atom while electron displacement was taking place.

DR. DE DUVE: With respect to the acid phosphatase, have you tried any other substituents of the carbon, such as cyclohexyl? Or what about benzyl phosphate–has that been active?

DR. NATH: No.

DR. HORECKER: I wonder if it isn't just a bulky group that is able to form Van der Walls interactions with the protein.

DR. NATH: Might be. Enzyme is such an unknown thing; we know very little about it. But whatever evidence we've got, we're just trying to give some relation.

I. B. WILSON (*University of Colorado, Boulder, Colo.*): I'd just like to comment that it is not true that your Michaelis-Menten constants would not really be binding constants, especially if there is a phosphoryl enzyme intermediate in which the treatment–any kind of treatment of the enzyme–might change the ratio of rates of phosphorylation to dephosphorylation. And this would immediately change the K_m. So it might just be a formal kind of thing.

DR. NATH: There may be disturbances, no doubt. But what we have found is just an enzyme reaction connected to the substituents of the benzene where we find some good correlation of the substituent constants. So we want to equalize it.

DR. WILSON: I'm not really arguing against the correlation, although, since it takes two points to make a straight line, I'm not really impressed that four falls someplace within a straight line.

DR. NATH: In response to this question I'd like to comment that in this hydrolytic process by phenylphosphatases and alkyl phosphatase, K_m is actually the dissociation constant, but it does not involve the decomposition of the ES to the products. So one can correlate this dissociation constant to the constant in a substrate.

DR. WILSON: But it was determined kinetically.

DR. NATH: Yes, but the condition that was used is the dissociation constant, and it does not involve the decomposition for the ES complex. Is this K_m value quite isolated from the decomposition? It is the dissociation constant and just for the formation of the complex.

DR. HORECKER: I think this point is going to have to be debated in private. Are there any other comments or questions? If not, thank you very much Dr. Nath.

ZINC AND COBALT ALKALINE PHOSPHATASES*

Robert T. Simpson†
and
Bert L. Vallee
Biophysics Research Laboratory, Department of Biological Chemistry, Harvard Medical School
and the
Division of Medical Biology, Peter Bent Brigham Hospital, Boston, Mass.

Alkaline phosphatase of *Escherichia coli* has proved to be particularly valuable in studying the mechanism of enzymatic cleavage of phosphate esters. Perhaps owing to its ready availability, this particular bacterial phosphatase has served as a prototype for studies of a large number of other phosphomonoesterases of nonbacterial origin. It has long been suspected that phosphatases may be metalloenzymes (Cloetens, 1942; Roche, 1946). However, thus far, the most extensive data concerning metal content have been recorded for the phosphatase of *E. coli.* This enzyme, initially identified by Horiuchi *et al.* (1959) and by Torriani (1960), and first prepared and characterized by Garen and Levinthal (1960), was found to be markedly inhibited by a variety of metal chelating agents, and was later shown to contain significant amounts of zinc (Plocke *et al.*, 1962). A reexamination of the zinc content of the protein will be presented briefly.

Plocke and Vallee (1962) showed that the native zinc atoms of alkaline phosphatase can be replaced by cobalt, resulting in a new, active enzyme. Owing to its intrinsic properties, e.g., absorption and electron paramagnetic resonance spectra, cobalt can serve as a probe for the environment of the metal atom at the active site and for its role in enzymatic function (Dennard & Williams, 1966; Vallee and Williams, 1968a; 1968b). The studies of cobalt phosphatase to be detailed comprise both kinetic and physicochemical investigations of this new metalloenzyme.

Isolation and Zinc Content of Alkaline Phosphatase

The stoichiometry of the zinc content of this phosphatase has not been settled with finality, a fact apparently related to some extent to the methods by which it has been isolated. Different preparative methods have resulted in enzymes of nearly comparable specific activities, but containing from 1,600 to 3,100 μg of zinc/gram of protein; equivalent to 2.3 to 4.2 gram atoms of zinc per mole of protein of molecular weight 89,000 (Plocke *et al.*, 1962; Harris & Coleman, 1968; Simpson *et al.*, 1968; Reynolds & Schlesinger, 1969).

The studies of Neu and Heppel (1965) and Malamy and Horecker (1964a) have localized phosphatase in *E. coli* among the proteins located in the region between the cellular membrane and the cell wall. Such proteins are easily separated from the major cellular constituents by an osmotic shock procedure (Neu & Heppel, 1965). This finding has led to a convenient starting material for the isolation of the enzyme. The water extract obtained by osmotic shock of washed cells of *E. coli,* strain C-90, is applied to a column of DEAE cellulose.

* This work was aided by grants-in-aid HE-07297 and GM-15,003 from the National Institutes of Health, Department of Health, Education and Welfare.

† Fellow of the National Institute of General Medical Sciences, National Institutes of Health, 1964–1968.

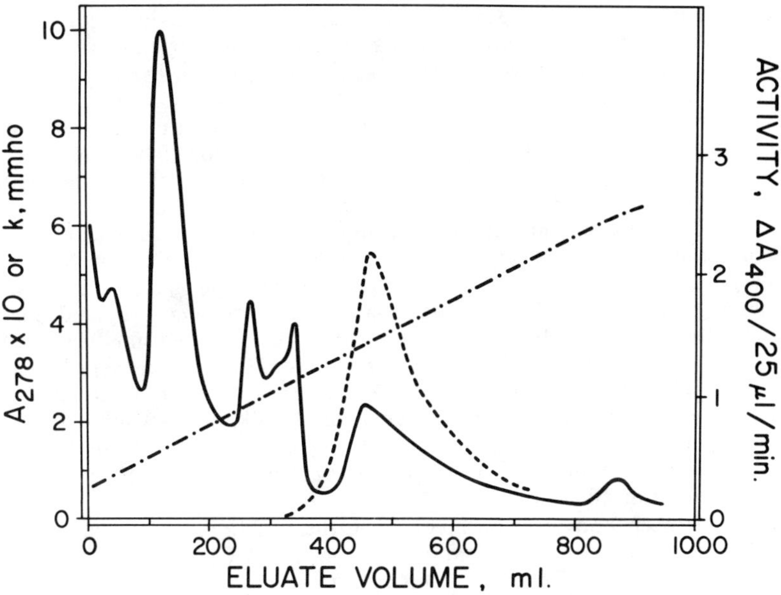

FIGURE 1. Purification of alkaline phosphatase of *E. coli.* The water extract from a 3-liter culture of *E. coli.* strain C-90, was applied to a 0.9 × 30 cm column of DEAE cellulose, equilibrated with 0.01 M imidazole chloride at pH 7.1 (the starting buffer). After absorption of the protein, elution was carried out with a linear gradient consisting of 500 ml each of the starting buffer, and the starting buffer + 0.1 M NaCl. As a function of the eluate volume, protein, determined as absorbance at 278 mμ (——), enzyme activity (- - - -), and the conductivity of the eluting buffer (-·-·-·-) are plotted.

Elution with a linear salt gradient leads in a single step to the isolation of alkaline phosphatase (FIGURE 1) with a specific activity equal to that of the enzyme crystallized from ammonium sulfate (Malamy & Horecker, 1964b). Such enzyme is pure as judged by ultracentrifugal analysis and free boundary electrophoresis (FIGURE 2).

With purification, specific enzymatic activity and zinc content increase in parallel (TABLE 1). From the second to the third steps of the procedure, magnesium also accumulates while the iron content remains constant. The content of all other metals decreases progressively during purification. The essentiality of zinc for the function of this enzyme has been demonstrated previously (Plocke & Vallee, 1962). Magnesium, also found consistently in variable but stoichiometric proportions, has long been known to stabilize this alkaline phosphatase against various denaturing processes (Garen & Levinthal, 1960), but has not been shown to have a specific, singular role in enzymatic function thus far. The significance of the iron content, corresponding to about 0.8 gram atoms per molecular weight 89,000, is unknown.

Chemical and spectroscopic analyses of a number of preparations obtained by this preparative method indicate a zinc content from 2,500 to 3,100 μg/g of protein (TABLE 2), to be contrasted with that of about 1,600 to 2,300 μg/zinc/g protein for enzymes of equivalent activities obtained previously (Plocke *et al.*, 1962). When based on a molecular weight for the protein of 89,000 (Simpson *et al.*, in preparation), the averages of these zinc contents correspond to molar ratios of zinc to protein of 3.8 and 2.3. These variations require comment. High concentrations of ammonium sulfate were added to preparations analyzed previously, either to precipitate or to crystallize the enzyme. Further, in most methods, 0.01 M magnesium ion was added at some stage to stabilize the protein. Either or both of these procedures could alter the metal content of the protein, displacing the native metals, or, alternatively, removing zinc through formation of the $Zn(NH_3)_4^{2+}$ complex (Sillen & Martell, 1964). Indeed, the metal content of preparations of enzyme obtained by ammonium sulfate crystallization of the pure protein prepared chromatographically suggests that, subsequent to exposure to ammonium sulfate, the average metal content falls from nearly four to about three gram atoms of zinc per mole of protein. The specific activity of such enzymes is equal to, or slightly lower than, that of enzyme prepared chromatographically (TABLE 2). In addition to the lower zinc content, the heat stability of enzymes prepared by us from ammonium sulfate is lower than that of the enzyme not exposed to this salt, as is their stability on storage in solution. When reporting the content and role of metal atoms in alkaline phosphatase, it would seem imperative to specify the method of preparation in detail. Further, the possibility cannot be eliminated, a priori that enzymes prepared by various methods may also differ in still other properties.

Zinc has been known to be involved in the function of this enzyme (Plocke *et al.*, 1962), and has been implicated in tertiary structure of the protein (Reynolds & Schlesinger, 1969). Our investigations indicate that zinc also plays a role in the maintenance of the quaternary structure of the native molecule. Thus 8 M urea and 40% dioxane, solvents that have little effect on the sedimentation behavior of native phosphatase (TABLE 3), dissociate the apoprotein into an ultracentrifugally homogeneous species, presumably the monomeric form of the enzyme previously observed following dissociation of alkaline phosphatase by acid (Schlesinger & Barrett, 1965) or by reduction and alkaylation in urea (Rothman & Byrne, 1963). The sedimentation constant and the molecular weight of the apoenzyme in dilute salt solutions are equal to those of the native

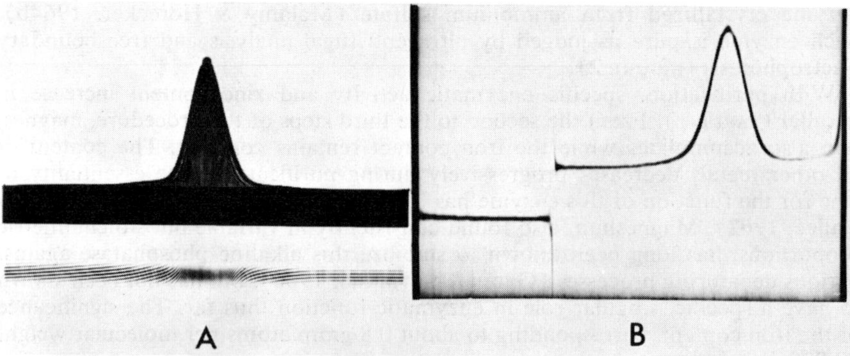

FIGURE 2A. Tiselius electrophoresis of alkaline phosphatase. The photograph was taken after 1100 minutes of electrophoresis at a gradient of 1.32 v/cm and a temperature of 1°. The concentration of protein is 6 mg/ml in 0.01 M Tris-Cl, 0.1 M KCl, pH 7.0. The direction of migration is from right to left.

FIGURE 2B. Ultracentrifugation of alkaline phosphatase. The photograph was taken 60 minutes after reaching maximal speed (59,780 rpm) at a phase plate angle of 70°. The protein concentration was 12 mg/ml in 0.01 M Tris-Cl, 0.1 M KCl, pH 7.0 The direction of sedimentation is from left to right.

TABLE 1

METAL CONTENT DURING PURIFICATION OF ALKALINE PHOSPHATE

Sample	Zn	Sr	Ba	Fe	Ca	Cr	Mn	Al	Ni	Mo	Mg
Washed Cells	350	—	9	>2500	510	>250	77	88	>770	95	1500
Water Extract	840	tr	14	520	300	10	25	65	tr	tr	125
Purified Enzyme	2500	—	5	500	100	—	45	29	tr	120	435

All results are the averages of duplicate analyses and are expressed as μg of metal/g of protein. Pb and Cd were not detected in any sample. tr = trace; — = not detected. Cu was not determined due to the method employed (Vallee, 1955).

TABLE 2

ACTIVITIES AND METAL CONTENTS OF PURIFIED ALKALINE PHOSPHATASE

Preparation	Specific Activity	Zn		Mg		Fe		Ba	Ca	Cr	Mn	Al	Ni	Mo
		μg/g	g atom/mole	μg/g	g atom/mole	μg/g	g atom/mole	μg/g						
Chrom. I	39	2500	3.5	430	1.6	500	.7	5	100	—	45	29	tr	120
Chrom. II	43	3100	4.2	tr	—	700	1.0	6	—	—	33	41	tr	—
Chrom. III	40	2800	3.9	560	2.0	N.D.	—	7	tr	N.D.	135	74	N.D.	tr
Chrom. IV	39	2600	3.7	480	1.8	500	.7	—	150	74	tr	75	—	70
Chrom. V	42	2700	3.8	520	1.9	400	.6	tr	350	tr	tr	55	—	100
Cryst. I	36	2200	3.0	760	2.8	570	.8	6	270	38	28	66	280	tr
Cryst. II	40	2000	2.8	550	2.0	N.D.	—	4	75	N.D.	42	46	N.D.	tr

Chrom. = Enzyme prepared chromatographically.
Cryst. = Crystalline enzyme prepared by the method of Malamy and Horecker (1964b).
All results are the averages of duplicate analyses. tr = trace; — = not detected; N.D. = not determined. Activities are expressed as U/mg protein, assayed in 1 M Tris chloride. Elements not listed were not detected, save for Cu, which cannot be measured due to the system employed (Vallee, 1955).

TABLE 3

SEDIMENTATION OF NATIVE AND APOALKALINE PHOSPHATASE

Solvent	$S_{20,w} \times 10^{13}$ Native	$S_{20,w} \times 10^{13}$ Apo
Water	6.1	6.1
5 M Guanidine HCl	1.2	1.2
8 M Urea	5.8	1.4
40% Dioxane	5.9	1.8

Experiments were performed at 20°, pH 7.0, 0.05 M Tris-Cl, 0.1 M. KCl, plus indicated additions.

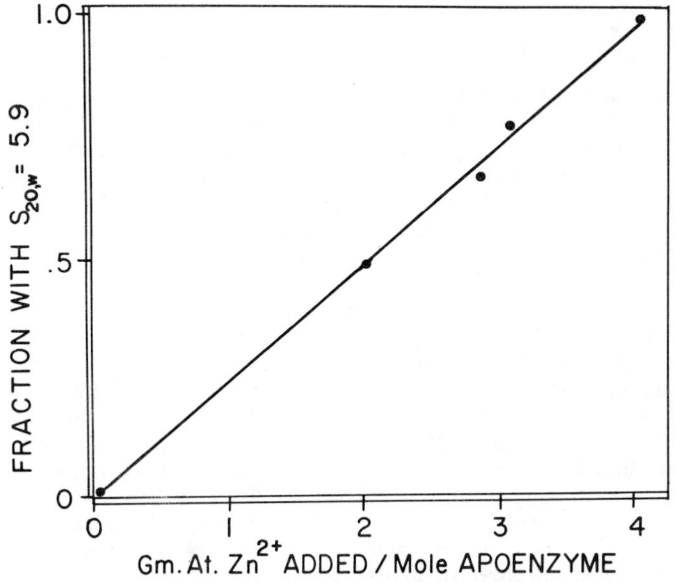

FIGURE 3. Reconstitution of the native, quaternary structure of alkaline phosphatase. The increments of zinc indicated were added to apophosphatase, prior to sedimentation of the resultant fractionally reconstituted protein in 0.01 M Tris-Cl, 0.1 M KCl, 40% dioxane, pH 7.0. The percent of the total sedimenting material moving with a sedimentation constant of 5.9 Svedbergs is plotted.

enzyme (TABLE 3). Thus, while metal protein interactions are not the only ones involved in polymerization, they do contribute significant stabilizing energy to the maintenance of the native quaternary structure.

When increments of zinc are added to the apoprotein, followed by sedimentation of the resultant, partially reconstituted enzyme, two boundaries are observed in the presence of 40% dioxane. In this solvent system, the more rapidly sedimenting species has a sedimentation constant equal to that of the native molecule, while that of the slower moving species is equal to that of the apoprotein. The relative proportions of these two boundaries vary as a function of the molar excess of zinc added to the apoprotein (FIGURE 3). Readdition of four gram atoms of zinc is necessary to restore fully the stability of the native molecule to the apoprotein, and thus, all four gram atoms of zinc would seem to serve in stabilizing quaternary structure in some manner.

TABLE 4

KINETIC PROPERTIES OF ALKALINE PHOSPHATASE

All phosphomonoesters hydrolyzed at equal rates.
V_{max} increases with $pK_b = 7.1$; $\Delta H_i = 6.6$ kcal.
K_m increases with $pK_a = 8.6$; $\Delta H_i = 17.5$ kcal.
$k_{H_2O}/k_{D_2O} = 2$
K_i for phosphate = K_m for substrate
k_3 rate limiting at pH <7
k_2 rate limiting at pH >7

Kinetics of Cobalt Alkaline Phosphatase

All four zinc atoms of the native phosphatase molecule can be replaced by cobalt to form a new, functionally active, enzymatic species. Such replacements of functional metals constitute one of the mildest and most specific of chemical modifications of active enzymatic sites. Owing to the differing properties of zinc and cobalt in ligand shell reactions, and as Lewis acids (Dennard & Williams, 1966), kinetic differences between the cobalt and zinc proteins might be expected in steps that directly involve the metal ion. Cobalt alkaline phosphatase bears many similarities to the native enzyme; yet, as detailed below, it differs significantly from the native protein in certain critical kinetic parameters.* Further, it does not exhibit transferase activity (Tait & Vallee, 1966).

The mechanism of the nonspecific phosphatases has been shown to involve a particularly reactive seryl residue that is phosphorylated by inorganic phosphate at low pH or during the course of enzymatic activity by substrate at neutral pH (Schwartz & Lippman, 1961; Engstrom, 1962). Careful kinetic studies of the steady-state hydrolysis of 4-NPP† by Lazdunski and Lazdunski (1966), and of the presteady-state hydrolysis of 5-MeUP,† 2-NPP† and 2,4-DNPP† by various workers (Fernley & Walker, 1966; Fife, 1966; Ko & Kezdy, 1967) have led to findings summarized in TABLE 4. These must be considered for inclusion in any kinetic scheme devised for alkaline phosphatase.

Like the native zinc enzyme, cobalt phosphatase hydrolyses a wide variety of phosphoester bonds with approximately equal facility (TABLE 5), although the rate for the cobalt enzyme is only about 15% of that for the zinc protein. Thus, varying the leaving group from glycerol to dinitrophenol is without significant effect on the overall rate of enzymatic hydrolysis. Similarly, the cleavage of the thio analogue of a phosphomonoester is nearly as rapid as the hydrolysis of more normal substrates (TABLE 5).

Again, as with the zinc enzyme, the substrate concentration dependent hydrolysis of both 4-NPP and 2,4-DNPP by the cobalt enzyme is anomalous. At high ionic strength, the Lineweaver-Burk plot is linear over a broad substrate range, while at low ionic strength, substrate activation is prominent at concentrations of substrate greater than 10^{-4} M. At both ionic strengths, substrate inhibition is observed at high substrate concentration, e.g., $> 10^{-2}$ M (FIGURE 4).

* The kinetic studies reviewed here will be published in detail in a separate communication (M. M. Gottesman, R. T. Simpson & B. L. Vallee, in preparation).

† Abbreviations for the various substrates employed are: 4-NPP = 4-nitrophenyl phosphate; 2,4-DNPP = 2,4-dinitrophenyl phosphate; 2-NPP = 2-nitrophenyl phosphate; 5-MeUP = 5-methylumbelliferyl phosphate; C-S-P = cysteamine-S-phosphate; β-G-P = β-glyceryl phosphate.

TABLE 5

RATES OF HYDROLYSIS OF DIFFERENT SUBSTRATES BY COBALT P'ASE

Substrate	Velocity, min^{-1}
4-nitrophenyl phosphate	310
2,4-dinitrophenyl phosphate	360
β-glycerol phosphate	340
Cysteamine-S-phosphate	240

Activities were determined at substrate concentrations of 1×10^{-2} M, in 0.01 M. Tris-HCl, 1 M NaCl, pH 8.0, 25°.

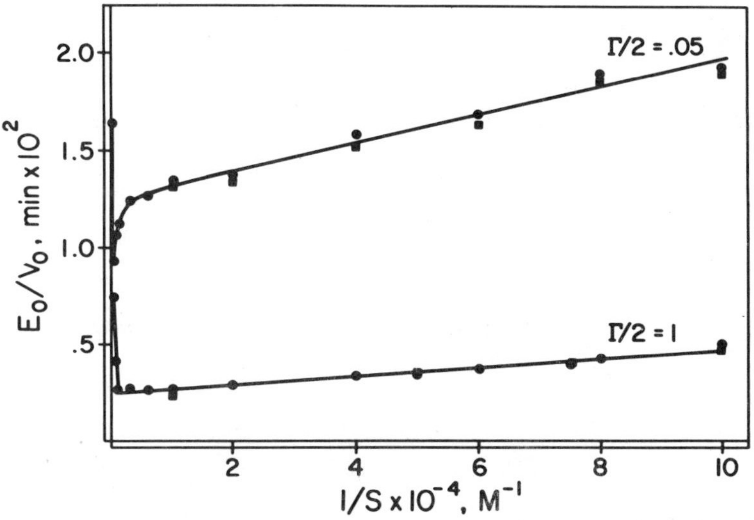

FIGURE 4. Substrate concentration dependence of the activity of cobalt alkaline phosphatase. The activity of cobalt alkaline phosphatase was determined at the indicated substrate concentrations with either 4-nitrophenyl phosphate (●), or with 2,4-dinitrophenyl phosphate (■) as substrates, at low and high ionic strengths as indicated. The buffer employed at low ionic strength was 0.01 M Tris-Cl, pH 8.0, while at high ionic strengths, 1.0 M NaCl was added.

Both at high and at low ionic strengths, K_m and V_{max} for 4-NPP, C-S-P and 2,4-DNPP are nearly identical for all three substrates for the linear portions of such plots (TABLE 6). Similar data demonstrating identity among these parameters for the reconstituted zinc enzyme have been obtained (TABLE 6). The maximal activity of cobalt phosphatase is about 15% of the activity of zinc phosphatase in all instances. Finally, inhibition constants for competitive inhibition of hydrolytic activity by phosphate, arsenate, and phenylphosphonate are nearly identical for the two metalloenzymes (TABLE 7).

The pH dependence of the activity of cobalt phosphatase differs from that of the native or reconstituted zinc enzymes. Log V_{max} (FIGURE 5) and pK_m (FIGURE 6) for both 4-NPP and 2,4-DNPP as substrates were determined over the linear portions of Lineweaver-Burk plots at pH's varying from 4.5 to 12. Although the pK's of the leaving groups of these two substrates vary by more than three, the behavior of the two species is indistinguishable over the entire pH range investigated.

TABLE 6

KINETIC PARAMETERS: ZINC AND COBALT PHOSPHATASES

Substrate	Cobalt Phosphatase K_m, M × 10^6	Cobalt Phosphatase V_{max}, min^{-1}	Zinc Phosphatase K_m, M × 10^6	Zinc Phosphatase V_{max}, min^{-1}
4-nitrophenyl phosphate	6	310	7	2180
2,4-dinitrophenyl phosphate	6	360	8	2300
Cysteamine-S-phosphate	7	240	7	2140

Determined in 0.01 M Tris-Cl, 1.0 M NaCl, pH 8.0, 25°.

TABLE 7

INHIBITION OF COBALT AND ZINC ALKALINE PHOSPHATASES

Inhibitor	K_I, M Cobalt Phosphatase	K_I, M Zinc Phosphatase
Phosphate	1×10^{-5}	1×10^{-5}
Arsenate	2×10^{-5}	3×10^{-5}
Phenylphosphonate	5×10^{-3}	6×10^{-3}

Determined with 4-nitrophenyl phosphate as substrate in 0.0-1 M Tris-Cl, 1.0 M NaCl, pH 8.0, 25°.

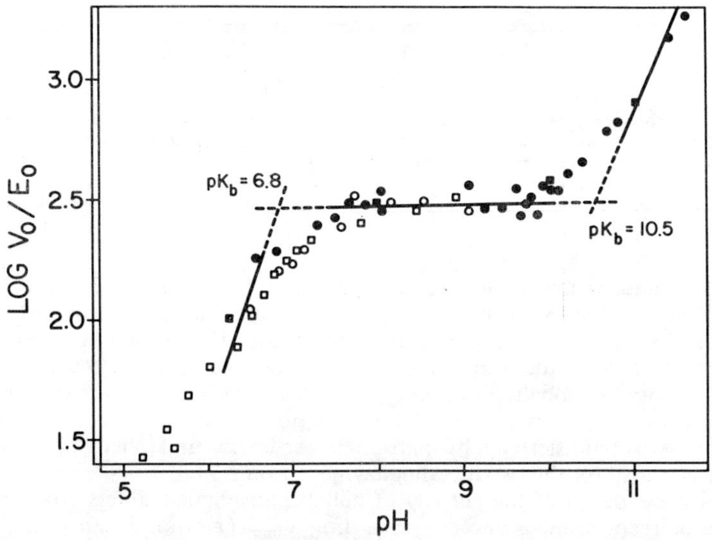

FIGURE 5. pH dependence of log V_{max} for cobalt alkaline phosphatase. Activities were determined at the indicated pH values with either 4-nitrophenyl phosphate (○, ●) or 2,4-dinitrophenyl phosphate (□, ■) as substrates in 0.01 M buffers containing 1 M NaCl, at 25°. The data presented are either extrapolated maximal velocities (●, ■), or alternatively, activities determined at a single concentration of substrate 100 times greater than the K_m (○, □).

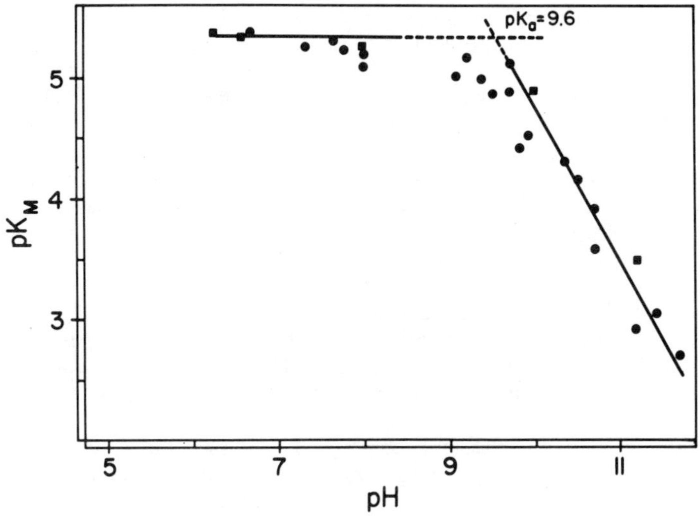

FIGURE 6. pH dependence of pK_m for cobalt alkaline phosphatase. The Michaelis constants for either 4-nitrophenyl phosphate (●) or 2,4-dinitrophenyl phosphate (■) were determined in 0.01 M buffers containing 1 M NaCl at 25° and the indicated pH values.

Like the zinc enzyme, the activity of cobalt phosphatase increases with a pK near neutrality, 6.8 in the case of the cobalt enzyme (FIGURE 5). In addition, the activity of the cobalt enzyme increases markedly above pH 10. The slope of this linear increase is unity, enabling the tentative assignment of the pK involved in the altered rate of activity as 10.5. The lower pK for the increase in V_{max} has a heat of ionization of 6,600 cal/mole, a value similar to that for the zinc enzyme and, based on models, could be consistent with the involvement of a histidyl residue in this ionization. (Lazdunski & Lazdunski, 1966).

As is the case for the zinc enzyme, K_m increases at alkaline pH values. However, the increase for the cobalt enzyme is displaced a full pH unit toward the alkaline pH range, i.e., $pK_a = 9.6$ (FIGURE 6), as compared to the $pK_a = 8.6$ for zinc phosphatase (Lazdunski & Lazdunski, 1966). Similar to the zinc species, the heat of ionization for the upper pK_a's is very large, i.e., about 15 kcal per mole. Based on models, no groups known to occur in proteins that ionize within this range are characterized by heats of ionization near this magnitude. This circumstance, together with the effect of the metal species present on the observed pK, suggests that it may be related to an ionization occurring at or very near to the metal atom itself, perhaps even within its hydration sphere.

Studies of the inhibition of the zinc enzyme by various phosphorous-containing compounds are relevant to the assignment of this pK. Phosphate ion and phenylphosphonate both inhibit the hydrolytic activity of alkaline phosphatase in a competitive fashion (FIGURE 7, A and B). In contrast, phenylphosphinate, and a phosphodiester, while both inhibiting the activity of the enzyme, do so in a noncompetitive fashion (FIGURE 7, C and D). These latter two compounds only possess one ionizable hydroxyl substituent on the phosphorous atom, while the two former species both have two ionizable oxygens. Thus, only compounds that form phosphorous oxydianions interact in a manner similar to that of substrates. Jointly with the above kinetic data, these findings suggest that the phosphate of the substrate might possibly interact with the enzyme through bidentate chelation of the phosphorous oxydianion with the metal ion at the active site.

A further difference between the cobalt and zinc enzymes arises from their relative effectiveness in the catalysis of phosphate transfer. In the presence of high concentrations of a variety of α-amino or α-hydroxy alcohols, the zinc enzyme catalyses the transfer of phosphate to the alcohol, with the formation of a new phosphoester (Wilson *et al.,* 1964). This transfer increases k overall at pH 8.0, 1 to 2-fold and 3 to 4-fold at pH's of less than 6, as might be expected from the known magnitudes of the various rate constants at these pH values (Trentham & Gutfreund, 1968). In contrast, the cobalt enzyme fails to catalyze phosphate transfer to several acceptor species at pH 8 (Tait & Vallee, 1966). The present investigations have confirmed this finding and have further failed to detect transferase activity to glycerol and Tris over the pH range from pH 4.5 to 11.0. The mechanistic basis for these findings remains unknown at the present.

At acidic pH values, the zinc enzyme shows an initial burst of hydrolytic activity, with a 1:1 molar stoichiometry of the release of the alcohol moiety of the substrate 2,4-DNPP (Ko & Kezdy, 1967; see also FIGURE 8). While such a transient phase in the kinetics of the hydrolysis of 4-NPP or 2,4-DNPP could not be demonstrated for the cobalt enzyme at 25°, and pH's from 4.8 to 11.0, it is noteworthy that, thus far, the extrapolation of the steady state rate to zero time in all cases, led to an intercept different from that due to the substrate alone (FIGURE 8). In fact, the difference approximates one mole of substrate transformed per mole of enzyme, consistent with an initial burst of activity that

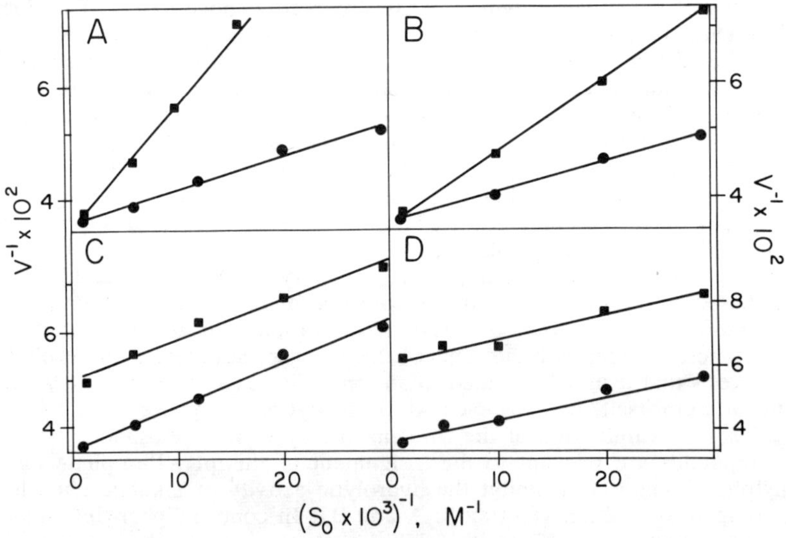

FIGURE 7. Inhibition of zinc alkaline phosphatase. The inhibition kinetics of various inhibitors with 4-nitrophenyl phosphate as substrate in 0.01 M Tris-Cl, 1 M NaCl, pH 8.0, 25°, are presented. In all cases, the lower line in the figure represents the uninhibited substrate concentration dependence, while the upper line presents the results obtained in the presence of the inhibitors. Inhibitors and their concentrations are: A, phosphate, 1×10^{-4} M; B, phenylphosphonate, 2×10^{-2} M; C, phenylphosphonate, 1.6×10^{-2} M; and D, bis-nitrophenyl phosphate, 5×10^{-3} M.

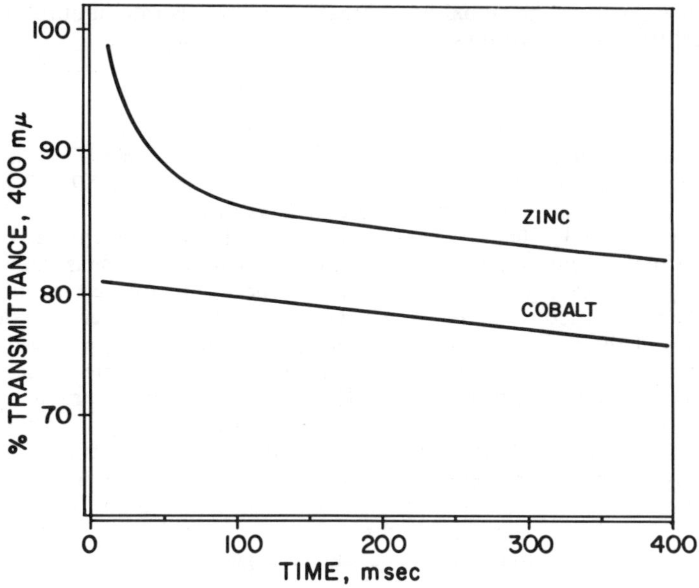

FIGURE 8. Stopped flow kinetics of zinc and cobalt phosphatase hydrolysis of 2,4-dinitrophenyl phosphate at pH 5.7, 0.05 M Tris acetate, 25°. The data were obtained with a Durrum-Gibson stopped flow apparatus, having a mixing time of about 2 to 3 msec and a path length of 2 cm. The instrument was zeroed on equal volume mixtures of substrate and distilled water. The concentrations of enzyme employed were: $Zn_4P'ase = 0.23$ mg/ml; and $Co_4P'ase =$ 0.46 mg/ml.

would be too fast to be observed in the stopped flow instrument under conditions where the transient kinetics of zinc phosphatase have been evaluated. Such reasoning suggested that the cobalt enzyme might indeed exhibit an initial burst of activity, but that its rate might exceed the capacity of the instrument under the conditions employed.

Indeed, lowering the temperature of the assay to 5° has demonstrated a transient phase in the kinetics of hydrolysis of 4-NPP by the cobalt enzyme (FIGURE 9). The rate constant for the transient phase of hydrolysis of this substrate by cobalt phosphatase is very rapid, with a half-time of about 15 msec, even though the low temperature and low ionic strength represent suboptimal conditions. Similar values of the rate constant for phosphorylation of the enzyme by substrate for the zinc protein, estimated from the data of Fernley and Walker (1966) and Ko and Kezdy (1967), indicates that this rate constant for the cobalt protein is nearly ten times greater than that expected for zinc phosphatase. The present data demonstrate that dephosphorylation is rate limiting for the hydrolysis of phosphomonoesters by the cobalt enzyme at pH 8. Comparison with the zinc enzyme, and other considerations (*vide supra*) suggest that, for the cobalt protein, dephosphorylation of the phosphoryl enzyme is rate limiting at all pH values from 4.8 to 11.0, provided that the usual mechanistic scheme used to describe hydrolysis by phosphatase is assumed to be applicable.

Further, despite marked dissimilarities in their leaving groups, all phosphoesters tested are hydrolyzed at approximately equivalent rates by the cobalt enzyme (*vide supra*). These observations are consistent with the supposition that a step subsequent to the actual bond breaking process is rate limiting for the enzymatically mediated hydrolysis.

Physicochemical Studies of Cobalt Phosphatase

Experiments previously discussed indicated that alkaline phosphatase, prepared so as to avoid removal of metals from the native molecule, appears to contain approximately four gram atoms of zinc per mole of 89,000 molecular weight. This enzyme has been thought to have two identical subunits (Rothman & Byrne, 1963). Thus, it would seem likely that the protein has two active sites, and presumably one metal ion located at each of these sites. Other studies indicate that all four gram atoms of zinc are necessary for full stabilization of the quaternary structure of the protein (*vide supra*). The present physicochemical studies of the zinc and cobalt enzymes suggest that this apparent dichotomy arises from the fact that phosphatase contains two differentiable classes of metal ions. One pair apparently serves only to stabilize quaternary structure and will be referred to as the "structural" metal ions. The second pair, while also involved in structural stabilization, primarily functions in substrate binding and or hydrolysis, and will be referred to as "catalytic" metal ions. When zinc is replaced by cobalt, the spectral properties of these two pairs of cobalt atoms differ significantly and suggest that the two types of metal atoms form complexes with apophosphatase that may have different geometries (Simpson & Vallee, 1968).

A kinetic analysis of the rate of removal of zinc from native phosphatase provided first indications of the two classes of metal atoms in this protein. Incubation of the enzyme with a 50-fold molar excess of the chelating agent, 8-hydroxyquinoline-5-sulfonic acid, indicates two different rates of zinc removal. One pair of zinc ions is removed rapidly, i.e., in 30 minutes, with kinetics that

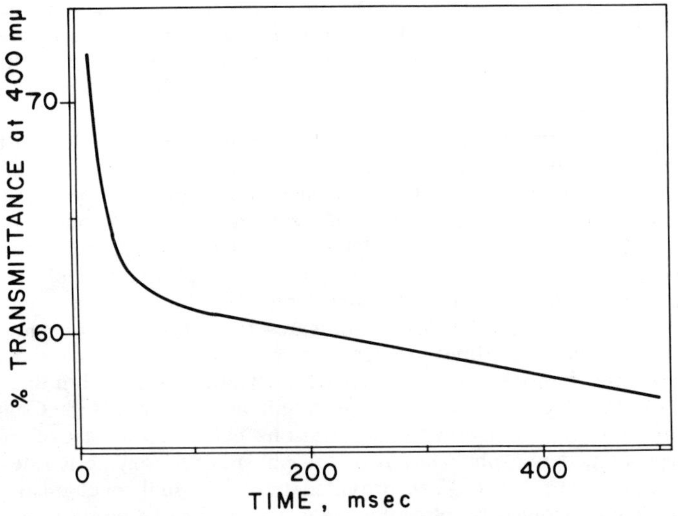

FIGURE 9. Stopped flow kinetics of cobalt phosphatase hydrolysis of 4-nitrophenyl phosphate at pH 8.0, 0.01 M Tris-Cl, pH 8.0, 5°. The data were obtained in a Durrum-Gibson stopped flow apparatus which was zeroed on distilled water, at an enzyme concentration of 0.46 mg/ml.

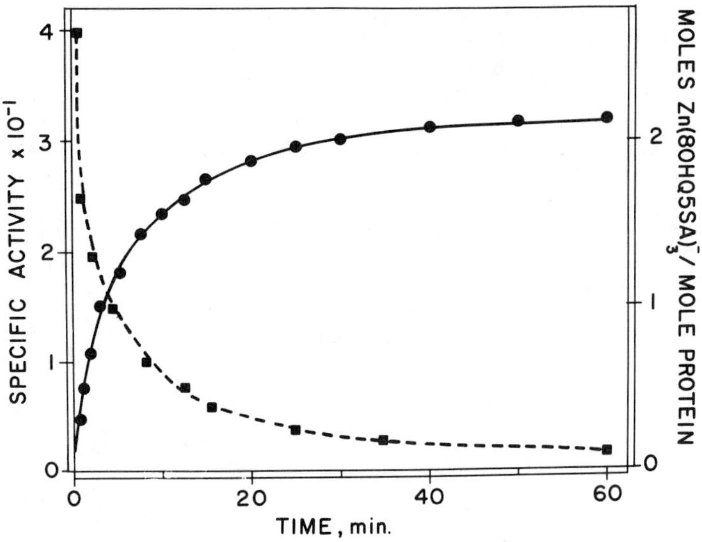

FIGURE 10. Removal of zinc from alkaline phosphatase by 8OHQ5SA. Enzyme, 1.33×10^{-5} M, was incubated with 6.66×10^{-4} M 8OHQ5SA in 0.1 M Tris-Cl buffer, pH 8.0, 25°. Zinc removal (———) was quantitated by absorbancy at 370 mμ, the maximum for the 3:1 complex of zinc with 8OHQ5SA. Activity (– – –) was determined on aliquots.

are pseudo first order in enzyme concentration. The second pair of zinc atoms are removed only in the course of about 24 hours under the conditions noted (FIGURE 10). Activity is lost to less than ten percent of the control activity concurrent with the removal of the rapidly reacting pair of metal ions (FIGURE 8). These data, together with the results demonstrating the stabilization of quaternary structure by the second pair of zinc atoms, strongly suggested the presence of the postulated two classes of metal ions in phosphatase concerned with catalysis and structure, respectively.

Addition of increments of metal ions to the apoprotein confirms the hypothesis that only two of the four metal ions that bind to the enzyme are directly involved in catalytic function. Addition of two gram atoms of zinc to apophosphotase generates 85% of the activity characteristic of the native molecule (FIGURE 11). Further addition of zinc restores activity fully but does not increase it to values higher than that of the control. In contrast, the addition of two gram atoms of cobalt to the apoprotein induces little activity. Further addition of another pair of cobalt ions, however, generates the activity characteristic of the cobalt enzyme (FIGURE 11). In the case of both zinc and cobalt, the incorporation of metal ion into the protein, measured subsequent to removal of unbound metal by gel filtration, increases linearly from 0 to 4 gram atoms of metal added, but not beyond. Similarly, studies indicate that both metal ions may occupy the same pairs of binding loci in the enzyme, since they compete for binding to the apoprotein (TABLE 8).

Cobalt, the only metal other than zinc known thus far to form an active alkaline phosphatase, is also an excellent physical probe. Thus, the absorption and electron paramagnetic resonance spectra of cobalt complexes can be indicative of the geometry of the metal binding site.

The visible absorption spectra associated with the structural and catalytic pair of metal atoms in cobalt phosphatase differ strikingly. The first two moles of cobalt added to the apoprotein result in a simple spectrum centered at about 500 mμ, with a molar absorptivity, based on protein concentration, of about 50 M^{-1} cm^{-1} (FIGURE 12). The appearance of this spectrum correlates with the binding of cobalt ions which serve in stabilization of quaternary protein structure but do not participate directly in the enzymatic mechanism.

In contrast, the absorption spectrum generated by the complex of the enzyme with the second pair of cobalt atoms is much more complex, extending from 700 to 450 mμ. Well defined maxima at 640, 555 and 510 mμ are detected, with a shoulder at 610 mμ. Moreover, the absorptivities, expressed per mole of protein, of these bands, 250, 350, 280 and 210 M^{-1} cm^{-1}, respectively, are much higher than those of the first pair of cobalt atoms (FIGURE 12).

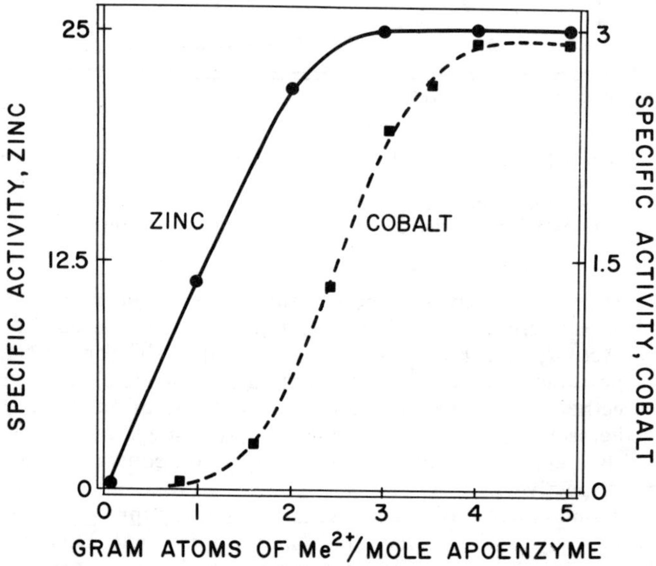

FIGURE 11. Activities of zinc and cobalt phosphatases. Apoenzyme, 1 × 10^{-5} M, was reconstituted by addition of the noted molar excesses of zinc (——) or cobalt (- - -) and assayed immediately.

TABLE 8

COMPLEMENTARITY OF ZINC AND COBALT BINDING TO ALKALINE PHOSPHATASE

Zinc Added	Cobalt Bound	Zinc + Cobalt
0	4.0	4.0
1.0	2.8	3.8
2.0	2.0	4.0
3.0	1.2	4.2
4.0	—	—

All results are expressed as g atoms of metal/mole of protein. Zinc, in the molar excess indicated, was added to the apoprotein prior to the addition of a 5.0-fold molar excess of $^{60}Co^{2+}$. Cobalt incorporation was measured following removal of unbound metal by gel filtration. In all cases, the amount of zinc bound after gel filtration was equal to that added to the protein.

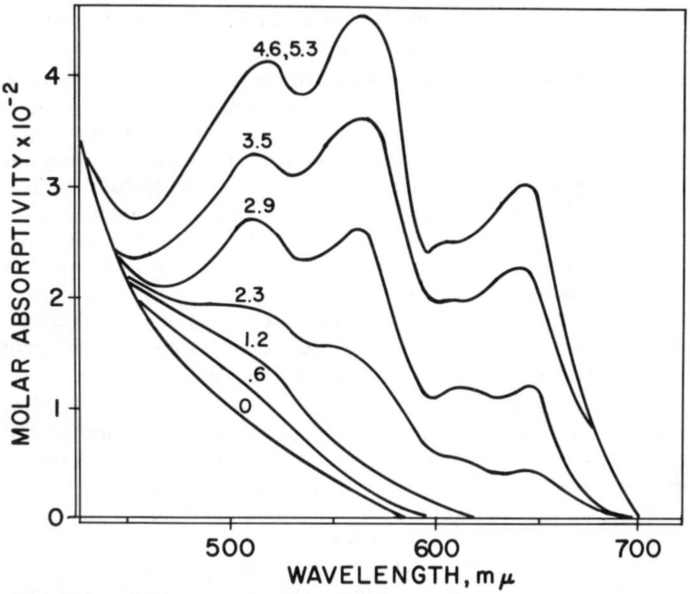

FIGURE 12. Absorption spectra of cobalt phosphatase. Apoenzyme, 2×10^{-4} M, in 0.01 M Tris-Cl, pH 8.0, was titrated by addition of the molar excesses of cobalt indicated above the spectral curves. In this and all succeeding spectra, the featureless curve at the lower left represents end absorption due to the protein itself, since the spectra were obtained with water as a reference. Absorptivity refers to the molar concentration of protein, not the metal species.

To the best of our knowledge, the generation of at least two different types of absorption spectra on addition of cobalt to an apoprotein is without precedent in enzyme chemistry, thus precluding comparison with analogous systems studied previously. The occurrence of two types of spectra is all the more intriguing since functional capacity seems to be associated only with the second pair of cobalt ions bound to the protein. Thus, the correlation of activity with the binding of the second pair of cobalt ions, their preferential displacement by zinc and the effects of phosphate ions on their characteristic spectrum (*vide infra*) suggest that the cobalt ions giving rise to it are at the active site of the enzyme. In contrast, the first pair of cobalt atoms bound do not appear to relate to activity directly, but seem to stabilize quaternary structure instead. Their absorption spectrum resembles that associated with cobalt (II) in an octahedral environment of nitrogen and/or oxygen donor groups in simple ligands, with maxima at about 500 mμ, and absorptivities of 5 to 40 M^{-1} cm^{-1} (Dennard & Williams, 1966). On the assumption that such cobalt-protein spectra can be compared directly with those of cobalt complex ions, the cobalt atoms that give rise to these spectra in alkaline phosphatase may well occupy an octahedral coordination environment.

While the spectrum generated by the second pair of cobalt ions, which are associated with catalytic activity, also invites comparisons with those of cobalt complex ions, it would seem much more difficult to arrive at similar analogies in this instance. The absorptivities are significantly higher than those of known octahedral cobalt complexes, but well below those of tetrahedral cobalt complexes previously studied with $\epsilon = 800$ M^{-1} cm^{-1}. The location of the maxima corresponds neither to those of simple octahedral nor of simple tetrahedral cobalt complexes (Vallee & Williams, 1968a; 1968b).

It might be considered that the spectrum generated by the second pair of cobalt atoms is the complex summation of two simpler spectra, each generated by a single cobalt atom, occupying different sites, but with approximately equal binding constants. In that case, interaction with inhibitors or substrate might alter each of these two hypothetical spectra in unique fashion. However, the spectrum associated with the catalytically essential cobalt ions behaves as a single entity, both on titration with H^+ and with phosphate ion (*vide infra*). These facts militate against this view, but do not rule it out. Further it may be recalled that cobalt carbonic anhydrase exhibits a spectrum closely similar to that of the catalytically active cobalt atoms of alkaline phosphatase, through cobalt carbonic anhydrase contains only one cobalt atom/mole of protein that could give rise to such spectra (Lindskog & Nyman, 1964).

In the absence of any unusual features in the geometry of binding of the cobalt atoms, this type of spectrum might conceivably arise from the diversity of ligand species present in proteins. Alternatively, it has been suggested that such unusual spectra associated with enzymatically active cobalt enzymes might be the consequence of unusual geometries of metal binding (Vallee & Williams, 1968a; 1968b), an interpretation consistent with recent studies of pentacoordinate cobalt (II) complexes.* Thus, the absorption spectrum of the enzymatically active cobalt ions could even reflect such unusual coordination as a pentacoordinate binding geometry in the protein, a geometry only described recently in the inorganic chemistry of cobalt. Other geometries are of course equally as possible, and cannot be ruled in or out as possible alternatives.

If the absorption spectrum of the enzymatically active cobalt atoms reflects a geometry required for function, conditions that alter activity might also alter the spectrum. The activity of cobalt phosphatase progressively decreases on lowering the pH to 6, with an apparent pK of 6.8 at 25° (*vide supra*). Simultaneously, the absorptivities of the spectral peaks decrease markedly, even though the general shape of the spectrum remains constant. Absorptivity at 640 mμ, characteristic of the spectrum of the enzymatically active cobalt atoms, exactly parallels hydrolytic activity (FIGURE 13).

Phosphate ion, the product of the energetically favored hydrolysis of phosphomonesters, inhibits hydrolysis and can also serve as substrate for the reverse reaction. Addition of phosphate to cobalt phosphatase markedly alters the absorption properties of the catalytic cobalt ions (FIGURE 14). The maxima associated with the cobalt protein itself are abolished, and a simpler spectrum with maximal absorption at 550 ($\epsilon = 280$) and 475 mμ ($\epsilon = 175$) develops. Two moles of phosphate interact with each mole of cobalt phosphatase to produce this spectral change (FIGURE 14, insert). This is to be compared to a value of one phosphate binding site obtained by equilibrium dialysis with the native enzyme (Reynolds & Schlesinger, 1969). Whether these differences relate to

* Recently, a number of five coordinate complexes of cobalt and other transition metals metals have been prepared. These are of the general formula bis-(R_2-aminoethyl)ZX_2 where R is methyl or ethyl, X is one of the halides, and Z is –O–, –NH–, –NR– (Ciampolini & Nardi, 1966; 1967; Ciampolini & Speroni, 1966; Dori & Gray, 1966). The visible band positions and absorptivities for the five coordinate models and the protein are quite similar, although there is a higher degree of splitting within the absorption envelope in the case of the proteins. Such increased splitting would accompany a reduction in symmetry that might be expected upon progressing from the relatively simple organic ligands to the more complex coordination site likely to be generated by the metal binding site of a protein.

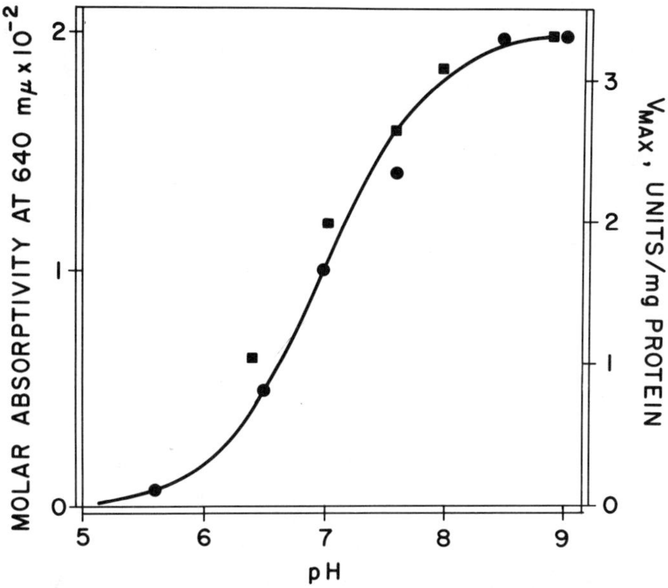

FIGURE 13. pH dependence of enzymatic activity and absorptivity at 640 mμ of cobalt phosphatase. Apoenzyme, 1×10^{-4} M, in water, was adjusted to pH 6 after addition of a five-fold molar excess of cobalt. The solution was titrated with dilute NaOH and A_{640} (●) determined as characteristic of the presence of the spectrum associated with enzymatically active cobalt. Enzymatic activity of cobalt phosphatase in the V_{max} (■) for hydrolytic activity.

methodology, the metal present, or as yet unknown features of the interaction of protein and substrate, remains to be established. The spectrum of the cobalt phosphatase-phosphate complex resembles that of an octahedral complex in band position and complexity, but its absorptivity is greater by an order of magnitude. Such an increase in absorptivity could arise from a distorted octahedral environment of cobalt ions at the active site when interacting with phosphate.

The circular dichroism of the cobalt enzyme further reinforces the deductions concerning the distinctive nature of the cobalt atoms at the active sites of this enzyme. Model complexes of cobalt (II) are not known to exhibit optical activity. In contrast, cobalt phosphatase exhibits four ellipticity bands within the absorption region of the two shorter wavelength transitions (FIGURE 15). The major band is positive, centered at 510 mμ, while minor bands are present at 570 mμ, 480 mμ, and 460 mμ. In the presence of phosphate ion, the geometry of the cobalt is altered and the dichroic bands of the protein are abolished with the substitution of two bands, at 550 and 505 mμ (FIGURE 15). In case of the E·S complex, the sign of the major band is reversed when compared to the protein itself.

Relation of These Studies to the Entatic State Hypothesis

Recent efforts to understand the mechanistic basis for the activity of metalloenzymes have noted dissimiliarities between the spectral properties of chromophoric metal ions at the active sites of metalloenzymes, and of these same metal ions when present either in simple model complexes, or in enzymatically inactive

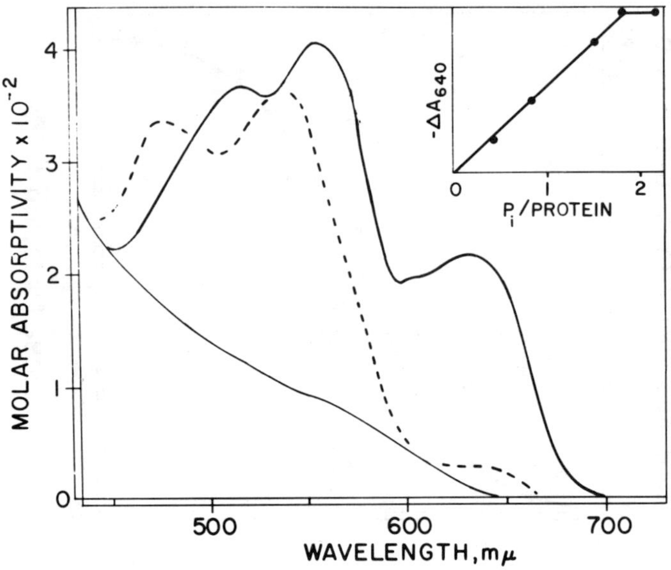

FIGURE 14. Effect of phosphate on the spectrum of cobalt phosphatase. Apoenzyme, 1.5×10^{-4} M, was reconstituted with a fivefold molar excess of cobalt (——), and then titrated with increments of phosphate ion to a final molar excess of 2.5 moles of phosphate per mole of enzyme (– – –). The insert presents the loss of absorptivity at 640 mμ as a function of the molar excess of phosphate added to the cobalt protein.

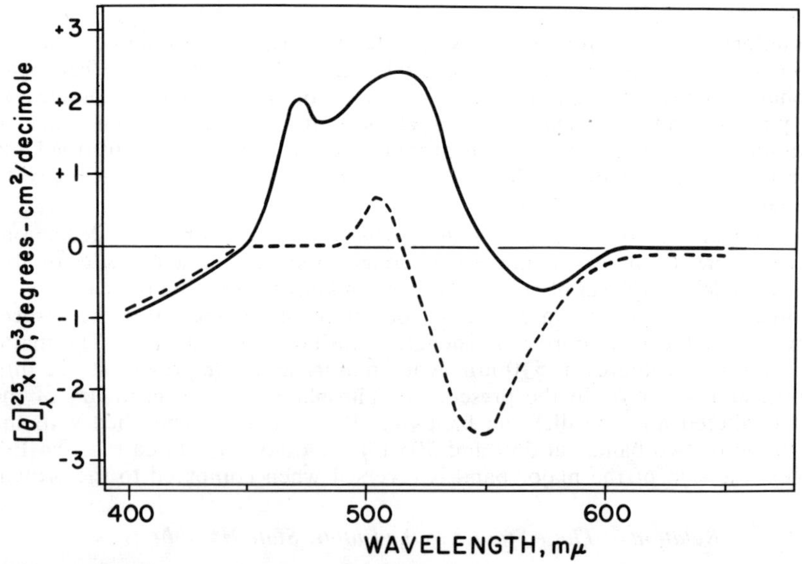

FIGURE 15. Circular dichroism of cobalt phosphatase and the phosphate cobalt phosphatase complex. The circular dichroism of apophosphatase reconstituted with a fivefold molar excess of cobalt (——), and the same sample plus a threefold molar excess of phosphate (– – –), were determined. Protein concentration was 2×10^{-4} M in a 2 cm pathlength cell, 0.01 M Tris-Cl, pH 8.0.

metalloproteins (Vallee & Williams, 1968a; 1968b). In general, the spectra associated with catalytically active metal ions in metalloenzymes are thought to reflect an irregular coordination environment of low symmetry. This irregularity, in turn, may confer a higher energy state upon the metal atom at the active site, thus placing it in a catalytically poised state. This state has been called "entatic," literally "in a state of tension" or under "stretch." In contrast, the spectra of enzymatically inactive metalloproteins can resemble those of simple model complexes.

Alkaline phosphatase of *E. coli* has provided the first opportunity to examine this hypothesis in a single protein that apparently contains two classes of metal ions. The two metal atoms that serve solely to stabilize quaternary structure exhibits spectra similar to those of simple model octahedral complexes. In contrast, the spectrum associated with the catalytically essential cobalt ions is unlike those of either octahedral or tetrahedral model complexes. The spectrum of the cobalt ions demonstrably involved in catalysis is altered by conditions that alter enzymatic activity. Thus, the present data are consistent with, and support, the entatic site hypothesis.

References

CIAMPOLINI, M. & N. NARDI. 1966. Inorg. Chem. **5:** 41.
CIAMPOLINI, M. & N. NARDI. 1967. Inorg. Chem. **6:** 445.
CIAMPOLINI, M. & G. P. SPERONI. 1966. Inorg. Chem. **5:** 45.
CLOETENS, R. 1942. Biochem. Z. **310:** 42.
DENNARD, A. E. & R. J. P. WILLIAMS. 1966. *In* Transition Metal Chemistry. R. Carlin, Ed. **2:** 116. M. Dekker, Inc., New York, N. Y.
DORI, Z. & H. B. GRAY. 1966. J. Amer. Chem. Soc. **83:** 1394.
ENGSTROM, L. 1962. Biochim. Biophys. Acta **56:** 606.
FERNLEY, H. N. & P. G. WALKER. 1966. Nature (London) **212:** 1435.
FIFE, W. K. 1966. Biochem. Biophys. Res. Comm. **28:** 309.
GAREN, A. & C. LEVINTHAL. 1960. Biochim. Biophys. Acta **38:** 470.
HARRIS, M. I. & J. E. COLEMAN. 1968. J. Biol. Chem. **243:** 5063.
HORIUCHI, T., S. HORIUCHI & D. MIZUNO. 1959. Nature (London) **183:** 1529.
KO, S. H. D. & F. J. KEZDY. 1967. J. Amer. Chem. Soc. **89:** 7139.
LAZDUNSKI, C. & M. LAZDUNSKI. 1966. Biochim. Biophys. Acta **113:** 551.
LINDSKOG, S. & P. O. NYMAN. 1964. Biochim. Biophys. Acta **85:** 462.
MALAMY, M. H. & B. L. HORECKER. 1964a. Biochemistry (Wash.) **3:** 1889.
MALAMY, M. H. & B. L. HORECKER. 1964b. Biochemistry (Wash.) **3:** 1893.
NEU, H. C. & L. A. HEPPEL. 1965. J. Biol. Chem. **240:** 3685.
PLOCKE, D. J., C. LEVINTHAL & B. L. VALLEE. 1962. Biochemistry (Wash.) **1:** 373.
PLOCKE, D. J. & B. L. VALLEE. 1962. Biochemistry (Wash.) **1:** 1039.
REYNOLDS, J. A. & M. J. SCHLESINGER. 1969. Biochemistry (Wash.) **8:** 588.
ROCHE, J. 1946. Helv. Chim. Acta **29:** 1253.
ROTHMAN, F. & R. BYRNE. 1963. J. Molec. Biol. **6:** 330.
SCHLESINGER, M. J. & K. BARRETT. 1965. J. Biol. Chem. **240:** 4284.
SCHWARTZ, J. H. & F. LIPPMAN. 1961. Proc. Nat. Acad. Sci. U.S.A. **47:** 1996.
SILLEN, L. G. & A. MARTELL. 1964. *In* Stability Constants of Metal Ion Complexes. Special Publication No. 17, The Chemical Society, London.
SIMPSON, R. T., J. L. BETHUNE & B. L. VALLEE. (In preparation.)
SIMPSON, R. T. & B. L. VALLEE. 1968. Biochemistry (Wash.) **7:** 4343.
SIMPSON, R. T., B. L. VALLEE & G. H. TAIT. 1968. Biochemistry (Wash.) **7:** 4336.
TAIT, G. H. & B. L. VALLEE. 1966. Proc. Nat. Acad. Sci. U.S.A. **56:** 1247.
TORRIANI, A. 1960. Biochim. Biophys. Acta **38:** 460.
TRENTHAM, D. R. & H. GUTFREUND. 1968. Biochem. J. **106:** 445.
VALLEE, B. L. 1955. *In* Advances in Protein Chemistry. M. L. Anson, V. Bailey & J. T. Edsall, Eds. **10:** 317–384. Academic Press, Inc., New York, N. Y.
VALLEE, B. L. & R. J. P. WILLIAMS. 1968a. Proc. Nat. Acad. Sci. U.S.A. **59:** 498.
VALLEE, B. L. & R. J. P. WILLIAMS. 1968b. Chem. in Britain **4:** 397.
WILSON, I. B., J. DAYAN & K. CYR. 1964. J. Biol. Chem. **239:** 4182.

Discussion of the Paper

C. DE DUVE: There appeared to be two catalytic sites. Is this consistent with the number of seryl residues phosphorylated and also with the rapid, instantaneous spectral change you saw when you titrated the enzyme?

DR. SIMPSON: No. The number of seryl residues phosphorylated is difficult to evaluate since the phosphorylation occurs at acid pH where the enzyme denatures. The highest value obtained, I believe, was by Pigretti and Milstein, who got something like 1.3 or 1.4 in trying to evaluate the downward trend due to denaturation and the upward trend due to lowered pH. The stopped-flow analyses that have been done have indicated the presence of one active site per mole. Dr. Schlesinger presented data obtained by Dr. Reynolds and himself that indicate one phosphate-binding site per mole for the zinc enzyme by equilibrium dialysis.

The present data indicate that two moles of phosphate per mole of enzyme are required to completely alter the spectrum. This could indicate that two moles interact with two active sites. However, this cannot be stated definitively until binding studies have been done. And whether these apparent differences arise from different metals, different methodology, or differences that are unknown in terms of the protein and the way it interacts with its substrate, is completely uncertain at this point.

D. SCHLESINGER (*Washington University, St. Louis, Mo.*): I was very interested in the fact that when you only have two zincs on the phosphatase, it is a more heat labile protein. When you take your zincless molecule and put back two, what type of heat stability do you see?

DR. SIMPSON: I'm not sure that I remember the numbers. There is another problem in this, and that is that the intrinsic magnesium appears to have a role also. If a remember correctly, one can keep the native enzyme at 91° C for an hour with the loss of 10% activity. With a two zinc enzyme under the same conditions, it will diminish to less than 10% in a period of two minutes, the four zinc enzyme will require 8 or 10, and the four zinc plus two magnesium enzyme will need about 30 minutes for the same degree of inactivation. These studies were done long ago, and I'm afraid I don't remember the actual numbers.

DR. SCHLESINGER: Actually, in the study of some mutants that I discussed previously, our data certainly confirmed the fact that the metal does stabilize the dimer. Because if you fool around with chelators, the zinc from one of those mutants falls apart. This is also true with the protein in which canavanine residues have been substituted.

B. L. HORECKER: With respect to the metal content of the native enzyme, you say you avoid ammonium sulfate and heat?

DR. SIMPSON: We set out with the idea of trying to set up a single-step preparation that would avoid these things, as we were concerned about the possible effects of these on the metal content. This problem has become apparent from a number of other studies (not yet published) on three other proteins that have highly variable metal contents as a function of the method of preparation.

B. L. HORECKER: Well, the question I had is that in the Neu and Heppel procedure, the very first step involves treatment of the cells with a chelating agent.

DR. SIMPSON: Yes, we've attempted to avoid it wherever possible. Unfortunately, one can't, to my knowledge, manage in any way that does not involve chelating agent. But what we have found is that if one uses the Neu and Heppel procedure–if anyone is not familiar with it–it involves incubation of washed cells in 20% sucrose and 10^{-3} M EDTA. These cells are then spun down and resuspended in distilled water, and the spheroplasts are formed by this procedure. If one takes cells grown to stationary phase, and then does the sucrose EDTA procedure for variable lengths of time, approximately 4 or 5 minutes is the minimum for full spheroplast formation. And if one does this for times varying from 2 minutes up to about an hour, the total zinc content of the water extract, which contains the phosphatase, decreases steadily with the time. The back extrapolated value in terms of zinc and activity seems to go back to about 4. This is certainly a possible cause for the average value of 3.8 as opposed to an integral number of 4.

DR. WILSON (*University of Colo., Boulder, Colo.*): I would like to point out, with regard to the labeling of alkaline phosphatase by P_{32} inorganic phosphate, that, first of all, you probably know the precision of these measurements is really terrible, and values all over the lot have been reported.

Secondly, it seems to be rather glibly accepted that this proves that phosphoryl enzyme is formed as an intermediate in catalysis. I'd like to tell you that this is not at all true, although I do think a phosphoryl enzyme intermediate is formed. The labeling experiments are a matter of thermodynamics and have nothing whatsoever to do with mechanism.

The second thing about this is that the phosphoprotein that is found in labeling experiments is extremely unusual. It has a dissociation, an energy of hydrolysis that is very different from ordinary phosphate esters. This enzyme phosphate ester is a million times more stable than simple phosphate esters or any known phosphate esters.

DR. SIMPSON: Yes, it is also, as you have pointed out previously, very kinetically labile.

DR. VALLEE: Since Dr. Wilson is here, I think it is particularly germane to point out that there is one more difference between the zinc and cobalt enzyme that has been possible to identify as a consequence of his studies on the transferase activity of the zinc enzyme.

As you know, the alkaline phosphatase of *E. coli* possesses both hydrolase and transferase activities. The cobalt enzyme, in contrast, is only a hydrolase, and has no transferase activity; that's one more feature of the peculiarity of the interaction of that atom as opposed to others.

N. K. GHOSH: I was very interested in your statement that ammonium sulfate could remove the metal atom from the enzyme molecule. In recent studies on placental enzymes, we have noticed that when the enzyme achieves a high purity, together with a large concentration of ammonium sulfate, it loses activity to a great extent. And that's the reason why we had to change the method of crystallization for ammonium sulfate to equilibrium dialysis. Do you think this is due to the removal of zinc by ammonium sulfate?

DR. SIMPSON: The analytic data demonstrate that, consequent to crystallization from ammonium sulfate and magnesium, the zinc content is decreased. Whether this is causal or not, I can't state. However, there are a number of analyses that indicate this, and now three other proteins that may behave similarly.

The Zn $(NH_3)_4^{2+}$ complex is fairly stable. The overall stability constant is 10^9, and one can easily calculate that at pH 8.0, there are quite high concentrations of ammonia in 70% ammonium sulfate.

DR. HORECKER: I think that Dr. Sussman has a few comments to make on the placental enzyme.

H. H. SUSSMAN (*Columbia University, New York, N. Y.*): We have been interested in the alkaline phosphatase of human placenta. At this time, I would like to present some of the data that we have obtained in studies of this enzyme. These data are the result of studies performed with Dr. Emil Laga and Dr. Arlan Gottlieb.

The initial objective was: (a) to obtain a relatively purified preparation of the enzyme, and then, subsequent to that, (b) to determine some of the enzymic properties of this enzyme.

The preparation we used was obtained from pooled placentae that were homogenized, extracted with *n*-butyl alcohol, isolated by 50% acetone precepitation, chromatographed on DEAE cellulose, and then filtered through Sephadex G-200. The resultant preparation was homogeneous by electrophoresis at several values of pH on polyacrylamide gel, and gave a linear pattern in sedimentation equilibrium studies. FIGURE 1 is a plot of ln c vs. radius squared of one of those studies. The molecular weight was calculated to be 116,000 in this preparation.

The molecule dissociated in 6.0-molar guanidine as shown by the ln c vs r^2 plot, which was linear, indicating homogeneity, and was of molecular weight

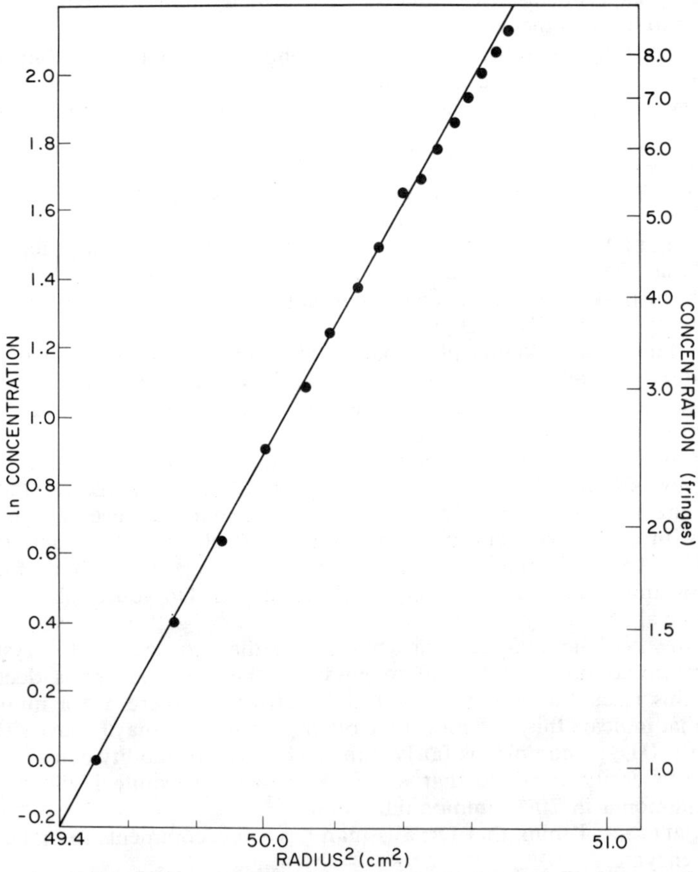

FIGURE 1. Sedimentation equilibrium experiment with placental alkaline phosphatase: plot of ln c vs. r^2 in 0.06 M glycine-NaOH, 0.05 M NaCl (pH 10.3). The experiment was conducted at 20°; rotor speed was 16,000 rev/min; dln c/dr^2 was 1.82.

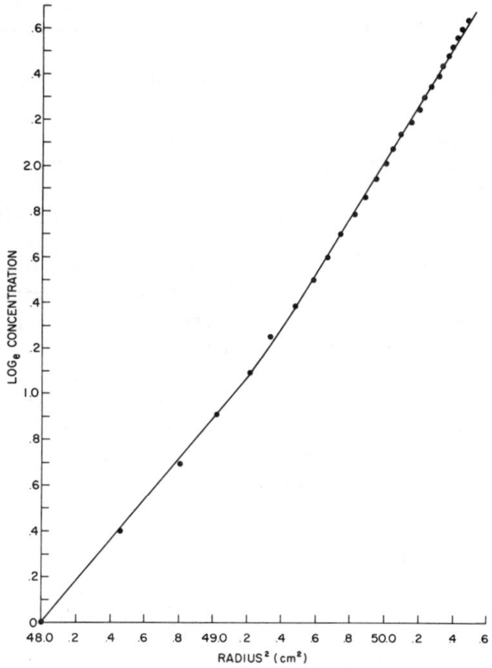

FIGURE 2.

58,000. From these experiments, we concluded that the placental enzyme, like the *E. coli* enzyme, is a dimer.

We then performed a series of sedimentation equilibrium experiments with enzyme that had been dialyzed to equilibrium at 4° C overnight. The results of these experiments indicated that between pH 4.7 and pH 10.3, the enzyme was stable as a dimer with molecular weights in the range of 116,000.

At pH 2.3, however, the molecule dissociated irreversibly, and gave a curvilinear plot in sedimentation equilibrium studies indicating molecular weight heterogeneity.

At pH 11.5 (FIGURE 2), the slope of the plot of ln c vs. radius $(\text{cm})^2$ was also nonlinear, giving a two-component plot. The molecular weight, calculated from the slope of the meniscus plot, gave a value of 57,000 to 61,000, suggesting that this component represents monomer. We then used a curve-peeling technique to calculate the molecular weight of the material at the bottom of the cell. This plot is shown by the diagonal line drawn to the right of the experimentally obtained points. This heavier component comprised approximately 10% of all of the material in the column and had a molecular weight of 240,000.

After completion of the sedimentation equilibrium studies, polyacrylamide disc-gel electrophoresis was performed using aliquots of the solution in the centrifuge cell.

These electrophoresis experiments are consistent with the ultracentrifuge studies and show dissociation of the enzyme at alkaline pH. As shown in FIGURE 3, the native enzyme is a single protein peak, which was coincident with enzyme activity. The cylinders were incubated in *p*-nitrophenyl phosphate, and the region of enzyme activity was marked with a cut, and then the cylinder was stained with amido-black dye. At pH 2.3, no activity is present and one sees a continuum of protein. When enzyme is dialyzed to pH 11.5, one sees the major protein band, which coincides with the native enzyme, plus a faster migrating component or components.

However, when enzyme is dialyzed from pH 11.5 back to pH 7.4, there is a diminution of these faster migrating heterogeneous components.

Also of interest regarding the dissociation phenomenon was that it was not affected by the presence of substrate. Sedimentation equilibrium experiments conducted at pH 11.5 in the presence of 0.01 M inorganic phosphate showed the same two-component, non-linear plot as that observed without substrate. Likewise, electrophoresis of these solution showed the same major enzyme-protein band and faster migrating bands as were seen without substrate.

We then conducted experiments of the enzymic properties of placental alkaline phosphatase. We were interested primarily in comparison of the hydrolytic and phosphoryl transfer reactions catalyzed by this enzyme. Initially, however, we studied only the hydrolytic activity with a series of mono-, di-, and tri-ester phosphates. We found that reactions with each of these substrates had different pH optima, and that all of the optima were above the dissociation constant for the second phosphoryl–oxy–anion.

The results showed that with placental alkaline phosphatase the relative enzyme activity is considerably greater with *p*-nitrophenyl phosphate than with any

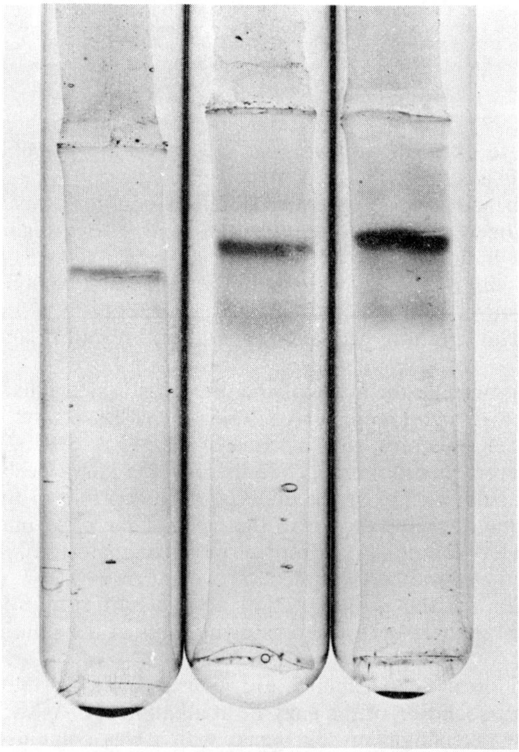

FIGURE 3.

of the other substrates. (ATP, AMP, UDP, phosphoryl ethanolamine, phosphoryl serine).

We then conducted a series of studies in which both hydrolytic activity and transferase activity were evaluated simultaneously. The substrates used were *p*-nitrophenyl phosphate and inorganic pyrophosphate, and the acceptors used were glycerol and glucose. The hydrolytic products measured were *p*-nitrophenol or inorganic phosphate; the transfer products measured were alpha-glycerophosphate or glucose-6-phosphate. We also conducted phosphoryl transfer reactions using inorganic phosphate as a substrate.

An interesting observation was that the ratio of phosphoryl transfer activity, comparing *p*-nitrophenyl phosphate and inorganic pyrophosphate each at its pH optimum, is in the range of 13:1, whereas the ratio of the hydrolytic reactions with each is about 40:1. Since the optimum with PP is in the region pH 7.5-pH 8.5 and the optimum with *p*-nitrophenyl phosphate is pH 11.5, we evaluated the percent transphosphorylation with each over a pH range from pH 6.0 to pH 11.5. We hoped that evaluation of these ratios over the entire pH spectrum would minimize any differences arising from the various pH optima with each substrate. The results showed that the percent of phosphoryl transfer was considerably greater in the pH range 6.0 to 7.5, independent of the substrate. This was interpreted to imply a separate pH optimum for each of these reactions.

DISCUSSION PAPER: SOME CONSIDERATIONS ON ALKALINE PHOSPHATASE

B. K. Bachhawat

Neurochemistry Laboratory, Christian Medical College Hospital, Vellore, S. India

The role of alkaline phosphatase in the degradation of pyridoxal phosphate in brain has already been established by earlier work from our laboratory.[1]

But I wish to discuss our recent work on the role of sialic acid in the heterogeneity of alkaline phosphatase in brain. Dr. Saraswathi in my laboratory has been working on the concept that the brain alkaline phosphatase is a sialoprotein and the difference in the sialic acid content may be one of the bases of the heterogeneity of alkaline phosphatase in brain.

In our earlier studies, we have shown that sheep brain contains two alkaline phosphatase fractions that differ in their elution pattern from DEAE-cellulose as well as in some of their properties, such as substrate affinity.[2]

We have also shown that one of the alkaline phosphatase fractions (ENZ-II) is associated with a higher amount of sialic acid than the other fraction (ENZ-I); sialic acid can be removed from the alkaline phosphatase by neuraminidase digestion and gel filtration on Sephadex G-200 to get rid of the free sialic acid and neuraminidase. The desialo ENZ-II on DEAE-cellulose column chromatography is eluted at a lower salt concentration than ENZ-II, but retains its original kinetics.[3]

Using this desialo alkaline phosphatase fraction, we have attempted to reconstitute the sialo alkaline phosphatase using the active form of sialic acid, i.e., CMP-sialic acid and rat liver microsomes as the source of transferase enzyme.[4] The transfer of sialic acid was followed by studying the elution pattern from DEAE-cellulose.

FIGURE 1 shows the elution pattern from DEAE-cellulose column of the (1) complete transferase system, (2) system where CMP-sialic acid was omitted and (3) system where microsomes were omitted from the incubation mixture and added before the chromatography.

The desialo alkaline phosphatase was prepared by incubating sialo enzyme with vibrio cholerae neuraminidase and gel filtration on Sephadex G-200. The desialo enzyme was separated from the sialo enzyme by chromatography on DEAE-cellulose and gradient elution with increasing concentration of sodium chloride as described in our earlier work.[3]

The incubation system for the transfer of sialic acid consisted of 1 mg of desialo alkaline phosphatase, 0.1 μmole of CMP-NANA, 3 μmoles of $MgCl_2$ and 3 mg of rat liver microsomes suspended in 0.3 ml of 0.01 M Tris-Maleate buffer at pH 7.4 in a total volume of 0.6 ml. Incubation was done for two hours, and the incubation mixture was dialyzed overnight against 0.02 M Tris-HCl at pH 7.4. Two control experiments were done–one where CMP-NANA was omitted from the incubation mixture and the other one, where microsomal suspension was added before the chromatography on DEAE-cellulose.

The transfer of sialic acid was followed by DEAE-cellulose column chromatography and gradient elution. The alkaline phosphatase activity was assayed using *p*-nitrophenyl phosphate as substrate, as described in our earlier paper.[1]

It is seen that in the complete system, nearly 50% of the alkaline phosphatase is eluted at a higher salt concentration. The system where CMP-sialic acid was

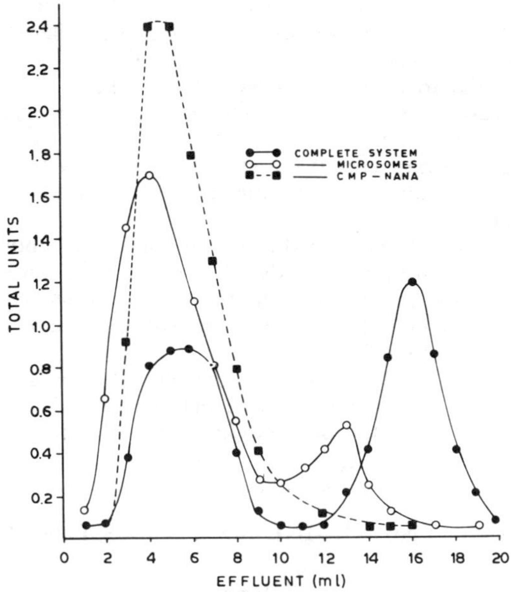

FIGURE 1. Elution pattern from DEAE-cellulose column of three systems: the complete transferase system; the system in which CMP-sialic acid was omitted; and the system in which microsomes were omitted from the incubation mixture and added before the chromatography.

omitted the entire alkaline phosphatase activity was eluted at peak-I and where microsomes was omitted, about 10% of the activity was recovered in peak-II.

These results indicate that there has been transfer of sialic acid to the desialo alkaline phosphatase in the presence of microsomes and CMP-sialic acid. This experimental system thus forms a good model for further studies on the formation of artificial isoenzymes by the successive removal of the carbohydrate portion of the alkaline phosphatase glycoprotein.

Since the alkaline phosphatase used in our studies was not highly purified, we are not in a position to suggest the exact mode of linkage of sialic acid to the alkaline phosphatase. However, based on the generally known structure of glycoproteins we have made some assumptions.

It is well known that in a glycoprotein sialic acid occupies a terminal position and is linked to the protein through an oligosaccharide chain, the sialic acid being linked to the galactose, N-Ac galactosamine or N-Ac glucosamine by a 2→6 or 2→3 glycosidic linkage. Two types of linkage between the carbohydrate and protein are known in glycoproteins: (1) N-glycosidic linkage between the amino group of asparagine, and C-1 of N-Ac glucosamine; (2) O-glycosidic linkage involving the hydroxyl group of serine or threonine.

Now, if we can achieve the sequential degradation of the carbohydrate chain by glucosidases, we would have a system to create heterogeneous alkaline phosphatase by successive removal of the carbohydrates in the oligosaccharide chain.

We did some experiments by treating the desialo alkaline phosphatase with galactose oxidase and studying the transfer of CMP-sialic acid to the galactose oxidase-treated desialo alkaline phosphatase. However, there was no inhibition of the transfer of NANA as shown by elution pattern in DEAE-cellulose.

These are some of the methods we are employing to see whether we can create the so-called heterogeneity by removing or blocking a particular carbohydrate in the oligosaccharide chain.

Finally I would like to state that various studies, especially in brain, have shown that during the development of the brain, the rate of incorporation of various carbohydrate into glycolipids varies with the brain development. Thus, the nature of oligosaccharide chain of the glycoprotein may depend on the stages of the brain development and, as such, may contribute to the heterogeneity of the alkaline phosphatase.[5]

We have heard some discussions during this conference about the blood group specificity of alkaline phosphatase. Also, Dr. Watkins has shown that specificity of blood group substances depends on the nature of the carbohydrate chain; thus, it may be possible that, depending on the nature of the blood group, different transferases may be present.[6]

Thus, one can assume that since alkaline phosphatase is a glycoprotein, the heterogeneity of the alkaline phosphatase may be related to the developmental process or due to disease states, or it may be genetically determined.

Acknowledgment

(Supported by Grant No. NIH-IND–6X4324, U. S. Public Health Service).

References

1. Saraswathi, S. & B. K. Bachhawat. 1963. J. Neurochem. **10:** 127.
2. Saraswathi, S. & B. K. Bachhawat. 1966. J. Neurochem. **13:** 237.
3. Saraswathi, S. & B. K. Bachhawat. 1968. Biochem. J. **107:** 185.
4. O'Brien, P. J., M. Canady, C. W. Hall & E. F. Neufeld. 1966. Biochim. Biophys. Acta **117:** 331.
5. Burton, R. M., M. A. Sodd & R. O. Brady. 1958. J. Biol. Chem. **233:** 1053.
6. Watkins, W. M. 1966. *In* Glycoproteins. A. Gottschalk, Ed. p. 462. Elsevier Press, Inc., Houston, Tex.

SOME PROPERTIES AND POSSIBLE PHYSIOLOGICAL FUNCTIONS OF PHOSPHOTRANSFERASE ACTIVITIES OF MICROSOMAL GLUCOSE-6-PHOSPHATASE*

Robert C. Nordlie

Guy and Bertha Ireland Laboratory, Department of Biochemistry, University of North Dakota Medical School, Grand Forks, N. Dak.

Blood glucose levels normally are maintained within rather narrow, constant limits by two opposing mechanisms operative in liver: glucose phosphorylation by kinase action and glucose release through the hydrolysis of the hexose phosphate ester.[1,2] Since 1949, the latter process has been known to be catalyzed in gluconeogenic tissues by a specific enzyme—glucose-6-phosphatase[3,4] (EC 3.1.3.9; Reaction 1). Because of the importance of glucose in energy metabolism throughout the body, the biological control of both phosphorylative and hydrolytic processes involving this compound has been a matter of continuing interest to the biochemist. The discovery in 1964, both in our own laboratory[5] and in that of Marjorie Stetten,[6] that glucose-6-phosphatase is a multifunctional enzyme capable not only of degrading glucose-6-P, but also of synthesizing this important metabolic intermediate *via* inorganic pyrophosphate (PP_i)-glucose phosphotransferase activity† (Reaction 2), was therefore of particular interest, and prompted continued investigations by us over the past five years. Some of these studies by Nordlie and Arion[8] have revealed that after detergent-treatment the enzyme also can utilize a variety of nucleoside tri- and diphosphate compounds as phosphoryl donors in the synthetic reaction (see Reaction 3). A number of sugar phosphate esters also have been found to act as phosphoryl donors[9,10] (Reaction 4) with this enzyme, which also catalyzes the hydrolysis of PP_i[5,6,9] (Reaction 5) and various nucleotides[8] (Reaction 6). The multifunctional nature of the enzyme from liver,[5–8] kidney,[11] and small intestine[12] has now been established. Some catalytic properties of the various hepatic activities are given in TABLE 1. K_m values and pH optima are listed both for untreated and deoxycholate-treated preparations, since detergents have a rather marked effect, particularly on phosphotransferase activities of the enzyme (see, for example, References 13 through 15). Whether observations with untreated microsomes or with detergent-treated preparations more nearly represent the properties of the enzyme in its natural state in intact, unfragmented endoplasmic reticulum in the cell is not yet clear.[13]

$$\text{Glucose-6-P} + H_2O \longrightarrow \text{glucose} + P_i \quad (1)$$

$$PP_i + \text{glucose} \longrightarrow \text{glucose-6-P} + P_i \quad (2)$$

$$\text{Nucleoside tri- or diphosphate} + \text{glucose} \longrightarrow \text{glucose-6-P} + \text{nucleoside di- or monophosphate} \quad (3)$$

$$\text{Sugar (or polyol)-phosphate} + \text{glucose} \rightleftarrows \text{glucose-6-P} + \text{sugar (or polyol)} \quad (4)$$

$$PP_i + H_2O \longrightarrow 2\,P_i \quad (5)$$

$$\text{Nucleoside tri- or diphosphate} + H_2O \longrightarrow P_i + \text{nucleoside di- or monophosphate} \quad (6)$$

* Work described in this paper was supported in part by grants from the Hill Family Foundation; the National Institute of Health, U.S. Public Health Service (AM07141); the National Science Foundation (B6–0823R), and the American Diabetes Association.

† PP_i-glucose phosphotransferase originally was described by Rafter[7] as a mouse mitochondrial enzyme. Its true microsomal nature and common identity with classical microsomal glucose-6-phosphatase were first recognized by Nordlie and Arion[5] and M. Stetten.[6]

TABLE 1

CATALYTIC PROPERTIES OF HYDROLYTIC AND SYNTHETIC ACTIVITIES OF HEPATIC GLUCOSE-6-PHOSPHATASE*

Activity	Without Detergent			Deoxycholate-Treated Preparation†		
	K_m (mM)	pH Optimum	V_{max}‡	K_m§ (mM)	pH Optimum	V_{max}‡
Glucose-6-P Phosphodydrolase	1.8	6.0	0.76	1.2	6.5	0.98
PP_i Phosphohydrolase	3.1	5.0	0.80	2.0	6.0	1.1
PP_i-Glucose Phosphotransferase						
PP_i:	2.9	4.5	0.55	1.3	6.0	1.2
Glucose:	127			90–100		
ATP-Glucose Phosphotransferase[50]						
ATP:	—	4.5	—	4.7	5.2–5.5	
Glucose:				90.		—
CDP-Glucose Phosphotransferase[8] (partially purified preparation)						
CDP	—	—	—	3.8	5.2–5.5	—
Glucose:				90.		

* Unless otherwise indicated, data presented, are from Reference 15, and were obtained with liver homogenates or microsomal suspensions from normal, fed rats. K_m values somewhat lower than those recorded have been observed with partially purified preparations.[5,9,12] K_m values were observed at the following pH values: glucose-6-P phosphohydrolase, pH 6.5; PP_i phosphohydrolase, pH 5.5; PP_i-glucose phosphotransferase, pH 5.5; nucleotide-glucose phosphotransferase, pH 5.2.

† Homogenates or microsomal suspensions were supplemented with neutral sodium deoxycholate to 0.2%, w/v, prior to assay.

‡ V_{max} values are expressed as 10 × Δ μmoles glucose-6-P formed or phosphate substrate hydrolyzed/min/mg liver protein.

§ K_m values for PP_i as low as 0.96 mM[12] have been observed with partially purified enzyme preparations, and values of 3.3×10^{-4}M have been noted in the presence of 0.3% cetrimide.[51] K_m values of 80 mM have been obtained for glucose with partially purified preparations.[9]

The reaction mechanism for this enzyme, depicted in FIGURE 1 is supported by kinetic studies of both glucose-6-P phosphohydrolase[9,10,16] and various other hydrolytic and synthetic activities.[9] In this scheme, which involves both binary enzyme-phosphoryl substrate and phosphoryl-enzyme complexes, glucose-6-P phosphohydrolase activity is described by Reactions 4 + 3 + 5; PP_i or nucleotide phosphohydrolase is depicted by Reactions 1 + 2 + 5; and phosphotransferase activities involve Reactions 1 + 2 + 3 + 4.

Control of Net Glucose Release

Glucose-6-phosphatase previously has been shown to be responsive to various hormonal and nutritional factors.[17] A consideration of the mechanistic scheme in FIGURE 1 reveals a number of interesting new possibilities for biological control of blood-sugar levels based on the recently characterized additional synthetic and hydrolytic activities of the enzyme. These additional possible control mechanisms include: (A) Net synthesis of glucose-6-P *via* phosphotransferase activity of glucose-6-phosphatase (Reaction 1); (B) Apparent noncompetitive inhibition of glucose-6-P hydrolysis by glucose, which actually involves glucose-6-P-glucose phosphotransferase (exchange) activity (Reaction 4a, below):

$$\text{Glucose-6-P} + \text{glucose*} \rightleftarrows \text{glucose*-6-P} + \text{glucose} \qquad \textbf{(4a)}$$

(see Reference 8); and (C) Competitive inhibition of glucose-6-P phosphohydrolase activity by PP_i[4,5,9] and various nucleoside tri- and diphosphates.[18]

During the past five years, the effects of a rather large number of factors—hormonal and nonhormonal—on synthetic and hydrolytic activities of this enzyme have been investigated in this laboratory with the ultimate objective of better-defining the enzyme's physiological roles and biological regulation. Factors studied are listed, and effects noted are briefly summarized, in TABLE 2 along with pertinent literature references. The complete list is much too extensive for detailed consideration here. We will, however, consider the three general addi-

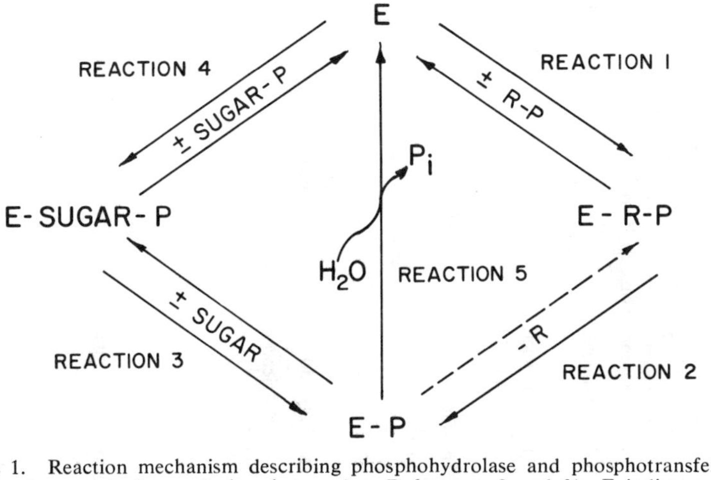

FIGURE 1. Reaction mechanism describing phosphohydrolase and phosphotransferase activities of microsomal glucose-6-phosphatase (see References 8 and 9). E indicates enzyme and R–P represents PP_i, nucleoside di- or triphosphate, or sugar phosphate ester.

TABLE 2

SOME FACTORS AFFECTING SYNTHETIC AND HYDROLYTIC ACTIVITIES OF GLUCOSE-6-PHOSPHATASE*

Factors	References	Effects Noted
Hormonal Manipulations, ***In Vivo***:		
Glucocorticoids	13, 14, 19, 52	Activity increased, principally through activation of existing enzyme molecules and involvement of a shift in pH optimum of phosphotransferase activity.
Alloxan Diabetes	8, 13, 53, 54	Two- to three-fold increase in all activities, apparently involving increased synthesis of enzyme. pH optima unchanged, but K_m values for phosphate substrates increased.[53,54]
Insulin	8, 13, 53, 54	Reverses effects of experimental diabetes.
Fasting	15, 29	Differential response, involving an increase in phosphatase, but not phosphotransferase, activities, as noted in the absence of detergent supplementation. All activities increased in a parallel manner when assayed in the presence of detergent.
Metabolites and other Factors, ***In Vitro***:		
Krebs' Tricarboxylic Acid Cycle Intermediates	21	Significant inhibition of all activities, below pH 7, by citrate for which a K_i value of 5.2 mM has been observed at pH 6.5. *Iso*citrate much less effective; only minor effects noted with *cis*-aconitate, *l*-malate, succinate, α-ketoglutarate, and oxalate. Malonate, tartrate, *L*-glutamate, glutarate, adipate, β-hydroxy-β-methyl glutaryl-Co A, and β-hydroxybutyrate also found ineffective as "instantaneous" inhibitors.
Glycolytic Intermediates	55	Slight activation by pyruvate; fructose-1,6-diphosphate is without effect; phosphopyruvate, 2-phosphoglycerate, 3-phosphoglycerate, glyceraldehyde-3-phosphate, and dihydroxyacetone phosphate inhibit slightly but $K_i > 36$ mM in all cases in absence of detergents.
Glycogen	53	No effects noted.
Varous Sugars and Polyols	8, 9, 56	Inhibit phosphatase activities by serving as phosphoryl group acceptors in competition with water. K_i (K_m) values considerably higher than for glucose, except for *D*-mannose and 2-deoxy-*D*-glucose.

Amino Acids	57–59	*L*-cysteine, *o*-tyrosine, and *L*-leucine inhibit and also stabilize enzyme against thermal inactivation. A variety of other amino acids also are effective to some degree in the latter respect.
Lipids:		
Long-Chain Fatty Acyl-Co A Esters	20, 28	Micromolar to 10^{-4} M levels affect hydrolytic and synthetic activities in an activity-discriminating, pH- and concentration dependent manner.
Fatty Acids	60	Millimolar-10^{-2} M levels also exert activity-discriminating effects.
Other Phospholipids	12, 60 30, 61–63	The former activates all activities; the latter are necessary for enzymatic activity and appear to maintain enzyme in a stable, active conformational state.
Nucleotides	18, 20	Various nucleoside di- and triphosphate compounds inhibit glucose-6-P phosphohydrolase activity competitively over a broad range of pH (pH 5–8). Also function as phosphoryl donors in phosphotransferase reactions. Effects are markedly potentiated by various detergents.
P_i	10, 33, 62	Inhibits in a manner similar to that of nucleotides. Also inhibits phosphotransferase activity.
Bicarbonate	34	Inhibits both synthetic and hydrolytic activities competitively with respect to phosphoryl substrates. $K_i \cong 20$ mM in absence of detergents.
Detergents	8, 12, 13, 62, 64	Optimal concentrations of deoxycholate, cholate, Triton X-100, and cetyltrimethylammonium bromide activate, as does urea. Activation of phosphotransferase > that of phosphohydrolase. Supraoptimal levels inhibit, as do all tested concentrations of sodium lauryl sulfate and Tweens 20 and 80. (See also "lysolecithin," "fatty acids," and "long-chain fatty acyl-Co A esters," above).
Metal-Binding Agents	21, 57, 58	Oxalate, citrate, 1,10-phenanthroline, azide, diethyldithiocarbamate, cyanide, and 8-hydroxyquinoline inhibit, suggesting the metalloenzyme nature of the catalyst.
Phlorizin	49	Inhibits noncompetitively both phosphodydrolate and phosphotransferase activities; inhibition potentiated by cetrimide and abolished or significantly ameliorated by deoxycholate, cholate, Triton X-100, or digitonin treatment of microsomes.

* An earlier review of factors affecting glucose-6-P phosphohydrolase activity has appeared.[17]

tional mechanisms for control of glucose-6-phosphatase activity described in items (A), (B) and (C), above, and will illustrate each with data from some of our more recent studies.

(A) Net Synthesis of Glucose-6-P by Phosphotransferase Activity

The phosphotransferase activities of the enzyme are characterized by rather acidic pH optima and high K_m values for glucose (see TABLE 1). A synthetic role for these activities cannot be excluded from consideration on this basis alone, however,[8] for a rather marked shift in activity-pH profiles toward neutrality is produced by various detergents (see TABLE 1, and FIGURES 2 and 6), and it has been demonstrated[8] that in the untreated diabetic animal, glucose concentrations are sufficiently high to allow for significant amounts of phosphotransferase activity. The administration of glucocorticoids to animals[19] also produces an alteration in pH-activity profiles of phosphotransferase activity, resulting in a relative increase in activity between pH 5.5 and 7 (see FIGURE 2). The effects of varied pH on glucose-6-P phosphohydrolase and PP_i-glucose phosphotransferase activities, and on K_m values for glucose-6-P and PP_i, are compared for detergent-treated preparations in FIGURE 3. It is apparent from these data that a lowering of pH will selectively favor the phosphotransferase activity (FIGURE 3 A), since the K_m value for PP_i is much more pH-sensitive in the range studied than is the K_m value for glucose-6-P (FIGURE 3 B). Indeed, in certain situations, phosphotransferase activity actually exceeds that of hydrolase. Thus, we[8,20] have suggested that phosphotransferase activity of this enzyme may play a physiologically significant compensatory role in glucose phosphorylation in the absence of insulin-dependent glucokinase in the diabetic animal. Acidosis, dehydration, hyper-

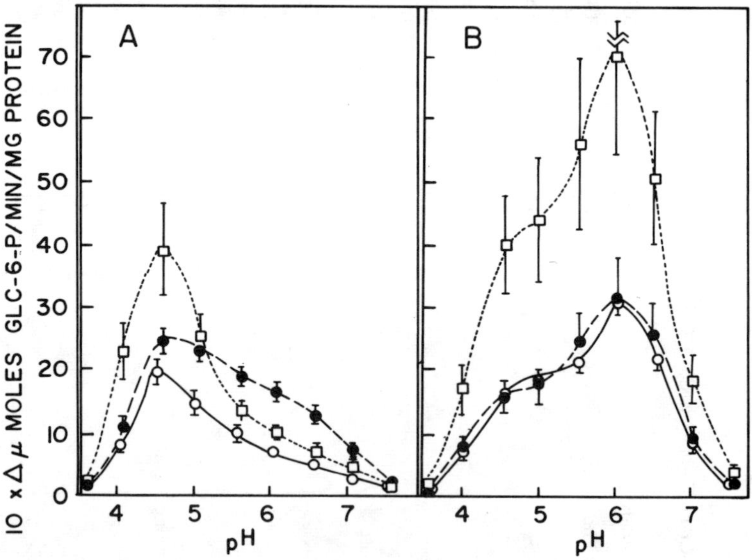

FIGURE 2. PP_i-glucose phosphotransferase activity-pH profiles assayed with (A) untreated and (B) deoxycholate-supplemented (to 0.2%, w/v) microsomal suspensions. Preparations were from normal (○), alloxan-diabetic (□), and cortisone-treated (●) animals. Further details are given in Reference 19.

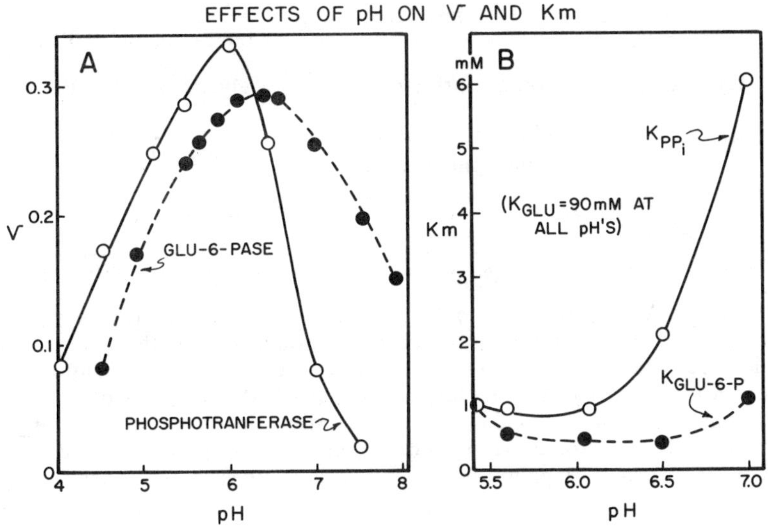

FIGURE 3. Effects of pH on (A) activity and (B) K_m values for glucose-6-P phosphohydrolase (●) and PP_i-glucose phosphotransferase (○) activities of partially purified enzyme preparations. In A, phosphate substrate concentrations were 10 mM and glucose was 180 mM (transferase). Buffer (40 mM) was sodium acetate, between pH 4 and 5, and sodium cacodylate, above pH 5. Further details regarding A are given in Reference 11; data in B are based on values given in Reference 21.

glycemia and increased enzyme formation (see FIGURES 2 and 4) in such animals all would favor such a situation. A comparison is made in FIGURE 4 of the relative ability of hexokinase, glucokinase, and PP_i-glucose phosphotransferase activities of livers of normal and diabetic animals to synthesize glucose-6-P at various pH values.[21] Concentrations of glucose employed in the calculations of the latter two activities were essentially the same (100 mM and 120 mM, respectively). It is apparent that PP_i-glucose phosphotransferase is *potentially* the most active glucose-phosphorylating system in the liver. Further, this activity is more than doubled in diabetes (FIGURE 4), while glucokinase essentially disappears.[22-24] A consideration of intracellular pH values compiled from the literature by Caldwell[25] indicates that significant amounts of phosphotransferase activity exist within observed cellular hydrogen ion concentrations (see double arrow and vertical dashed lines in FIGURE 4). Weinhouse and coworkers[26] recently have concluded that the combined action of hexokinase plus glucokinase is insufficient to account for the phosphorylation of administered glucose traditionally believed a prerequisite* to its incorporation into glycogen in the liver of the glucagon-treated, alloxan-diabetic animal, and have suggested that PP-glucose phosphotransferase activity may be involved in this overall process. They indicate that the PP_i produced in the UDPG synthetase reaction (Reaction 7) may serve as phosphoryl donor for glucose phosphorylation according to Reaction 2. The complete process may be envisioned to occur as follows:

* Some recent, preliminary studies[27] suggest, however, that glucose-6-P may not be a compulsory intermediate in the conversion of glucose to glycogen in liver.

$$\text{UTP} + \text{glucose-1-P} \xrightarrow{\text{UDPG synthetase}} \text{UDP-glucose} + \text{PPi} \quad (7)$$

$$\text{UDP-glucose} + \text{glycogen primer} \xrightarrow[\text{synthetase}]{\text{glycogen}} \text{glycogen} + \text{UDP} \quad (8)$$

$$\text{PP}_i + \text{glucose} \xrightarrow[\text{phosphotransferase}]{\text{glucose-6-phosphatase-}} \text{glucose-6-P} + \text{P}_i \quad (2)$$

$$\text{Glucose-6-P} \underset{}{\overset{\text{phosphoglucomutase}}{\rightleftarrows}} \text{glucose-1-P} \quad (9)$$

$$\text{Net: UTP} + \text{glucose} + \text{glycogen primer} \longrightarrow \text{glycogen} + \text{UDP} + \text{P}_i \quad (10)$$

In addition to alterations in pH and glucose concentrations, certain other factors have recently been found to exert differential effects on the synthetase and hydrolase activities of this enzyme. Micromolar to 10^{-4} M concentrations of long-chain fatty acyl-Co A esters and millimolar to 10^{-2} M levels of fatty acids, for example, have been found, in *in vitro* studies, to exert rather striking discriminatory effects on these two types of activity of the enzymes[20,28] (see FIGURES 5 and 6). For example, palmitoyl-Co A concentrations in the range 1 to 3 ×

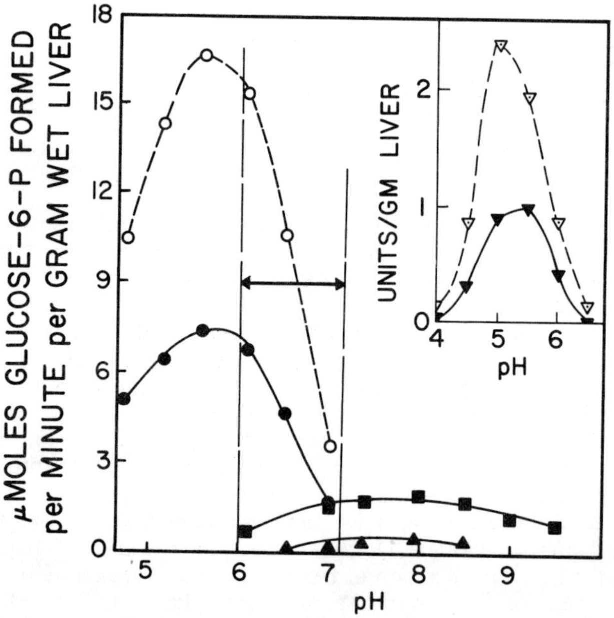

FIGURE 4. Larger drawing shows comparison of relative ability of liver hexokinase (▲), glucokinase (■), and PP_i-glucose phosphotransferase (circles, ○ and ●) activities to phosphorylate glucose at various pH values. All closed symbols indicate values for normal animals while the open circles depict phosphotransferase activity in diabetic animals, in which glucokinase essentially disappears and hexokinase is unaltered. Values are calculated for 5 mM ATP or PP_i, and 100 mM (glucokinase) or 120 mM (phosphotransferase) glucose. The horizontal double arrow indicates predominant intracellular pH values tabulated by Caldwell.[25] Further details are given in Reference 21. The inset indicates ATP-glucose phosphotransferase activity[50] for normal (▼) and diabetic (▽) animals. Glucose concentration was 120 mM and ATP concentration 10 mM. Units of activity are expressed on the axis of ordinates as in the larger drawing.

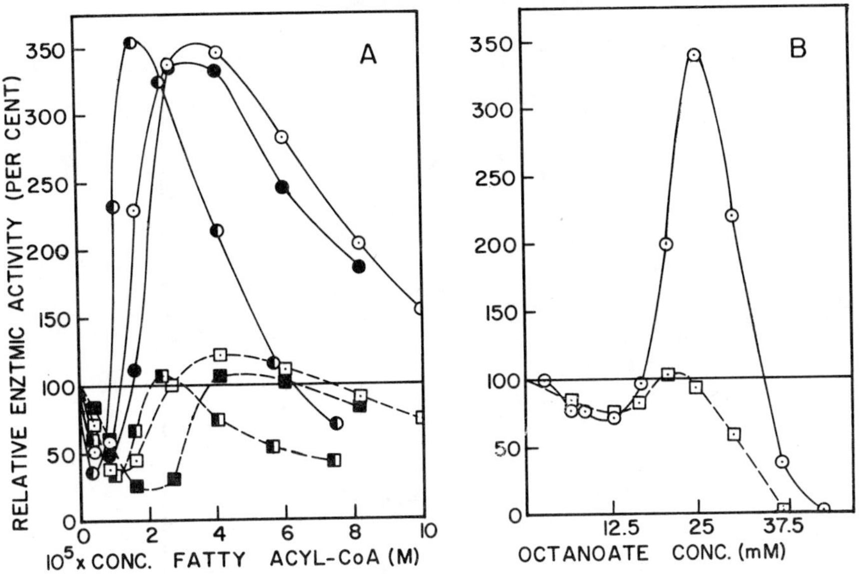

FIGURE 5. Effects of varied concentrations of (A) long-chain fatty acyl-Co A esters and (B) octanoate on glucose-6-P phosphohydrolase (squares on dashed lines) and PP_i-glucose phosphotransferase (circles on solid lines) activities. Assays were at pH 6.0. In A, results are those obtained with palmitoyl-Co A (⊙, ⊡), stearoyl-Co A (●, ■), and oleoyl-Co A (◐, ◧). Further details are given in References 18 (A) and 60 (B). Oleoyl-Co A was a gift of Dr. W. E. M. Lands.

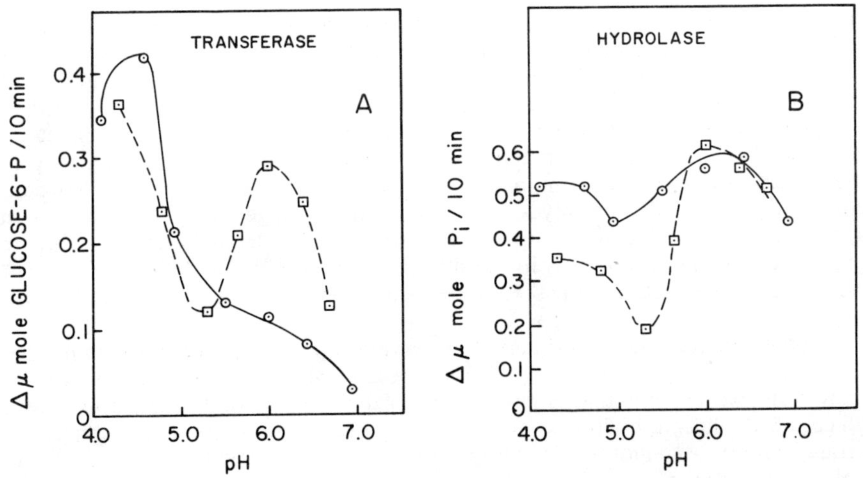

FIGURE 6. Effect of stearoyl-Co A on (A) PP_i-glucose phosphotransferase and (B) glucose-6-P phosphohydrolase activities as a function of pH. Circles indicate activity values observed in the absence of added detergent while squares depict values obtained with 41 μM stearoyl-Co A in assay mixtures. Additional details are given in References 18 and 60.

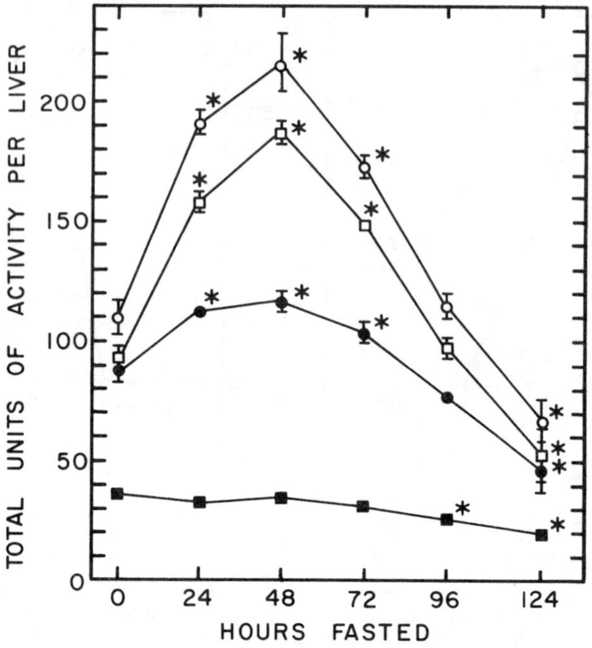

FIGURE 7. Effects of fasting on glucose-6-P phosphohydrolase (circles) and PP_i-glucose phosphotransferase (squares) activities. Assays were carried out with both untreated liver homogenates (closed symbols) and homogenates that had been supplemented with sodium deoxycholate to 0.2% w/v. Asterisks (*) indicate that differences between control values (zero hours fasted) and indicated values are statistically significant ($p < 0.05$). Further details are given in References 15 and 29.

10^{-5} M markedly stimulate phosphotransferase activity while significantly inhibiting glucose-6-P phosphohydrolase activity (FIGURE 5 A). Much higher concentrations of fatty acids exhibit similar effects (FIGURE 5B). A significant shift in phosphotransferase pH optimum toward neutrality also is observed in the presence of 41 μM palmityl-Co A (FIGURE 6 A), although this effect on glucose-6-P phosphohydrolase activity is minimal (FIGURE 6 B). This ability of these naturally occurring compounds to "turn on" synthetase activity and concomitantly "turn off" hydrolytic activity has been suggested to be involved in a mechanism for placing an upper limit on the (accelerated) rate of glucose production *via* gluconeogensis in the diabetic animal.[20,28] This hypothesis is considered in greater detail in the section on general conclusions, near the end of this paper.

Another interesting experimental observation implying, perhaps somewhat indirectly, the physiological significance of phosphotransferase activity of the enzyme is that enzyme that is newly synthesized in response to fasting manifests glucose-6-P phosphohydrolase activity but possesses only latent phosphotransferase activity[15,29] (FIGURE 7). Suppression of the latter activity appears to involve a transfer of the phosphoryl group from the phosphoryl-enzyme intermediate, since kinetic studies[15] indicate that altered affinity of the enzyme for phosphate substrates is not a factor. Hydrolysis of gluconeogenically generated glucose-6-P would appear to be the all-important function of this enzyme in the fasted animal in contrast to the fed diabetic. However, since blood-sugar levels of the former animals are quite low, it would seem that, unless phosphotransferase activity were able to function significantly under these conditions, it would be unnecessary to have this activity suppressed in enzyme molecules synthesized in response to fasting. By implication, then, it may be concluded tentatively that the synthetic activity of this enzyme may function significantly even at normal (or, indeed, subnormal) blood-sugar levels. Localized concentrations of glucose in the vicinity of the enzyme may conceivably be considerably higher than in the whole liver or in blood; and water in the immediate vicinity of this enzyme, which is a part of, or strongly associated with, the lipoprotein of the endoplasmic reticulum,[30] may have very limited access to the active enzymic site. Since water and glucose compete as phosphoryl group acceptors,[9] such situations would favor phosphotransferase activity.

(B) *Inhibition by Glucose of Glucose-6-P Phosphohydrolase Activity*

According to the mechanism in FIGURE 1, glucose may compete with water as alternate acceptor of a phosphoryl group from the phosphoryl-enzyme intermediate. Further, as predicted from this scheme and as experimentally observed,[9,16] the effects of glucose on the glucose-6-P phosphohydrolase reaction are identical kinetically with those of a noncompetitive inhibitor, although the actual phenomenon involved is transphosphorylation as indicated in Reaction 4a, above. The reduction in net glucose-6-P hydrolysis by varying concentrations of glucose is described in FIGURE 8. Data have been calculated with the aid of Rate Equation 8 in Reference 9. Although inhibitions noted at physiological blood-sugar levels are quite modest (< 10%), inhibition rises quite markedly with increasing

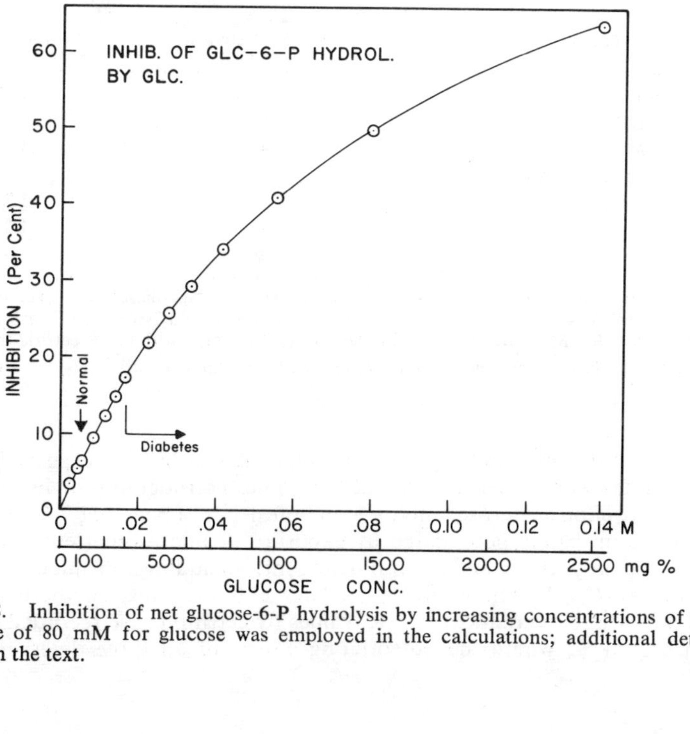

FIGURE 8. Inhibition of net glucose-6-P hydrolysis by increasing concentrations of glucose. A K_i value of 80 mM for glucose was employed in the calculations; additional details are presented in the text.

glucose concentrations and may be quite significant in the diabetic animal in which blood-sugar levels of 300 to 600 mg/100 ml or higher[8] are observed (see FIGURE 8). This inhibition by elevated glucose concentrations of the enzyme catalyzing the terminal step in gluconeogenesis may be a significant, built-in mechanism for self-regulation of liver glucose release in the diabetic animal, and may help to prevent uncontrolled depletion of liver noncarbohydrate percursors with an accompanying loss of much of the excess generated glucose in the urine. Glucose-6-phosphatase appears, on the basis of its relative abundance, to function as a "pace-maker" enzyme,[31] and its control, in the absence of glucokinase in the diabetic, would appear to be essential if constant, but higher-than-normal plateau levels, of blood glucose[1] are to be maintained. Recent observations by McCraw *et al.*[32] suggest the auto-regulation of glucose production in perfused livers.

(C) Inhibition of Glucose-6-P Hydrolysis by PP_i, Nucleotides and Anions

According to the scheme depicted in FIGURE 1, PP_i and various nucleoside tri- and diphosphates should compete with glucose-6-P for the active enzymic site. Competitive inhibition of glucose-6-P phosphohydrolase activity has been observed both with PP_i[5,6,8] and with various nucleotides.[18] K_i values for PP_i and adenine nucleotides are listed in TABLE 3. Inhibitions of glucose-6-P phosphohydrolase by these compounds are of particular interest in two respects:[18] (a) Potent inhibitions were observed even at pH values considerably higher than those at which phosphotransferase activity is manifest (i.e., above pH 7.5) and (b) inhibitions are markedly potentiated by exposure of microsomal enzyme preparations to various synthetic and natural detergents, including cetrimide, lysolecithin, and palmitoyl-Co A. These effects of detergents are apparent both from data in TABLE 3, where the reduction in K_i values by cetrimide are recorded, and from data in FIGURE 9, where the potentiating effects of all three detergents on the

TABLE 3

K_i VALUES FOR INHIBITION OF GLUCOSE-6-P PHOSPHOTRANSFERASE ACTIVITY BY ADENINE NUCLEOTIDES, PP_i, P_i, AND BICARBONATE*

Inhibitor	K_i Values (mM) Without Detergent Treatment	With Cetrimide Supplementation†
ATP	19.	2.0
ADP	14.	3.1
AMP	46.	14.
3′, 5′-cyclic AMP	76.	—
PP_i	12.	1.2
P_i	13.	1.9
$HC\bar{O}_3$	20.	—

* All K_i values, observed at pH 7.5, are from the work of Nordlie *et al.*,[18] except for $HC\bar{O}_3$ (pH 6.5) which is taken from the work of Dyson, Anderson and Nordlie.[34] The K_m value for glucose-6-P was 3.8 mM in the absence of detergent and 1.1 mM with 0.1% cetride treatment.

† Microsomal suspensions were supplemented with cetrimide to 0.1%, w/v, one-half hour prior ot assay.

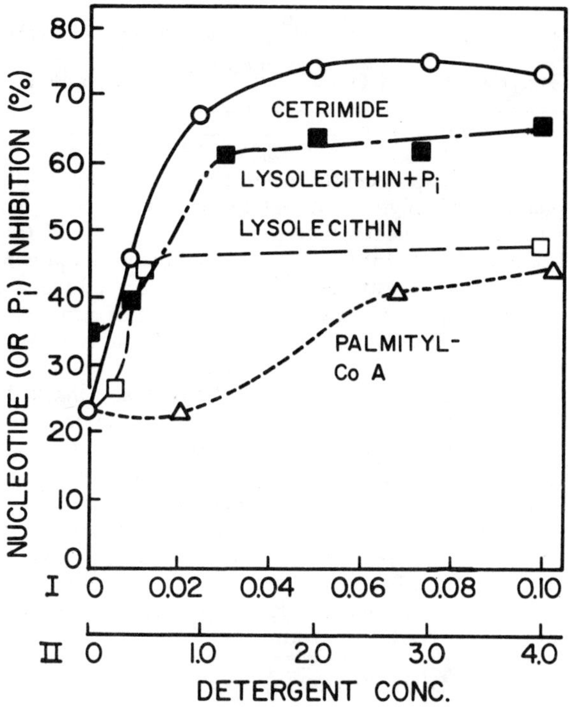

FIGURE 9. Potentiation by various detergents of inhibition by ATP plus ADP, and by P_i of glucose-6-P phosphohydrolase activity at pH 7.5. All data are for inhibition by nucleotides, except where specifically noted otherwise. Axis of abscissas I indicates cetrimide concentration (%, w/v) in microsomal suspension, while II describes palmitoyl-Co A concentration ($M \times 10^5$) or lysolecithin concentration ($M \times 10^4$) in assay mixtures. In calculations, described in detail in Reference 18, physiological levels of substrate and inhibitors were assumed to be as follows: glucose-6-P, 0.13 mM; ATP plus ADP, 6 mM; and P_i, 10 mM.

inhibition of glucose-6-P phosphohydrolase by physiological levels of ATP plus ADP (6 mM) are described.

The anions P_i and bicarbonate also have been found in recent studies to inhibit both synthetic and hydrolytic activities of the enzyme[33,34] (see TABLE 3 and FIGURES 9, 10, and 11). Inhibitions by P_i of glucose-6-P phosphohydrolase activity also were significantly potentiated by detergents (TABLE 3 and FIGURES 9 and 10 A), although little effect of this sort on the phosphotransferase was noted (FIGURE 10 B).

As Stadtman[35] has pointed out, the net effect of the combined action of hexokinase and glucokinase (Reaction 11) plus glucose-6-P phosphohydrolase (Reaction 1) would be the energetically wasteful hydrolysis of ATP to ADP plus P_i (Reaction 12). It is now apparent that inhibition by ATP of the hydrolysis reaction may be an important factor in preventing this nonsense cycling. It may be of particular significance that when the conservation of ATP is most essential (i.e., when ATP/ADP ratios are low), two molecules of effective inhibitor—ADP and P_i are present for each original ATP molecule. And the K_i values for the latter two compounds approximate that for ATP (see TABLE 3).

$$\text{ATP} + \text{glucose} \xrightarrow{\text{kinase}} \text{glucose-6-P} + \text{ADP} \qquad (11)$$

$$\text{Glucose-6-P} + H_2O \xrightarrow{\text{phosphatase}} \text{glucose} + P_i \qquad (1)$$

$$\text{Net: ATP} + H_2O \longrightarrow \text{ADP} + P_i \qquad (12)$$

Bicarbonate ion has also recently been found to inhibit all activities of glucose-6-phosphatase.[33,34] Significant inhibitions were observed within the generally accepted limits of bicarbonate ion concentrations—10 to 50 mM (FIGURE 11) (see Reference 34). Inhibition was kinetically of the competitive type with respect to phosphate substrates and was noncompetitive with respect to glucose in the phosphotransferase reaction. A K_i value of approximately 20 mM was calculated for added HCO_3^- with all activities. These observations, together with our earlier ones on the differential effects of bicarbonate on glucose-6-P dehydrogenase (inhibition) and glucose dehydrogenase (marked stimulation) activities,[36] offer an attractive rationale for the observations of Hastings and coworkers (see Reference 37) that elevated bicarbonate levels lead to increased conversion of glucose to glycogen in liver slices. Inhibition of glucose-6-P phosphohydrolase and glucose-6-P dehydrogenase[36] activities would impede two of the four principal pathways for removal of generated glucose-6-P in liver; and an increase in metabolic flow in the direction of glycogen formation might reasonably be expected to result. Concomitant stimulation by this anion of glucose dehydrogenase activity of glucose-6-P-dehydrogenase may provide for some continuance of NADPH production.[36]

Some General Conclusions

As a result of discovering the multiplicity of functions of classical microsomal glucose-6-phosphatase, as well as studying the factors to which the several activities respond in various ways, it has become apparent that the biological regulation of glucose release through the terminal action of this enzyme in the gluconeogenic process must be much more complex than had previously been thought. Extrapolations of observations made with an enzyme studied in the test tube to control of this catalyst in the intact cell are always speculative. However, several interesting and potentially physiologically important mechanisms for control of the release of blood glucose under a variety of conditions are suggested by the experimental observations described above and elsewhere (see references in TABLE 2), and appear worthy of note. For example, the following series of adjustments in the control of enzymic activities may be envisioned to occur as accompaniments to the development of the diabetic state:

1. Liver glucokinase activity (K_m for glucose = 10-40 mM) decreases to almost zero as insulin production ceases.[22-24]
2. Levels of key gluconeogenic enzymes – phosphoenolypyruvate carboxykinase[38,39] and fructose-1,6-diphosphatase[40] as well as glucose-6-P phosphohydrolase[8,13,17,19]–rise.
3. Glycolysis may be inhibited by increased levels of fatty acids acting on hexokinase, phosphofructokinase and pyruvate kinase.[41]
4. Net glucose production *via* accelerated gluconeogenesis is thus increased and is further favored by activation of pyruvate carboxylase[42], by accumulated acetyl-Co A,[43] and by inhibition of citrate synthetase[44] and glucose-6-P dehydrogenase[45] activities by elevated levels of long-chain fatty acyl-Co A esters (see Reference 20 for more detailed discussion).

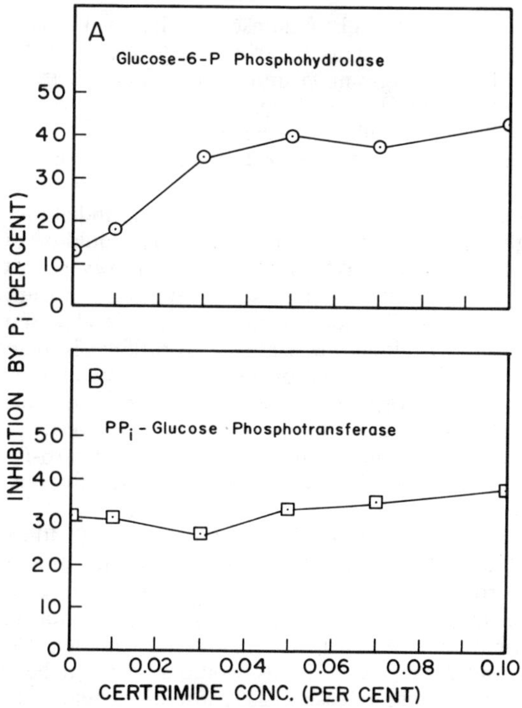

FIGURE 10. Effects of cetrimide on the inhibition by P_i of glucose-6-P phosphohydrolase (pH 7.5) and PP_i-glucose phosphotransferase activities (pH 6.5).[33] P_i concentrations were 8 mM; glucose-6-P or PP_i, 2 mM; and glucose (phosphotransferase), 135 mM. Cetrimide concentrations indicated are those (%, w/v) in microsomal suspensions.

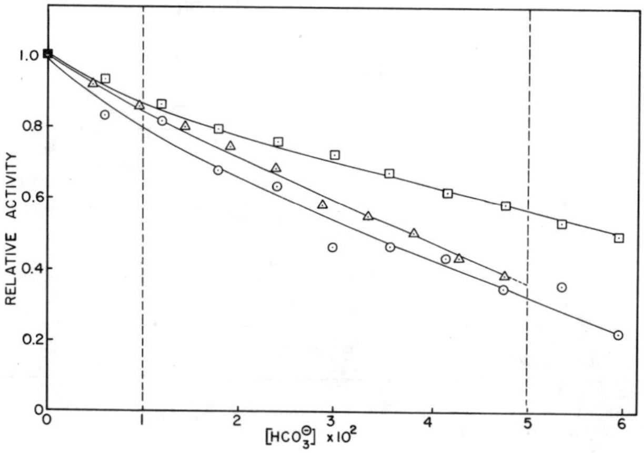

FIGURE 11. Inhibitions by bicarbonate of PP_i-phosphohydrolase (△), glucose-6-P phosphohydrolase (⊡), and PP_i-glucose phosphotransferase (⊙) activities. Relative activity = (activity without bicarbonate − activity with bicarbonate)/activity without bicarbonate. Details are given in Reference 34.

5. Inhibition of glucose-6-phosphatase activity by bicarbonate ion (see FIGURE 11) is partially relieved as bicarbonate levels fall[46] in diabetic acidosis.

6. The net effect of phenomena described in items 1 through 5 is a marked increase in the rate of release of glucose from the liver into the blood; elevated blood-glucose levels thus effected appear necessary for the continuance of carbohydrate metabolism in peripheral tissues in the absence of insulin (see Reference 1).

7. Were the above processes allowed to procede indefinitely without control, the release of glucose from the liver (and kidney) would be expected to procede in an ever increasing, autocatlytic manner.[20,28] However, as Cahill *et al.*[1] have pointed out, ". . . in all but the most severe states of insulin deficiency, a new equilibrium with essentially normal rates of periferal assimilation—albeit obtained at much higher blood-glucose concentrations—is reached." We suggest (see also Reference 20) that some or all of the following mechanisms involving activities of glucose-6-phosphatase may contribute to the plateauing of blood-glucose concentrations at these higher-than-normal levels:

a. Progressively increasing inhibition of net glucose-6-P phosphohydrolase activity by rising levels of blood glucose to which liver is freely permeable (see FIGURE 8).

b. Replacement of glucokinase (K_m for glucose = 10–40 mM[24,47] with PP_i- or nucleotide-glucose phosphotransferase activity (K_m for glucose = 80–90 mM[9]) as a mechanism for glucose phosphorylation. High blood-glucose levels, acidosis and dehydration in diabetes would tend to favor phosphotransferase activity of glucose-6-phosphatase (see FIGURES 2, 3, and 4). The net rate of glucose release from the liver under these conditions would appear to be determined by the opposing action of glucose release *via* glucose-6-phosphohydrolase activity, and glucose phosphorylation by phosphotransferase activity of glucose-6-phosphatase (see FIGURE 12) in place of glucokinase.[1]

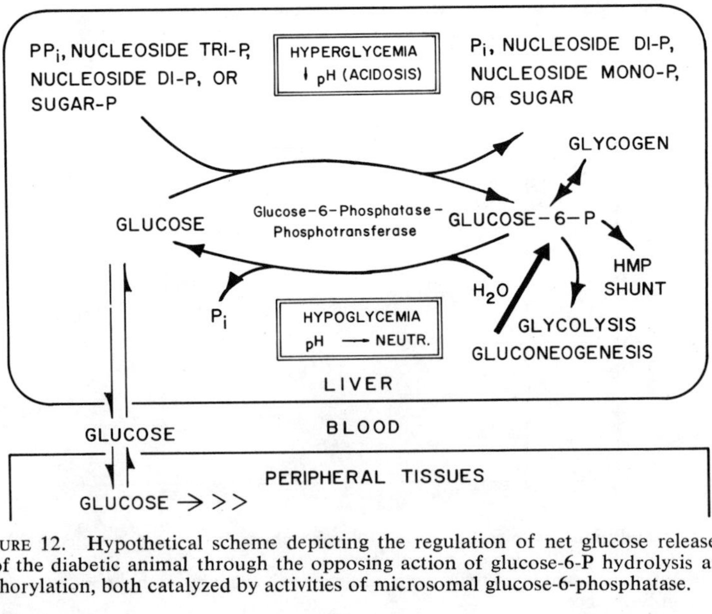

FIGURE 12. Hypothetical scheme depicting the regulation of net glucose release from the liver of the diabetic animal through the opposing action of glucose-6-P hydrolysis and glucose phosphorylation, both catalyzed by activities of microsomal glucose-6-phosphatase.

c. Preferential activation of phosphotransferase activity of glucose-6-phosphatase and inhibition of glucose-6-P phosphohydrolase activity (or only modest stimulation of the latter) by long-chain acyl-Co A esters and, possibly, fatty acids (see FIGURES 5 and 6), which increase their concentration in the liver in diabetes.[43,48]

d. Increased inhibition of glucose-6-P phosphohydrolase activity by (a) elevated levels of ADP plus P_i (TABLE 3), formed at the expense of ATP, and (b) potentiation of nucleotide and P_i inhibition of hydrolytic activity by elevated levels of natural detergents (see FIGURES 9 and 10, and Reference 18).

e. The possible involvement of kidney glucose-6-phosphatase-phosphohydrolase in the conservation of glucose through promotion of its tubular reabsorption in the diabetic animal has also been suggested,[49] and may contribute to the overall picture.

These concepts presently constitute a working hypothesis that serves as a basis for the design of further experiments in this laboratory relating to the physiological roles and regulation of this interesting and important biological catalyst.

Summary

Classical microsomal glucose-6-phosphatase of liver, kidney and small intestine has been shown to possess potent synthetic activities involving the transfer of a phosphoryl group from PP_i, various nucleoside di- and triphosphates, and certain sugar phosphate esters to glucose (or other sugars and polyols). The enzyme also catalyzes the hydrolysis of PP_i and nucleoside di- and triphosphates. A large number of hormonal and nonhormonal factors have been tested for *in vivo* or *in vitro* effects on these enzymic activities. Factors studied include glucocorticoids, alloxan diabetes and insulin, fasting, tricarboxylic-acid-cycle intermediates, glycolytic intermediates, glycogen, various sugars and polyols, amino acids, lipids (including fatty acids, long-chain acyl- Co A esters, lysolecithin and various other phospholipids), nucleotides, P_i, bicarbonate, detergents and phlorizin. Activity-discriminating inhibitory and stimulatory effects of some of these factors are described, and the possibility of their playing physiologically significant roles in the regulation of net hepatic glucose release in normal and diabetic animals is discussed with respect to (a) net synthesis of glucose-6-P *via* phosphotransferase activity and (b) control of glucose-6-P hydrolysis.

Acknowledgments

The author is indebted to Drs. J. E. D. Dyson, A. L. Vianna, W. J. Arion, T. L. Hanson, J. F. Soodsma, D. G. Lygre, and W. B. Anderson, as well as to R. E. Snoke, P. T. Johns, J. F. Gilsdorf, R. N Horne, R. J. Paur, S.M. Huang, P. M. Setness and R. Tello who, as postdoctoral associates or students, collaborated in the studies described.

References

1. CAHILL, G. F. JR., J. ASHMORE, A. E. RENOLD & A. B. HASTINGS. 1959. Amer. J. Med. **26:** 264.
2. NEWSHOLME, E. A. & W. GEVERS. 1967. Vitamins Hormones (N. Y.) **25:** 1.
3. DE DUVE, C., J. BÊRTHET, H. G. HERS & L. DUPRET. 1949. Bull. Soc. Chim. Biol. (Paris) **31:** 1242.
4. SWANSON, M. A. 1950. J. Biol. Chem. **184:** 647.
5. NORDLIE, R. C. & W. J. ARION. 1964. J. Biol. Chem. **239:** 1680.
6. STETTEN, M. R. 1964. J. Biol. Chem. **239:** 3576.

7. Rafter, G. W. 1960. J. Biol. Chem. **235:** 2475.
8. Nordlie, R. C. & W. J. Arion. 1965. J. Biol. Chem. **240:** 2155.
9. Arion, W. J. & R. C. Nordlie. 1964. J. Biol. Chem. **239:** 2752.
10. Hass, L. F. & W. L. Byrne. 1960. J. Amer. Chem. Soc. **82:** 947.
11. Nordlie, R. C. & J. F. Soodsma. 1966. J. Biol. Chem. **241:** 1719.
12. Lygre, D. G. & R. C. Nordlie. 1968. Biochemistry (Wash.) **7:** 3219.
13. Nordlie, R. C. & R. E. Snoke. 1967. Biochim. Biophys. Acta **148:** 222.
14. Nordlie, R. C., W. J. Arion & E. A. Glende, Jr. 1965. J. Biol. Chem. **240:** 3479.
15. Nordlie, R. C., W. J. Arion, T. L. Hanson, J. R. Gilsdorf & R. N. Horne. 1968. J. Biol. Chem. **243:** 1140.
16. Segal, H L. 1959. J. Amer. Chem. Soc. **82:** 947.
17. Ashmore, J. & G. Weber. 1959. Vitamins Hormones (N. Y.) **17:** 91.
18. Nordlie, R. C., T. L. Hanson, P. T. Johns & D. G. Lygre. 1968. Proc. Nat. Acad. Sci. U.S.A. **60:** 590.
19. Nordlie, R. C., J. R. Gilsdorf, R. N. Horne & R. J. Paur. 1968. Biochim. Biophys. Acta **158:** 157.
20. Nordlie, R. C. 1968. *In* Control of Glycogen Metabolism. W. J. Whelan, Ed. : 153. Universitetsforlaget, Oslo.
21. Nordlie, R. C. & D. G. Lygre. 1966. J. Biol. Chem. **241:** 3136.
22. Sharma, C., R. Manjeshwar & S. Weinhouse. 1963. J. Biol. Chem. **238:** 3840.
23. Salas, M., E. Viñuela & A. Sols. 1963. J. Biol. Chem. **238:** 3535.
24. Viñuela, E., M. Salas & A. Sols. 1963. J. Biol. Chem. **238:** PC1175.
25. Caldwell, P. C. 1956. Int. Rev. Cytol. **5:** 229.
26. Friedmann, B., E. H. Goodman, Jr. & S. Weinhouse. 1967. Endocrinology **81:** 486.
27. Das, I., H-G. Sie & W. H. Fishman. 1968. American Chemical Society, 156th National Meeting, Atlantic City, N. J. (Abstract Biol. 42).
28. Nordlie, R. C., T. L. Hanson & P. T. Johns. 1967. J. Biol. Chem. **242:** 4144.
29. Arion, W. J. & R. C. Nordlie. 1965. Biochem. Biophys. Res. Comm. **20:** 606.
30. Ernster, L., P. Siekevitz & G. Palade. 1962. J. Cell Biol. **15:** 541.
31. Weber, G. 1963. Advances Enzyme Regulat. **1:** 1.
32. McCraw, E. F., M. J. Peterson & J. Ashmore. 1967. Proc. Soc. Exp. Biol. Med. **126:** 232.
33. Nordlie, R. C. & A. L. Vianna. 1968. American Chemical Society, 156th National Meeting, Atlantic City, N. J. (Abstract Biol. 41).
34. Dyson, J. E. D., W. B. Anderson & R. C. Nordlie. 1969. J. Biol. Chem. **244:** 560.
35. Stadtman, E. R. 1966. Advances Enzym. **28:** 41.
36. Anderson, W. B. & R. C. Nordlie. 1968. Biochemistry **7:** 1479.
37. Hastings, A. B. & W. J. Longmore. 1965. Advances Enzyme Regulat. **3:** 147.
38. Shrago, E., H. A. Lardy, R. C. Nordlie & D. O. Foster. 1963. J. Biol. Chem. **238:** 3188.
39. Nordlie, R. C., F. E. Varricchio & D. D. Holten. 1965. Biochim. Biophys. Acta **97:** 214.
40. Weber, G., R. L. Singhal, N. B. Stamm, E. A. Fisher & M. A. Mentendiek. 1964. Advances Enzyme Regulat. **2:** 1.
41. Weber, G., H. J. H. Convery, M. A. Lea & N. B. Stamm. 1966. Science **154:** 1357.
42. Utter, M. F. & D. B. Keech. 1963. J. Biol. Chem. **238:** 2603.
43. Tubbs, P. K. & P. B. Garland. 1964. Nature (London) **211:** 1192.
44. Wieland, O. & L. Weiss. 1963. Biochem. Biophys. Res. Comm. **13:** 26.
45. Taketa, K. & B. M. Pogell. 1966. J. Biol. Chem. **241:** 720.
46. Bland, J. H. 1956. Disturbances of Body Fluids. 2nd edit. : 106. Saunders, Philadelphia, Pa.
47. DiPietro, D. L., C. Sharma & S. Weinhouse. 1962. Biochemistry **1:** 455.
48. Tarrant, M. E., R. Mahler & J. Ashmore. 1964. J. Biol. Chem. **239:** 1714.
49. Soodsma, J. F., B. Legler & R. C. Nordlie. 1967. J. Biol. Chem. **242:** 1955.
50. Horne, R. N. & R. C. Nordlie. (Unpublished observation.)
51. Soodsma, J. F. 1968. Ph.D. Dissertation. University of North Dakota, Grand Forks, N. Dak.
52. Arion, W. J. & R. C. Nordlie. 1967. J. Biol. Chem. **242:** 2207.
53. Hanson, T. L. & R. C. Nordlie. (Unpublished observations.)
54. Segal, H. L. & M. E. Washko. 1959. J. Biol. Chem. **234:** 1934.
55. Paur, R. J. 1968. Masters thesis. University of North Dakota, Grand Forks, N. Dak.
56. Stetten, M. R. 1965. J. Biol. Chem. **240:** 2248.
57. Nordlie, R. C. & P. T. Johns. 1967. Biochem. J. **104:** 37P.
58. Nordlie, R. C. & P. T. Johns. 1968. Biochemistry **7:** 1473.

59. Nordlie, R. C. & S. M. Huang. (Unpublished observations.)
60. Hanson, T. L. 1968. Ph.D. Dissertation. University of North Dakota, Grand Forks, N. Dak.
61. Snoke, R. E. & R. C. Nordlie. (Unpublished observations.)
62. Beaufay, H., H. G. Hers, J. Berthet & C. de Duve. 1954. Bull. Soc. Chim. Biol. (Paris) **36:** 1539.
63. Duttera, S. M., W. L. Byrne & M. C. Ganoza. 1968. J. Biol. Chem. **243:** 2216.
64. Snoke, R. E. & R. C. Nordlie. 1967. Biochim. Biophys. Acta **132:** 190.

Discussion of the Paper

C. de Duve: Assuming that the enzyme does play a role in phosphorylation of glucose, what do you regard as the most likely substrate donor? In the data you showed for the activity where pyrophosphate is the substrate, what about the nucleotide?

Dr. Nordlie: The nucleotides merit considerably more consideration. Or rather, they've been given a lot of consideration but not a lot of data has been published. A problem with pyrophosphate is that all pyrophosphate might be destroyed as soon as it's formed. I would suggest there may be, on the basis of differential pH and availability of magnesium plus compartmentalization, a possibility that pyrophosphate can funnel into the system. But this is only speculation. I don't think I've convinced anyone else. I certainly have not completely convinced myself. There is potential for producing pyrophosphate in tissues, however. A lot of pyrophosphate is produced, but my first argument will be that there is enough ATP present to work with the system. Then I think it's up to me to demonstrate that the pyrophosphate can be coupled in its production with this system to drive glucose-6-phosphate synthesis—a very complicated answer to a simple question, I guess.

I. Das (*Tufts University, Boston, Mass.*): I'd like to know one thing. It is obvious that glucose-6-phosphatase, phosphotransferase, will transfer to 6 position. But I would like to know whether you have any experimental evidence that the 6 position—phosphorylation in the 6 position—is the only product for transferase reactions?

Dr. Nordlie: In the phosphorylation of glucose, glucose-6-phosphate is the product. We explored this in great detail when we first worked with the activity. There is no evidence whatever that glucose-1-phosphate, for instance, could be produced, and that, then, through the action of the phosphoglucomutase, glucose-6-phosphate was formed.

The possibility of putting phosphoryl groups on other hydroxyl groups, on the molecule, I would say is ruled out, because we have used radioactive tracers and chromatographic means of separation. The product of this reaction travels exclusively with glucose-6-phosphate.

With other compounds, ribose for instance, it can put it on the 5 position.

C. de Duve: Have you tried any other acceptor besides glucose for this phosphotransferase reaction?

Dr. Nordlie: Yes, many compounds have been tried as possible acceptors. The obvious reason for using glucose is that we have a very nice assay for it and study it in detail. But we, and particularly Dr. Marjorie Stetten, have been quite interested in specificity. Indeed, she published a paper in which she described about 25 or 30 sugars and polyols as potential acceptors. Mannose is about as effective as glucose, the K_m being about the same; 2-deoxy-glucose is approximately as effective a receptor as glucose. All of the compounds studied had K_m's of 300 mM, 500 mM, or, essentially, infinity—very little activity. We've found nothing that works anywhere near as well as glucose as an acceptor of phosphoryl groups with the enzyme, except mannose and 2-deoxy-glucose.

DR. DE DUVE. One more question. Is there a relationship between the order in which these sugars accept the phosphoryl group and the rate at which the phosphorylated sugar is dephosphorylated by the enzyme?

DR. NORDLIE: I would suspect there is. I was interested in exploring this whole area at one time, and initiated some detailed kinetic studies in which we evaluated V_{max} and K_m's, feeling that this is the way to study such phenomena. Dr. Stetten published a paper on specificity in the JBC while these studies were underway, and I went on to other things. We found that nucleotides worked, and we're pretty excited about that. So I couldn't answer you directly. I would suspect that there is a correlation, and this should be worked out someday.

OLIGO- AND POLYSACCHARIDE INHIBITION OF MUSCLE TRANSFERASE *D* PHOSPHATASE*

C. Villar-Palasi

Department of Biochemistry, School of Medicine, University of Minnesota, Minneapolis, Minn.

Introduction

Glycogen synthesis in animal cells is catalyzed by UDP-glucose α-1,4-glucan α-4-glucosyltransferase (glycogen synthetase, transferase, E.C. 2.4.1.11). In skeletal muscle, this enzyme is present in two interconvertible forms, namely transferase *I*, stimulated by glucose 6-phosphate but active in the absence of this activator, and transferase *D*, totally dependent on the presence of glucose 6-phosphate for activity.[1,2] The interconversion of the two forms of the transferase involves a phosphorylation by ATP-Mg^{+2} of the *I* form in the presence of a kinase to yield the *D* form, and in the opposite direction, a dephosphorylation of the transferase *D* by a phosphatase, transferase *D* phosphatase, resulting in the formation of transferase *I*.[3] Measurements of the amount of glycogen synthesized *in vivo* by skeletal muscle,[4] as well as *in vitro* studies on the effect of muscle metabolites on the activity of the two forms of the transferase,[5] indicate that transferase *D* is essentially inactive under normal physiological conditions.

The relative proportion of the two forms of transferase is under hormonal control. Insulin, either *in vivo*,[6,7] or in isolated rat diaphragm preparations,[1,8] produces an increase in the percentage of transferase in the *I* form, while epinephrine[4,8] decreases the levels of transferase *I*. These hormonal effects appear to be mediated by modifications of the transferase *I* kinase activity, either through an increase in the concentration of its activator, 3′5′ cyclic adenylate (epinephrine)[9,11] or through alteration of the transferase *I* kinase to a form more dependent on this activator (insulin).[7]

A different type of control of the transferase activity is exerted by the final product of the reaction, glycogen. Danforth[4] has shown that in mouse skeletal muscle *in vivo*, and in rat diaphragm *in vitro*, there is an inverse relationship between glycogen concentration of the tissue and percentage of transferase in *I* form; this relationship appears to be independent and superimposed on any changes of transferase activity due to the action of hormones. An identical glycogen effect has been found under a large variety of conditions in the isolated rat heart. In a previous communication,[10] data were presented indicating that one possible mechanism of control by glycogen of transferase *I* levels could be the inhibition of transferase phosphatase by oligo- and polysaccharides.

In the present paper, the purification and properties of skeletal muscle transferase phosphatase are described, with particular emphasis on the inhibitory effects of glycogen and other oligo- and polysaccharides.

Experimental Procedure

Materials

Enzymes. Purified rabbit skeletal muscle transferase *D* (1.8 to 2.2 u/mg protein), free of phosphorylase, transferase *D* phosphatase and transferase *I* kinase, and contaminated with only traces of transferase *I* (1 to 2%), was obtained by

* Supported in part by a fellowship of the Public Health Service, U.S.A. No. 5F3AM-35-199-02, and a grant (AM-09071) from the National Institute of Arthritis and Metabolic Diseases of the U. S. Public Health Service.

a modification of the method of Villar-Palasi *et al.*[11] Transferase and transferase *I* kinase were eluted together from the DEAE cellulose column (Step 4) with 300 mM NaCl–50 mM Tris-HCl–50 mM mercaptoethanol–5 mM EDTA at pH 7.8 (TME buffer). To this column fraction, rabbit liver glycogen (8% solution) was added to a final concentration of 1 mg/ml, and transferase and transferase *I* kinase were precipitated by the addition of cold 95% ethanol to a final concentration of 30%. ($-2°$ to $5°$). The precipitated material was collected by centrifugation at $-10°$ for 10 minutes at $27{,}000 \times g$ and resuspended in 50 mM Tris-HCl–5 mM EDTA at pH 7.8, using about 0.1 the volume of the column fraction. To this solution, 0.1 volume of 80 mM ATP–150 mM $MgCl_2$–0.01 mM 3′5′ cyclic adenylate, pH 7.8, was added, and the mixture was incubated overnight at 3° to 5°. Transferase *D*, free of transferase *I* kinase, was precipitated by the addition of cold 95% ethanol to a final concentration of 15% ($-7°$ to $-10°$), the enzyme was collected by centrifugation at $-10°$ at $27{,}000 \times g$ for 10 to 15 minutes, and the precipitate dissolved in a minimum volume of 50 mM Tris-HCl–5 mM EDTA, pH 7.8. These preparations were found to retain activity for two to three months when stored frozen in small aliquots at $-80°$.

Rat muscle transferase *D* was obtained following essentially the same procedure, starting with fresh muscle of four to six rats. The enzyme obtained had a specific activity of 1.85 to 2 u/mg protein, and the final recovery was about 20%.

Crystalline rabbit skeletal muscle phosphorylase *a* was obtained as described by Cori *et al.*[12]

Other materials. UDPG (uridine diphosphate glucose), ^{14}C uniformly labeled in the glucose residue, was prepared by the method described by Thomas *et al.*[13] Rabbit liver glycogen was obtained from Nutritional Biochemical Co. Before use, it was purified by passage of 8–10% solutions over a mixed bed ion exchange column (Amberlite MB-3, 50 ml bed volume/g of glycogen), reprecipitated with ethanol and air-dried. Samples of cold-water-extracted glycogens, characterized structurally as well as with regard to sedimentation coefficient (TABLE 3), were a generous gift of Dr. E. Bueding. Phosphorylase limit dextrin (from alkali-extracted rabbit liver glycogen, 34.5% degradation) and waxy maize amylopectin were prepared by Dr. J. Larner. Highly purified oligosaccharides were prepared by Dr. T. E. Nelson, of this laboratory, who kindly supplied the amounts required for the present study.

Methods

Transferase activity was measured either as described by Villar-Palasi *et al.*[11] or by the filter paper method developed by Thomas *et al.*[13] Transferase *D* phosphatase activity was determined by the extent of conversion of transferase *D* into transferase *I* activity. The usual reaction mixture contained: 0.1 ml of purified muscle transferase *D*, [diluted immediately before assay with 50 mM Tris-HCl–50 mM mercaptoethanol–5 mM EDTA (TME buffer), pH 7.0, to a concentration of 0.8 to 1 u/ml, preincubated for 30 minutes at 30° and then chilled in ice bath]; 0.2 ml of transferase preparation, and 0.1 ml of additions or TME buffer. The assay mixture was incubated at 30°, and aliquots (30–50 μl) were taken at 0 time and after 5 to 15 minutes for determination of transferase *I* and total transferase activity (+ glucose 6-phosphate). In order to stop transferase *D* phosphatase activity during the assay for transferase, the transferase text mixture contained 25 mM KF in addition to the usual components.

Protein concentrations were determined either by the biuret method or by the optical densities of the samples at 280 and 260 mμ.[14] Oligo- and polysaccharide concentration were determined by the phenol-sulfuric acid method.[15]

One unit of transferase activity has been defined as the amount of enzyme that catalyzes the incorporation of 1 μ*mole* of glucose from UDP-glucose into glycogen in 1 minute at 30°.[11]

RESULTS

Proportionality of the Transferase D *Phosphatase Assay*

From previous work, it was known that transferase *D* phosphatase activity was relatively unstable under the conditions of assay (30° at pH 7.0), and also that the amount of substrate, transferase *D*, would probably be limiting. It was therefore necessary to study the limits of proportionality of the assay before attempting further studies.

Conversion of transferase *D* into transferase *I*, catalyzed by transferase *D* phosphatase, was proportional to time during the first 15 minutes of incubation at 30°, the rate of conversion decreasing rapidly after this point (FIGURE 1). Utilization of substrate was not responsible for the decrease in activity. Phosphatase was apparently more stable at 20°, and consequently the activity was found to be proportional to time up to 30 minutes, but the rate of conversion of transferase *D* into *I* was nearly halved. For convenience, the assays were carried at 30° for no more than 15 minutes.

Under these assay conditions, transferase *D* phosphatase activity was proportional to the amount of phosphatase in the test (FIGURE 2). The limiting factor

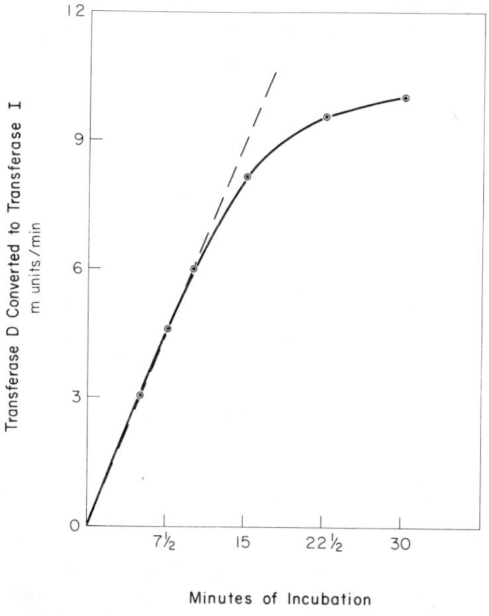

FIGURE 1. To 0.1 of transferase *D* (diluted to an activity of 2.08 U/ml), 0.2 ml of transferase *D* phosphatase and 0.1 ml of TME buffer were added, and at 0 time and after the indicated times of incubation at 30°, samples of 50 μl were taken for the determination of transferase *I* and total transferase activity.

in this case was the substrate utilization. The concentration of transferase *D* in the ordinary test mixture was of the order of ½ the Km for phosphatase; consequently, when the utilization of substrate was larger than 15% of the total transferase *D,* the assay was no longer proportional. As will be shown in this paper, glycogen inhibits transferase *D* phosphatase activity. Purified transferase *D* is more stable when stored in the presence of glycogen (about 1%) and to use a more concentrated solution of transferase *D* would require the removal of this glycogen, not practical for routine assays of phosphatase activity. The final dilutions of purified transferase *D* were of the order of 1:40 to 1:60 in the phosphatase test mixture.

Under these conditions, a unit of transferase *D* phosphatase activity is defined as the amount of enzyme that catalyzes the conversion of one unit of transferase *D* into transferase *I* in one minute at 30°.

Purification of Transferase D *Phosphatase*

Fed male Holzman rats of 300 to 350 grams in weight were decapitated while under seconal anesthesia and bled, and muscle of the hind legs was removed rapidly, chilled and roughly trimmed free of fat. Three to four animals were used to obtain 100 to 130 grams of muscle. The rest of the procedure was carried out at 2 to 4°.

The muscle was homogenized in a Waring blendor for 1½ minutes with 7 volumes (w/v) of 50 mM Tris-HCl–5 mM EDTA, pH 7.8, and the homogenate was centrifuged at 16,000 × *g* for 20 minutes. The supernatant fluid was filtered through glass wool. The filtrate, pH 7.1 to 7.2 was centrifuged at 78,000 × *g* for three hours, and the supernatant was applied to a DEAE cellulose column (5 ml bed volume per gram of muscle) equilibrated with TME buffer. After applying the enzyme, the columns were washed overnight with 7 to 10 times their

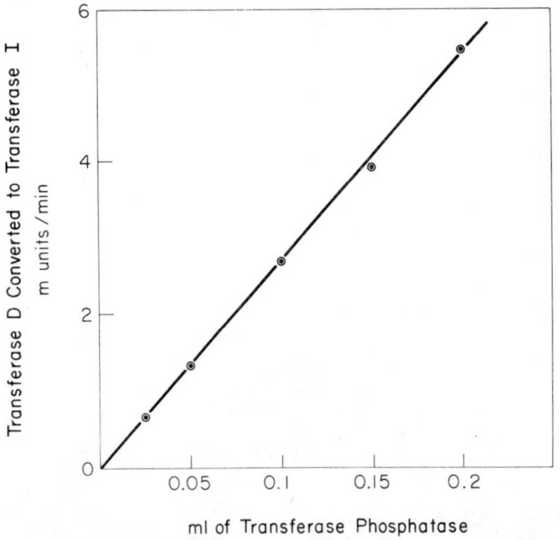

FIGURE 2. To 0.1 ml of purified rabbit skeletal muscle transferase *D* (as in FIGURE 1), the indicated volumes of partially purified transferase *D* phosphatase (free of transferase) were added, and the volume was adjusted to 0.4 ml with 50 mM Tris–50 mM mercaptoethanol–5 mM EDTA, pH 7.0. Samples of 50 μl of each assay mixture were taken at 0 times and after 10 min of incubation at 30° to determine transferase *I* and total transferase activity.

TABLE 1

PURIFICATION OF TRANSFERASE *D* PHOSPHATASE

Procedure	Volume (ml)	Protein (mg/ml)	Total Activity (units)	Specific Activity (m units/mg)	Recovery (%)
Extract	690	9.7	7.94	1.48	100
78,000 × *g* Supernatant	625	8.4	6.3	1.2	63
0.1 M NaCl	69	0.48	0.44	13.4	4.4
0.150 M NaCl	53	0.51	0.21	7.6	2.2
0.25 M NaCl	54	0.86	0.32	6.8	3.2

volume of TME buffer. Transferase *D* phosphatase was eluted from the column using TME buffer containing increasing concentrations of NaCl. Traces of activity appeared in the effluent obtained with 0.05 M NaCl, while most of the recoverable activity was eluted with solutions containing 0.1 M to 0.25 M NaCl, the 0.1 M NaCl peak having the highest specific activity. The effluent peaks were dialyzed against TME buffer for 6 to 18 hours before assay. An example of the purification is shown in TABLE 1.

The enzyme eluted with 0.1 M NaCl was free of transferase, phosphorylase, and transferase *I* kinase activities. However, it had phosphorylase phosphatase activity.

Attempts to further purify transferase *D* phosphatase were unsuccessful. Ethanol (20%), which in the presence of 1 mg of glycogen/ml precipitates transferase *D* phosphatase activity in the crude extract, inactivates the enzyme either in the 78,000 × *g* supernatant or in the column fractions.

Transferase *D* phosphatase activity appeared to be partially bound to sedimentable materials. Between 20 and 25% of the activity was recovered in the precipitate after centrifugation for three hours at 78,000 × *g*, and from 30 to 40% of the transferase *D* phosphatase was recovered in the precipitate after centrifugation at 158,000 × *g* for three hours. (TABLE 2).

Stability

Transferase *D* phosphatase activity was found to be unstable at all stages of purification. Freezing of the enzyme produced total inactivation in minutes. No activity was obtained from muscle stored frozen over 7 to 10 days. Transferase *D* phosphatase activity was lost after 30 minutes of incubation at 30° and pH 7.0; maximum stability was found at pH 7.6 to 7.8. Glycogen appeared partially to protect the enzyme against inactivation. Mercaptoethanol (50 mM) protected, and sometimes increased, the activity of the phosphatase.

Affinity of the Transferase D *Phosphatase for Transferase* D

The K_m of transferase *D* phosphatase for its substrate was determined using either crude rat muscle extracts or the partially purified transferase *D* phosphatase preparations described and purified muscle transferase *D*, either from rabbit or rat. In all cases, the K_m was found to be 0.45 to 0.5 units of transferase *D*/ml (FIGURE 3). No effect of transferase I on the K_m for transferase *D* was observed.

TABLE 2

FRACTIONATIONS OF TRANSFERASE *D* PHOSPHATASE ACTIVITY BY ULTRACENTRIFUGATION*

Procedure	Recovery Transferase Pase.	Recovery Transferase
Crude extract	100	100
Precipitate, 78,000 × *g*	23	70
Precipitate, 158,000 × *g*	13	16
Supernatant, 158,000 × *g*	63	14

* Fresh rat muscle was homogenized 1:10 (w/v) with 50 mM Tris and 5 mM EDTA, pH 7.8 (final pH 7.2), and centrifuged at 16,000 × *g* for 20 min. The extract was then centrifuged for three hours at 78,000 × *g*. The precipitated material was resuspended in 50 mM Tris–50 mM mercaptoethanol–5 mM EDTA, pH 7.2; the supernatant fluid was then centrifuged at 158,000 × *g* for three hours, the precipitate resuspended as above, and the supernatant fluid dialyzed against 50 mM Tris–50 mM mercaptoethanol–5 mM EDTA, pH 7.2, for three hours.

Effect of Phosphorylase a *on the* K_m *for Transferase* D

No distinct separation of transferase *D* phosphatase and phosphorylase phosphatase activities was achieved during the purification of either enzyme. In view of the identical amino acid sequence of the hexapeptide around the serine phosphate group in transferase and phosphorylase,[16] there was the possibility that both phosphatase activities were due to a single enzyme. To test this hypothesis, the K_m of transferase *D* phosphatase for transferase *D* was determined in the presence of 2,200 Cori units of crystalline muscle phosphorylase *a* (FIGURE 3). No effect on the K_m was observed upon the addition of phosphorylase *a*.

pH Optimum

Maximal transferase *D* phosphatase activity was observed between pH 6.5 and 7.3. The concentration and the type of buffers used, however, have a marked effect on the activity. Imidazole and tris (8.5 mM) produced an activation of over twofold, while maleate (8.5 mM) inhibited between 70 and 90%. EDTA was also found to be an activator, a concentration of 10 mM in the assay resulting in an increase of 2.5- to 3-fold in the phosphatase activity.

Effect of Glycogen on the Transferase D *Phosphatase Activity*

Highly purified alkali-extracted rabbit liver glycogen was found to inhibit the conversion of transferase *D* into transferase *I* in fresh rat skeletal muscle extracts supplemented with purified transferase *D*. The degree of inhibition was proportional to the concentration of glycogen present in the assay (FIGURE 4). The concentration of glycogen present in these extracts did not exceed 400 mg/ml, and the final concentration during the assays was less than 200 μg/ml (170 to 200 μg/ml).

No effect of glycogen (in excess of that present in the transferase assay mixture) was observed on the transferase activity.

Type of Inhibition Produced by Glycogen

The effect of glycogen on the kinetic constants of transferase *D* phosphatase was tested in fresh muscle extracts supplemented with different concentrations of transferase *D* with and without added glycogen (FIGURE 5). It was found that

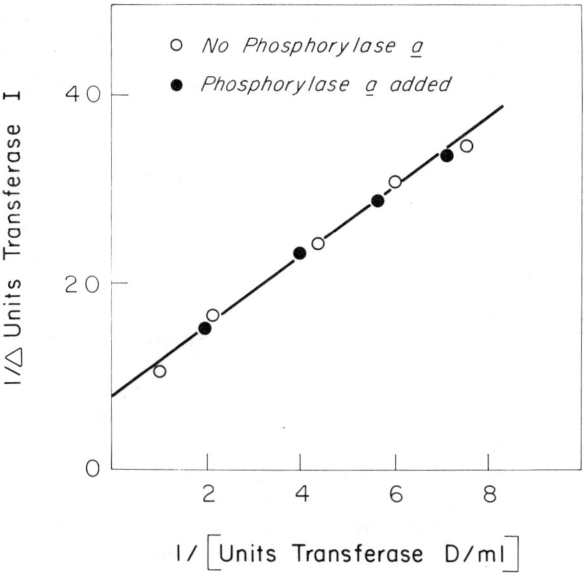

FIGURE 3. K_m of transferase *D* phosphatase for transferase *D,* and effect of phosphorylase *a.* The test mixtures consisted of: 0.2 ml of partially purified rat muscle phosphatase, 0.1 ml of transferase *D* at the different concentrations, and 0.1 ml of 50 mM Tris–HCl–50 mM mercapto-ethanol–5 mM EDTA, pH 7.0 (TME buffer), or 2,200 Cori units of three-times crystalized rabbit muscle phosphorylase *a,* dissolved and preincubated 10 minutes at 30° C in TME buffer. The reaction mixtures were incubated at 30°, and aliquots were taken at 0 and 10 min for assay of transferase (± G6P).

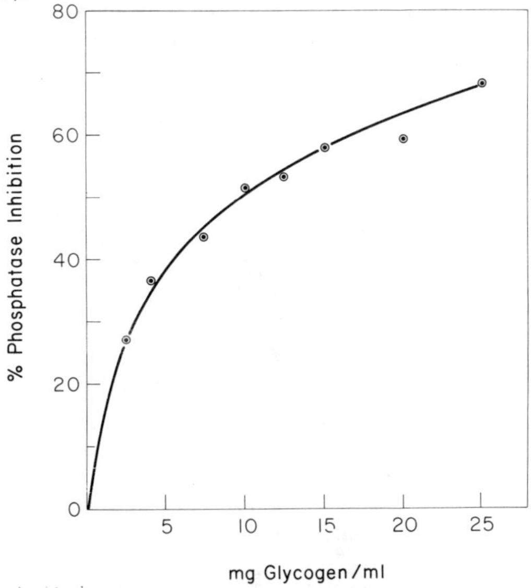

FIGURE 4. Inhibition of transferase *D* phosphatase by glycogen. Fresh rat muscle extract (0.2 ml) was supplemented with 0.1 ml of purified rabbit muscle transferase *D* (1 U/ml) and 0.1 ml of water or rabbit liver glycogen, alkali-extracted.

the inhibition of the transferase *D* phosphatase produced by glycogen could be decreased in a reversible manner by increasing the concentration of transferase *D*.

No inhibition of phosphorylase phosphatase activity by alkali-extracted rabbit liver glycogen was found, as already indicated by Cori and Cori.[17]

Inhibition of Transferase D *Phosphatase Activity by Oligosaccharides*

The series of linear oligosaccharides ranging from maltose to maltoheptaose was tested in the transferase *D* phosphatase system in order to determine the influence of the chain length of glucose residues on the inhibitory effect. The results obtained are presented in FIGURE 6. The extent of inhibition of the phosphatase increased, and the amount required for a given percent inhibition decreased from maltose to maltotetraose. However, no apparent further increase in inhibitory potency was found when maltopentaose, maltohexaose, or maltoheptaose were tested. Alkali-extracted rabbit liver glycogen was assayed simultaneously, and it is apparent that, notwithstanding the large difference in molecular weight, the inhibition produced was no larger than that obtained with a similar concentration (on a weight base) of maltotetraose.

As previously indicated in the case of the inhibition produced by glycogen, when no purified transferase *D* was added to the assay, the inhibition of transferase *D* phosphatase activity obtained with these oligosaccharides was significantly larger; therefore, it would appear that the inhibition produced by oligosaccharides is reversed by an increase in transferase *D* concentration, as is the inhibition produced by glycogen.

Effect of Water-Extracted Glycogen on the Transferase D *Phosphatase Activity*

Samples of undegraded glycogen of increasing sedimentatious coefficients, isolated and characterized by Dr. Bueding using a water-extractions procedure[18] were tested as inhibitors of the transferase *D* phosphatase activity. It was found that the inhibitory effects increase proportionally with the sedimentation co-

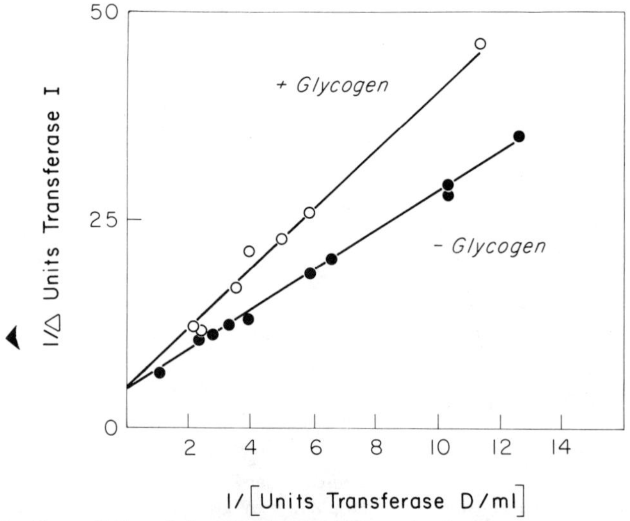

FIGURE 5. Reversibility of the glycogen inhibition. Fresh rat muscle extract (0.2 ml) was incubated with 0.1 ml of purified rat muscle transferase *D*, at several dilutions, and 0.1 ml of water or a 10 mg/ml solution of alkali-extracted rabbit liver glycogen.

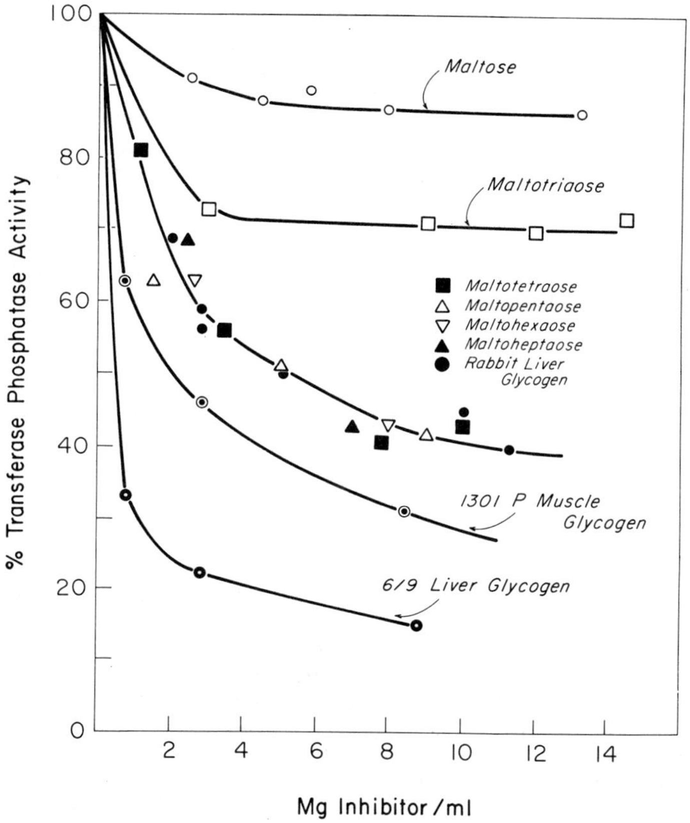

FIGURE 6. Effect of oligo- and polysaccharides on the transferase *D* phosphatase activity. Fresh rat muscle extract (0.2 ml in TME buffer) was mixed with 0.1 ml of purified rabbit muscle transferase *D* (1 U/ml) and 0.1 ml of distilled water, or water solutions of the oligo- and polysaccharides.

efficient (TABLE 3) and was in all instances larger than the inhibitory effects found using alkali-extracted glycogen. The increase in inhibition with sedimentation coefficient found in these undegraded glycogen samples is in contrast with the essentially identical inhibitions found with the oligosaccharides larger than maltotetraose and with alkali-extracted glycogen.

Effect of Polysaccharides of Short and Long Outer Chains

The effects of purified waxy maize amylopectin and of liver glycogen phosphorylase limit dextrin on the transferase *D* phosphatase activity were compared with the effect produced by alkali-extracted liver glycogen. Amylopectin at concentrations from 2 to 10 mg/ml. was found to have no, or very little, inhibitory effect (95% of residual phosphatase activity at 10 mg amylopectin/ml). In contrast, limit dextrin was found to be a more effective inhibitor than glycogen. At concentrations of 7.5 and 10 mg limit dextrin/ml, the residual phosphatase activities were, respectively, 25% and 5% of the original.

TABLE 3

EFFECT OF WATER-EXTRACTED GLYCOGEN ON THE PHOSPHATASE ACTIVITY

Type of Glycogen	S*	% Branch Points	% Outer Branches	50% Inhibition (mg/ml)
1301 P, Muscle	100	8.0	36.4	2.0
6/9 Liver	250	8.75	40.8	0.15
10/13 Liver	650	8.65	40.7	0.08
14/19 Liver	1200	8.8	39.4	0.045
20/25 Liver	1700	9.0	40.1	0.025
26/23 Liver	2500	8.9	39.8	0.018

* Average sedimentation coefficient.

Lability of the Inhibitory Effect of Glycogen

No inhibition by glycogen was found when its effect was assayed on purified preparations of transferase *D* phosphatase. The disappearance of the inhibitory effect would be due either (a) to removal of a substance present in the fresh extracts during the chromatography and/or subsequent dialysis of the enzyme or (b) to an alteration of the phosphatase molecule.

In order to test the first hypothesis, fresh rat muscle extracts were chromatographed through Sephadex G-25 in order to remove low molecular weight substances. It was found that the phosphatase present in the effluent was inhibited by glycogen to the same extent as the enzyme present in the extracts.

Also, ethanol-precipitated (20%, $-5°$) transferase *D* phosphatase from crude extracts was inhibited by glycogen. Overnight dialysis of fresh extracts resulted in loss of phosphatase activity (about 60%), and the remaining enzyme was no longer inhibited by glycogen. Samples of the same muscle extract, stored in identical conditions but not dialyzed, also lost activity and the residual activity was not affected by glycogen. Therefore, it would appear that an alteration of the transferase *D* phosphatase molecule is the most likely reason for the disappearance of the inhibitory effect.

Muscle phosphatase from young rats (250 to 300 g) is inhibited by glycogen; however, the phosphatase of rats over 500 grams, from the same litter, was very little or not at all inhibited by glycogen. This (preliminary) observation would apparently agree with the hypothesis that only a certain structure of transferase *D* phosphatase is susceptible to inhibition by glycogen.

DISCUSSION

Glycogen levels in muscle are controlled by the relative activities of transferase and phosphorylase. It has been shown by Krebs *et al.*[19] that physiological concentrations of glycogen can produce an increase in phosphorylase *a* by (1) stimulating nonactivated phosphorylase kinase, and (2) by stimulating the activation of nonactivated phosphorylase kinase. However, this mechanism can only account for the control of the degradation of glycogen. It would appear that a second mechanism–inhibition of glycogen synthesis by high levels of glycogen–would be required, or else part of the glucose 1-phosphate formed by the action of phosphorylase would be recycled to glycogen.

The inhibition of transferase *D* phosphatase by glycogen appears to be a possible feed-back control of the levels of activity of the glycogen-synthesizing enzyme, transferase. Physiological concentrations of glycogen were found to inhibit the conversion of transferase *D* into the active transferase *I*. To what extent this inhibition can be effective *in vivo* may perhaps be calculated from data presented in this paper. Transferase activity in rat skeletal muscle is equivalent to nearly 2 u/g wet weight of tissue, and the glycogen concentration varies in normal rats between 2 and 20 mg/g of wet tissue. Assuming that all the transferase is present in the *D* form, 2 mg of glycogen/g would inhibit transferase *D* phosphatase activity only to the extent of 7 to 10%; however, 20 mg of glycogen/g would result in over 80% inhibition of the phosphatase.

Furthermore, when glycogen is being actively degraded by phosphorylase, an increase in the inhibition of transferase *D* phosphatase would perhaps be produced by the formation of phosphorylase limit dextrin, or, at least, of short outer-chain types of glycogen, apparently more effective than normal glycogen as phosphatase inhibitors. An increase in size of the glycogen molecules would also result in a higher inhibition, but muscle glycogen does not appear to vary in size to any large extent.

The lability of the glycogen inhibition of muscle transferase *D* phosphatase offers several possibilities for further investigation. It would be interesting to relate muscle glycogen concentrations in animals at different stages of development with the extent of the phosphatase inhibition produced by glycogen. Glycogenosis due to a lack of control of transferase *D* phosphatase by glycogen may perhaps be found. And, finally, it has been found[20] that human muscle, after heavy, exhausting exercise can accumulate up to 50 mg of glycogen per gram, if provided with an adequate supply of carbohydrates; this extremely high glycogen concentration could perhaps be explained if the structure of the transferase *D* phosphatase molecule were altered as a result of the exercise to a form no longer inhibited by glycogen.

References

1. Villar-Palasi, C. & J. Larner. 1960. Biochem. Biophys. Acta **39:** 171.
2. Rosell-Perez, N., C. Villar-Palasi & J. Larner. 1962. Biochemistry **1:** 763.
3. Friedman, D. C. & J. Larner. 1963. Biochemistry **2:** 669.
4. Danforth, W. H. 1965. J. Biol. Chem. **240:** 588.
5. Piras, R., L. B. Rothman & E. Cabib. 1967. Biochem. Biophys. Res. Comm. **28:** 54.
6. Goldberg, N. D., C. Villar-Palasi, H. Sasko & J. Larner. 1967. Biochem. Biophys. Acta **148:** 665.
7. Villar-Palasi, C. & J. J. Wenger. 1967. Fed. Proc. **26:** 563.
8. Craig, J. W. & J. Larner. 1964. Nature (London) **202:** 971.
9. Huijing, F. & J. Larner. 1966. Proc. Nat. Acad. Sci. U.S.A. **56:** 647.
10. Villar-Palasi, C. & J. Larner. 1966. Fed. Proc. **25:** 583.
11. Villar-Palasi, C., M. Rosell-Perez, S. Hizukuri & F. Huijing & J. Larner. 1966. *In* Methods in Enzymology. E. F. Neufeld & V. Ginsburg, Eds. **8:** 374. Academic Press, Inc., New York, N. Y.
12. Cori, G. T., B. Illingworth & P. J. Keller. 1955. *In* Methods in Enzymology. S. P. Colowick & N. O. Kaplan, Eds. **1:** 200. Academic Press, Inc., New York, N. Y.
13. Thomas, J. A., K. K. Schlender & J. Larner. (In press.)
14. Kalckar, H. M. 1947. J. Biol. Chem. **167:** 461.
15. Dubois, M., K. A. Gilles, J. K. Hamilton, P. A. Rebers & F. Smith. 1956. Anal. Chem. **28:** 350.
16. Larner, J., C. Villar-Palasi, N. D. Goldberg, J. S. Bishop, F. Huijing, J. I. Wenger, H. Sasko & N. B. Brown. 1968. *In* Control of Glycogen Metabolism. 1–18, Universitetsforlaget, Oslo.
17. Cori, G. T. & C. F. Cori. 1945. J. Biol. Chem. **158:** 321.
18. Bueding, E. & S. A. Orrell. 1964. J. Biol. Chem. **239:** 4018.
19. Krebs, E. G., D. S. Love, G. E. Bratvold, K. A. Trayser, W. L. Meyer & E. H. Fischer. 1964. Biochemistry **3:** 1022
20. Hultman, E. 1967. Circ. Res. Suppl. to **20, 21:** 99.

Discussion of the Paper

C. de Duve: I think it is an extraordinary, fascinating combination. You are inhibiting one enzyme by adding the substrate of the substrate of this enzyme—because glycogen is a substrate for the transferase, which is a substrate for the enzyme you inhibit. And so I wonder can you explain the kinetics of this phenomena by removing the binding of the substrate, which is your transferase, by the inhibitor, which is glycogen, the inhibition being the simple removal of the substrate?

Dr. Villar-Palasi: Yes, we have thought of that—or even something perhaps a little more involved—which is the following: that the inhibitor was a complex molecule consisting of transferase *I* bound to glycogen, this possibly being a competitive inhibitor of the free transferase.

I think we can rule this out because the inhibition disappears with aging, but the complex doesn't disappear. We have transferase, we have glycogen; why should not the same compound transferase and glycogen be formed when the phosphatase is aged or when the phosphatase is obtained from old animals? If it is a substrate inhibitor complex, you have the added components exactly the same, and therefore you would have the same inhibitor.

B. L. Horecker: Don't you have more particulate glycogen in old animals? You showed this to be a very powerful inhibitor.

Dr. Villar-Palasi: No, or yes, whatever you want. The whole thing is that in muscle the glycogen is of relatively low and constant molecular weight, no matter what the age is. So you may have more glycogen, but no more particulate glycogen or no larger species of glycogen.

Dr. de Duve: Is there any influence of age on the Michaelis constant of the transferase *I* phosphatase for glycogen? If the affinity of the enzyme for glycogen is decreased with age, then you could explain the lack of inhibition.

Dr. Villar-Palasi: We added large amounts of glycogen up to 100 miligrams, and it did not inhibit. Therefore, if the K*m* has increased, then it has increased very much.

SUMMATION OF THE SESSION ON BIOCHEMISTRY

Bernard L. Horecker

Albert Einstein College of Medicine,
Bronx, N. Y.

I have been particularly intrigued by a number of things that have developed in these discussions.

One aspect I found most interesting was the suggestion that possibly some enzyme variants may be interchangeable. Apparently, this may be true even of genetic variants, and we may have to revise our notions about the role of genetics in the production of these modified proteins. The brief comments of Dr. Bachhawat were particularly pertinent. It is apparent that a glycoprotein can be modified genetically without changing any of the amino acids in the primary structure. Thus while there are genetic effects that cause changes in the genetic code, resulting in substitutions of amino acids, there may also be genetic changes such as we see in the blood-group substances, where polysaccharide side chains would be different. These would also be expressed as genetic variants.

It is also apparent that we must be very cautious about the use of terms such as alkaline and acid phosphatases. This property may be related not necessarily to the enzyme or its physiological function, but to the particular substrate used to assay its activities. Dr. Moss showed us that the "alkaline" phosphatase he was studying was not an alkaline phophatase if you considered its pyrophosphatase activity. This reminded me of the work with our own enzyme, the fructose diphosphatase, which would also be classified as an alkaline phosphatase, except that such is probably not the case *in vivo*.

Turning to the latter parts of the session, we've seen some very exciting and fascinating studies on the mechanism of action and the regulation of these phosphatases. We have two beautiful examples of assays in which probes could be used to define the catalytic site and the catalytic mechanism. Dr. Nath illustrated this by changing the substrates permitting him to make some deductions about the nature of the catalytic site. On the other hand, it was demonstrated by Dr. Simpson's presentation that this can by no means be developed as a generalized method, because, in the case of the *E. coli* alkaline phosphatase, one can make any change one pleases in the substrate without affecting the catalytic activity. And in that case, it was necessary to use a different kind of probe, changing the metal in order to gain some information about the nature of the mechanism and the catalytic site.

In the discussions of phosphatases, it has been rather common to conclude that the metals that we frequently find as cofactors for these phosphatases are involved in the binding of the substrate at the catlytic site. The paper by Dr. Simpson showed very clearly that in *E. coli* alkaline phosphatase, this might be true for half of the metal associated with the protein, but the remainder was involved in maintaining the three-dimensional structure of the protein. This seems to be true also for the fructose diphosphatase, where the substrate can be bound in the absence of the divalent cation, and where the divalent cation can be shown to be specifically required for hydrolysis of the substrate, not for binding. The reports published earlier suggesting that the presence of the metal changed the affinity of this enzyme for AMP, the allosteric effector, can be explained in terms of the formation of an Mg^{++}–AMP complex.

With respect to the possible function of phosphatases, we have seen a number of examples that suggest that a phosphatase may have some other function. Dr.

Moss described a new type of activity for his enzyme. Dr. Nordlie has suggested that glucose-6-phosphatase may actually have a more important role as an enzyme for the phosphorylation of glucose rather than for its dephosphorylation.

We have, I believe, entered a completely new area of phosphatases when we consider specific phosphatases that are involved in the removal of phosphate groups from proteins, involved directly in the regulation of the activity of these proteins. Phosphorylase has been an example of this, and now we have seen a similar kind of control in the case of the glycogen synthetase. This has also been suggested for a number of other enzymes; fructose diphosphatase has been reported to react with ATP to form an inactive phosphorylated protein. That remains to be confirmed, but it may be that here, too, we may have a protein phosphorylation and dephosphorylation as a control mechanism.

It is evident that the biochemistry will advance very rapidly once the enzymes are available in soluble, and it is to be hoped, eventually in pure form. The difficult step that must be taken in the case of many of the membrane-bound phosphatases is, somehow, to get them off in water-soluble form. Here, nature may have pointed the way. If we can attach sugars to make these enzymes water-soluble, then we may be able to study their activity and to purify them without necessarily having them membrane-associated.

I would like to thank all the speakers today for their excellent presentations.

PART V. CLINICAL ENZYMOLOGY

PLACENTAL ALKALINE PHOSPHATASE AND PREGNANCY*

Solomon Posen, Coralie J. Cornish, Michael Horne and Parmesh K. Saini

Departments of Medicine and Biochemistry, University of Sydney, Sydney, Australia

Human placental alkaline phosphatase† resembles other mammalian alkaline phosphatases by its close association with the surface membrane of epithelial cells. The maternal surfaces of the syncytiotrophoblastic cells are especially rich in alkaline phosphatase,[3] and there is reason to believe that placental microvilli project into the maternal uterine sinusoids in much the same fashion as intestinal microvilli project into the intestinal lumen. Some particulate trophoblastic material is shed into the maternal circulation[4] in the same way as particulate matter from the intestinal wall is desquamated into the gut lumen.[5]

The structure of human placental alkaline phosphatase was studied by Harkness, who concluded that human placental alkaline phosphatase has a molecular weight of approximately 125,000,[6] and that, like other alkaline phosphatases, it is a zinc metalloenzyme.

As yet, no physiological function has been established for placental, or indeed for any other, mammalian alkaline phosphatase. The assumption that this group of enzymes is somehow connected with active transport rests on their location within the cell, on their ability to bind inorganic phosphate,[7] and on evidence obtained with bacterial alkaline phosphatases.[8] Placental alkaline phosphatase injected into human subjects has no measurable effect on the metabolism of the recipients,[9] and L-phenylalanine a known inhibitor of intestinal alkaline phosphatase is without effect on the absorption of glucose or inorganic phosphate from the everted gut loop.[10]

Placental alkaline phosphatase shares with nonplacental alkaline phosphatases the ability to hydrolyze a large number of substrates,[11,12] including inorganic pyrophosphate[13] and 4-methylumbelliferyl phosphate.[14] Harkness,[12] who determined the rates of hydrolysis of a number of substrates at the same substrate concentration in the same buffer, at the same buffer strength, and at the same pH found that, mole for mole, slightly more beta-glycerophosphate than para-nitrophenylphosphate was hydrolyzed per unit of time by placental alkaline phosphatase.

Human placental alkaline phosphatase differs from nonplacental alkaline phosphatases[15] by its remarkable resistance to heat denaturation (TABLE 1). Some of this heat stability is lost during butanol extraction, acetone precipitation and dialysis (TABLE 2) but even crystalline human placental alkaline phosphatase has been shown to be relatively heat resistant.[12] The heat resistance of human placental alkaline phosphatase appears to be species-specific. All nonhuman placental alkaline phosphatases examined so far have been denatured to varying degrees at 56° C. (TABLE 3).

Heat stability is accompanied by a resistance to denaturation during pre-incubation with urea.[16,17] Human placental alkaline phosphatase may be pre-

* This work was supported by the National Health and Medical Research Council of Australia, the N.S.W. State Cancer Council and the Post-Graduate Medical Foundation, University of Sydney.

† Throughout this paper, placental alkaline phosphatase will be treated as if it were a single enzyme. There is, as yet, no evidence that the various placental isoenzymes[1,2] differ from one another in any parameter other than their electrophoretic migration.

TABLE 1
MEAN ALKALINE PHOSPHATASE ACTIVITIES OF HUMAN TISSUE EXTRACTS AFTER 15 MINUTES' PREINCUBATION AT 56° C*

Tissue	No. of Specimens	Mean Initial Activity (K.A. Units/ g Wet Wt.)	Mean Percentage Activity Remaining	Range of Percentage Activities Remaining
Bone	5	3.4	11.6	3.6– 28.2
Liver	4	0.6	16.4	8.0– 24.8
Intestine	8	15.2	31.9	17.3– 56.6
Placenta	8	19.3	100	92.2–105.4

* The tissues were homogenized with approximately twice their volume of 0.01 M Tris-HCl at pH 7.4. The extracts were filtered, and the filtrates were suitably diluted with Tris HCl buffer to bring their alkaline phosphatase activities within the range of the recording apparatus. Enzyme assay was performed by an automated phenylphosphate method[29] before and after each specimen had been heated at 56° for 15 minutes.

TABLE 2
EFFECT OF BUTANOL EXTRACTION, ACETONE PRECIPITATION AND DIALYSIS AGAINST DISTILLED WATER FOR 48 HOURS[17] ON THE HEAT STABILITY OF ALKALINE PHOSPHATASE FROM VARIOUS HUMAN TISSUES*

Tissue	Mean and Ranges of Percentage of Activities Remaining After 15 Min Preincubation at 56° C.	
	Crude Aqueous Extracts	Purified Extracts
Bone	11.6 (3.6– 28.2)	10.6 (5.0–14.8)
Liver	16.4 (8.0– 24.8)	20.9 (8.3–32.8)
Intestine	31.9 (17.3– 56.6)	89.9 (82.4–95.2)
Placenta	100.0 (92.2–105.4)	87.2 (80.0–97.7)

* The increase in the heat stability of intestinal alkaline phosphatase is believed to be due to the loss of heat labile material during purification.

incubated in 7 M urea at 37° for 30 minutes, by the end of which time only 10% of the original activity has disappeared. Skeletal alkaline phosphatase, preincubated with this concentration of urea at this temperature, has a half life of less than one minute. (This time-dependent, irreversible denaturation with urea must not be confused with the instantaneous, reversible, noncompetitive inhibition seen when urea is incorporated in the assay system. This inhibition is found with all alkaline phosphatases examined.[16])

Heat stability and urea stability are accompanied by a relative resistance to acid inactivation.[18] Human placental alkaline phosphatase may be preincubated at pH 4.0 at 37° for 30 minutes with only 35% loss of activity. Human skeletal alkaline phosphatase, under similar circumstances, loses 74% of its original activity.

Preincubation with ethylenediaminetetraacetic acid (EDTA) leads to a loss of enzyme activity in all alkaline phosphatases.[19] This loss is time-dependent and only partially reversible with divalent cations or substrates. Placental alkaline phosphatase is more resistant to preincubation with EDTA than the other alkaline phosphatases, so that its half-life at a given EDTA concentration is very much longer than that of skeletal alkaline phosphatases under similar conditions. The effect of EDTA on human placental alkaline phosphatase in the presence of substrate depends on the substrate concentration. At low substrate concentrations, there is a time-dependent fall in enzyme activity.[12] In the presence of excess substrate, EDTA in concentrations of up to 10^{-1}M causes a 20% enhancement of placental alkaline phosphatase activity.[19]

In all these respects, placental alkaline phosphatase is more resistant to physical and chemical denaturation than other alkaline phosphatases. The nature of the intramolecular forces responsible for this resistance is at present unknown.

The resistance to denaturation by physical and chemical agents is associated with a relative "resistance" to enzymatic activity. Placental alkaline phosphatase requires and tolerates a more "unnatural" pH for optimum activity than other alkaline phosphatases assayed with the same substrate and at the same substrate concentrations.[20] Placental alkaline phosphatase has a "worse" (i.e., a higher) K_m than other alkaline phosphatases assayed at a similar pH with the same substrate, the same buffer, and at the same buffer concentration.[16,20] Placental alkaline phosphatase, like intestinal alkaline phosphatase, is inhibited by L-phenylalanine in the assay system[17,20] at concentrations that leave the more unstable alkaline phosphatases relatively unaffected.

Placental alkaline phosphatase also differs from other human alkaline phosphatases in its magnesium requirements. When skeletal alkaline phosphatase (obtained from fetal ribs, femurs and tibias) is extracted with butanol, precipitated with acetone, dialyzed against distilled water for 48 hours[17] and assayed for enzymatic activity in a system containing low substrate concentrations, the time courses of the enzymatic reaction are not linear (FIGURE 1). Moreover, if

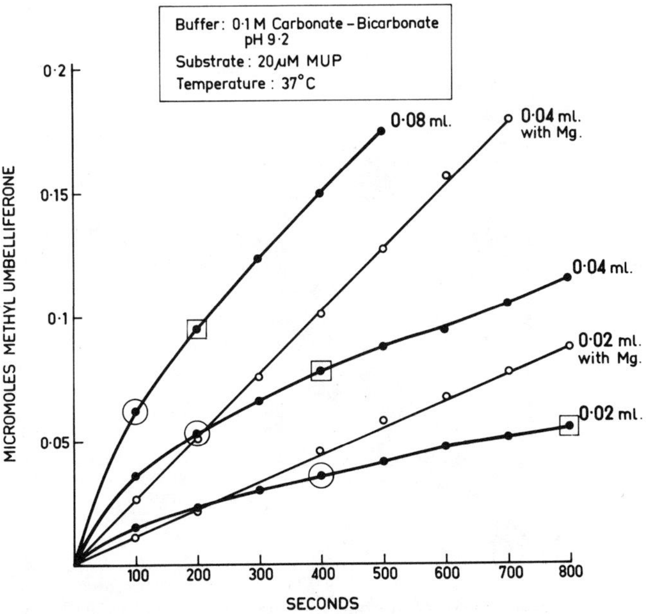

FIGURE 1. The nonlinear time course of skeletal alkaline phosphatase when enzyme activity is assayed at low substrate concentrations. If this nonlinearity were due to substrate depletion or product inhibition, the three points marked with circles and the three points marked with squares should lie on straight lines parallel to the horizontal axis. The fact that they do not, suggests enzyme denaturation during assay.[21] Magnesium (10^{-4} M) linearizes the time courses for skeletal alkaline phosphatase. Plecental alkaline phosphatase, in this system, displays linear time courses even in the absence of added magnesium.

several enzyme concentrations are used, the reaction product is not constant for a constant time × enzyme concentration product,[21] suggesting enzyme denaturation during assay. Magnesium in the assay system linearizes the time courses, presumably by protecting the enzyme against denaturation. Placental alkaline phosphatase treated in the same manner and assayed in the same system shows linear time courses regardless of the presence of added magnesium.

The electrophoretic migration of placental alkaline phosphatase has been intensively studied since Boyer's initial publication, which demonstrated the heterogeneity of human placental alkaline phosphatases on starch gel.[1] A multiplicity of placental alkaline phosphatase bands has been described by Robson and Harris,[22] Beckman *et al.*[23] and Blake *et al.*,[24] who all used slightly different electrophoretic techniques and studied different populations. Ghosh and Fishman,[25] who used pooled placentas, found only two electrophoretic zones in their purified preparation. These two zones were thought to contain alkaline phosphatases of different molecular weights, the slow-moving material with its high molecular weight representing a polymer of the more rapidly moving material with the lower molecular weight. Harkness,[6] who used a large number of placentas, as his starting material, found that his crystalline enzyme migrated in a single electrophoretic band on polyacrylamide gel.

On cellulose acetate, human placental alkaline phosphatase migrates as a single band, just cathodally to the alpha$_2$ globulin fraction. This rate of migration is somewhat slower than that of bone alkaline phosphatase, but considerably

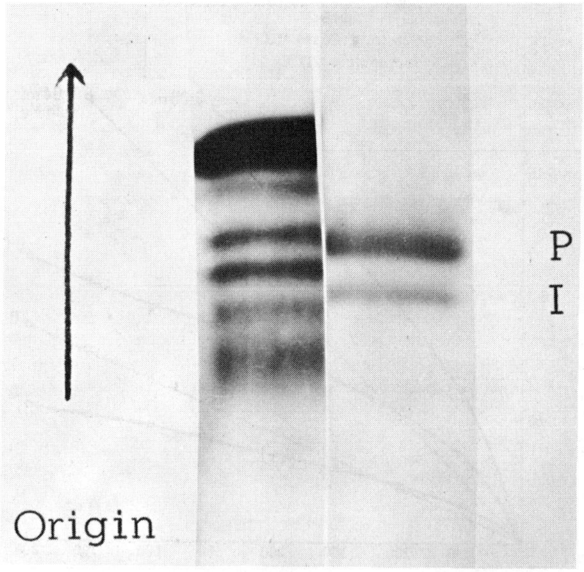

FIGURE 2. Electrophoresis of normal, nonpregnant serum to which placental (P) and intestinal (I) alkaline phosphatase had been added. A faint area of activity may be seen anodal to the placental band. This area is seen in all sera. The supporting medium was "Cellogel" (Chemetron, Milan, Italy), the buffer was 0.375 M Tris-HCl at pH 8.8, and a constant current of 30 ma was applied at room temperature for three hours. The plasma proteins are on the left of the photograph, the phosphatases are on the right. Maternal serum contains an alkaline phosphatase that migrates in the same position as placental alkaline phosphatase added *in vitro*.[29]

TABLE 3

THERMAL INACTIVATION OF NONHUMAN PLACENTAL ALKALINE PHOSPHATASES (30 MINUTES AT 56° C.)

Species	No. of Animals (Mothers)	Mean Initial Activity (K.A. Units/ g wet wt.)	Mean Residual Activity (K.A. Units/ g wet wt.)
Rat	3	11.7	0.15
Mouse	3	16.6	0.19
Guinea Pig	3	11.5	0.32
Rabbit	3	10.8	0.41
Sheep	1	16.9	1.03
Horse (Uterus)	1	9.3	0.09
Horse (Chorion)	1	0.2	0.03

more rapid than that of intestinal alkaline phosphatase. (FIGURE 2). Preincubation with bacterial neuraminidase causes placental alkaline phosphatase to migrate more cathodally, both on cellulose acetate[26] and on starch gel.[22]

Alkaline phosphatase in the maternal circulation in the later stages of pregnancy resembles placental alkaline phosphatase in a number of ways. It is resistant to heat denaturation.[27] The heat-resistant moiety in pregnancy sera is precipitated by an antihuman placental alkaline phosphatase antibody (FIGURE 3), which is without effect on sera from nonpregnant individuals.[28] The heat-

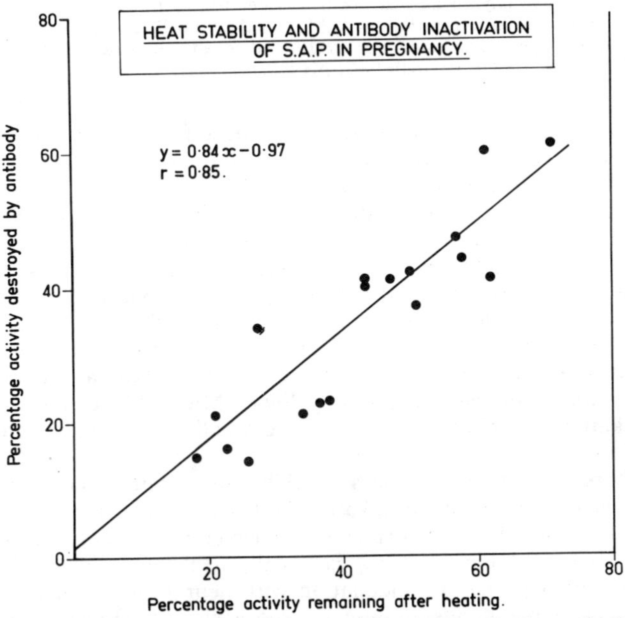

FIGURE 3. The correlation between the heat stability and antibody sensitivity of alkaline phosphatase activity in 18 maternal sera in the last month of pregnancy. The horizontal axis shows the heat stability, expressed as the percentage activity remaining after 30 minutes' preheating at 56° C. The vertical axis shows the percentage enzyme activity lost during 96 hours' preincubation with antihuman placental alkaline phosphatase antibody. The greater the proportion of heat stable alkaline phosphatase in maternal serum, the greater the proportion of alkaline phosphatase precipitated by antihuman placental alkaline phosphatase antibody.[28]

resistant fraction is inhibited by L-phenylalanine to the same extent as the placental enzyme.[17]

The heat-resistant fraction of the maternal serum alkaline phosphatase is also resistant to urea denaturation.[17] This heat-stable, urea-stable fraction disappears from the maternal circulation after confinement at a rate similar to that of placental alkaline phosphatase after infusion into nonpregnant subjects.[9] Prolonged dialysis of the heat-stable alkaline phosphatase fraction in maternal sera against distilled water causes no loss in enzyme activity, even when substrate concentrations of 2 μM of methylumbelliferyl phosphate is used in the assay system. Nonpregnant sera, when similarly dialyzed, lose up to 60% of their activity unless the assay system contains magnesium or greater concentrations of substrate (TABLE 4).

TABLE 4

EFFECT OF MAGNESIUM OF ALKALINE PHOSPHATASE ACTIVITIES OF DIALYZED SERA*

Source of Serum	Alkaline Phosphatase Activity (Percentage Activity of Undialyzed Serum)		
	No Mg	6×10^{-5} M Mg	3×10^{-4} M Mg
Normal Subject	12.5	250	300
Patient with Pagets Disease	22.5	124	163
Patient with Cholestasis	41.9	158	184
Pregnant Subject (Serum Preheated)	320	320	320

* Representative sera dialyzed against distilled water for 72 hours and assayed for enzyme activity at low substrate concentrations (2 μM 4-methylumbelliferyl phosphate) at different magnesium concentrations. The assay was performed in an automated fluorometric system[14] in ammediol-HCl buffer, ionic strength 0.02, pH 9.0.

The K_m of the heat-stable alkaline phosphatase fraction in the circulation of pregnant women resembles that of placental alkaline phosphatase (0.033 mM phenylphosphate) when the assay is performed in 0.05 Tris-HCl buffer at pH 9.0 in the absence of added magnesium. The determination of Michaelis constants for the identification of the tissue sources of other circulating alkaline phosphatase is fraught with difficulties because of the different magnesium requirements of non-placental alkaline phosphatases at different substrate concentrations. If no magnesium is used, Lineweaver-Burk plots are obtained that are concave upwards because of the loss of activity by nonpregnancy sera at low substrate concentrations. If magnesium is used in the assay system, nonplacental alkaline phosphatases in the circulation have apparently lower Michaelis constants than either placental alkaline phosphatase or heat-stable alkaline phosphatase in the maternal circulation.

Electrophoresis of pregnancy sera on cellulose acetate shows a characteristic band cathodal to normal serum alkaline phosphatase and in the same position as purified placental alkaline phosphatase subjected to the same treatment.[29] This band, which is heat-stable, migrates cathodally to the heat labile alkaline phosphatase in pregnancy sera. Preincubation with neuraminidase causes both heat-labile and heat-stable bands to migrate more slowly. However, they change position during this process, so that after neuraminidase incubation, the heat-stable band is cathodal to the heat-labile fraction.[26]

In all these respects, maternal serum alkaline phosphatase resembles placental alkaline phosphatase. Alkaline phosphatase in cord serum displays none of the placental characteristics (TABLE 5).

TABLE 5

SOME CHARACTERISTICS OF ALKALINE PHOSPHATASE OBTAINED FROM HUMAN PLACENTAS, MATERNAL SERA AND FETAL SERA

Procedures	Placenta	Maternal Serum	Fetal Serum
Heat[27]	Stable	Stable	Unstable
Urea[16,17]	Stable	Stable	Unstable
EDTA[19,29]	Stable	Stable	Unstable
Phenylalanine[17]	Inhibited	Inhibited	Not Inhibited
Biological Half-Life[9,29]	7 Days	7 Days	Not Known
Antiplacental Alkaline Phosphatase Antibody[28]	Precipitated	Precipitated	Not Affected
Mg at Low Substrate Concentrations[14]	No Effect	No Effect	Enhances Activity

Conclusions

Two conclusions arise out of this work–one speculative, the other of practical importance. The resistance of alkaline phosphatase to denaturation, and its relative resistance to enzymatic activity, are best explained by an extension of Fernley and Walker's[30] postulate that alkaline phosphatases exist in several conformational states. The "natural" state is stable but enzymatically inactive, possibly because of the inability of the phosphatases in this state to release inorganic phosphate. The second conformational state (with which the first is in equilibrium) is enzymatically active but, while in this state, the enzyme is liable to undergo a time-dependent, irreversible denaturation, possibly by dissociating into monomers. The most diverse substances (substrates, competitive inhibitors or divalent cations) may prevent the assumption of the second conformational state and thereby act as enzyme inhibitors. These same substances are liable to prevent denaturation of the enzyme before or during the enzymatic reaction. Placental alkaline phosphatase, more stable than other alkaline phosphatases, is less likely to assume the active conformational state, and therefore has a higher K_m, a higher pH optimum, and a smaller magnesium requirement than other alkaline phosphatases.

The practical conclusion lies in the evidence that serum alkaline phosphatase elevation in pregnancy is due to placental alkaline phosphatase in the maternal circulation. Statements regarding serum alkaline phosphatase in pregnant subjects are not very meaningful unless this fact is taken into account.

When the heat-stable moiety is subtracted from the total alkaline phosphatase activity of the serum of women in the third trimester of pregnancy, the calculated, "nonplacental" activity (mean $= 9.5 \pm 2.3$ K.A. units per 100 ml) is still significantly higher than that of nonpregnant women (mean $= 7.0 \pm 1.6$ K.A. units per 100 ml.[29]) This elevation may be due to impaired hepatic function in the third trimester of pregnancy in some women, though no qualitative studies of the heat-labile alkaline phosphatase fraction in the serum of pregnant women have as yet appeared in the literature.

Summary

Human placental alkaline phosphatase differs from other human alkaline phosphatases in a number of respects. The placental enzyme is more resistant to denaturation by physical or chemical agents. It is relatively resistant to preincubation with high concentrations of ethylenediaminetetraacetic acid. It has its own immunological characteristics. Its K_m for various substrates is higher than the K_m of other human alkaline phosphatases tested with the same substrates under similar conditions. It requires no magnesium for linear time-courses at low substrate concentrations.

On cellulose acetate, placental alkaline phosphatase travels more anodally than intestinal alkaline phosphatase, though not as anodally as skeletal and hepatic phosphatases. Placental alkaline phosphatase, like intestinal alkaline phosphatase, is inhibited by L-phenylalanine in the assay system. Unlike intestinal alkaline phosphatase, placental alkaline phosphatase is slowed in its electrophoretic migration on starch gel and cellulose acetate by preincubation with neuraminidase.

Alkaline phosphatase in the maternal circulation in the last three months of pregnancy resembles placental alkaline phosphatase in all these respects. In addition, alkaline phosphatase disappears from the maternal circulation after confinement at the same rate as injected alkaline phosphatase disappears from the circulation of nonpregnant subjects. Alkaline phosphatase in the fetal circulation shares none of the characteristics of placental alkaline phosphatase. It is concluded that placental alkaline phosphatase enters the maternal, but not the fetal, circulation.

The biological function of placental alkaline phosphatase is unknown. This function is believed to be unrelated to the hydrolysis of phosphate esters at pH 10.6.

Acknowledgment

The interest of Drs. F. C. Neale and W. J. O'Sullivan is gratefully acknowledged. Miss Dilys Ward gave valuable secretarial assistance.

References

1. Boyer, S. H. 1961. Alkaline phosphatase in human sera and placentae. Science **134:** 1002–1004.
2. Robson, E. B. & H. Harris. 1965. Genetics of the alkaline phosphatase polymorphism of the human placenta. Nature (London) **207:** 1257–1259.
3. Wachstein, M., J. G. Meagher & J. Ortiz. 1963. Enzymatic histochemistry of the term human placenta. Amer. J. Obstet. Gynec. **87:** 13–26.
4. Attwood, H. D. & W. W. Park. 1961. Embolism to the lungs by trophoblast. J. Obstet. Gynaec. Brit. Comm. **68:** 611–617.
5. Bertalanffy, F. D. 1962. Cell renewal in the gastrointestinal tract of man. Gastroenterology **43:** 472–475.
6. Harkness, D. R. 1968. Studies on human placental alkaline phosphatase. 1. Purification and crystallization. Arch. Biochem. **126:** 503–512.
7. Engstrom, L. 1961. Studies on calf-intestinal alkaline phosphatase. 2. Incorporation of inorganic phosphate into a highly purified enzyme preparation. Biochim. Biophys. Acta **52:** 49–59.
8. Torriani, A. 1960. Influence of inorganic phosphate on the formation of phosphatases by *Escherichia coli*. Biochim. Biophys. Acta **38:** 460–469.
9. Clubb, J. S., F. C. Neale & S. Posen. 1965. The behavior of infused placental alkaline phosphatase in human subjects. J. Lab. Clin. Med. **66:** 493–507.
10. Saini, P. K., M. Horne & S. Posen. 1968. (Unpublished.)
11. Ahmed, Z. & E. J. King. 1960. Kinetics of placental alkaline phosphatase. Biochim. Biophys. Acta **45:** 581–592.
12. Harkness, D. R. 1968. Studies on human placental alkaline phosphatase 2. Kinetic properties and studies on the apoenzyme. Arch. Biochem. **126:** 513–523.
13. Sussman, H. H. & E. Laga. 1968. Inorganic pyrophosphatase activity of human placental alkaline phosphatase. Biochim. Biophys. Acta **151:** 281–283.
14. C. J. Cornish, F. C. Neale & S. Posen. 1969. An automated alkaline phosphatase micro-assay with 4-methyl-umbelliferyl phosphate as a substrate. (Submitted for publication.)
15. Neale, F. C., J. S. Clubb, D. Hotchkis & S. Posen. 1965. The heat stability of human placental alkaline phosphatase. J. Clin. Path. **18:** 359–363.

16. Birkett, D. J., R. A. J. Conyers, F. C. Neale, S. Posen & J. Brudenell-Woods. 1967. Action of urea on human alkaline phosphatases: with a description of some automated techniques for the study of enzyme kinetics. Arch. Biochem. **121:** 470–479.
17. Horne, M., C. J. Cornish & S. Posen. 1968. The use of urea denaturation in the identification of human alkaline phosphatases. J. Lab. Clin. Med. **72:** 905–915.
18. Posen, S., D. J. Birkett, R. A. J. Conyers, C. J. Cornish & F. C. Neale. 1968. Automated methods in the study of enzyme kinetics. *In* Automation in Analytical Chemistry : 583–585. Mediaid Inc., White Plains, N. Y.
19. Conyers, R. A. J., D. J. Birkett, F. C. Neale, S. Posen & J. Brudenell-Woods. 1967. The action of EDTA on human alkaline phosphatases. Biochim. Biophys. Acta **139:** 363–371.
20. Fishman, W. H. & N. K. Ghosh. 1967. Isoenzymes of human alkaline phosphatase. Advances Clin. Chem. **10:** 255–370.
21. Selwyn, M. J. 1965. A simple test for inactivation of an enzyme during assay. Biochim. Biophys. Acta **105:** 193–195.
22. Robson, E. B. & H. Harris. 1967. Further studies on the genetics of placental alkaline phosphatase. Ann. Hum. Genet. (Lond.) **30:** 219–232.
23. Beckman, L., G. Beckman, C. Christodoulou & A. Ifekwunigwe. 1967. Variations in human placental alkaline phosphatase. Acta Genet. (Basel) **17:** 406–412.
24. Blake, N. M., R. L. Kirk & V. Osathanondh. 1968. Placental alkaline phosphatase types in Thailand. Med. J. Aust. **2:** 1042–1045.
25. Ghosh, N. K. & W. H. Fishman. 1967. Characterization of human placental alkaline phosphatase isozymes. Fed. Proc. **26:** 558.
26. Posen S. 1966. Studies in human alkaline phosphatases. M.D. Thesis (p. 173 and 178). University of Adelaide, Australia.
27. McMaster, Y., R. Tennant, J. S. Clubb, F. C. Neale & S. Posen. 1964. The mechanism of the elevation of serum alkaline phosphatase in pregnancy. J. Obstet. Gynaec. Brit. Comm. **71:** 735–739.
28. Birkett, D. J., J. Done, F. C. Neale & S. Posen. 1966. Serum alkaline phosphatase in pregnancy: An immunological study. Brit. Med. J. **1:** 1210–1212.
29. Kitchener, P. N., F. C. Neale, S. Posen & J. Brudenell-Woods. 1965. Alkaline phosphatase in maternal and fetal sera at term and during the puerperium. Amer. J. Clin. Path. **44:** 654–661.
30. Fernley, H. N. & P. G. Walker. 1967. Studies on alkaline phosphatase. Inhibition by phosphate derivatives and the substrate specificity. Biochem. J. **104:** 1011–1018.

Discussion of the Paper

W. H. Fishman: The results of our own work supports the conclusion of Dr. Posen's and of earlier workers, that placental alkaline phosphatase progressively enriches the blood with the advance of pregnancy.

Together with Dr. Bardawil at St. Margaret's Hospital, we have studied 125 consecutive pregnancies, 76 of which were considered normal in every respect. The definition of the placental isoenzyme unit follows: 1 unit equals 1 milligram of phenol liberated from 72 mM phenylphosphate in the presence of bicarbonate buffer at pH 10.7 per 100 millimeter of serum, an aliquot of which had been heated previously in a water bath for 60 minutes at 55° C.

Figure 1 represents a composite curve of the 76 normal pregnancies in which serum placental isoenzyme units are plotted against weeks of pregnancies. You will notice that the term value of 40 units shows a wide variation. A good deal of this variation can be explained by the parity and blood type of the mother. As a rule, primipara shows a higher term value, whereas multipara often exhibit a prepartum fall in the serum value. Term values were higher in women with blood type A as compared to B, O and AB. This difference can be traced to the placental output of isoenzyme.

The exponential nature of the curve permits one to extrapolate the values at midterm to the expected term value, and may thereby provide an independent basis for predicting the day of delivery.

In figure 2, three observed values (black circles) provide the basis for extrap-

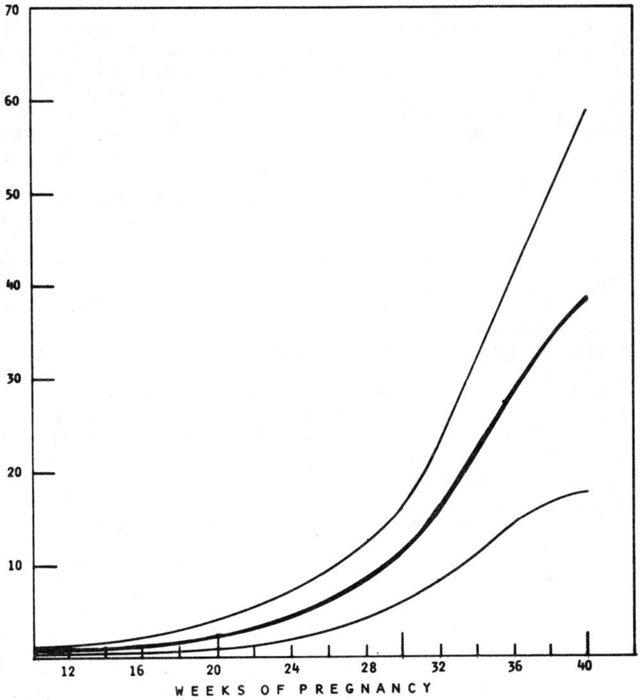

FIGURE 1.

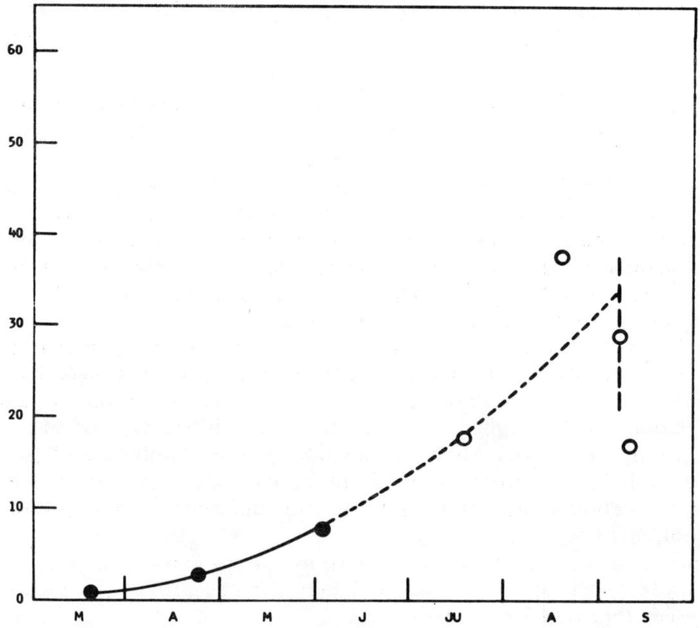

FIGURE 2.

olating the slope of the curve to a term level. The later observations (open circles) indicate a prepartum fall, but the dotted vertical line was the delivery day.

Finally, a case of a diabetic pregnancy terminating in a stillborn is illustrated in FIGURE 3. The placental isoenzyme values fell below the expected curve.

Thus it appears that a simple automated biochemical measurement can provide an exact titer of the placental alkaline phosphatase.

O. BODANSKY: Thank you very much. Are there any other questions for Dr. Posen?

L. BECKMAN: In all these exercises, in an attempt to identify the component in serum with that of the placenta, I think we should not forget the work by Dr. Boyer in 1961, which showed that electrophoretic patterns in extracts of placenta always agreed with those in serum. We confirm that in 300 cases. This is another way of attacking the problem.

I think it is interesting to understand the relationship between blood type in the child and the blood type of the mother. Because everything so far found in the placenta is controlled by the genotype of the child, you might expect to have some relation of the serum alkaline phosphatase in pregnancy to the blood type of the child rather than to that of the mother.

O. BODANSKY: Dr. Posen, could we save these questions? Dr. Schwartz, you had a question.

M. K. SCHWARTZ: What was the source of the bone enzyme?

DR. BODANSKY: Are there any other questions, maybe you could answer them all at once. Yes?

M. ETZLER: I should like to ask Dr. Posen how he can account for the changing places of the intestinal and placental isoenzymes in treatment with neuraminidase.

DR. BODANSKY: Any other questions? Then we'll have Dr. Posen answer the two questions that were asked of him and then Dr. Fishman can answer the question directed to him.

DR. POSEN: First of all, in answer to Dr. Fishman's remarks, we have not investigated the babies' blood groups. In relation to the maternal blood groups, we were unable to show a difference, between group O and group A individuals. We couldn't convince ourselves there was a significant relationship between the maternal blood groups, the parity of the mother, the type of delivery or the sex of the infant, and the amount of phosphatase circulating.

However, I must state we've only done a fifth of the number that Dr. Fishman and his group have investigated.

In relation to Dr. Beckman's question, certainly Boyer showed that alkaline phosphatase in the maternal circulation resembled placental phosphatase in this particular respect. You seem to be the only one who's been able to reproduce the placental phenotypes in the maternal circulation, because other people, including Dr. Harris in London, were able to confirm this work.

The source of our bone enzyme was fetal bone, Dr. Schwartz, largely from premature infants. We ground up femurs, tibias and ribs. We have not been able to use adult bone because our yield has been very low, nor have we been able to purify bone phosphatase sufficiently to inject into animals to make an antibody, because as we start purifying it, we lose activity. So that after some days of dialysis there is almost no activity in bone phosphatase.

Dr. Etzler's question was, why do intestinal and placental alkaline phosphatases change place after neuranindase treatment. I don't know the answer. Dr. Fishman has considered that the sialic acid content of the placental enzyme is higher than

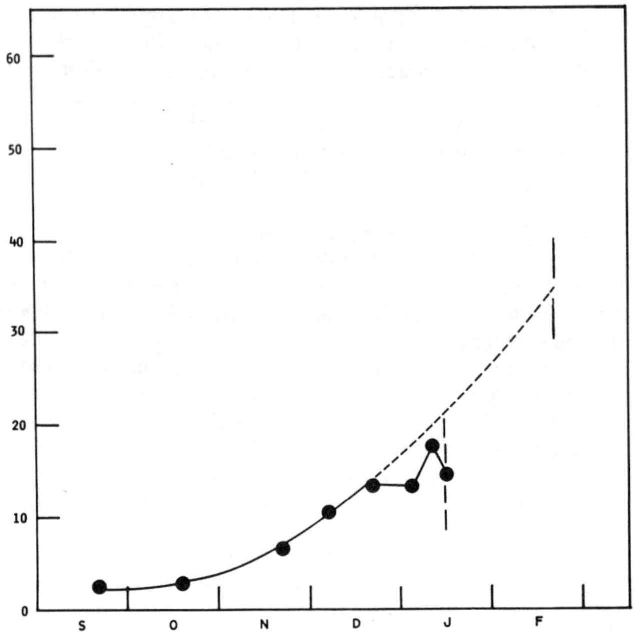

that of intestinal alkaline phosphatase. This may, of course, be due to the fact that what sialic acid there is in intestinal alkaline phosphatase, has previously been removed, as was suggested in one of the former presentations.

DR. ETZLER: Do I understand you correctly, then as saying that because these intestinal and placental isozymes change places, the mobility of the intestinal enzyme should increase. I don't understand how you could account for this.

DR. POSEN: No, the intestinal material doesn't advance, but the placental phosphatase is closer to the origin. The mobility of intestinal alkaline phosphatase doesn't change.

DR. FISHMAN: In answer to Dr. Beckman, the blood type of the infant could be ascertained in our series so far only in those infants that were products of RH difficulty. In this small number of cases, the infants with blood type O correlated with the lowest output of placental alkaline phosphatase. And together with Dr. Bardawil, we are collecting the desired information on fetal blood type.

IMMUNOLOGIC AND BIOCHEMICAL APPROACHES TO ALKALINE PHOSPHATASE ISOENZYME ANALYSIS: THE REGAN ISOENZYME*

William H. Fishman

Tufts University School of Medicine
and the
New England Medical Center Hospitals
Boston, Mass.

Introduction

Our approach to the study of isoenzymes of alkaline phosphatase has been to develop an understanding of their organ-specific differences based on biochemical characteristics and immunologic properties. These properties, in turn, provide useful analytical tools for evaluating the mixture of isoenzymes that are found in the serum and for identifying the organ source of individual zones on gel electrophoresis. We have adopted for the present a working definition of an isoenzyme, i.e., a catalytically-active protein that is biochemically distinguishable from other proteins of the same enzyme species whether or not it has the same or different electrophoretic variants. Thus, we can deal with the confusion of molecular variants that these isoenzymes may have by using biochemical and immunologic reagents that have an organ specificity in automated analytical systems and by starch gel electrophoresis.

Brief reference is made here to advances in our knowledge of certain organ-associated isoenzymes in which this laboratory, along with others around the world, has participated. Thus, there is the contribution of intestinal alkaline phosphatase to the circulating blood, its recognition by means of L-phenylalanine inhibition[1-4] and its association with ABH blood groups and secretor status.[5-14] The possibility has been raised that much of the alkaline phosphatase migrating to the liver position or starch gel electrophoresis may represent modified intestinal alkaline phosphatase.[15] The great heat sensitivity of bone alkaline phosphatase has been documented. In recent times, we have been able to distinguish between placental and intestinal alkaline phosphatases,[16] (both of which are inhibited by L-phenylalanine) on the basis of neuraminidase action and differences in optimum pH. The placental alkaline phosphatase has been shown to consist of molecular weight variants,[17] one of which was crystallized. Purified rat and human intestinal alkaline phosphatases exhibit uncompetitive, homosteric inhibition by L-phenylalanine.[19,20] Metal and sulfhydryl sites appear to be requirements in the enzyme molecule for this type of inhibition.[18] Finally, mention has been made earlier in this session of a biochemical assay of the placental isoenzyme in serum as an index of placental status.[21]

This brings us to our main current interest in an isoenzyme uncommon by association with certain human cancer patients.[22]

The Regan isoenzyme[23] was named after the first patient, Peter Regan, in whose tumor tissue and serum it was discovered. Its properties at that time were indistinguishable from the ones known for placental alkaline phosphatase. This finding was interpreted as an instance of the derepression of the genome of the cancer cell, a mechanism that is frequently used to explain ectopic polypeptide hormone production in an ever-increasing number of cases of human cancer.[23]

* This study was supported in part by a research grant (P–106) from the American Cancer Society Inc., New York, and by grants-in-aid (CA–07538 and K6–CA–18453) of the National Cancer Institute, National Institutes of Health, U.S.P.H.S., Bethesda, Md.

Perhaps Regan isoenzyme is qualified to be known as an example of ectopic isoenzyme production.

The work to be reported today represents essentially our new findings since the publication of our previous paper in August, 1968 following a review of methods.[23]

Methods

A description will first be given in FIGURE 1 of the method by which we determine the biochemical isoenzyme profile of the serum alkaline phosphatase. The serum is here assumed to be a mixture of liver, bone, intestine, placenta and Regan isoenzymes. One aliquot is passed through the Auto-Analyzer and its activity is measured[24] at pH 9.8 in 18 mM phenylphosphate in the presence separately of D-phenylalanine and L-phenylalanine. The differences in the two activities is that portion inhibited by L-phenylalanine, and is referred to as L-phenylalanine-sensitive alkaline phosphatase or LPSAP.

A second aliquot of serum is heated for 16 minutes at 55° C prior to measurement of enzyme activity at pH 9.8 in 18 mM phenylphosphate in the presence of D- and L-phenylalanine. The bone isoenzyme is almost completely inactivated, whereas liver and intestine are only partially inactivated. Placental and Regan isoenzymes are unaffected by these conditions of heat inactivation. The computation of the percent heat inactivation is shown for the total alkaline phosphatase, the latter being defined as the activity measured in the presence of 0.005 M D-phenylalanine.

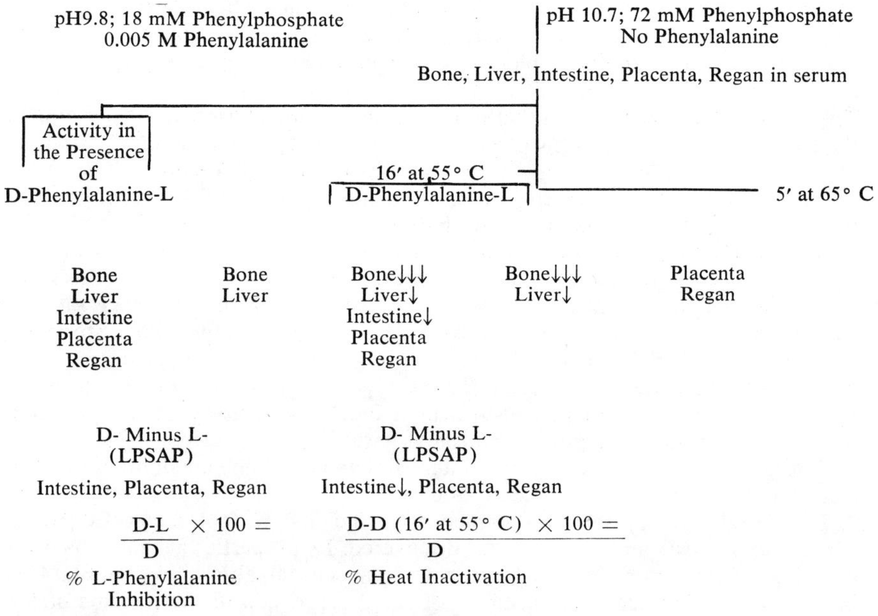

FIGURE 1. System of establishing the biochemical profile of isoenzymes of alkaline phosphatase where the mixture contains the bone, liver, intestine, placenta and Regan types. The left side of the chart refers only to the determinations done in the presence of D- and L-phenylalanine according to Fishman and Green.[24] No phenylalanine is required for the placental and Regan isoenzymes since the enzyme that survives 5′ at 65° C is presumably completely inhibited by L-phenylalanine. Downward arrow signifies loss of activity.

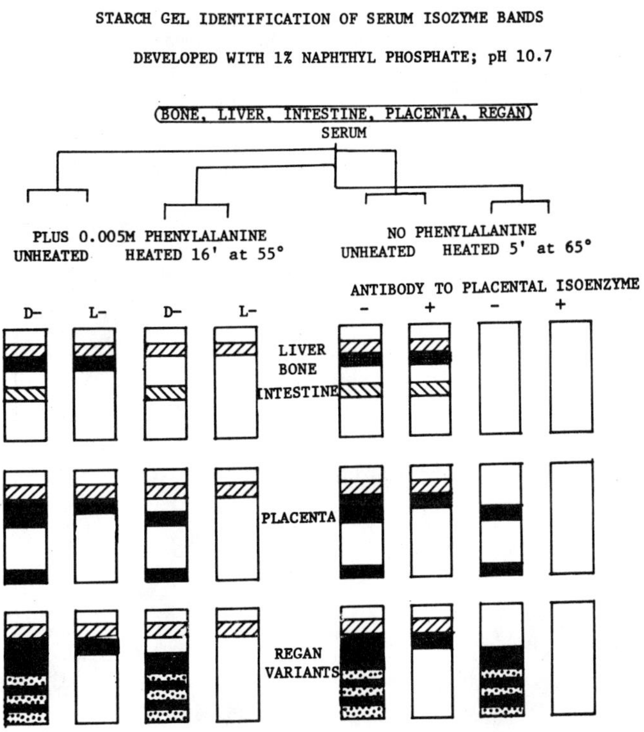

FIGURE 2. System of identifying serum isozyme bands according to organ origin. After electrophoresis of unheated or heated serum, as indicated on the left side of the figure, the isozyme bands are developed with filter paper soaked with 1% naphthyl phosphate in carbonate buffer at pH 10.7 and in either 0.05 M D- or L-phenylalanine. On the right side of the figure, unheated and heated sera were mixed with an appropriate dilution of antiserum to placental alkaline phosphatase before electrophoresis on starch gel. Placenta and Regan variants failed to migrate.

The third aliquot of serum is heated for 5 minutes at 65° C to destroy the isoenzymes other than placenta and Regan. The surviving alkaline phosphatase activity is now measured at pH 10.7 in the presence of 72 mM phenylphosphate, conditions that favor the activity of placental and Regan isoenzymes.[21]

A similar approach, which included in addition the use of antibody to placental isoenzyme, has been fashioned for the starch gel identification of serum isoenzyme bands. These are all developed following electrophoresis with a solution of 1% naphthyl phosphate at pH 10.7 as described earlier (FIGURE 2). In the starch gel pattern to the left, obtained with unheated serum and serum heated 16 minutes at 55° C, the intestine, placenta, and Regan variants* all fail to appear at their expected locations when the substrate contains L-phenylalanine. The heat-sensitive bone band is missing in the gels after electrophoresis of the heated sera.

On the right side of FIGURE 2, the use of a 1 to 1000 dilution of antibody to

* Variation in the number of isozyme bands and the extent of diffuse areas have been encountered in the sera of patients showing the Regan isoenzyme of alkaline phosphatase.

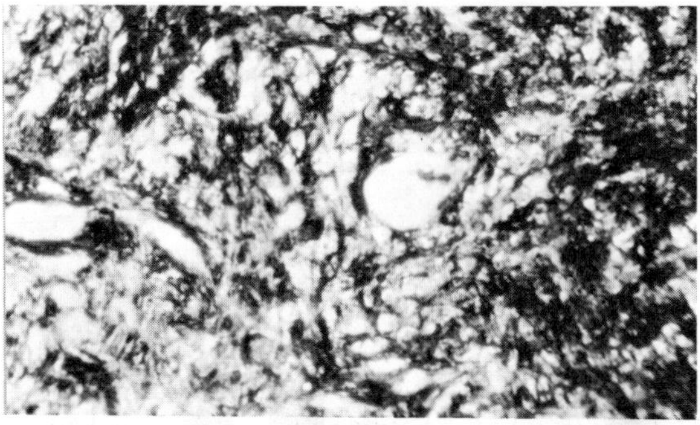

FIGURE 3. Tumor in lung showing positive sites for alkaline phosphatase ×400. (Reproduced by permission of Cancer Research.[22])

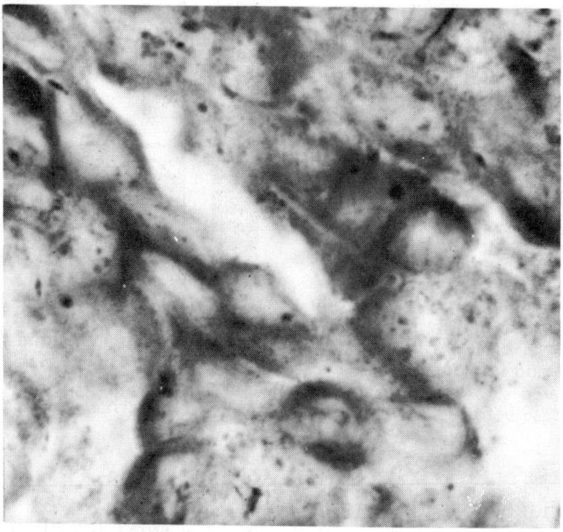

FIGURE 4. High power magnification of enzyme-positive sites for alkaline phosphatase-nuclei are negative ×1000. (Reproduced by permission of Cancer Research.[22])

placental alkaline phosphatase (A + B + Albumin†) reacts with only placenta and Regan isoenzyme variants, and the antigen-antibody complex fails to migrate. This phenomena is most striking in the starch gel, in which the serum was first heated 5 minutes at 65° C, because nonplacental isoenzymes of alkaline phosphatase are absent.

A third technique, which is applied to the tumor tissue itself, is the use of Watanabe and Fishman's procedure[25] for demonstrating L-phenylalanine-sensitive Regan isoenzyme. FIGURE 3 shows the appearance of the staining reaction for alkaline phosphatase in the primary tumor done in the presence of D-phenyl-

† The antigen was a preparation of placental alkaline phosphatase with a specific activity of 10.0 that contained molecular weight variants A and B and placental albumin. It was mixed with Freunds adjuvant and falba oil, and the emulsion was injected into the foot pad of the rabbit at regular intervals according to Reif and Norris.[23]

TABLE 1

COMPARISON OF SOME BIOCHEMICAL PARAMETERS OF PLACENTAL AND NEOPLASTIC ALKALINE PHOSPHATASES

Parameters	Placenta	Neoplastic	
		MO†	N†
1. K_m (pH 9.6)	0.51 mM	0.55 mM	1.00 mM
2. Optimum pH (18 mM Phenylphosphate)	10.6	10.9	10.7
3. Ratio of Activity at pH 10.7 vs 9.8 (9.0 mM Phenylphosphate)	1.19	2.11	2.70
4. Interval in which the Enzyme Obeys Zero Order Kinetics	40 Min	20 Min	20 Min
5. L-Phenylalanine Inhibition at pH 9.8 (18 mM Phenylphosphate)	78.0	78.3	76.3
6. N*	1.43	1.57	1.64

* The number of L-phenylalanine molecules combining with one molecule of alkaline phosphatase.

† MO refers to a patient whose pleural fluid contained Regan isoenzyme and N, to a patient from whom a lymph node replaced by tumor of the Regan isoenzyme type was removed. These were purified to the extent possible with this limited amount of material. The N preparation showed a specific activity of 3.8.[17]

TABLE 2

INHIBITION CONSTANTS OF SOME REAGENTS ACTING ON HUMAN PLACENTAL AND NEOPLASTIC ALKALINE PHOSPHATASES

	Inhibitor Constants (K_I) (M)		
Reagent	Placenta	Neoplastic MO*	Neoplastic N*
O-Phenanthrolene	6.30×10^{-4}	2.00×10^{-4}	1.51×10^{-3}
PHMB	5.62×10^{-3}	5.37×10^{-3}	5.25×10^{-3}
HCHO-Acetamide	2.57	1.66	3.81
50% Inactivation by:			
L-Phenylalanine	1.58×10^{-3}	7.41×10^{-4}	2.24×10^{-3}
Urea	6.76	1.05	3.38

* Preparations were those explained in TABLE 1.

alanine and FIGURE 4 represents the staining reaction as seen in metastasis to the adrenal. A negative reaction is obtained in the presence of L-phenylalanine (not shown).

Enzyme Kinetics

It is of some importance to ascertain to what extent Regan isoenzyme prepared from several tumor tissues are the same or different from theoretical and practical points of view. To this end, we are now reporting a comparison of two preparations of Regan isoenzyme with one of placenta in regard to enzyme kinetics and immunologic properties. These kinetic studies have been done with purer preparations, and have been executed more carefully and critically than the earlier one reported by Dr. Ghosh at this conference.

TABLE 1 lists a variety of kinetic constants that characterize the catalytic reaction, and TABLE 2 contains information relating to the effect of reagents that block amino, sulfhydryl and metal sites in the enzyme. Included also are studies on the L-phenylalanine inhibition and urea inactivation.

The uncompetitive nature of the inhibition by L-phenylalanine is shown by the parallel curves[15] in FIGURE 5 for the three isoenzyme preparations. The urea inactivation data in FIGURE 6 shows a greater urea sensitivity of the Regan isoenzyme as compared to the placental isoenzyme.

From this study, one can state that the properties of the active site are quite similar for the placenta and Regan isoenzyme, but there is reason to consider that the three-dimensional structure may be appreciably different between these two as indicated from the urea inactivation study.

Immunology Studies

A convenient and rapid means of identifying the Regan isoenzyme has been the failure of the antigen-antibody complex of Regan isoenzyme to migrate during electrophoresis (the antibody is present in rabbit sera following immunization with placenta alkaline phosphatase preparation). FIGURE 7 illustrates our first experience with this technique.[23] The antiserum to placental alkaline phosphatase cross-reacts with the alkaline phosphatase of human cancer cells grown in culture. HeLa strain (FIGURE 8).

One of our first problems has been to develop convenient methods for detecting and measuring the activity of the Regan isoenzyme. Attempts were centered on

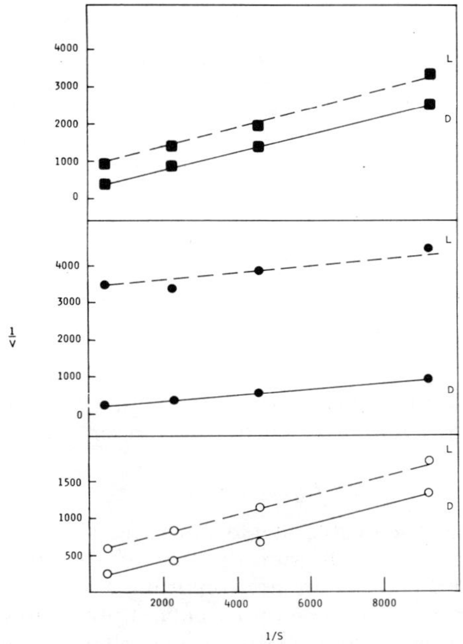

FIGURE 5. Uncompetitive inhibition of L-phenylalanine of alkaline phosphatase preparations of placenta, open circles (O), MO pleural fluid, black circles (●), N. lymph node metastasis, black squares (■).

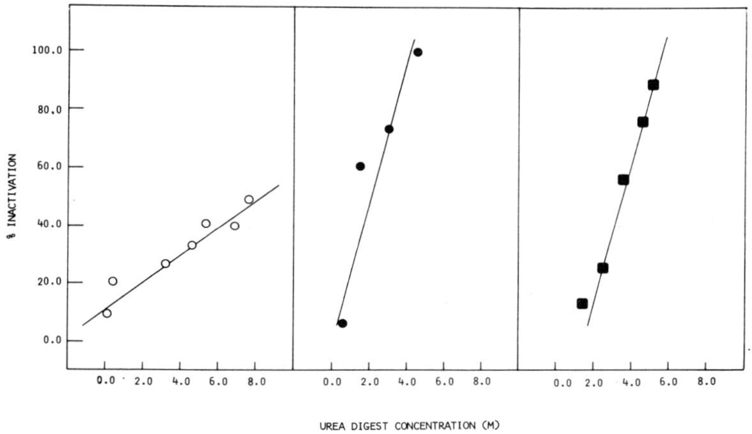

FIGURE 6. Degree of inactivation of placental alkaline phosphatase as a function of the concentration of urea in the digest (same symbols as in FIGURE 7).

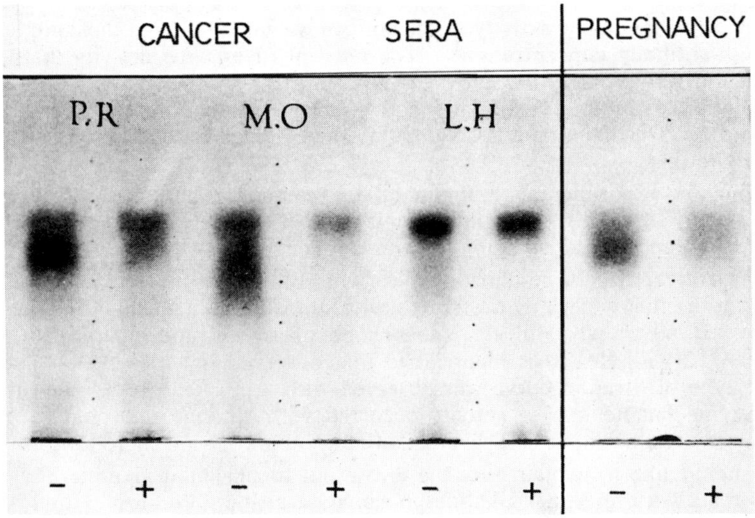

FIGURE 7. Electrophoretic study of migration of antigen (Regan or placental isoenzyme) (A + B + Alb.) and antigen-antibody complexes (Reproduced by permission of Nature, London).

the starch gel technique in which we have found, (FIGURE 9) than an end point can be defined as the highest dilution of antibody that will prevent the placental isoenzyme from traveling to the placental position. In FIGURE 10, the exclusion from the starch gel of the antigen-antibody complexes for Regan isoenzyme and serum placental isoenzyme is demonstrated for antisera to the SA 20 antigen which has a specific activity for alkaline phosphatase of 20.[17]

In studies of the antigen-antibody complex, we also included an experiment on antigen-antibody mixtures in solution. We found that approximately 50%

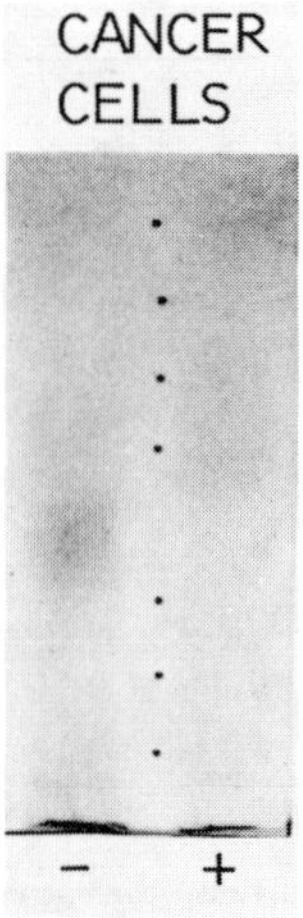

FIGURE 8. Cross-reaction of HeLa alkaline phosphatase with antiserum to placental alkaline phosphatase.

of the original enzyme activity of the antigen was missing from the complex made at high-antibody concentrations.* The amount of enzyme activity disappearing in the antigen-antibody complex is measured in the Auto-Analyzer as a function of dilution of antibody in heat inactivated, nonpregnancy serum, as shown in FIGURE 11. This experiment was done on the original antibody used in FIGURE 7, and its antigen.

Thus, the experimental results including reaction of antibody with Regan isoenzyme on starch gel (described in Nature),[23] have been confirmed in the experiments reported today using a purer antigen.

The antigen SA 20 contains only variants B and not molecular variants A + B, as in the first experiments and its antiserum is less potent than the one against (A + B albumin). However, the shape of the titration curve obtained in FIGURE 12 with SA 20 is identical to that observed in FIGURE 11. Finally, the same type of titration curve was observed with a purified preparation of Regan isoenzyme but no loss of activity occurred with alkaline phosphatase preparations of intestine, bone and liver alkaline in serum (FIGURE 13).

I should like to explain that the antiserum to placental alkaline phosphatase does react with intestinal alkaline phosphatase at the dilution of 1 to 150 of the antisera to A + B + albumin and in a dilution of 1 to 10 of antisera to SA 20, as shown by starch gel technique (FIGURE 14). However, in aqueous mixture, the intestinal enzyme in the antigen-antibody complex registers its full catalytic activity and, consequently, there is no disappearance of intestinal alkaline phosphatase activity as shown in FIGURE 13.

It is obvious that in a mixture of liver, intestine, bone and Regan isoenzymes, the presence of antibody to placental alkaline phosphatase can be expected to produce a loss in enzyme activity of only Regan isoenzyme.

The consequence of these experiments is that we now have in our possession

* It is known that when enzyme combines with its specific antibody the combination may show degrees of loss of enzyme activity ranging from zero to 100 per cent depending on the substrate employed.

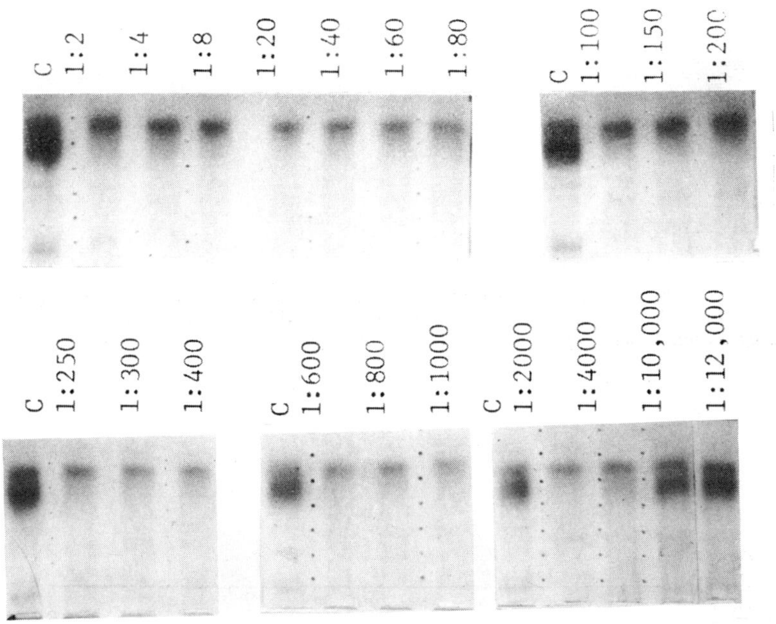

FIGURE 9. Titer of antiserum to placental alkaline phosphatase using pregnancy serum, rabbit antiserum and starch gel electrophoresis. Five separate experiments each included the pregnancy serum control (c) at the farthest position to the left and dilutions with rabbit antisera to the right as follows: (1) c, 1:2, 1:4, 1:8, 1:20, 1:60, 1:80 (2) c, 1:100, 1:150, 1:200 (3) c, 1:250, 1:300, 1:400, (4) c, 1:600, 1:800, 1:1000, (5) 1:2000, 1:4000, 1:10,000, 1:12,000.

a sensitive biochemical technique for detecting and measuring specifically placental and/or Regan isoenzymes in a mixture of isoenzymes of alkaline phosphatase that are encountered in the blood.

In summary, the biochemical and immunologic profiles of the interaction between Regan isoenzyme and antisera to placental alkaline phosphatase are indistinguishable from the interaction of the same antibody with molecular Variant B of placental alkaline phosphatase. This concordance is the strongest evidence for the derepression explanation of the ectopic isoenzyme production by tumor. The enzyme kinetic studies showed a close resemblance between the placenta

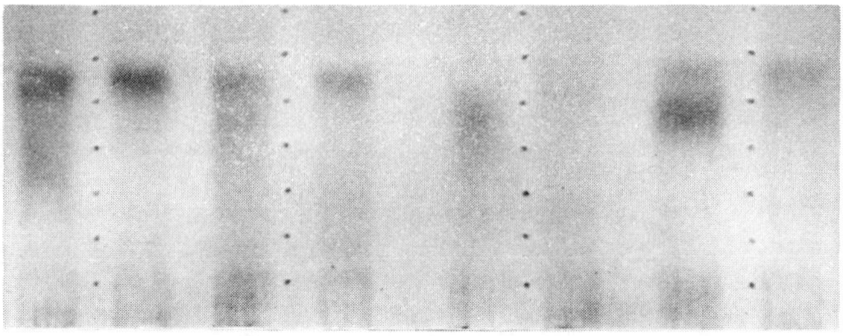

FIGURE 10. Ability of antiserum to SA 20 to react with Regan isoenzyme and placental isoenzyme. From left to right by pairs, serum (M.O.), fluid (A.N.), tumor (P.R.) and late pregnancy serum. Absence or presence of antiserum is indicated by minus or plus, respectively.

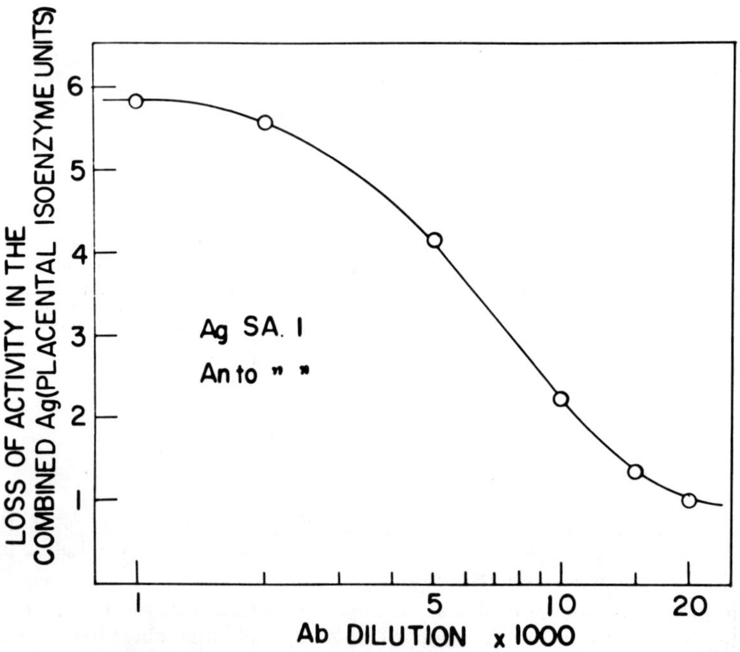

FIGURE 11. Plot of loss of enzyme activity of the antigen (A + B + Alb.) in the antigen-antibody complex as a function of dilution of antibody to A + B + Alb.[23]

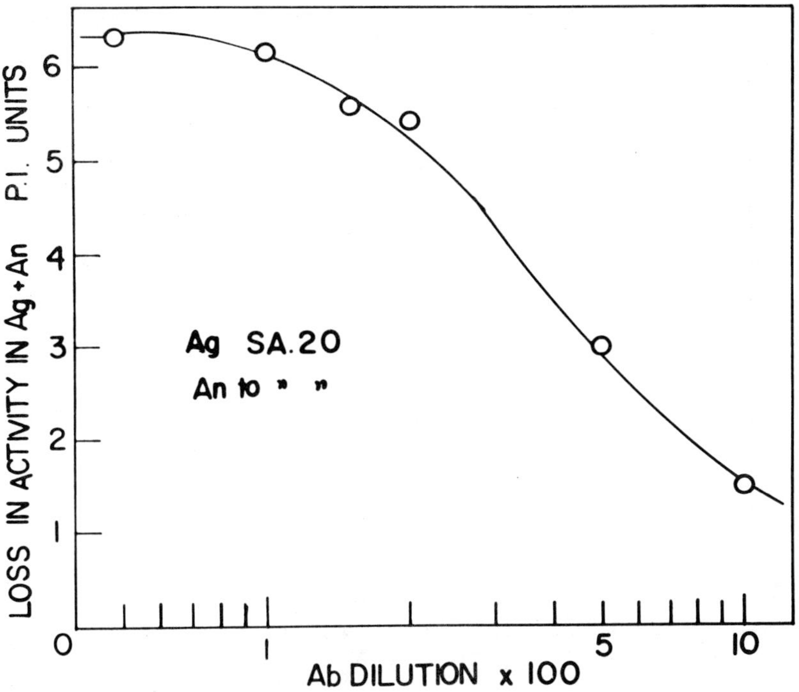

FIGURE 12. Plot of loss of enzyme activity of the antigen (SA 20) in the antigen-antibody complex in relation to dilution of antibody to SA 20, variant B.

and Regan isoenzyme, except for the experiment with urea, which reflected a difference in the three-dimensional structure.*

These findings illustrate how a combination of biochemical, electrophoretic and immunologic techniques have not only succeeded in characterizing the Regan isoenzyme in certain cancer patients but in providing an approach to isoenzymes of other tissues. With respect to cancer, it now seems logical to search in cancer patients for other enzymes whose counterpart in the placenta may have distinctive biochemical and immunologic properties.

Acknowledgments

This report is the product of the many coworkers whose names appear in the publications from this laboratory. In chronological order of their association with this study beginning in 1956 they are Sidney Green, Norma R. Inglis, Leo L. Stolbach, Claire L. Anstiss, J. H. Kreisher, K. Watanabe, M. J. Krant, N. K. Ghosh, R. Rustigian, A. E. Reif, E. Schaner and L. Kotowitz. Their cooperation is sincerely appreciated.

* Urea inactivation has been advanced as a means of distinguishing placental from non-placental isoenzymes of alkaline phosphatase, the placental isoenzyme being urea resistant. The reader is warned against the uncritical use of urea inactivation as a means for detecting Regan isoenzyme on the assumption that Regan isoenzyme has this placental characteristic in full measure.

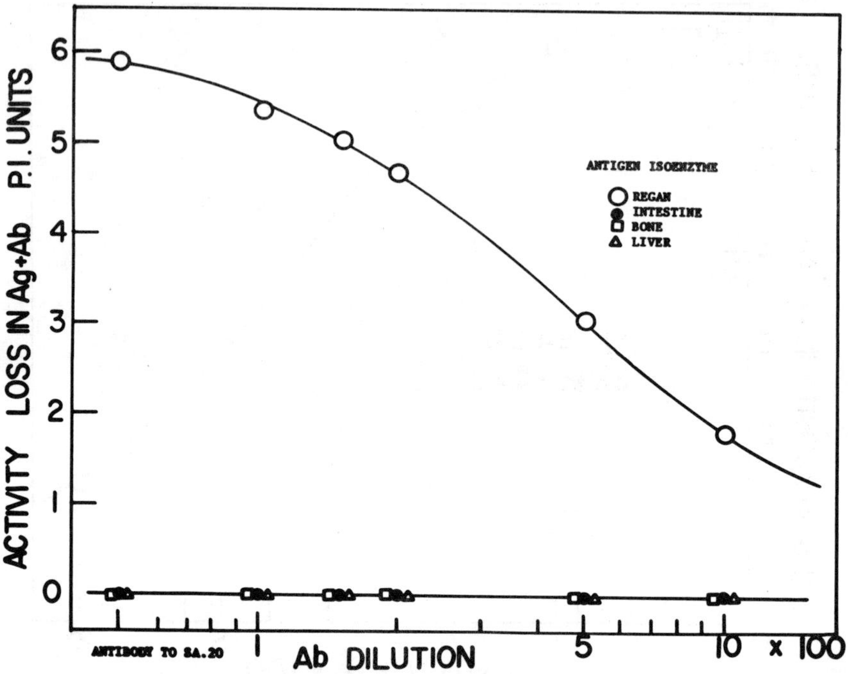

FIGURE 13. Relationship of loss of enzyme activity of the antigen (Regan isoenzyme prepared from Nowodworski's lymph node metastasis) to dilutions of antisera to SA 20, variant B.

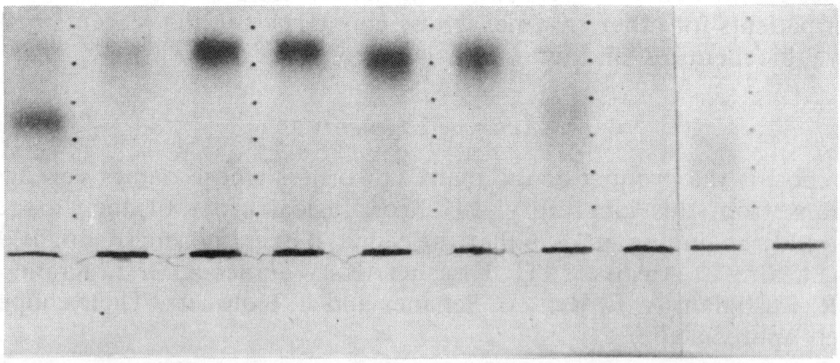

FIGURE 14. Ability of antiserum to SA 20 to react with various alkaline phosphatase preparations. From left to right by pairs; intestinal alkaline phosphatase, serum rich in liver alkaline phosphatase, serum rich in bone alkaline phosphatase, tumor tissue preparations of Regan isoenzyme and placental alkaline phosphatase antigen, SA 20. Note there was no cross reaction with liver and bone isoenzymes which migrated to their expected positions.

References

1. Fishman, W. H., S. Green & N. I. Inglis. 1963. L-Phenylalanine: an organ-specific, stereospecific, inhibitor of human intestinal alkaline phosphatase (EC 3.1.3.1). Nature (London) **198:** 685–686.
2. Fishman, W. H. & J. H. Kreisher. 1963. Stereospecific, organ specific inhibition of intestinal alkaline phosphatase. Ann. N. Y. Acad. Sci. **103:** 951–955.
3. Kreisher, J. H., V. A. Close & W. H. Fishman. 1965. Identification by means of L-phenylalanine inhibition of intestinal alkaline phosphatase components separated by starch-gel electrophoresis of serum. Clin. Chim. Acta **11:** 122–127.
4. Robinson, J. C. & J. E. Pierce. 1964. Differential action of neuraminidase on human serum alkaline phosphatases. Nature (London) **204:** 472–473.
5. Arfors, K. E., L. Beckman & L. G. Lundin. 1963. Genetic variations of human serum phosphatases. Acta Genet. **13:** 89–94.
6. Beckman, L. 1964. Associations between human serum alkaline phosphatase and blood groups. Acta Genet. **14:** 286–297.
7. Bamford, K. F., H. Harris, J. E. Luffman, E. B. Robson & T. E. Cleghorn. 1965. Serum alkaline phosphatase and the ABO blood groups. Lancet **I:** 530–531.
8. Fishman, W. H., N. I. Inglis & M. J. Krant. 1965. Serum alkaline phosphatase of intestinal origin in patients with cancer and with cirrhosis of the liver. Clin. Chim. Acta **12:** 298–303.
9. Shreffler, D. C. 1965. Genetic studies of blood group-associated variations in a human serum alkaline phosphatase. Amer. J. Hum. Genet. **17:** 71–86.
10. Stolbach, L. L., M. J. Krant, N. I. Inglis & W. H. Fishman. 1967. Correlation of serum L-phenylalanine sensitive alkaline phosphatase, derived from intestine, with the ABO blood group of cirrhotics. Gastroenterology **103:** 819–827.
11. Warnock, M. L. 1966. Characterization of tissue and serum alkaline phosphatases. Clin. Chim. Acta **14:** 156–165.
12. Newton, M. A. 1966. A distinctive fraction of alkaline phosphatase in health and disease. J. Clin. Pathol. **19:** 491–495.
13. Keiding, N. R. 1966. Intestinal alkaline phosphatase in human lymph and serum. Scand. J. Clin. Lab. Invest. **18:** 134–140.
14. Langman, M. J. S., E. Leuthold, E. B. Robson, J. Harris, J. E. Luffman & H. Harris. 1966. Influence of diet on the "intestinal" component of serum alkaline phosphatase in people of different ABO blood groups and secretor status. Nature (London) **212:** 41–43.
15. Fishman, W. H. & N. K. Ghosh. 1967. Isoenzymes of human alkaline phosphatase. Advances Clin. Chem. **10:** 255.
16. Fishman, W. H., N. R. Inglis & N. K. Ghosh. 1968. Distinctions between intestinal and placental isoenzymes of alkaline phosphatase. Clin. Chim. Acta **19:** 71.
17. Ghosh, N. K. & W. H. Fishman. 1968. Purification and properties of molecular-weight variants of human placental alkaline phosphatase. Biochem. J. **108:** 779.
18. Fishman, W. H. & N. K. Ghosh. 1967. Influence of reagents reacting with metal, thiol and amino sites on catalytic activity and L-phenylalanine inhibition of rat intestinal alkaline phosphatase. Biochem. J. **105:** 1163–1170.
19. Ghosh, N. K. & W. H. Fishman. 1966. On the mechanism of inhibition of intestinal alkaline phosphatase by L-phenylalanine. I. Kinetic Studies. J. Biol. Chem. **241:** 2516–2522.
20. Ghosh, N. K. & W. H. Fishman. 1968. L-phenylalanine inhibition of rat intestinal alkaline phosphatase: a homosteric phenomenon. Arch. Biochem. **126:** 700–706.
21. Fishman, W. H., N. K. Ghosh, N. R. Inglis & S. Green. 1968. Quantitation of the placental isoenzyme of alkaline phosphatase in pregnancy sera. Enzymologia **34:** 317–321.
22. Fishman, W. H., N. R. Inglis, L. L. Stolbach & M. J. Krant. 1968. A serum alkaline phosphatase isoenzyme of human neoplastic cell origin. Cancer Res. **28:** 150–154.
23. Fishman, W. H., N. R. Inglis, S. Green, C. L. Anstiss, N. K. Ghosh, A. E. Rief, R. Rustigian, M. J. Krant & L. L. Stolbach. 1968. Nature (London) **219:** 697–699.
24. Fishman, W. H. & S. Green. 1967. Automated differential isoenzyme analysis. I. L-phenylalanine-sensitive isoenzymes of human serum alkaline phosphatase. Enzymologia **33:** 89–99.
25. Watanabe, K. & W. H. Fishman. 1964. Application of the stereospecific L-phenylalanine inhibitor to the enzymorphology of intestinal alkaline phosphatase. J. Histochem. Cytochem. **12:** 252–260.

Discussion of the Paper

L. BECKMAN: This is indeed a very exciting discovery, and it is a dream for a geneticist to meet this situation, especially in a system where we do have a polymorphism that is rather well investigated. And I believe you have now found a number of individuals, a small series of them. And it would be extremely interesting to type them according to the polymorphism of six different types as described by Dr. Harris because you would expect to find a distribution rather similar to that in the general population. Or if you don't, if they all have one phenotype, it would mean that only individuals of a certain genotype develop malignancy.

Have you attempted to investigate genetic phenotypes of the individuals having the malignancy?

O. BODANSKY: I want to ask a question here for clarity. Are you talking about immunochemical methods?

DR. BECKMAN: I'm talking about the polymorphism by electrophoresis at alkaline and acid pH as reported by the Harris group.

DR. BODANSKY: Are there any other questions? Yes?

R. KEIDING: I might have missed the beginning of your talk. Could you tell me what was the histological diagnosis of that patient with lung cancer?

DR. BODANSKY: Shall we save these question? Dr. Schwartz has one.

M. K. SCHWARTZ: Dr. Fishman, I notice on your first slide you listed the phenylphosphate concentration as both 18.2 and 72 millimolar. If my memory serves me, the concentration of phenylphosphate in the King method and in the Kind and King modification, which is the one employed on the Auto-Analyzer, is 8.1 millimolar. I was wondering if your findings are substrate dependent.

S. POSEN: I wonder if Dr. Fishman could give us some of his techniques for preparation of his antibody, in particular did he have to use a second antibody, did he have to make antibody against rabbit γ-globulin, or anything like that, in order to precipitate the antibody-antigen complex? [The reader is referred to Ref. 23]

DR. BODANSKY: Are there any other questions, because I want to ask one of my own along those lines. Of course, in general, when you compare antibodies to enzymes, you may either use the criterion of inhibition, which is true for many enzymes, or precipitation. And I think each of these requires a certain care in technique.

For example, in the case of inhibition, that is usually a time-dependent thing. That is, you will not get the characteristic inhibition or maximal inhibition until you incubate for a certain period of time. With regard to precipitation, which is another technique, you may remove the enzyme by the antibody and get it into the precipitate, which isn't necessary for the inhibition technique. And there, as Heidelberger, Kabat, and many others have shown, time also is very important–you may incubate four hours or two days, or if you have very low concentrations of enzyme, that is the antigen, 14 days. So I'd like to ask a question about the technique here. Whether this is inhibition or precipitation and whether the time factor is taken into account?

DR. FISHMAN: With regard to Dr. Beckman's question about the phenotype and also perhaps, the blood type, and others of the parameters that one looks to from the genetic studies of the Harris and Beckman groups for guidance and interpretation–I think that Dr. Stolbach's experience was that the blood type wasn't pertinent, that no particular blood type characterized the patients with

Regan isoenzyme. I was excited, but he was not, with the fact that 16 of these 17 patients were secretors of ABH substance in their blood. But perhaps he will deal with that in his talk.

The Regan tumor had the histologic characteristics of a squamous cell carcinoma of the lung, which had metastasized to adrenal gland, lymph node, brain and kidney, but no metastases were discovered in the liver or in the skeletal system. The presence of the Regan isoenzyme is, therefore, not determined by the histologic type of tumor or its location.

Dr. Schwartz asked whether the use of higher substrate concentrations might have been the basis for determining the specificity of the results we've obtained. I don't think so. What we've always had to do was to strive for the greatest sensitivity for measuring a particular isoenzyme, and we've always controlled the newer substrate concentration used against the King-Armstrong conditions.

In the case of the 72-mM substrate at pH 10.7, the values that we measured there are four times the ones measured for placental alkaline phosphatase at 9.8 at 18-millimolar substrate concentration. And this is a very helpful consideration in the analyses.

With regard to the immunologic characteristics of this antigen-antibody reaction, Dr. Bodansky has dealt very well with the types of reactions that one may encounter. We have observed a practically instantaneous combination of antigen and antibodies as described in my paper both with electrophoretic technique and the Auto-Analyzer measurements of decrease in enzyme activity. And we simply haven't had the time to wait and see if any precipitates have formed in the Auto-Analyzer cups before coming to the conference. Perhaps when we get back, we may find some precipitates in the tubes.

DR. BODANSKY: Thank you, Dr. Fishman.

DR. NAUGHETY (*Ohio State University, Columbus, Ohio*): It may be pertinent to mention that we found that this phenomenon is not species specific, at least completely. We found this in the dog also. We have one case so far. This may be important because . . .

DR. BODANSKY: Which particular phenomenon?

DR. NAUGHETY: The Regan isoenzyme in a reticulum cell sarcoma. In the serum, its activity was increased to over 10 times the normal amount. The serum and the tumor had characteristics similar to those Dr. Fishman has mentioned for Regan. If hamsters and rats have these same characteristics, then this could open up a wide area for immediate exploitation.

DR. BODANSKY: Thank you very much. Yes, Dr. Beckman.

DR. BECKMAN: I'm afraid Dr. Fishman misunderstood my question. I didn't ask for blood types. I meant that if you already have 17 individuals, you are bound to find at least three of the common phenotypes among them. So now you already have in your hands the information necessary to find out if this indeed is placental alkaline phosphatase. I would be glad to type them for you. And if they are all having the same electrophoretic mobility, this is not placental alkaline phosphatase. Because if the individual starts to make an enzyme that he normally would do in fetal stage, he should do it according to his genotype. Do you see my point now?

CLINICAL APPLICATION OF ALKALINE PHOSPHATASE ISOENZYME ANALYSIS*

Leo L. Stolbach†

Lemuel Shattuck Hospital, and Tufts University School of Medicine, Boston, Mass.

In the past, an elevated alkaline phosphatase has usually been taken as evidence of either bone or liver disease. However, with the development of the isoenzyme techniques described in detail by other participants in this symposium, it has become possible to differentiate with a fair degree of accuracy not only the isoenzymes of bone and liver but also those originating in intestine, placenta and tumor.

A combination of isoenzyme analysis techniques have been used in our laboratory to study the serum alkaline phosphatase of patients with various diseases. The use of one or more of these techniques will be described for the following clinical situations: (1) patients with cirrhosis; (2) patients with tumor in bone or liver; and (3) patients with malignancy whose serum and/or tumor contains the Regan isoenzyme.[1] These studies have made it clear that isoenzyme analysis can result in more accurate interpretations of serum alkaline phosphatase values.

TABLE 1 summarizes the characteristics of the alkaline phosphatases originating in the various tissues known to be sources of serum alkaline phosphatase. The alkaline phosphatases of liver and bone are only minimally inhibited by L-phenylalanine, whereas intestinal and placental alkaline phosphatase and Regan isoenzyme are inhibited 77 to 79%. Heat inactivation at 55° C for 16 minutes causes 90 to 100% inhibition of bone alkaline phosphatase but no inhibition of placental or Regan isoenzyme, whereas liver and intestinal alkaline phosphatase are inhibited 50 to 70% under these conditions. A more drastic condition of heat inactivation at 65° C for five minutes causes complete inhibition of bone, liver, and intestinal alkaline phosphatase but no inhibition of Regan or placental isoenzyme. As has been previously shown, both Regan and placental isoenzyme migrate after starch gel electrophoresis to a position between the bone-liver band and the intestinal band. This band disappears after mixing with antiserum to placental alkaline phosphatase.[1] These isoenzyme characteristics have diagnostic applicability, since the percent inhibition by L-phenylalanine helps to identify patients whose sera contain intestinal alkaline phosphatase, Regan isoenzyme or placental isoenzyme; heat inactivation at 55° C is a useful aid in diagnosing bone or liver disease; and heat inactivation at 65° C identifies patients whose sera contain Regan or placental isoenzyme. At present, all of these determinations are carried out on each serum tested in our laboratory.

Hepatic Cirrhosis

In the past, it has usually been assumed that a rise in alkaline phosphatase in patients with cirrhosis is due to enzyme originating in the liver. Our findings in a

* This work was supported in part by grants CA–07190 from the National Cancer Institute, National Institutes of Health; DRG–988 from the Damon Runyon Memorial Fund for Cancer Research, Inc., New York and P–106 from the American Cancer Society, Inc., New York, N.Y.

† Research Physician, Oncology Division, Lemuel Shattuck Hospital, and Assistant Professor of Medicine, Tufts University School of Medicine, Boston, Mass. Requests for reprints should be addressed to Dr. Leo L. Stolbach, Oncology Division, Lemuel Shattuck Hospital, 170 Morton Street, Boston, Mass.

TABLE 1

BIOCHEMICAL AND IMMUNOLOGICAL CHARACTERISTICS OF VARIOUS HUMAN ISOENZYMES OF ALKALINE PHOSPHATASE

Conditions for Alkaline Phosphatase Measurement						
	Phenylphosphate (mM)	18	18	72		
	pH	9.8	9.8	10.7		
			Heat inactivation			
Tissues		% Inhibition by L-Phenylalanine	16′ at 55° %	5′ at 65° %	Order of Anodal Migration on Starch Gel	Reaction With Antiserum to Placental Isoenzyme SA20
Liver		7.7	50–70	100	1	0
Bone		10.3	90–100	100	2	0
Intestine		77.0	50–60	100	4	0
Placenta		79.0	0	0	3	+
Regan Isoenzyme		79.0	0	0	3 (diffuse)	+

group of 139 patients with cirrhosis have shown that this is not necessarily the case, since in a significant number of these patients, a major portion of the total serum alkaline phosphatase was found to be of intestinal origin.[2] The presence of this isoenzyme in the serum of these patients is genetically associated with the ABO blood type of the individual in a manner similar to that described by Beckman for normal individuals.[3] The intestinal contribution to the serum content of alkaline phosphatase was indicated by the levels of L-phenylalanine-sensitive alkaline phosphatase (abbreviated LPSAP), and the finding of a slow-moving intestinal band after starch gel electrophoresis of serum. Since enzyme from nonintestinal sources may be slightly inhibited by L-phenylalanine,[4] and since purified intestinal alkaline phosphatase is not totally inhibited by this amino acid,[4] it is usually impossible to ascertain the exact amount of enzyme of intestinal origin present in a given serum from the L-phenylalanine inhibition values. For these reasons, we report our results in terms of LPSAP rather than as intestinal alkaline phosphatase.

The diagnosis of cirrhosis in these 139 patients was based on clinical and laboratory findings and in many cases was confirmed by liver biopsy or autopsy. The ratio of LPSAP to total alkaline phosphatase was calculated for each patient's serum, and the distribution of these ratios according to blood type is shown in FIGURE 1. The dotted line separates ratios of less than 0.3 from those of 0.3 and greater. Ratios of 0.3 and over are found uncommonly in patients with blood types A and AB and with significant frequency in patients with types B and O. It should be noted that all sera with ratios greater than 0.3 that were subjected to starch gel electrophoresis showed a slow-moving enzyme band. Therefore, it can be assumed that as the ratios increase above 0.3, a greater percentage of

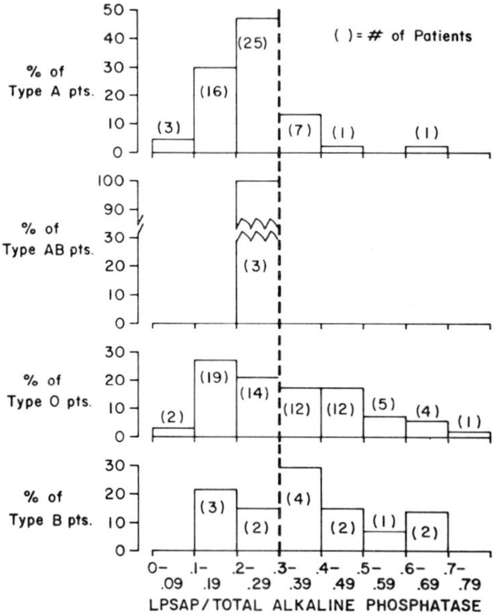

FIGURE 1. Distribution of ratios of L-phenylalanine-sensitive alkaline phosphatase (LPSAP) to total alkaline phosphatase. The bars represent the percentage of patients, and the numbers in parentheses are the numbers of patients, of each blood type occurring in each ratio range. (Published with the permission of L. L. Stolbach and *Gastroenterology* 1967, **52**: 819–827.)

TABLE 2

PATIENTS WITH LPSAP/TAP > 0.30

Blood Groups	Patients
O	34/69 = 49%
A	9/53 = 17%
B	9/14 = 64%
AB	0/3 = 0%

p values: O vs. A and B vs. A; $p = < 0.001$.

intestinal alkaline phosphatase is present in the serum. TABLE 2 summarizes our results in these patients. Thirty-four of 69 patients with type O and 9 of 14 patients with type B were found to have ratios of greater than 0.3, whereas only 9 of 53 and 0 of 3 patients with types A and AB, respectively, had ratios of over 0.3. These differences in ratio are independent of whether the total alkaline phosphatase level is normal or elevated.[2]

The physiopathology underlying the elevation of LPSAP in the serum of patients with cirrhosis is not understood at this time, and no correlation could be made with such factors as increased portal pressure, as manifested by esophageal varices, or the presence of ascites.[2] However, some of the highest LPSAP levels and ratios were found in patients with a portacaval shunt. Thus, while the mechanism causing the increase in a specific isoenzyme in cirrhosis needs to be investigated further, it would appear that the potential to express the enzyme elevation is genetically determined.

Tumor in Bone or Liver

Whether bone or liver is the source of an elevated serum alkaline phosphatase in a patient with malignancy is often uncertain, even after careful physical examination and routine x-ray and laboratory studies. Moss[5] had previously described differences in the heat inactivation of bone and liver alkaline phosphatase and Posen[6] and Chang[7] demonstrated that heat inactivation of serum alkaline phosphatase can be of value in differentiating patients with liver disease from those with bone disease. To evaluate the usefulness of this technique in patients with malignancy, we initiated a retrospective study to correlate the heat inactivation of serum alkaline phosphatase with the presence of bone and/or liver disease in a group of 63 patients with tumor in bone or liver as well as in a group of 33 patients with nontumor liver disease.

Only patients with an elevated total serum alkaline phosphatase were included in the present study. All patients with a diagnosis of malignancy had pathological confirmation of this diagnosis as well as clinical, biochemical, or x-ray evidence of tumor in either bone or liver. If both liver and bone disease were present at the time that the initial elevated serum alkaline phosphatase value was obtained, the patient was eliminated from the study. The presence of tumor in bone was determined roentgenologically by a skeletal survey. Evidence of liver disease was based on one or more of the following criteria: (1) elevated serum glutamic oxaloacetic transaminase (SGOT) or serum glutamic pyruvic transaminase (SGPT) greater than 50 units, or bilirubin greater than 1.0 mg%; (2) enlarged or nodular liver; (3) liver scan compatible with metastatic disease or (4) tumor in the liver found by liver biopsy or at laparotomy. If a patient, after being included in either the tumor in bone or tumor in liver group, subsequently developed disease in the other organ, he remained in the study. The charts of all patients who were found to have an elevated alkaline phosphatase and who had heat inactivation determinations carried out during the two-year interval of this study were reviewed independently by a physician who had no knowledge of the heat inactivation data. The reviewer then classified these patients according to whether bone or liver disease was present.

Serum alkaline phosphatase determinations were initially carried out by a modification of the manual method of Shinowara,[8] but more recently we have been utilizing an autoanalyzer technique.[9] The upper limit of normal in our laboratory for the manual method is 5.0 Shinowara units and for the autoanalyzer method, 15.0 King-Armstrong units. Heat inactivation was carried out for 16 minutes at 55° C.

TABLE 3 shows the site of the primary tumor for the 31 patients with tumor in bone. In most of the cases the tumor had metastasized to bone, but the series does include three patients whose tumor arose primarily in bone, namely the two patients with multiple myeloma and one patient with an osteogenic sarcoma. TABLE 4 shows the site of the primary tumor for the 32 patients with tumor in liver. Liver involvement in most of these cases was due to tumor that had metastasized, but in two cases the tumor arose in the liver, one being a hepatoma and the other a biliary carcinoma. The diagnoses of the 33 patients with nontumor liver disease are shown in TABLE 5. Most of these patients had cirrhosis, but several patients with various types of hepatitis were also included in the study.

The distribution of heat inactivation results in these three groups of patients is shown in FIGURE 2. The mean heat inactivation of 80.7% in the 31 patients with tumor in bone (Group A) was significantly higher than the 61.5% mean heat inactivation found in the 32 patients with tumor in the liver (Group B)

TABLE 3

TUMOR IN BONE

Primary Site of Tumor	No. of Patients
Breast	14
Prostate	8
Lung	2
Colon and Rectum	2
Multiple Myeloma	2
Osteogenic Sarcoma	1
Miscellaneous	2

TABLE 4

TUMOR IN LIVER

Primary Site of Tumor	No. of Patients
Lung	7
Colon and Rectum	5
Lymph Nodes (Hodgkin's, Retic Cell)	4
Ovary	2
Breast	3
Stomach	2
Miscellaneous	6
Unknown	3

TABLE 5

NONTUMOR LIVER DISEASE

Disease	No. of Patients
Cirrhosis	24
Chronic Hepatitis	3
Infectious Hepatitis	2
Drug Hepatitis	1
Lupoid Hepatitis	1
Reiter's Disease	1
Granuloma Involving Liver	1

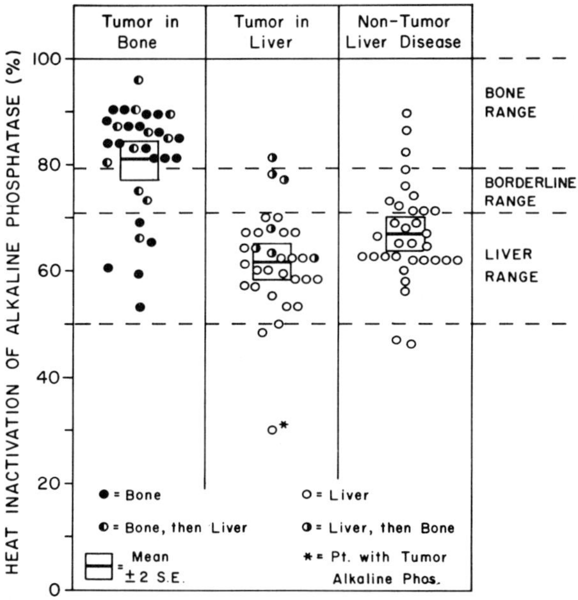

FIGURE 2. Distribution of alkaline phosphatase heat inactivation values (% activity lost after heating for 16 minutes at 55° C). Tumor in bone = Group A; tumor in liver, Group B; non-tumor liver disease, Group C. Patients in Groups A or B who subsequently were found to have disease in the other organ are designated by split circles.

(p value$<$0.01). The values for nontumor liver disease (Group C) were in an intermediate range with a mean heat inactivation of 66.8%.

Of 31 patients in Group A, 23 were found to have heat inactivations of 80% or greater, 2 were found to have values between 71 and 79%; and 6 were found to have values of 70% or less. Eleven patients shown as having "Bone, then Liver" were subsequently found to have liver disease on the basis of surgery, autopsy, physical examination, or laboratory data.

In Group B, 29 of 32 values were found to be 70% or less, 2 were between 71 and 79%, and 1 had a value greater than 80%. Seven patients in Group B who subsequently were found to have bone metastases on the basis of x-ray or autopsy, are shown as "Liver, then Bone." The 3 patients with values over 70% were all found to have bone metastases within two months after the heat inactivation determination. One case classified as having tumor in the liver, on the basis of an enlarged liver and an elevated SGOT, was found to have a heat inactivation of only 30%. This patient was subsequently found to have in her serum a significant amount of Regan isoenzyme[1] originating from her tumor cells in addition to alkaline phosphatase probably arising from liver. The presence of this tumor isoenzyme resulted in the low heat inactivation.

In Group C, 22 of 33 patients had values below 70%, 8 were found to have values between 71 and 79%, and 3 were found to have values above 80%. In 2 of these last 3 patients, no clinical evidence of bone disease was found; the third had advanced rheumatoid arthritis.

It has been suggested by a number of investigators that an elevated alkaline phosphatase is a more sensitive indicator of liver metastases than other parameters such as bilirubin, SGOT, SGPT, bromsulfalein excretion or liver enlargement, and that such elevations may occur when relatively small amounts of tumor are present. The findings in our patients with tumor in liver are compatible with the "regurgitation theory" of serum alkaline phosphatase elevation, which states that in such patients the enzyme is mainly due to reflux of bile alkaline phosphatase into the circulation. As has been previously shown, this isoenzyme has heat inactivations of 50 to 70%.[6] Since, as has been suggested by Posen[6,10] and other investigators,[11] the liver most likely does not contribute significantly to the excretion or metabolism of alkaline phosphatase present in the serum, the bile alkaline phosphatase remains in the circulation and is metabolized in the same manner as other serum proteins. In contradistinction, bilirubin, which also refluxes into the circulation as a result of local intrahepatic biliary obstruction, will be excreted when recirculated to other portions of the liver. Elevations of SGOT and SGPT require damage to liver cells, and this may be minimal when only small amounts of tumor are present. Even though the bile regurgitation theory is appealing, we cannot rule out the possibility that modified intestinal alkaline phosphatase[12] and/or other hepatic isoenzymes contribute to serum enzyme levels in these patients.

In patients with tumor in bone and an elevated alkaline phosphatase, the heat inactivation values of 80% and greater are probably due to bone alkaline phosphatase that has entered the circulation. This assumption is based on the fact that bone alkaline phosphatase is heat inactivated 90 to 100% under the conditions of our study. In addition, supporting evidence comes from the studies of Yong,[13] who utilized agar gel electrophoresis to demonstrate that bone alkaline phosphatase is present in the serum of patients with osteoblastic disease but absent in the serum of normal adults. We have, however, observed heat inactivation values of 80% or greater in some normal individuals and in cancer patients with normal total serum alkaline phosphatase levels. The cause of these high heat inactivation values remains to be determined. A discussion of this point by Fishman and Ghosh has appeared.[12] In our patients with bone metastases and heat inactivation values of 70% or less, undetected liver metastases may have been present or other unknown factors may have played a role.

To summarize the results of this study, heat inactivation of alkaline phosphatase is a simple modification of an enzyme test available in most clinical laboratories that can be useful in clarifying the cause of an elevated serum alkaline phosphatase in patients with malignancy. Our data suggests that in cancer patients with heat inactivation levels of 80% and greater, bone disease should be strongly suspected. On the other hand, heat inactivation levels of 70% or less indicate liver disease. A change in heat inactivation from the bone to liver range, or vice-versa, in patients with definite tumor in one of these organs should suggest the development of metastases in the other organ. Heat inactivation values below 40% in patients with malignancy usually indicate the presence of Regan isoenzyme.

Regan Isoenzyme

During the past two years, we have studied a number of patients whose serum and/or tumor contained Regan isoenzyme. The clinical, pathological and biochemical data regarding these patients are presented below. Heat inactivation at 65° C and the immunological techniques described by Fishman *et al.*[1] have been in use for only the past eight months. However, sera previously suspected of containing Regan isoenzyme on the basis of the initial biochemical analysis were retested utilizing these newer techniques to prove that Regan isoenzyme was present. Sera were kept frozen until retested.

Since the original case of Mr. Regan was discovered two years ago, a study of the sera of 520 cancer patients has resulted in the finding of 15 additional cases whose sera contained the Regan isoenzyme. Starch gel electrophoresis of the sera from these 16 patients revealed a band in the placental position, but in 10 of these 16 cases, the sera had to be concentrated threefold to demonstrate the Regan isoenzyme. The serum levels of Regan isoenzyme in these 16 patients ranged from 0.14 to 210 placental isoenzyme u/100 ml. In one additional case, the presence of Regan isoenzyme was suspected on the basis of finding 0.42 placental isoenzyme units of activity/100 ml in the serum. Starch gel electrophoresis of this patient's serum did not reveal a band in the appropriate location, even after concentration. However, a butanol extract of a node obtained at autopsy contained Regan isoenzyme. The incidence of Regan isoenzyme in our patient population was therefore 3.3%. TABLE 6 summarizes the tumor cell types and values for total alkaline phosphatase and Regan isoenzyme in this group of patients. The primary tumor site and the number of patients with elevated total serum alkaline phosphatase, as well as the number of patients with bone and/or liver metastases for each primary tumor site, are shown in TABLE 7. It is of some interest that only 12 of the 17 patients had an elevated alkaline phosphatase by our criteria, and in many of these, a large portion of the total alkaline phosphatase was apparently due to enzyme originating in bone or liver and reflected metastases in these organs. As shown in TABLE 6, two patients (A.S. and D.P.) had unusually low alkaline phosphatase values. It is apparent, therefore, that the level of Regan isoenzyme is independent of the total alkaline phosphatase value.

In 6 of the 17 patients (see TABLE 6), we subsequently had the opportunity to analyze tumor tissue obtained at autopsy. In each case, butanol extracts of tumor were found to contain the isoenzyme at levels ranging from 2 to 130 placental isoenzyme u/g of tissue. We also carried out isoenzyme analyses on the butanol extracts of tumor from 23 other patients whose sera did not reveal Regan isoenzyme. The primary tumor site of these patients are shown in TABLE 8. In none of these 23 cases could Regan isoenzyme be identified in the tumor tissue.

The changes in levels of total alkaline phosphatase and Regan isoenzyme observed in a patient during chemotherapy are shown in FIGURE 3. This patient (P.V.) is a 58-year-old male with a diagnosis of carcinoma of the colon with liver metastases. When first seen, the patient's liver was markedly enlarged, extending 10 cm below the right costal margin. The patient was treated with 5-Fluorouracil (5-FU), 500 mg/day by mouth given in seven-day courses. The liver decreased in size and the total alkaline phosphatase dropped as did the level of

TABLE 6

CLINICAL, BIOCHEMICAL AND PATHOLOGICAL CHARACTERISTICS OF PATIENT'S WITH REGAN ISOENZYME

Patient	Diagnosis	Sites of Metastases	Total Alkaline Phosphatase (K-A Units)			Regan Isoenzyme (Placental Isoenzyme Units*)			Starch Gel and Antibody	Tumor Tissue and/or Malignant Effusion Fluid
			Initial	Maximum	Minimum	Initial	Maximum	Minimum		
1. P.R.	Poorly differentiated squamous carcinoma of lung	Brain, Adrenal, Nodes, Kidney, Spleen	37.0	37.0	22.8	30.0	—	—	+	Tumor tissue positive
2. A.P.	Adenocarcinoma of endometrium	Liver, Lung, Nodes	125.4	145.0	125.4	42.3	—	—	+	
3. M.O.	Papillary cystadeno-carcinoma of ovary	Liver, Peritoneum, Pleura	26.9	213.0	26.9	37.2	—	—	+	Pleural fluid and cells positive
4. M.J.	Adenocarcinoma–primary in endometrium or lung	Lung, Bone	23.6	23.6	8.1	3.86	—	—	+	
5. T.J.	Undifferentiated carcinoma of lung	Bone, Adrenal	21.6	25.8	11.0	1.82	—	—	+[a]	Tumor tissue positive
6. J.R.	Undifferentiated carcinoma–primary of testicular origin	Lung, Kidney, Nodes	16.2	95.7	16.2	0.86	—	—	+[a]	
7. A.N.	Poorly differentiated squamous carcinoma of lung	Bone, Adrenal, Epicardium, Pericardium, Nodes, Liver, Kidney, Small Intestine	33.5	122.0	33.5	20.42	—	—	+	Tumor tissue and pericardial effusion fluid positive

8. P.V.	Adenocarcinoma, colon	Liver	34.4	34.4	13.0	8.4	8.4	0	+	
9. E.I.	Mucoepidermoid carcinoma of lung	Lung, Adrenal, Kidney, Nodes, Jejunum	27.4	27.4	19.1	0.9	1.9	0.9	+[a]	Tumor tissue positive
10. A.S.	Papillary adenocarcinoma of ovary or uterus	Nodes, Uterus, Vagina, Cervix	3.8	11.4	2.6	0.8	0.8	0.37	+[a]	
11. M.W.	Papillary adenocarcinoma of ovary	Peritoneum, Bladder, Sigmoid, Omentum	6.5	—	—	0.14	—	—	+[a]	Omental node positive
12. D.P.	Scirrhous carcinoma of breast	No clinical or lab. evidence of metastases	4.8	5.4	4.6	0.42	0.73	0.28	+[a]	
13. M.B.	Adenocarcinoma of sigmoid	Liver, Lung, Omentum, Nodes	59.1	131.0	59.1	0.24	0.42	0.24	—	Omental node positive
14. D.K.	Papillary cystadenocarcinoma of ovary	Breast, Nodes, Omentum	6.82	—	—	1.49	—	—	+[a]	
15. W.H.	Adenocarcinoma of colon	Liver, Nodes	36.2	48.4	34.1	0.53	0.68	0.06	+[a]	
16. T.C.	Multiple myeloma	Bone	11.1	11.1	8.14	0.80	0.80	0.44	+[a]	
17. L.F.	Adenocarcinoma of colon	Liver, Nodes	80.0	145.2	57.0	0.29	1.05	0.13	+[a]	

a = concentrated 3-fold.
* mg/phenol/100 ml/15 minutes.

Regan isoenzyme, which reached 0 placental-isoenzyme units. As the time between courses of 5-FU was increased, the levels of both total alkaline phosphatase and Regan isoenzyme rose, and the liver enlarged again. As illustrated in this case, measurement of Regan isoenzyme can be of value in assessing response to antitumor therapy in a manner similar to the use of urinary gonadotropin measurement in following response to therapy in patients with choriocarcinoma.

The value of measuring Regan isoenzyme in malignant effusions is demonstrated by two of our patients (M.O. and A.N.). The malignant nature of the effusions in these two patients was verified by the discovery of Regan isoenzyme in the effusion fluid at a concentration greater than that found in the serum. In patient M.O., who had metastatic carcinoma of the ovary, and in whom both ascites and bilateral pleural effusions were present, malignant cells were readily found in the pleural fluid. However, in the case of A.N., a man with carcinoma of the lung, the malignant nature of a pericardial effusion could not initially be determined since pericardiocentesis on two occasions did not reveal malignant cells. Malignant cells were identified in subsequent fluids. The malignant cells in the effusion fluid of both patients were found histochemically to be rich in an alkaline phosphatase that could be inhibited by L-phenylalanine. This finding strongly suggests that the malignant cells were indeed the source of the alkaline phosphatase present in the effusion fluids.

As has been mentioned earlier, when a patient with malignancy is found to have an elevated serum alkaline phosphatase, it is usually assumed that bone or liver metastases are present. This is not necessarily the case as shown by our first patient, P.R. This 30-year-old male with carcinoma of the lung was found

TABLE 7.

PATIENTS WITH REGAN ISOENZYME IN SERUM AND/OR TUMOR TISSUE

Primary Site of Tumor	No. of Patients	Total Alkaline Phosphatase > 15 K-A units	No. Patients With Metastasis to: Bone	Liver
Lung	4	4	2	1
Colon	4	4	0	4
Ovary	3	1	0	1
Endometrium	1	1	0	1
Breast	1	0	0	0
Multiple Myeloma	1	0	1	0
Primary Unknown	3	2	1	0
Total	17	12	4	7

TABLE 8

TUMOR TISSUE WITH NO REGAN ISOENZYME (BUTANOL EXTRACTS)

Primary Tumor Site	No. of Patients
Lung	6
Lymphoma	5
Colon	4
Kidney	3
Breast	2
Prostate	1
Bile Duct	1
Uterus	1

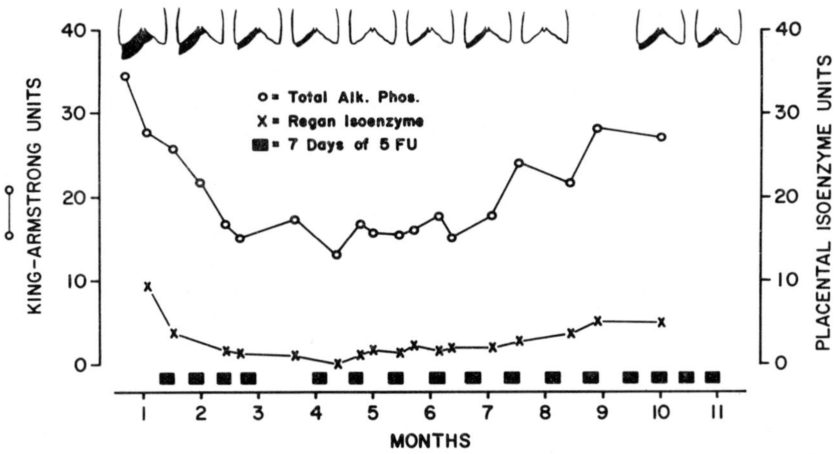

FIGURE 3. Levels of total alkaline phosphatase (in King-Armstrong units) and Regan isoenzyme (in placental isoenzyme units) in patient P.V. during therapy with 5-Fluorouracil. Changes in liver size during therapy are depicted at the top of the figure.

to have an elevated alkaline phosphatase when he was first admitted to the hospital and on that basis was suspected of having bone and/or liver metastases. However, the results of several bone surveys and liver chemistries (SGOT, SGPT, bilirubin, prothrombin time) remained within normal limits. At autopsy, no tumor could be found in the liver or spine. Even though this patient was found to have metastases to numerous organs, including adrenal, kidneys, spleen, brain and lymph nodes, there was no involvement of the organs usually implicated when an elevated serum alkaline phosphatase is present. Even though we have not yet found a patient with a localized malignancy whose serum alkaline phosphatase elevation is due only to Regan isoenzyme, it is quite probable that cases of this kind will be identified in the future, and that in such cases, removal of the tumor by surgery or treatment by radiation could result in cure.

An additional possible application of the measurement of Regan isoenzyme is in the study of patients who have no obvious residual tumor following surgery. To date, we have found one patient (D.P.), who had a radical mastectomy for carcinoma of the breast and who presently has no evidence of metastases by physical examination, metastatic bone survey and routine blood work, but whose serum contains Regan isoenzyme. We plan to observe this patient in order to correlate any rise in levels of Regan isoenzyme with the development of metastases, if and when they occur.

To summarize, the areas where measurement of Regan isoenzyme in serum can be useful are: (1) in following the course of disease in cancer patients, both with and without therapy; (2) in the identification of malignant pleural effusions; and (3) in clarifying the nature of unexplained elevations of serum alkaline phosphatase and possibly determining that patients may be curable by surgery even in the face of an elevated serum alkaline phosphatase.

In broader biologic terms, the presence in the tumor of an alkaline phosphatase isoenzyme that has the characteristics of placental alkaline phosphatase suggests that this is an additional example of the "ectopic" synthesis by tumor cells of a normal protein not usually produced by the tissue of tumor origin. In addition to the numerous examples of the "ectopic" synthesis by tumors of polypeptides, such as ADH, ACTH, parathormone, etc., there are now at least two examples of synthesis by malignant cells of proteins normally produced by fetal tissue but absent in later life. The first of these proteins is the carcinoembryonic antigen described by Gold[14] to be present in the tumor and serum of patients with carcinoma of the gastrointestinal tract, liver and pancreas. Normally an identical protein is present in these tissues in the fetus but disappears after birth. A second example of a fetal protein produced by tumor is that of the alpha fetoglobulin reported by Abelev *et al.*[15] to be present in the serum of certain patients with hepatoma or testicular tumors. Again, an identical protein is found in fetal liver but is absent in liver after birth. It is of some interest that Regan isoenzyme is not limited to just a few tumor types as is the case for these other proteins. In addition, it should be mentioned that placental alkaline phosphatase, which is the normal protein analogous to the Regan isoenzyme in tumors, is produced not by the fetus but rather by the placenta, and is present in the maternal rather than the fetal circulation.[16] The synthesis of each of the tumor proteins discussed is most likely the result of a common mechanism, namely, derepression of specific genomes in the tumor cell.

Summary

A combination of isoenzyme analysis techniques have been of considerable value in more accurately defining the sources of serum alkaline phosphatase in various diseases. One or more of these techniques has been useful in the following clinical situations:

1. Inhibition of alkaline phosphatase activity by L-phenylalanine, combined with the finding of a slow-moving enzyme band after starch gel electrophoresis, is characteristic of intestinal alkaline phosphatase. In a number of patients with hepatic cirrhosis, a significant amount of the total serum alkaline phosphatase can be identified as being of intestinal origin, and its presence was found to be genetically determined as it is in normal individuals.

2. Heat inactivation (55° C for 16 minutes) of serum alkaline phosphatase was determined in a group of patients with an elevated total serum alkaline phosphatase and tumor in bone or liver. In cancer patients with heat inactivation values of 80% or greater, bone disease should be strongly suspected, whereas heat inactivation levels of 70% or less suggest liver disease.

3. An isoenzyme originating in tumor cells (Regan isoenzyme) can be identified by (a) its heat stability (65° C for 5 minutes), (b) inhibition by L-phenylalanine, (c) characteristic migration location after starch gel electrophoresis, and (d) inhibition of electrophoretic migration by preincubation with a specific antiserum to placental alkaline phosphatase. Regan isoenzyme has been identified in the serum, effusion fluids and tumors of a number of patients with various malignancies.

References

1. FISHMAN, W. H., N. I. INGLIS, S. GREEN, C. L. ANSTISS, N. K. GHOSH, A. E. REIF, R. RUSTIGIAN, M. J. KRANT & L. L. STOLBACH. 1968. Immunology and biochemistry of Regan isoenzyme of alkaline phosphatase in human cancer. Nature (London) **219:** 697–699.

2. STOLBACH, L. L., M. J. KRANT, N. I. INGLIS & W. H. FISHMAN. 1967. Correlation of serum L-phenylalanine-sensitive alkaline phosphatase, derived from intestine, with the ABO blood group of cirrhotics. Gastroenterology **52:** 819–827.

3. BECKMAN, L. 1964. Associations between human serum alkaline phosphatases and blood groups. Acta Genet. (Basel) **14:** 286–297.
4. FISHMAN, W. H., S. GREEN & N. I. INGLIS. 1963. L-phenylalanine: an organ specific stereospecific inhibitor of human intestinal alkaline phosphatase. Nature (London) **198:** 685–686.
5. MOSS, D. W. & E. J. KING. 1962. Properties of alkaline phosphatase fractions separated by starch gel electrophoresis. Biochem. J. **84:** 192–195.
6. POSEN, S., F. C. NEALE & J. S. CLUBB. 1965. Heat inactivation in the study of human alkaline phosphatases. Ann. Intern. Med. **62:** 1234–1243.
7. CHANG, C., G. S. FISHER & J. VANDERLUGT. 1966. Alkaline phosphatase heat stability. J. Grace Hosp. **7:** 70–74.
8. FISHMAN, W. H., N. I. INGLIS & M. J. KRANT. 1965. Serum alkaline phosphatase of intestinal origin in patients with cancer and with cirrhosis of the liver. Clin. Chim. Acta **12:** 298–303.
9. FISHMAN, W. H. & S. GREEN. 1967. Automated differential isoenzyme analysis. I. L-phenylalanine-sensitive isoenzymes of human serum alkaline phosphatase. Enzymologia **33:** 89–99.
10. CLUBB, J. S., F. C. NEALE & S. POSEN. 1965. The behavior of infused human placental alkaline phosphatase in human subjects. J. Lab. Clin. Med. **66:** 493–507.
11. HILL, P. G. & H. G. SAMMONS. 1967. An interpretation of the elevation of serum alkaline phosphatase in disease. J. Clin. Path. **20:** 654–659.
12. FISHMAN, W. H. & N. K. GHOSH. 1967. *In* Advances in Clinical Chemistry. O. Bodansky & C. P. Stewart, Eds. **10:** Academic Press, Inc., New York, N. Y.
13. YONG, J. M. 1967. Origins of serum alkaline phosphatase. J. Clin. Path. **20:** 647–653.
14. GOLD, P. 1968. Carcinoembryonic antigens of the human digestive system. Cancer **20:** 1663–1667.
15. ABELEV, G. I., I. V. ASSECRITOVA, N. A. KRAEVSKY, S. D. PEROVA & N. I. PEREVODCHIKOVA. 1967. Embryonal serum globulin in cancer patients: diagnostic value. Int. J. Cancer **2:** 551–558.
16. MCMASTER, Y., R. TENNANT, J. S. CLUBB, F. C. NEALE & S. POSEN. 1964. The mechanism of the elevation of serum alkaline phosphatase in pregnancy. J. Obstet. Gynaec. Brit. Comm. **71:** 735–739.

Discussion of the Paper

B. K. BACHHAWAT: What I'd like to ask is, is it not possible that only a slight change in the carbohydrate portion of your alkaline phosphatase will give rise to all these variants? Will it not be possible to assess that way rather than to say there is a different type of protein involved? Because, as you know, if you have sialic acid-containing proteins, you'll get a different type of antigen, depending on the sugar present. I'll just suggest that the isoenzyme may be considered as a varient of alkaline phosphatase, the parent enzyme being the same.

D. HSIA (*Northwestern University, Chicago, Ill.*): I just wanted to make one comment. In the course of doing some surveys on polymorphisms in various genetically-determined diseases, we had the opportunity of surveying alkaline phosphatase in cystic fibrosis of the pancreas. And in this disease, which has an absorption defect, we found a marked deficiency of intestinal alkaline phosphatase in serum when the patients were on a normal diet as compared with controls. And the ABO blood group and secretor statuses of the cystic fibrosis patient were identical or similar, comparable to that of the normal controls in which we did these studies.

J. J. FENNELLY: Just a few comments. First of all, about the liver disease, there is one correlation we may find here between phenylalanine inhibition and liver disease. This is in relation to the lipid levels . . . because the highest phenylalanine inhibition I got was in a patient with a condition called Zieve's syndrome where the cholesterol is very high. The patient had a cholesterol of 900, and a very high phenylalanine inhibition.

I just wonder, in relation to this Regan isoenzyme, since you have so many essential resemblances in relation to the placental phosphatase, have you done chorionic gonadotrophins on the patients studied?

O. BODANSKY: We'll have these three questions answered.

L. L. STOLBACH: In regard to the first question about the sialic acid content in the explanation of the variance, it looks to us as if placental alkaline phosphatase and Regan isoenzyme have a number of similarities. The sialic acid content of the placental alkaline phosphatase and Regan isoenzyme, we believe, are probably the same. Now, whether this occurs because sialic acid is added to alkaline phosphatase that is already circulating is a possibility, but we would doubt it. And I think the immunologic data certainly does suggest that there is a derepressed protein rather than something that is formed subsequently. This is not an absolute thing, but this is our present working hypothesis.

In regard to some of the trophoblastic malignancies, we had the opportunity to study the tissue of one choriocarcinoma patient that did not contain the Regan isoenzyme. It did contain a heat labile alkaline phosphatase that was not inhibited by the antibody against placental alkaline phosphatase. And we've also had the opportunity to study the serum of one patient with choriocarcinoma and a few patients with testicular choriocarcinomas. And in none of these cases did we find the Regan isoenzyme.

I would say that I won't be surprised to find it in some cases, but it doesn't seem to be a universal phenomenon in patients with trophoblastic disease.

S. POSEN: I wonder if I could just make one plea, Sir. Out of this conference, one term is going to arise and get into the literature. I wonder whether we, as a group, ought to perpetuate this term, particularly in the singular, to talk about Regan isoenzyme, when almost certainly this is not going to be a single enzyme. Should we perhaps rather talk about placental-like alkaline phosphatase circulating in patients with tumors, rather than add yet another eponym to an already abundant collection?

DR. BODANSKY: I think we'll discuss that later. Personally, I agree with you.

CLINICAL APPLICATION OF PHOSPHOHYDROLASE MEASUREMENTS IN CANCER*

Morton K. Schwartz, Martin Fleisher and Oscar Bodansky

Sloan-Kettering Institute for Cancer Research and Memorial Hospital for Cancer and Allied Diseases, New York, N. Y.

The measurement of phosphohydrolase activity in body fluids and tissues of patients with cancer has been of interest for many years. Assays of serum acid and alkaline phosphatase and 5′-nucleotidase are useful tools in the diagnosis of certain forms of cancer and in following the course of the disease. In addition to determining total serum phosphohydrolase activity, attempts have been made to define more clearly the tissue of origin of these enzymes by utilizing specific chemical inhibitors, chromatographic or electrophoretic techniques, immunochemical reactions, heat denaturation and other physicochemical or kinetic properties. The purpose of this presentation is to review the clinical role of phosphohydrolase assays and to present additional data concerning means of differentiating phosphohydrolases of various normal and cancerous tissues.

Acid Phosphatase

Acid phosphatase measurements in serum have been used for many years as aids in the diagnosis of prostatic carcinoma. An earlier review of the literature by Bodansky[1] indicated that, in 282 of 349 cases of prostatic carcinoma with bony metastases, the serum acid phosphatase was elevated. In only 42 of 218 cases without metastases were abnormal values observed.

When β-glycerophosphate is used as substrate, elevations have rarely been observed in other than prostatic disease. In a series of 878 patients without prostatic disease, Woodard[2] reported elevations of serum acid β-glycerophosphatase activity in only seven patients; three with osteogenic sarcoma, two with plasma cell myeloma, one with Paget's disease and one with a nonspecific inflammatory bone disease. Bases[3] has reported serum β-glycerophosphatase levels as high as 5 times the upper limit of normal in 9 of 16 patients with chronic granulocytic leukemia or myeloid metaplasia. The values appeared to be correlated with the white cell or platelet count.

When orthophosphate esters other than β-glycerophosphate, such as phenylphosphate, are used as substrate, elevations in nonprostatic disease are more common. Reynolds *et al.*[4] found elevations in 74% of patients with metastatic breast disease and about 25% of patients with nonneoplastic disease. When the same substrate was used, 11 of 12 patients with Gaucher's disease showed elevated acid phosphatase, but only 3 of these patients had elevated activity when β-glycerophosphate was used.[5]

In an effort to define the elevations of serum acid phosphatase more specifically, Fishman and Lerner[6] have utilized the finding of Abdul-Fadl and King[7] that L-tartrate inhibits acid phosphatase from prostate, but not from other tissues. In early studies, Fishman *et al.*,[8,9] reported that 21 of 26 patients without metastases, or 81% had elevations of the "prostatic" fraction, but only 4, or 15%, of these patients had elevations of the total serum acid phosphatase. In a more

* This work was supported in part by grant CA–08748 from the National Cancer Institute, National Institutes of Health, and grant T–431J from the American Cancer Society.

recent study by Green *et al.*,[10] 44 of 45 cases of prostatic carcinoma demonstrated elevated "prostatic" acid phosphatase, whereas only 24 of the 45 cases had elevated total activity. Green *et al.*[11] evaluated L-tartrate-sensitive serum acid phosphatase determinations done routinely in a series of 918 patients. Of 454 patients in this series whose medical history was available for review, 14 of 34 patients with prostatic carcinoma, 2 of 90 with benign prostatic hypertrophy, 15 of 76 with other forms of cancer and 23 patients without cancer had elevations of serum-tartrate-sensitive acid phosphatase.

Babson *et al.*[12] have recommended the use of α-naphthyl phosphate as substrate for acid phosphatase assays. Their suggestion is based on studies of the relative velocity of activity of prostatic and erythrocytic acid phosphatase with phenylphosphate, phenolphthalein phosphate, *p*-nitrophenyl phosphate, β-naphthyl phosphate, β-glycerophosphate and α-naphthyl phosphate.[13]

These authors found that the ratio for the activities of prostatic to erythrocytic acid phosphatase was highest when α-naphthyl phosphate was used as substrate. This ratio was twice as high as that obtained when β-glycerophosphate was used, and 40 to 100 times that with the other substrates. Green *et al.*[10] utilized this finding and compared in serum the ratio of serum acid phosphatase activity

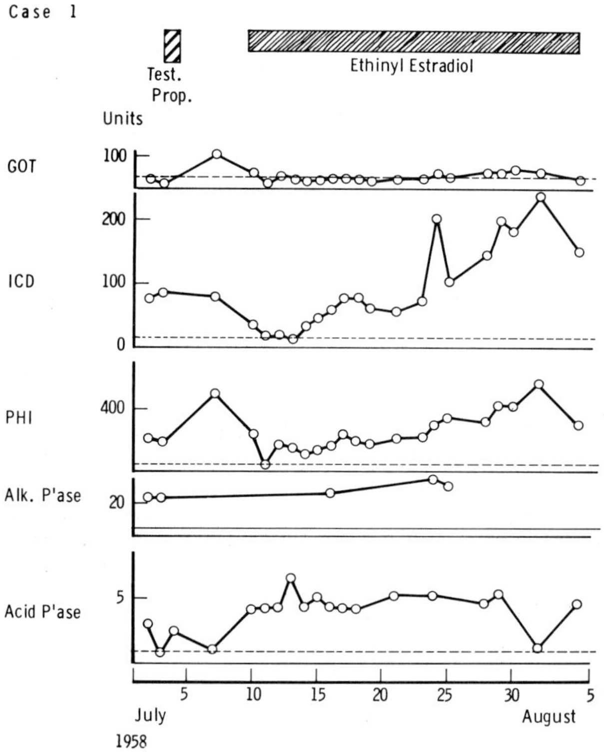

FIGURE 1. Sequential determinaiton of serum acid phosphatase (bottom) and other enzymes in a patient with prostatic carcinoma. GOT = glutamic oxaloacetic transaminase; ICD = isocitric dehydrogenase; PHI = phosphohexose isomerase. (Reproduced, with permission, from Cancer **16:** 583.[14])

TABLE 1

EVALUATION OF SERUM ALKALINE PHOSPHATASE IN TUMORS OF BONE

Disease	Number of Cases	Percentage of Cases Having Values In:				
		Normal Range	1.1 to 1.9 × Normal Range	2.0 to 3.9 × Normal Range	4.0 to 6.0 × Normal Range	6.0 × Normal Range
Osteogenic Sarcoma[16]						
a) Blastic	18	0	39	39	11	11
b) Lytic	16	50	25	19	6	0
Parathyroid Cancer[20,21,40]	39	3	15	20	31	31
Metastatic Breast Cancer[15–17]	40	23	53	18	3	5
Metastatic Prostate Cancer[15–17]	29	14	35	17	10	24
Multiple Myeloma[15,19,20]	23	57	44	0	0	0

with α-naphthyl phosphate and phenylphosphate as substrates. Purified prostatic acid phosphatase gave a ratio of 1.36 and liver acid phosphatase, 0.63. Serum from patients with prostatic carcinoma had elevated ratios, i.e., between 1.16 and 1.56. Of 38 patients without prostatic carcinoma and elevated acid phosphatase, 7 showed elevated ratios and 24 had ratios in the liver range of 0.63 or lower.

Levels of serum acid phosphatase frequently do not represent the status of disease, and in many instances do not reflect the progression or regression of metastases.[14] This appears particularly true of patients receiving hormonal therapy. The lack of responsiveness of acid phosphatase to the extent and status of prostatic disease was reported by Schwartz *et al.*[14] FIGURE 1 shows the serum acid phosphatase data, and that of other serum enzymes, in a patient with prostatic carcinoma who had had a suprapubic prostatectomy and orchiectomy seven years before this study, and a hypophysectomy two months before. Despite widespread bony metastases, severe episodes of pain and a rapidly enlarging liver reflected by crescendo-like increases in isocitric dehydrogenase and phosphohexose isomerase, the acid phosphatase remained essentially at about 4 U during the entire period.

Alkaline Phosphatase

Total serum alkaline phosphatase activity has been elevated in the serum of patients with diseases of the bone and bone-forming tissues and those affecting the structural or functional integrity of the liver. Cancers involving bone include primary tumors, such as osteogenic sarcoma, parathyroid adenomas or carcinoma, and those neoplasms, such as carcinoma of breast or prostate, that metastasize to bone. Alkaline phosphatase levels in patients with bone disease are summarized in TABLE 1.

In primary tumors of the bone, serum alkaline phosphatase activity is elevated when the tumor is predominantly osteoblastic. In cases of osteogenic sarcoma of the osteoblastic type, the serum level appears to parallel the growth of the tumor, and has been reported elevated to levels as high as 40 times the upper limit of normal.[15,16] In other primary malignant tumors of the bone, such as Ewing's tumor, giant cell tumor and chondrosarcoma, normal or slightly elevated values are obtained, and normal values are found in benign tumors of the bone such as osteomas and chondromas.[16,17] In multiple myeloma, it has been reported that 13 of 45 cases had abnormal serum alkaline phosphatase, and most abnormal values were less than four times the upper limit of normal.[18,19]

Alkaline phosphatase was elevated in the serum of 38 of 39 patients (97%) with adenomas or carcinomas of the parathyroid.[20,21] These elevations in most patients were above 20 Bodansky units. Sixty percent of the patients had elevations greater than four times the upper limit of normal. In patients with carcinoma metastatic to bone, elevations in serum alkaline phosphatase are observed when the metastatic lesion is osteoblastic. Since most cases of bony metastases in breast carcinoma are chiefly osteolytic, alkaline phosphatase levels are usually in the normal range or slightly elevated.[22,23] In prostatic carcinoma, the opposite is true, and most bony metastatic lesions are osteoblastic. Hence, the serum alkaline phosphatase is usually elevated to values between 15 and 40 Bodansky units.[22]

In patients with carcinoma metastatic to bone and elevated alkaline phosphatase activity, there is occasionally an increase in activity following favorable response to therapy.[23] FIGURE 2 shows sequential alkaline phosphatase determinations in such a patient. This represents data on a 64-year-old man diagnosed as having carcinoma of the prostate 18 months prior to the present study. In that period, he had undergone a transurethral resection, bilateral orchiectomy and a hypophysectomy. On roentgenological examination, he showed generalized bone metastases to nearly all bones, primarily of an osteoblastic nature. He was admitted to the hospital at the time of the study because of weakness and increasing pain. Between early February and early March, the patient experienced clinical signs of remission, and, in general, the pain disappeared. During this period, the serum alkaline phosphatase rose and reached a level of 54 U. On March 4, the administration of ethinyl estradiol was started. The patient's condition worsened, and he experienced severe pain. The rise in alkaline phosphatase was interpreted as the initial phase of a reparative process of bone, and the latter

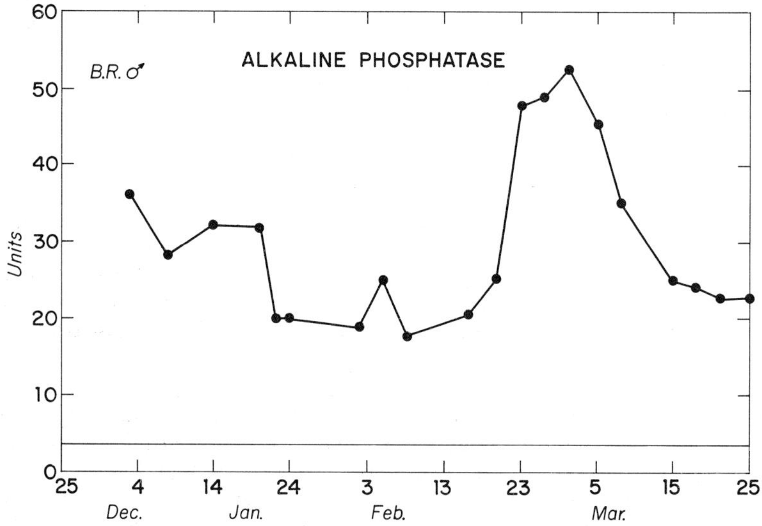

FIGURE 2. Sequential serum alkaline phosphatase determinations in a patient with prostatic carcinoma. The line at 4 U. indicates the upper limit of normal.

decrease indicative of the latter stages of skeletal healing. The fact that the serum alkaline phosphatase did not reach a lower level than 20 U. may be due to the presence and growth of liver metastasis at that time.

Elevations of serum alkaline phosphatase are often found in patients with extrahepatic obstruction of the biliary tract by carcinoma or carcinoma metastatic to the liver, regardless of the primary site of the tumor. Gutman[24] has reported elevations to more than twice the upper limit of normal in 141 of 150 cases of extrahepatic obstruction. Mendelsohn and Bodansky[25] found elevations in 39 of 50 patients with intrahepatic metastasis proved by direct visualization and biopsy. The highest value was 64.8 Bodansky units, or 16 times the upper limit of normal. The extent of elevation was directly related to the degree of intrahepatic involvement. Seventeen of the 50 patients who had a nonpalpable liver had a mean alkaline phosphatase of 4.8 U. Ten patients with livers palpable at the costal margin had a mean value of about 7 U. Twenty-three patients with liver palpable to the level of the umbilicus and below, had a mean alkaline phosphatase value of about 12 U.

In our laboratory, alkaline phosphatase activity in a number of normal and tumor tissues has been determined, and the isozyme pattern of these tissues examined using the starch gel technique of Smithies[26] and a diazotization staining technique with β-naphthyl phosphate as substrate.[27] The tissues were homogenized in a glass-teflon, motor-driven homogenizer in the proportion of one part by weight of tissue to nine parts of water and then the enzyme solubilized with *n*-butanol as described by Ahmen and King.[28] Enzyme activity was determined by measuring the inorganic phosphorus liberated in a reaction mixture containing, per ml: 5 μmoles of β-naphthylphosphate, 10 μmoles Mg^{++}, 100 μmoles Tris buffer adjusted to pH 9.4 and 0.1 ml of the phosphatase extract, equivalent to 10 mg extracted tissue. The unit of phosphatase activity was defined as the μmoles of β-naphthylphosphate hydrolyzed per minute at 37° under the above described conditions. The activity is that of 10 mg wet weight of tissue.

Starch gel electrophoresis was determined with 0.04 ml of the butanol extract of the tissue in each slot. The isozyme pattern of normal liver was utilized as a standard and was determined concurrently with the pattern of butanol-treated homogenates of other tissues. In general, the pattern of the normal liver was similar to that obtained by Moss *et al.*,[27] namely, two thin lines quite near the cathode and a rapidly migrating heavy anionic band. Some variability from day to day occurred in the pattern of the standard butanol extract of the normal liver, and this is understandable considering the inherent difficulty in preparing the same type of starch gel from day to day.

The problem of sensitivity of the starch gel technique is illustrated in FIGURE 3. The slots are at the bottom of the figure. In slot 1 was placed an aliquot of a butanol extract of normal human liver containing 5.31 U of phosphatase activity and three bands are visible, the very dark anionic band and two bands near the origin, the faster one being fainter. In slots 2 through 5 are water dilutions of the butanol extract containing 2.66, 1.33, 0.66 and 0.33 U of phosphatase activity. The bands become fainter; by slot 3, the third band is not visible, and by slot 5, the second band is barely visible. It is also of interest that the bands migrate more rapidly in the more dilute solutions.

The mean phosphatase activity of five specimens of normal adult human liver was 5.4 U with an average deviation of 0.72 U. Liver from a 30-hour-old infant had an activity of 1.5 U. TABLE 2 shows the activity of the normal liver tissues and various specimens of abnormal liver. The hepatoma, the poorly differentiated adenocarcinoma, and the normal liver from an infant all demonstrated such less activity than the other tissues.

FIGURE 4 shows the electrophoretic pattern of the normal liver standard and the liver specimen containing metastases from an insuloma. The activities of the extracts per 0.04 ml were as follows: normal liver (slot 1), 5.5 U; abnormal liver (slots 4 and 5), 6.0 U; parotid tumor (slots 2 and 3), 0.13 U. The activity of the parotid tumor was too low to permit visualization, and the patterns of the normal liver and the liver containing metastatic insuloma are quite similar.

A primary hepatoma, a poorly differentiated liver adenocarcinoma, and normal liver tissue from an infant demonstrated less activity than the adult normal liver (TABLE 2). On electrophoretic examination of butanol extracts of the hepatoma, the adenocarcinoma and the infant's liver, a rapidly moving anodic band similar

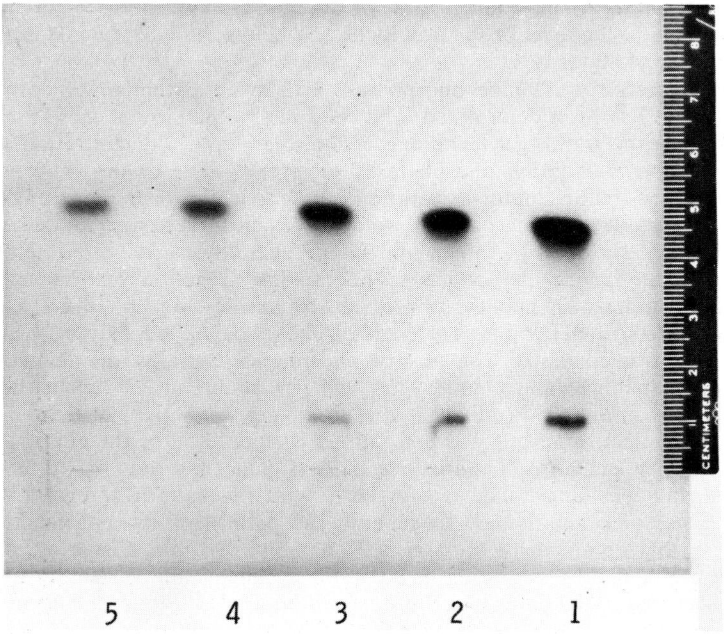

FIGURE 3. Starch gel electrophoresis of dilutions of a butanol extract of normal human liver. The activities are as follows: Slot 1, 5.31 U; slot 2, 2.66 U; slot 3, 1.33 U; slot 4, 0.67 U; and slot 5, 0.33 U.

TABLE 2

ALKALINE PHOSPHATASE IN NORMAL AND ABNORMAL HUMAN LIVER

Liver Tissue	Activity (Units)
Normal Adults	5.4 ± 0.72*
Newborn (30-hr) Infant	1.49
Metastatic Insuloma	7.52
Infiltrative Leukemia (1½-yr-old)	7.87
Primary Hepatoma	0.54
Adenocarcinoma	1.21

* Average deviation of five specimens.

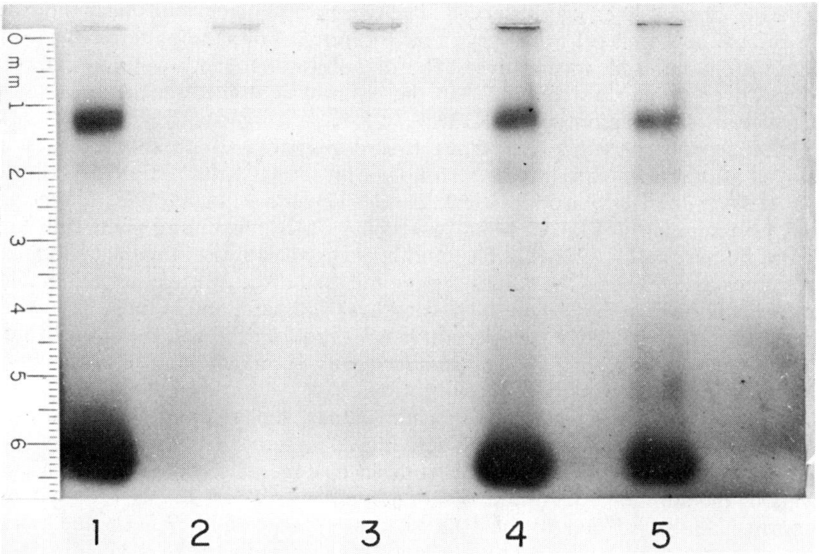

FIGURE 4. Starch gel electrophoresis of normal liver (slot 1), metastatic insuloma (slots 4 and 5), parotid tumor (slots 2 and 3).

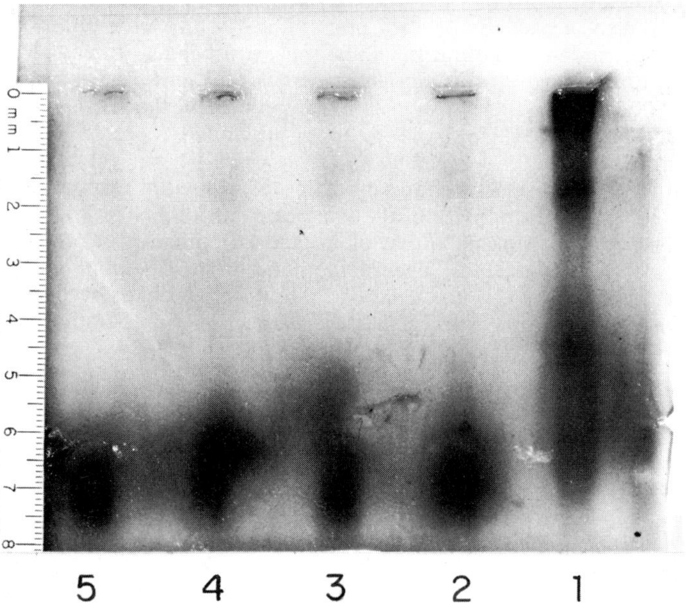

FIGURE 5. Starch gel electrophoresis of normal liver (slot 1), and, in the other slots, a poorly differentiated adenocarcinoma of the liver.

to that of normal liver was observed. The two normal liver bands near the cathodic end of the starch gel were very faint. FIGURE 5 shows the patterns of the liver adenocarcinoma and normal liver. The first slot contained a butanol extract of normal liver with an activity of 5.2 U; the last four contained the adenocarcinoma of the liver whose activity was 1.2 U.

The activities of other cancerous tissues prepared as butanol extracts and assayed as described earlier were as follows: breast (16), 0.42 ± 0.25 U; thyroid (4), 0.99 ± 0.16 U; parotid (3), 0.25 ± 0.17 cervix (1), 0.69 U; tongue (1), 0.68 U; rectum (1) 1.06 U; leiomyosarcoma (1), 0.76 U and giant cell tumor of the humerus (1), 5.26 U. The numbers in parentheses are the numbers of specimens assayed, and the values are the mean and the average deviation. These tumors had lower activity than the normal liver standard, and in those cases where there was sufficient activity to permit visualization on the gel, the broad anionic band similar to the normal liver standard was observed. However, the fainter cationic bands were usually not seen.

TABLE 3 shows the activity of normal kidney and adrenal, and three tumor tissues that gave outstandingly high activities. The tumor tissues included a specimen of lung containing metastases from an osteogenic sarcoma, 55 U; a carcinoma of the adrenal, 132 U, and a seminoma of the testes, 127 U. Adrenal from a normal adult had activity of 10.8 U; that from a child, 7.5 U; and normal kidney, a mean value of 1.8 U with an average deviation of 0.41 U.

The electrophoretic pattern of the osteogenic sarcoma metastatic to lung is shown in FIGURE 6. Slot 1 contained a butanol extract of normal human liver with an activity of 5.2 U; slots 2 and 3, and lung specimen with an activity of 55 U; and slots 4 and 5, a 1:1 water dilution of that specimen. The metastasis in lung showed an extra band midway between the two small cationic and the large anionic bands of the normal liver preparation. The lung tumor pattern was not similar to that of a partially purified preparation[29] of alkaline phosphatase from an osteogenic sarcoma that did not show the extra band. In an effort to characterize this tumor further, the inhibitory effects of L-histidine were studied. At pH 9.5, 0.002 M histidine showed 26% inhibition and 0.001 M histidine, 21% inhibition. These values are similar to those previously reported for the enzyme purified from bone.[29]

FIGURE 7 gives the electrophoretic pattern of a butanol extract from a seminoma of the testes. The activity of the seminoma in slot 2 is 24.4 U and in slot 3, 2.4 U. The pattern is similar to that of a standard human liver preparation with an activity of 6.9 U, in slot 1. The anodic band of the seminoma, which is very dense and large (slot 2), is not separated into different bands even when diluted tenfold (slot 3). Of further interest is the pattern of a preparation of fibroade-

TABLE 3

ALKALINE PHOSPHATASE IN HUMAN TISSUES

Tissue	Activity (Units)
Kidney (Normal)	1.8 ± 0.41*
Adrenal (Normal Adult)	10.8
Adrenal (Normal Child)	7.5
Osteogenic Sarcoma Metastasis to Lung	55
Adrenal Carcinoma	132
Seminoma Testis	127

* Average deviation of three specimens.

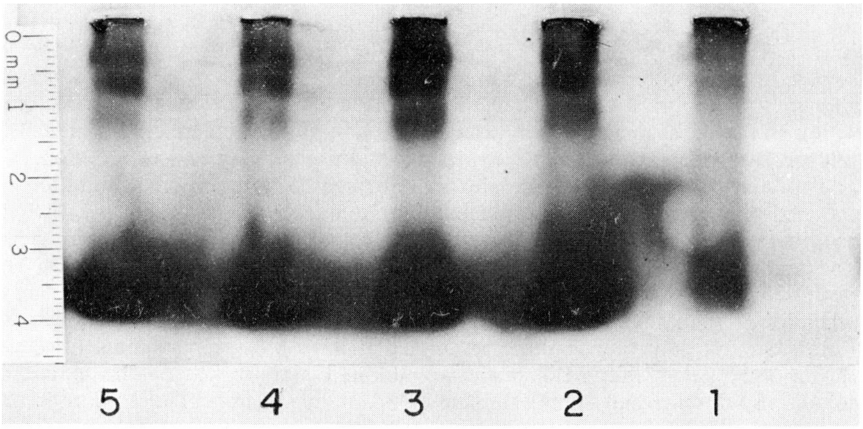

FIGURE 6. Electrophoretic pattern of normal liver (slot 1), of undiluted extract of osteogenic sarcoma metastasis in lung (slots 2 and 3), and of 1:1 water dilution of lung specimen (slots 4 and 5).

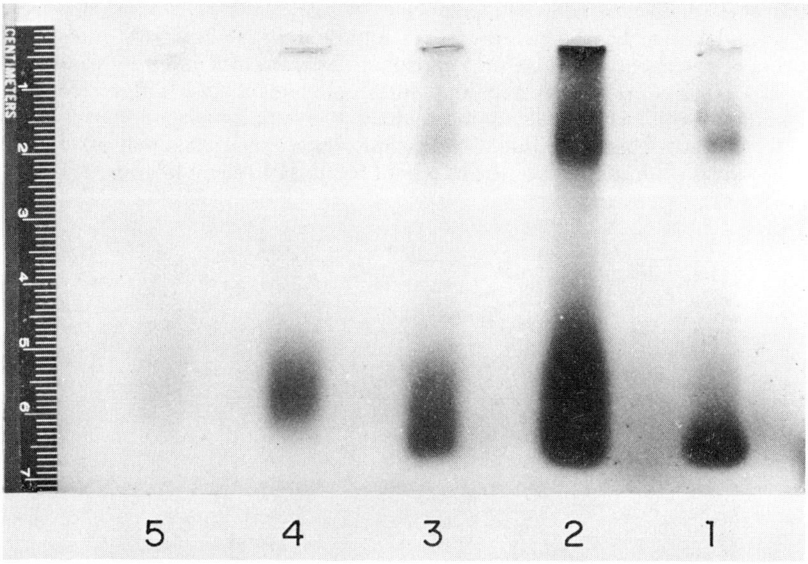

FIGURE 7. Starch gel electrophoresis of normal liver (slot 1), of seminoma of the testes (slots 2 and 3), of fibroadenoma of the breast (slot 4) and of parotid tumor (slot 5).

noma of the breast (1.8 U) in slot 4, and a tumor of the parotid (0.57 U) in slot 5. The cationic components are not visible in the patterns of these tissues. However, it must be kept in mind that the activity of these specimens was much lower than that of the standard.

The electrophoretic pattern of an unusual adrenal carcinoma with high phosphatase activity is shown in FIGURE 8.* The adrenal preparation at dilutions of

* We wish to thank Dr. Frederick L. Nichols of Hartford Hospital, Hartford, Conn., for making this tissue available to us.

44 U in slot 1, 13.2 U in slot 2 and 6.1 U in slot 3, was most similar to that of liver with an activity of 4.9 U in slot 5. The adrenal phosphatase did not resemble normal adult kidney with an activity of 2.2 U in slot 4. Other studies not shown in the figure indicated that the cancerous adrenal, which had more than 10 times the activity of normal adrenal, had a similar electrophoretic pattern to phosphatase preparations from normal adrenal tissue of a child or an adult.

The relationships of pH and L-histidine or sodium taurocholate inhibition on the phosphatase from the adrenal carcinoma were studied, and are shown in FIGURE 9. In order to compare these data with that obtained previously for other phosphatases, 0.015 M sodium β-glycerophosphate was used as substrate. The optimal pH of the adrenal carcinoma phosphatase, pH 8.7, seemed to be somewhat lower than that for other human tissue phosphatases.[29] Inhibition by L-histidine or sodium taurocholate resembled that with bone phosphatase.[29,30] At the optimal pH, 0.002 M L-histidine inhibited activity 40%. The extent of inhibition fell off rapidly on either side of this point. With 0.01 M sodium taurocholate at pH 8.7, 47% of the activity was inhibited. At the optimal pH, 0.002 M L-histidine has been reported to inhibit bone phosphatase about 45% and intestinal phosphatase, 19%.[29] Taurocholate inhibits human bone phosphatase about 38%, and human kidney phosphatase, about 31%, but has no effect on human intestinal phosphatase (TABLE 4).[30]

L-phenylalanine has been reported to inhibit phosphatase from intestine and placenta to the extent of 80%, and phosphatases from other sources to the extent of about 10 to 15%.[31] The fact that intestinal phosphatase differs from other phosphatases was demonstrated more than 30 years ago by Bodansky,[30] who found that bile acids inhibited bone phosphatase but not that of intestine. TABLE 4 gives a comparison of the effects of 0.005 M L-phenylalanine and 0.01 M

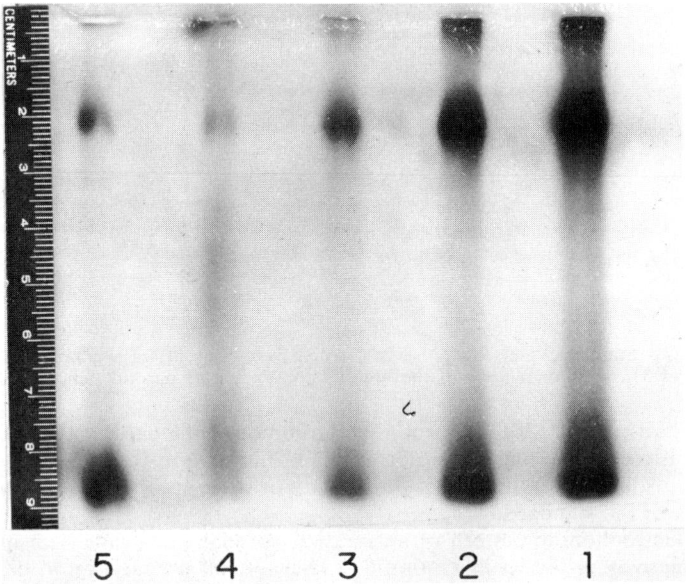

FIGURE 8. Electrophoretic pattern of normal liver (slot 5), of normal kidney (slot 4), and of an adrenal carcinoma (slots 1, 2 and 3).

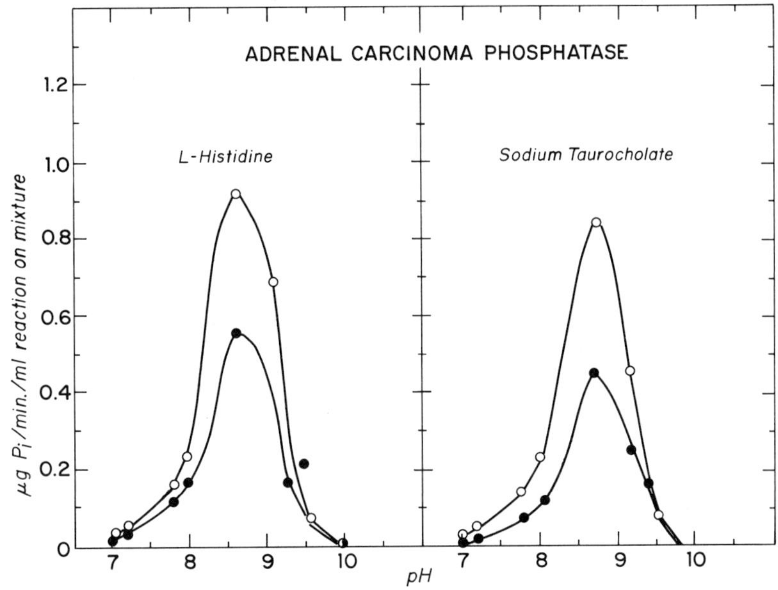

FIGURE 9. Influence of pH on the inhibition of adrenal carcinoma phosphatase by 0.002 M L-histidine (left side) and by 0.01 M sodium taurocholate (right side). The final concentrations were 0.015 M β-glycerophosphate, 0.01 M Mg^{++} and 0.08 M Tris buffer. Velocities without inhibitor are designated ○——○; those with 0.002 M L-histidine or 0.01 M sodium taurocholate are designated ●——●.

TABLE 4

EFFECTS OF L-PHENYLALANINE AND TAUROCHOLATE ON PURIFIED HUMAN PHOSPHATASES*

Tissue	0.005 M L-Phenylalanine (% Inhibition)	0.01 M Taurocholate (% Inhibition)
Kidney	38	31
Intestine	75	−7
Liver	—	50
Bone†	24	38
Normal Serums	28	37

* Values represent the averages of at least three replicate experiments.
† Osteogenic sarcoma.

sodium taurocholate on partially purified phosphatases from human tissues,[29] as well as on alkaline phosphatase in normal serum. Sodium β-glycerophosphate was used as substrate. It is of interest that L-phenylalanine and taurocholate inhibit human bone phosphatase 24% and 38%, respectively. This inhibition is almost identical to that observed in the serum of normal persons. Phenylalanine inhibition of intestinal phosphatase exhibits species differences. Human intestinal phosphatase was inhibited 75%, rat intestinal phosphatase, 60% and guinea pig intestinal phosphatase, only 32%.

As indicated in TABLE 4, the mean inhibition by 0.005 M L-phenylalanine of serum alkaline phosphate in 11 normal individuals was 28% (S.D. ± 6%) and that by 0.01 M taurocholate in 12 normal persons 37% (S.D. ± 5%). When limits of the mean ± 2.5 S.D. are used, the normal range of phenylalanine inhibition is 13 to 43% and that of taurocholate, 25 to 47%.

TABLE 5 lists inhibitions by both 0.005 M L-phenylalanine and 0.01 M sodium taurocholate of serum alkaline phosphatase activity in patients with cancer and elevated serum alkaline phosphatase. In 17 other patients not listed in the table, who presumably had liver disease indicated by clinical findings and elevations in both serum alkaline phosphatase and 5′-nucleotidase, the extent of phenylalanine inhibition ranged from 18 to 41% with a mean value of 27%. Our data indicate that the inhibition of alkaline phosphatase by L-phenylalanine or taurocholate in the serum of normal individuals and in the serum of patients with cancer and liver disease do not differ significantly.

5′-Nucleotidase

Serum 5′-nucleotidase, a specific phosphohydrolase that catalyzes the liberation of inorganic phosphorus from 5′-nucleotides, has been reported by several investigators to be elevated in various types of liver disease, but to remain within normal limits in skeletal disease.[32,33] We have previously reported that the determination of serum 5′-nucleotidase activity can be useful in determining the presence or absence of liver disease in a patient with an elevated serum alkaline phosphatase activity and in following the progression of liver metastases.[24]

We have determined serum 5′-nucleotidase in our laboratory by using Ni^{++} inhibition of 5′-nucleotidase according to a modification of the method proposed by Campbell.[35] The assumption upon which this method is based is that Ni^{++} inhibits 5′-nucleotidase but not the nonspecific phosphatases. This assumption is not completely justified in the sense that bone and liver phosphatases are inhibited about 70% by 0.01 M Ni^{++}, the concentration used in the assay. The activity of bone phosphatase at pH 7.5, the optimal pH of 5′-nucleotidase is 4% of that observed at the phosphatase optimal pH of 9.5.[36] A patient with an elevated alkaline phosphatase of 100 U, all of which came from bone, would contribute 4 U of activity at pH 7.5, and only 70% of this would be inhibited by Ni^{++}. Therefore, the contribution of nonspecific phosphatase activity in the 5′-nucleotidase assay would be 2.8 U. At pH 7.5, with 0.005 M adenosine 5′-phos-

TABLE 5

EFFECTS OF 0.005 M L-PHENYLALANINE AND 0.01 M TAUROCHOLATE ON SERUM ALKALINE PHOSPHATASE ACTIVITY IN PATIENTS WITH CANCER

Case	Primary Diagnosis	Alkaline Phosphatase Activity (Bodansky Units)	Percent Inhibition	
			L-Phenylalanine	Taurocholate
1	Primary Hepatoma	22	26	56
2	Breast	37	25	48
3	Breast	14	28	33
4	Colon	30	25	50
5	Prostate	27	19	39
6	Rectum	13	16	52
7	Colon	29	21	—
8	Testes	29	30	—
9	Colon	24	41	—
10	Breast	16	11	—
11	Common Bile Duct or Pancreas	17	11	—

TABLE 6

SERUM ALKALINE PHOSPHATASE AND 5′-NUCLEOTIDASE ACTIVITIES IN 117 SPECIMENS FROM PATIENTS WITH CLINICALLY DIAGNOSED LIVER INVOLVEMENT

Level of Serum		Number of Specimens Analyzed	Percent of Total
Alkaline Phosphatase	5′-Nucleotidase		
Normal	Normal	37	32
Elevated	Elevated	51	43
Elevated	Normal	6	5
Normal	Elevated	23	20
	Total	117	

phate as substrate, the following inhibitions of purified human phosphatases by 0.01 M Ni^{++} were observed: intestine, 0%; kidney, 0%; bone, 70%; liver, 75%.

Despite this limitation in the method, 5′-nucleotidase activity measured in this was elevated in the serum of cancer patients with hepatobiliary disease. There did not appear to be a strict correlation between 5′-nucleotidase and other biochemical parameters of liver involvement. Sequential determinations of 5′-nucleotidase were helpful in following the course of cancer metastatic to the liver.[34] The classical method of utilizing the serum 5′-nucleotidase assay is illustrated by the following data in a patient with metastatic cancer of the colon. Upon skeletal survey this patient had widespread bony metastases. His bromsulphalein retention was 7%; total bilirubin, 0.4 mg per 100 ml; alkaline phosphatase, 24 BU; and the liver was not plapable. However, his serum 5′-nucleotidase was elevated to 68 U, or 6 times the upper limit of normal. At autopsy, he was found to have metastases to the liver.

On numerous occasions we have noted elevations of serum 5′-nucleotidase in patients at a time when the alkaline phosphatase was within normal limits. During a period of two months. 117 specimens of serum were submitted to the Department of Biochemistry by physicians suspecting hepatic disease and requesting determinations of both serum alkaline phosphatase and 5′-nucleotidase. TABLE 6 shows that 37 specimens had normal values for alkaline phosphatase and 5′-nucleotidase, 51 had elevations of both enzymes, six had normal 5′-nucleotidase and elevated serum alkaline phosphatase, and 23 had an elevated 5′-nucleotidase and a normal alkaline phosphatase. Thus, of 80 patients with elevations of either or both enzymes, 23 (30%) had an elevation of 5′-nucleotidase when the alkaline phosphatase was normal.

It was possible to review the medical histories of 20 of these 23 patients, and their data is listed in TABLE 7. Four of these 20 patients had posttransfusion serum hepatitis, and two had drug-induced hepatitis. In addition to abnormal levels of 5′-nucleotidase, these six patients had elevations in glutamic oxaloacetic transaminase, and in four of the six patients, elevations in total bilirubin (cases 1, 2, 5 and 6). In cases 1 and 2, elevated alkaline phosphatase activity had been observed in earlier specimens, and it can be concluded that in these two patients the serum alkaline phosphatase returned to normal before the 5′-nucleotidase. In four of a group of five patients with reticulum cell sarcoma, lymphosarcoma, or Hodgkins disease the elevated 5′-nucleotidase value was the only biochemical indication of liver disease (patients 7, 8, 10 and 11, TABLE 7). In the fifth patient of this group

TABLE 7

5′-NUCLEOTIDASE ACTIVITY IN SERUM OF PATIENTS WITH NORMAL LEVELS OF ALKALINE PHOSPHATASE

Patient Number	Primary Diagnosis	Secondary Diagnosis	Alkaline Phosphatase (Units)	5′-Nuc. (Units)	GOT (Units)	Bilirubin (mg/100 ml)	BSP retention (%)	Enlargement of Liver*	Presence of Metastasis by Autopsy (A) or Biopsy (B)
1	Hodgkins	Serum Hepatitis	2.2	39	67	0.53	—	—	B
2	Vocal cord-tongue	Serum Hepatitis	3.4	15	1150	5.1	—	—	—
3	Conus Medularis	Serum Hepatitis	2.8	13	101	0.42	—	2+	Neg. B
4	Cervix	Serum Hepatitis	3.4	23	125	3.24	—	—	—
5	?	Drug-Induced Hepatitis	3.1	17	154	1.05	25	—	Neg. B
6	Acute Leukemia	Drug-Induced Hepatitis	1.9	18	51	1.33	—	1+	—
7	Reticulum Cell Sarcoma	—	3.4	15	36	0.33	4	2+	—
8	Reticulum Cell Sarcoma	—	3.5	15	44	0.37	—	—	A
9	Reticulum Cell Sarcoma	Porta Hepatitis Involvement	2.1	132	246	7.2	30	—	A-tumor porta hepatitis, partial obstruction, common bile duct 2° edema. No tumor in liver.

10	Lymphosarcoma	Bone Metastasis	3.1	16	26	0.23	—	2+	—
11	Hodgkins	—	3.9	14	48	0.33	—	—	—
12	Breast	—	1.9	20	50	—	11	2+	—
13	Breast	Pleural Effusion	2.6	40	45	1.26	21	3+	—
14	Breast	—	2.9	21	49	0.26	—	2+	—
15	Breast	Pleural Effusion	3.1	25	112	0.25	—	—	—
16	Ovary	—	3.4	37	—	—	—	—	A
17	Cervix	—	4.0	14	52	0.23	7	1+	—
18	Sigmoid	Acute Renal Failure	2.5	13	63	0.81	20	—	—
19	Ewing's Sarcoma	—	3.3	14	88	0.56	16	0	—
20	Lung	? Cirrhosis 2° alcohol	1.8	18	77	1.64	—	—	B

* In evaluating the chart notes of clinical enlargement of the liver, 1+ indicates enlargement down to 2 cm below the costal margin; 2+ is enlargement from 2 to 4 cm; 3+ is 4 to 6 cm; 4+ is enlargement beyond 6 cm. Dash (—) indicates that clinical examination of the liver was not recorded.

(9, TABLE 7), the 5′-nucleotidase was elevated to 11 times the upper limit of normal, and the patient had an elevation of transaminase, bilirubin and bromsulphalein retention. At autopsy, tumor was found in the porta hepatis, and there was partial obstruction of the common bile duct, presumably because of edema. No tumor was found in the liver.

Of the four patients with breast carcinoma, it is of interest that in two cases (13 and 15, TABLE 7) pleural effusion with possible compression of the liver was reported. In patient 14 of this group, jaundice and elevation of bilirubin to 8.0 mg per 100 ml, of transaminase to 414 U, and of alkaline phosphatase to 22.5 BU occurred three weeks after the first reported elevation of 5′-nucleotidase.

There have been several reports in the literature[33,37] that elevations of serum 5′-nucleotidase and alkaline phosphatase parallel each other in hepatic disease, and that alkaline phosphatase is more frequently elevated.[38,39] Our data indicate, in a patient population with hepatic disease as represented by that of Memorial Hospital, that 5′-nucleotidase is more frequently elevated than alkaline phosphatase. There is much greater frequency of 5′-nucleotidase elevation with normal alkaline phosphatase than of the reverse situation, elevated alkaline phosphatase with normal 5′-nucleotidase. However, to insure maximum diagnostic aid, both serum enzyme determinations should be carried out.

Summary

We have presented data concerning alkaline phosphatase activity in normal and cancerous human tissue and the possible differences in these tissue phosphatases when studied by starch gel electrophoresis or with specific inhibitors, including L-phenylalanine, L-histidine and sodium taurocholate. The clinical biochemical significance of the assay of total serum acid and alkaline phosphatases, and of 5′-nucleotidase, in patients with cancer has been reviewed.

References

1. BODANSKY, O. 1960. Enzymes in Tumor growth with special reference to serum enzymes in cancer. *In* Enzymes in Health and Disease. D. A. Greenberg & H. A. Harper, Eds. : 269–330. Charles C. Thomas, Springfield, Ill.
2. WOODARD, H. G. 1959. Clinical significance of serum acid phosphatase. Amer. J. Med. **27**: 902.
3. BASES, R. 1962. Elevation of serum acid phosphatase in certain myeloproliferative diseases. New Eng. J. Med. **266**: 538.
4. REYNOLD, M. D., H. M. LEMON & W. W. BYRNES. 1959. Copper resistant serum acid phosphatase. I. Method and values in health and disease. Cancer Res. **27**: 902.
5. TUCHMAN, L. R., G. GOLDSTEIN & M. CLYMAN. 1962. Studies on nature of increased serum acid phosphatase in Gaucher's disease. Amer. J. Med. **27**: 959.
6. FISHMAN, W. H. & F. LERNER. 1953. A method for estimating serum acid phosphatase of prostatic origin. J. Biol. Chem. **200**: 89.
7. ABDUL-FADL, M. A. M. & E. J. KING. 1949. Properties of acid phosphatase of erythrocytes and of human prostate gland. Biochem. J. **45**: 51.
8. FISHMAN, W. H., R. M. DART, C. D. BONNER, W. F. LEADBETTER, F. LERNER & F. HOMBURGER. 1953. A new method for estimating serum acid phosphatase of prostatic origin applied to the clinical investigation of cancer of the prostate. J. Clin. Invest. **32**: 1034.
9. FISHMAN, W. H., C. D. BONNER & F. HOMBURGER. 1956. Serum prostatic acid phosphatase and cancer of the prostate. New Eng. J. Med. **255**: 925.
10. GREEN, S., T. J. GIOVANNIELLO & W. H. FISHMAN. 1967. Automated differential analysis of several serum phosphatase isoenzymes. *In* Automation in Analytical Chemistry, Technicon Symposium, 1966. : 480–488. Mediad Inc., White Plains, N. Y.
11. GREEN, S., T. J. GIOVANNIELLO, R. A. COTE & W. H. FISHMAN. 1968. *In* Automation in Analytical Chemistry, Technicon Symposium 1967. : 563–570. Mediad Inc., White Plains, N. Y.

12. Babson, A. & P. A. Read. 1959. A new assay for prostatic acid phosphatase in serum. Amer. J. Clin. Path. **32**: 6.
13. Babson, A. L., P. A. Read & G. E. Phillips. 1959. The importance of the substrate in assays of acid phosphatase in serum. Amer. J. Clin. Path. **32**: 83.
14. Schwartz, M. K., E. Greenberg & O. Bodansky. 1963. Comparative values of phosphatases and other serum enzymes in following patients with prostatic carcinoma. Cancer **16**: 583.
15. Franseen, C. C. & R. McLean. 1935. Phosphatase activity of tissues and plasma in tumors of bone. Am. J. Cancer **24**: 299.
16. Woodard, H. Q. & N. L. Higinbotham. 1937. The correlation between serum phosphatase and roentgenographic type in bone disease. Am. J. Cancer **31**: 221.
17. Woodard, H. Q., G. H. Twombly & B. L. Coley. 1936. A study of serum phosphatase in bone disease. J. Clin. Invest. **15**: 193.
18. Bayrd, E. D. & F. J. Heck. 1947. Multiple myeloma. JAMA **133**: 147.
19. Adams, W. S., E. L. Alling & J. S. Lawrence. 1949. Multiple myeloma. Amer. J. Med. **6**: 141.
20. Gutman, A. B., T. L. Tyson & E. B. Gutman. 1936. Serum calcium, inorganic phosphorus and phosphatase activity. Arch. Intern. Med. (Chicago) **57**: 379.
21. Burk, L. B. 1948. Hyperparathyroidism. Amer. J. Surg. **76**: 404.
22. Woodard, H. Q. 1953. Changes in blood chemistry associated with carcinoma metastatic to bone. Cancer **6**: 1219.
23. Staubitz, W. J., O. J. Oberkircher & M. H. Lent. 1954. Clinical results of the treatment of prostatic carcinoma over a ten-year period. J. Urol. **72**: 939.
24. Gutman, A. B. 1959. Serum alkaline phosphatase activity in diseases of the skeletal and hepatobiliary systems. Amer. J. Med. **27**: 875.
25. Mendelsohn, M. L. & O. Bodansky. 1952. The value of liver-function tests in the diagnosis of intrahepatic metastases in the nonicteric cancer patient. Cancer **5**: 1.
26. Smithies, O. 1955. Zone electrophoresis in starch gels: Group variations in the serum proteins of normal human adults. Biochem. J. **61**: 629.
27. Moss, D. W., D. M. Campbell, E. Anagnostov-Kakaras & E. J. King. 1961. Characterization of tissue alkaline phosphatases and their partial purification by starch-gel electrophoresis. Biochem. J. **81**: 441.
28. Ahmed, Z. & E. J. King. 1960. Purification of placental alkaline phosphatase. Biochim. Biophys. Acta **40**: 320.
29. Bodansky, O. & M. K. Schwartz. 1963. Comparative effects of L-histidine on the activities of 5′-nucleotidase and alkaline phosphatase. J. Biol. Chem. **238**: 3420.
30. Bodansky, O. 1937. Are the phosphatases of bone, kidney, intestine and serum identical? J. Biol. Chem. **118**: 341.
31. Fishman, W. H. & N. K. Ghosh. 1967. Isoenzymes of human alkaline phosphatase. Advances Clin. Chem. **10**: 255.
32. Dixon, T. F. & M. Purdom. 1954. Serum 5′-nucleotidase. J. Clin. Path. **7**: 341.
33. Kowlessar, O. D., L. J. Haeffner, E. M. Riley & M. H. Sleisenger. 1961. Comparative study of serum leucine aminopeptidase, 5′-nucleotidase and nonspecific alkaline phosphatase in diseases affecting the pancreas, hepatobiliary tree and bone. Amer. J. Med. **31**: 231.
34. Schwartz, M. K. & O. Bodansky. 1965. Serum 5′-nucleotidase in patients with cancer. Cancer **18**: 886.
35. Campbell, D. M. 1962. Determination of 5′-nucleotidase in blood serum. Biochem. J. **82**: 34p.
36. Schwartz, M. K. & O. Bodansky. 1964. Properties of activity of 5′-nucleotidase in human serum and applications in diagnosis. Amer. J. Clin. Path. **42**: 572.
37. Young, I. I. 1958. Serum 5′-nucleotidase. J. Clin. Path. **7**: 341.
38. Wachstein, M. & R. Sigismondi. 1958. 5′-Nucleotidase activity and adenosine triphosphatase activity in human serum. Amer. J. Clin. Path. **30**: 523.
39. Eschar, J., C. Rudzki & H. J. Zimmerman. 1967. Serum levels of 5′-nucleotidase in disease. Amer. J. Clin. Path. **46**: 598.
40. Meyer, K. A., P. A. Rosi & A. B. Ragins. 1939. Carcinoma of the parathyroid gland. Surgery **6**: 190.

Discussion of the Paper

O. Bodansky: I think if we have questions from the audience, they will be noted by Dr. Schwartz and answered at one time. Dr. Fishman?

W. H. FISHMAN: Were the experiments with L-phenylalanine accompanied by controls containing D-phenylalanine at the same concentration?

L. WARNOCK (*University of Chicago, Chicago, Ill.*): I was particularly interested in your slide showing the extract of the hepatoma. Am I correct in assuming this is an extract of the tumor tissue within the liver, and if so, how do you explain the cell of origin for this phosphatase you found, the extract of which, apparently, has no liver cells?

And my second comment is that, well, a question: I wonder how many hepatomas have you studied, because I've now studied 10 hepatomas – hepatocellular carcinomas – and found in eight of them a faster moving anodic band that is just ahead of the normal liver phosphatase present in these extracts. I found this present in three of five serum samples from these patients. I wonder how many of them you have examined.

DR. NAUGETY (*Ohio State University, Columbus, Ohio*): This is more in the way of a comment. We've seen in the past many times, and today too, that an osteogenic sarcoma was used as a source of bone-type alkaline phosphatase. We were concerned, when the first reports of the Regan-type enzyme came out, about the possibility of osteogenic sarcomas having the characteristics of Regan isoenzyme rather than bone type. And indeed they are the opposite. The phenylalanine inhibition and the heat sensitivity, particularly, are direct opposite.

So we took a look at 20 different extracts of 20 different osteogenic sarcomas we had in dogs. And it may be encouraging to know that in each of the 20, the characteristics were identical to bone enzyme. In no instance, were the 20 like the Regan.

S. POSEN: Would it be appropriate to address one question to the last speaker from Ohio State. Do the various tissues in the dog or other species resemble those of human tissues in the various characteristics, such as electrophoresis or heating denaturation or phenylalanine sensitivity – any resemblance to what we see in clinical work?

DR. NAUGETY: I'm very glad you asked that because the work was just finished. Yes, the conclusion is that using heat and phenylalanine, urea and polyacrylamide gel disc electrophoresis, characteristics in dogs' kidneys, livers, intestines and bones are all extremely similar to that reported in man. And I think we've also seen the Regan enzyme in one case. We have increased intestinal enzyme in the patient with steatorrhea. So it appears to us that the dog is an excellent model animal to use in further studies on alkaline phosphatase, as they have proved so valuable in past years. The placenta we haven't looked at at all.

DR. SCHWARTZ: I'll start from the back and work forward. The question concerning the osteogenic sarcoma – we, of course, worried about the fact that our alkaline phosphatase came from osteogenic sarcoma and not from normal bone. We have compared the osteogenic sarcoma phosphatase with the cattle bone phosphatase, and in a publication of Dr. Bodansky's and mine in the Journal of Biological Chemistry several years ago, compared them quite critically. We evaluated the effects of various substrates, of pH and of histidine, and we determined Michaelis-Menten constants, inhibitor constants and various other parameters. We found that the cattle bone phosphatase and the phosphatase from our osteogenic sarcoma were similar.

As far as our hepatoma studies are concerned, unfortunately, the series only includes one hepatoma. The slide I showed was not a hepatoma but rather a poorly differentiated adenocarcinocarcinoma of the liver. But the fact of the matter is, because of variability in starch gel, it is extremely difficult in my opinion to compare speeds and extent of migration from specimen to specimen. Proper controls obviously are needed. In our study we used an extract of normal liver.

Concerning Dr. Fishman's comments, all of the studies I showed on L-phenylalanine were actually compared to D-phenylalanine LAPT. They represent data taken from experiments in which the entire pH curve was determined. The study was run with D- and L-phenylalanine from pH 7.5 to 11. Then we obtained the optimal pH for each of the tissues from the curve and calculated from that data the percentage seen on the table. This does not represent individual assays of all of the tissues at the same pH.

DR. FISHMAN: Your lack of success with L-phenylalanine may be due to not using phenylphosphate, as we did.

DR. WARNOCK: I see the normal liver component in the extract of the hepatomas as well as the fast band, which is inhibited by L-phenylalanine differentially and migrates on sephadex G-200 filtration a little bit different from the normal liver phosphatase.

DR. SCHWARTZ: Yes, I would think that in some of the studies with L-phenylalanine, it would be quite appropriate to include the bile acid. Here you have an agent – bile acid – that has no effect on the intestinal enzyme but has marked inhibition on the enzyme from the other sources. It seems to me it would be of great interest to see if you can use both of them together to obtain even a greater amount of information concerning the organ specificity of phosphatases.

L. BECKMAN: Just a few words. I don't think I've ever seen so many overloaded electrophoresis gels in my whole life. Of course it breaks down if you overload it, and then its not interpretable. There is a limit to what the gel can consume. So I would say if people agreed to use standard concentrations of enzymes prepared from standard tissues, we would be speaking the same language.

DR. BODANSKY: I think, Dr. Beckman, you will also notice that some of Dr. Schwartz's gels were underloaded. The question of sensitivity starch gel electrophoresis was discussed in the paper. The problem is how much enzyme must be applied to demonstrate minor bands.

G. MARTIN: A brief comment and question to Dr. Warnock. I think, in general, it is useful to do controls when one looks at various parameters wtih the neoplasms, suitable controls involving fetal tissues or regenerating tissues. I think all of us should keep that in mind if possible. In case of liver, one could study fetal liver and regenerating liver in experimental animals.

THE IMPORTANCE OF VARYING MOLECULAR SIZE, DIFFERENTIAL HEAT AND UREA INACTIVATION OF PHOSPHATASE IN THE IDENTIFICATION OF DISEASE PATTERNS*

James J. Fennelly, Joseph Dunne, Kevin McGeeney, Lee Chong, and M. FitzGerald

St. Paul's Chemotherapy Unit, and Department of Medicine and Therapeutics, University College, Dublin, Ireland

Our interest in alkaline phosphatase studies started in 1964 when we were using gel filtration techniques for many collateral studies. We studied serum in patients with various types of liver disease, and noted that an enzyme was present that was excluded from Sephadex G-200, i.e., it eluted mainly with the macroglobulins.[1,2] This suggested an enzyme of unusual size,[3] and prompted our subsequent investigations.

During this time, other methods of identifying patterns have been described, and we have used some of them, such as differential thermostability,[4,5] differential urea inactivation[6–8] and phenylalanine inhibition.[9] Our studies have been devoted mainly to patterns obtained in a variety of diseases involving the hepatobiliary and skeletal systems.

Materials and Methods

Sera were studied from (a) control subjects, i.e. laboratory personnel (aged 20 to 40 years) and blood donors (aged 40 to 60 years); (b) patients with skeletal diseases of various types, both malignant and nonmalignant, such as Paget's disease, hyperparathyroidism and osteomalacia; (c) hepatic diseases, both metastatic and nonmalignant, and extrahepatic obstructive biliary disease. Sera were studied fresh or were kept frozen at $-20°$ C. until time of study.

For gel filtration studies, Sephadex G-200 was allowed to swell over 72 hours in distilled water. The gel was mounted in a vertical column 52×2 cm, and equilibrated with 50 mM Tris buffer containing 1.0 M NaCl at pH 8.0. The serum sample (0.5 to 1.0 ml) was diluted 1 to 3 with buffer before being applied to the column. The column was eluted at 10 ml/hr and fractions of 2 ml were collected in an L.K.B. or Shandon-Jeffs fraction collector. The effluent was scanned in an L.K.B. Uvicord 11 at 280 nm, or fractions read on a Beckman spectrophotometer. Samples were assayed for alkaline phosphatase activity using a modification of the Bessey Lowry Brock method,[10] as already described.[1] The incubation mixture contained 3.96 mM *p*-nitrophenyl phosphate as substrate, 0.75 M 2-amino-2-methyl-1-propanol buffer (Sigma) and 5 mM Mg^{++} at pH 10.0. Enzyme activity was terminated following 15 to 30 minutes incubation at 37° C. by addition of a mixture containing 8 volumes of 0.5 M NaOH and 2 volumes of 0.1 M EDTA. Solutions were then read in a Beckman spectrophotometer at 410 nm. The three protein peaks obtained in order of their elution from the column are designated A, B and C respectively, and are used as reference points for the enzyme position in the profile. In some cases, beta lipoproteins were extracted from serum using dextran sulphate according to the method of Walton and Scott.[11]

* Tenovus (Wales) and the Irish Cancer Society provided financial support for this study.

Differential Thermostability

Serum for assay was heated for 10 and 20 minutes at 56° C. in an accurate incubation bath (type S.B. 2, Grant Instruments, Cambridge) following the method described by Posen, Neale and Clubb.[5] Temperature was checked constantly using a thermometer accurate to 0.01° C. (Grant Instruments, Cambridge). The heated sample was put on ice until assayed for enzyme. The enzyme activities of the 10- and 20-minute samples were taken as the representative samples and referred to as the percentage remaining enzyme.[12] Where very high enzyme concentrations were present, serum was diluted before testing. This did not affect the thermostability pattern.

Urea

Urea (Analar) was incorporated into the substrate to give a concentration ranging from 0.1 to 4 M, similar to the methods of Bahr and Wilkinson[6] and Birkett *et al.*[7] For the phosphatase assay, the method of Kind and King[13] was used with addition of magnesium chloride, 1.6 mM, to the 0.1 mM bicarbonate/carbonate buffer. The substrate was phenylphosphate.

These studies have been supplemented in some cases with observations on L-phenylalanine inhibition as studied by Fishman *et al.*[9] L-phenylalanine (Sigma) was used in concentration of 5 mM, and the results of L-phenylalanine inhibition were expressed as a percentage of the D-phenylalanine-treated enzyme.

Polyacrylamide Disc Electrophoresis

Polyacrylamide disc electrophoresis was carried out according to the method of Davis[14] using a Pleuger power pack. Ten to 50μl of serum were applied to the top of the gel, consisting of a spacer gel, 3% concentration, and a separation gel of 7.5% concentration. Separation took place over 45 minutes at 3 ma per tube. Gels were then stained with Naphthyl MX Phosphate (Sigma), using Fast Blue RR as coupling agent.

In many cases, separated peaks from gel filtration were subjected to heat inactivation and urea inhibition. Where tests were carried out on partially purified gel filtration peaks, the addition of magnesium was essential, as no enzyme activity was obtained without such addition.

Results

Gel Filtration

The protein peak on the left side of FIGURE 1, (i.e. peak A) is composed mainly of IgM protein with lesser amount of IgA, mostly of 19S sedimentation. The second peak (B) contains mostly gammaglobulins IgG and IgA of 7S sedimentation, while the peak on the right (ie., peak C) is mostly albumin (4S) in content.[3] In control serum, as shown in FIGURE 1, the phosphatase eluted as one peak in the peak B protein region. This was the case in almost all control subjects studied. except in a few where there was a trailing of activity into peak A or the excluded peak. In one control, this reached 7.5% of the total enzyme activity. We have not analyzed a large enough group to relate this to blood group.[15]

In sera of patients with skeletal disease of various types, the enzyme was eluted in a similar region, except that the peak was larger (FIGURE 2). This enzyme peak was particularly homogeneous in patients with primary skeletal conditions, such as Paget's disease of bone, and primary hyperparathyroidism. Little, if any, enzyme activity was found in the first protein peak A region. In patients with skeletal disease of a more complicated pattern, such as osteomalacia due to malabsorption, or metastatic malignant disease, the picture was not quite so clear. The enzyme peak B was of a broader nature, and there was also evidence of enzyme activity in the first peak A region.

Hepatobiliary Disease

In hepatobiliary disease, the pattern is in marked contrast, for, in addition to the peak already noted in the control group and those with skeletal disease, a peak is noted in protein peak A suggesting an enzyme complex of unusually large molecular size (FIGURE 3). This peak was present in all types of liver disease, whether it was metastatic liver disease, primary hepatoma or cirrhosis. The pat-

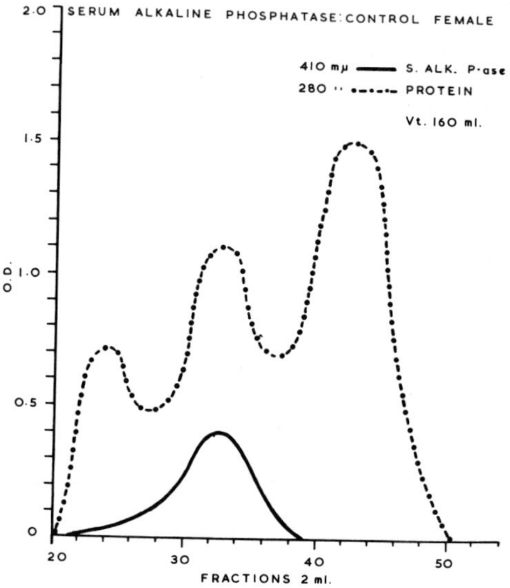

FIGURE 1. Gel filtration pattern of protein and phosphatase in control serum. Three protein peaks, left to right, are designated A, B and C in text.

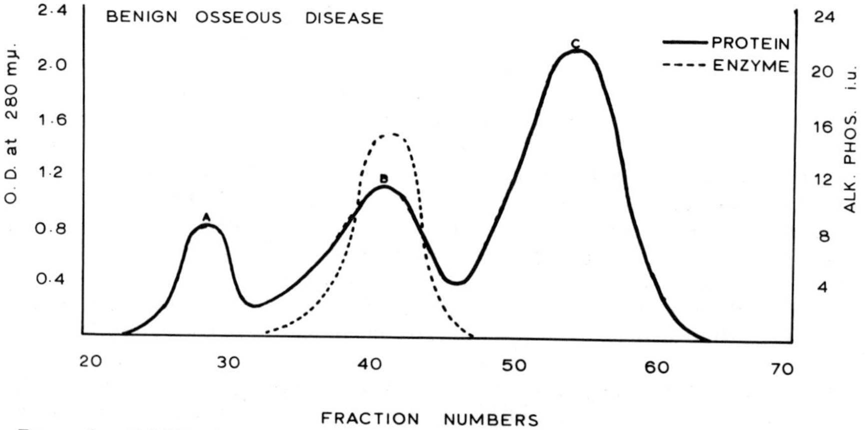

FIGURE 2. Gel filtration pattern of protein and phosphatase in a patient with osteomalacia.

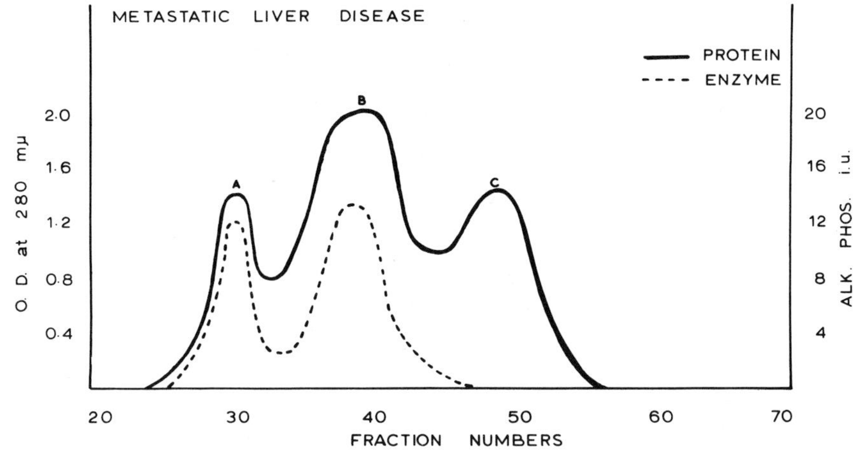

FIGURE 3. Gel filtration pattern of protein and phosphatase in a patient with metastatic liver disease.

terns described for intrahepatic disease were similar to those found in extrahepatic biliary obstruction where there was no evidence of intrahepatic disease. FIGURE 4 illustrates the case of a patient who, at laparotomy, proved to have a lymphoma of the duodenum, causing obstruction of the common bile duct. The first peak was particularly prominent, forming 60% of the total, and was also prominent in four other patients with extrahepatic obstruction, forming 35, 48, 33 and 33% of the total. The pattern noted in various subjects is not necessarily a function of the amount of circulating enzyme, as in FIGURE 5, where the pattern is shown for a patient with hepatic metastases, but of a normal total enzyme level. The enzyme is divided between the two peaks.

What of changing patterns? In a patient with Paget's disease of the bone, there was an associated episode of hepatic insufficiency that resulted in esophageal bleeding. At this time, gel filtration revealed the typical picture of liver disease with two peaks, 25% of the enzyme moving in peak A. The patient recovered, and his hepatic insufficiency improved so much that when checked 6 months later 99.5% of the enzyme was in peak B, i.e. it reflected the underlying Paget's disease of bone. When the figures are analyzed, as shown in TABLE 1, we find that the excluded enzyme peak A forms a mean of 1.73% ± 2.8 in controls, 1.4% ± 2.04 in those with nonmetastatic bone disease, 6.4% ± 5.73 in those with secondary malignant skeletal disease, 15.53% ± 8.30 in those with nonmalignant liver disease and 36.23% ± 11.82 in those with hepatoma and metastatic liver disease.

Polyacrylamide Disc Electrophoresis

In patients with liver disease, the enzyme moved in two, and sometimes three, regions, one being retained at the origin of the spacer gel, the second sometimes present was retained at the origin of the separation gel, while the third band moved well into the separation gel. In contrast, in patients with skeletal disease, the one enzyme disc present moved well into the separation gel to a site similar to that of the third band mentioned in liver disease.

Gel filtration as described here is really a research tool, and is not a practical

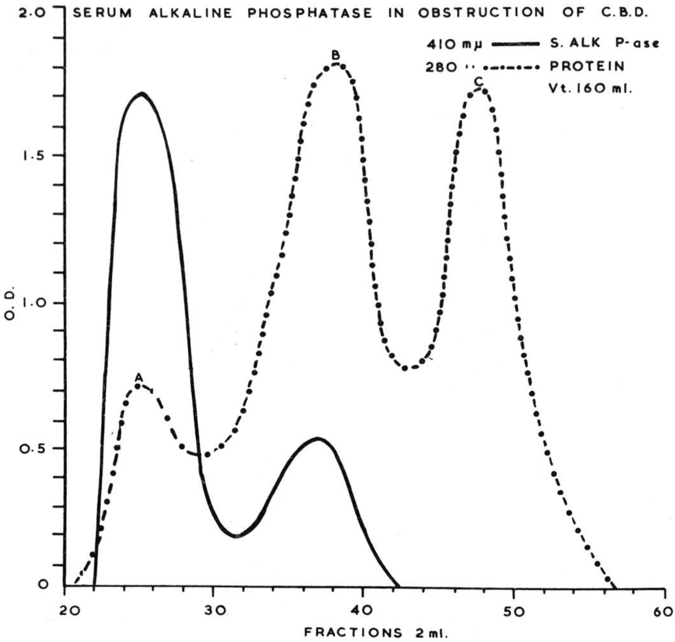

FIGURE 4. Gel filtration of protein and phosphatase in a patient with obstruction of the common bile duct.

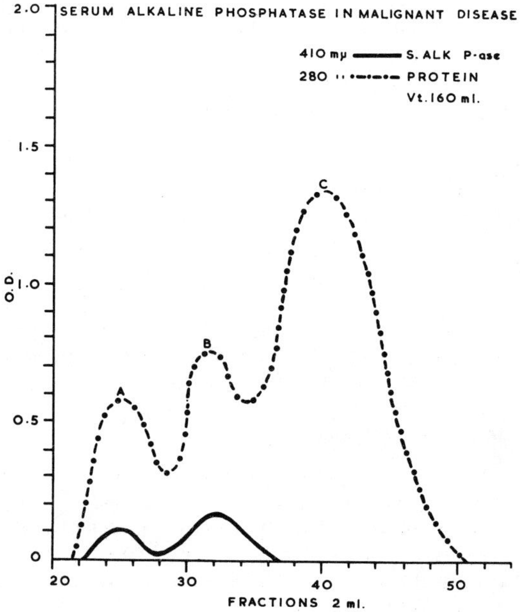

FIGURE 5. Gel filtration pattern of serum protein and phosphatase in a patient with metastatic liver disease and normal total enzyme level.

proposition for routine clinical work. In our routine studies, we rely on heat inactivation and urea inhibition.[12,16]

Differential Thermostability

FIGURE 6 illustrates the scatter of the 10-minute thermostable enzyme in the groups studied, while TABLE 2 gives an analysis of these. The 10- and 20-minute mean figures ± 1 standard deviation in control subjects are 27% ± 5.3 and 6.1% ± 5.5; in patients with nonmalignant skeletal disease, the remaining activity is 18% ± 5.6 and 6.5% ± 3.7; in metastatic bone disease, 23.9% ± 7.8 and 10% ± 6.5; in patients with nonmalignant hepatic disease, 51% ± 10 and 24% ± 6; and in those with metastatic liver disease, 43% ± 11 and 19.7% ± 8.5, respectively. The difference between the groups with skeletal and hepatic disease

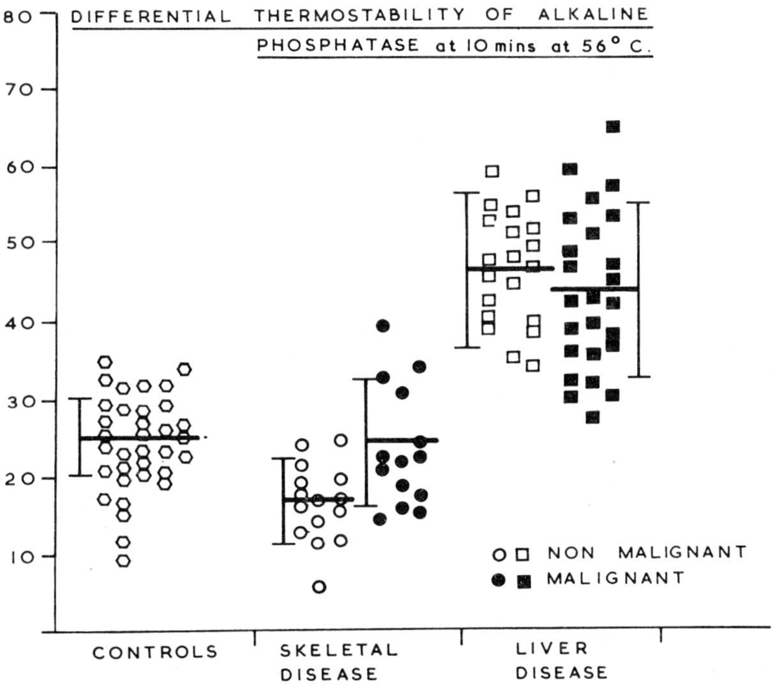

FIGURE 6. Scattergram of 10-minute thermostable phosphatase at 56° C. Transverse line represents mean with one standard deviation.

TABLE 1

PERCENTAGE ENZYME IN EXCLUDED PROTEIN PEAK A

Patients	No.	Mean	St. Dev.	S.E.M.
Control	11	1.73	2.8	0.84
Skeletal D.	11	1.4	2.04	0.62
Metastatic Skeletal D.	11	6.4	5.73	1.73
Liver D.	12	15.53	8.30	2.40
Metastatic Liver D.	13	36.23	11.82	3.30

TABLE 2

DIFFERENTIAL THERMOSTABILITY OF SERUM ALKALINE PHOSPHATASE

Conditions	No.	% Remaining at 10 Min at 56° C Mean, 10 Min	Mean, 20 Min
Control	19	27 ± 5.3	6.1 ± 5.5
Bone Disease	15	18 ± 5.6	6.5 ± 3.7
Bone Disease (Secondary)	15	23.9 ± 7.8	10.5 ± 6.5
Hepatic Disease	21	51 ± 10	24 ± 6
Hepatic Disease (Secondary)	36	43 ± 11	19.7 ± 8.5

$P < .001$ when comparing bone and liver disease.
Bone Disease (Secondary) = metastatic bone disease.
Hepatic Disease = hepatitis, cirrhosis, obstructive biliary disease.
Hepatic Disease (Secondary) = metastatic liver disease.

is highly significant, $p < .001$, but the patients in these groups were clear-cut examples of the disease. In the subgroups in skeletal disease, those with primary skeletal lesions, Paget's disease and hyperparathyroidism had an enzyme of greater sensitivity than that in patients with metastatic skeletal disease.

When patients with liver disease were studied further, we found that there was a great overlap between those with metastatic disease and those with hepatic, cirrhosis and extrahepatic obstruction. A few patients within the subgroup are worthy of comment.

Patient M.W. (TABLE 3) whose serum showed marked thermostability, was examined in 1966 when he had colon carcinoma with hepatic metastases and ascites. The serum enzyme was thermostable, particularly when checked at 20 minutes (between 41 and 58% remaining as compared to 19.7% in those with liver disease). The ascitic fluid examined also showed a similar marked thermostability. The 20-minute figure for serum and ascitic fluid phosphatase suggested a flattening in the decay curve resembling placental enzyme.[17] In the total group, the correlation between differential thermostability and total level was not as clear as anticipated. In some cancer subjects, the enzyme thermostability changed months before the total level or other sign, such as hepatic enlargement, appeared, while in others the increase in enzyme thermostability followed closely the rise in total serum enzyme activity.

Case J.F., TABLE 4, was a male with bronchogenic carcinoma who had skeletal and hepatic secondaries. The serum phosphatase was relatively thermostable. The enzyme in adjacent areas of bone was studied. While enzyme in normal bone was sensitive to heat, that in adjacent infiltrated bone was much more heat-resistant and resembled the enzyme in the tumor primary and liver secondary.

TABLE 3

MARKED THERMOSTABILITY OF SERUM AND ASCITIC FLUID ALKALINE PHOSPHATASE IN PATIENT WITH COLON CARCINOMA AND HEPATIC METASTASES

Total K.A.	% Remaining Phosphatase 10 Min	20 Min	
(Hepatic Disease)	43 ± 11	19.7 ± 8.5	
66.5	75	58	Serum
90	60	41	Serum
75	72	53	Serum
25	65	52	Ascites

Urea Inhibition

The effect of urea bears many qualitative resemblances to that of heat. The effect of urea is of a twofold nature, as pointed out by Birkett *et al.*[7] At low concentration, there is a low grade uncompetitive inactivation that is reversible, but at concentrations over 1 M urea, the rate of inactivation is much greater, is irreversible, and shows specific patterns for different tissues. FIGURE 7 illustrates

TABLE 4

THERMOSTABILITY OF SERUM AND TISSUE ENZYMES AT 10 AND 20 MIN IN A PATIENT WHO DIED WITH CARCINOMA OF THE LUNG

Enzymes	Lung Ca. % Remaining at 56° C	
	10 Min	20 Min
Serum	60	30
N. Bone	22	6
Bone (Secondary)	43	21
Lung (Primary)	55	35
Liver (Secondary)	52	31
Peak (Serum)	A (39%) 40	B (61%) 42.5

Bottom column represents thermostability at 10 min of peak A (gel filtration) and peak B, 39% and 61% of total, respectively.

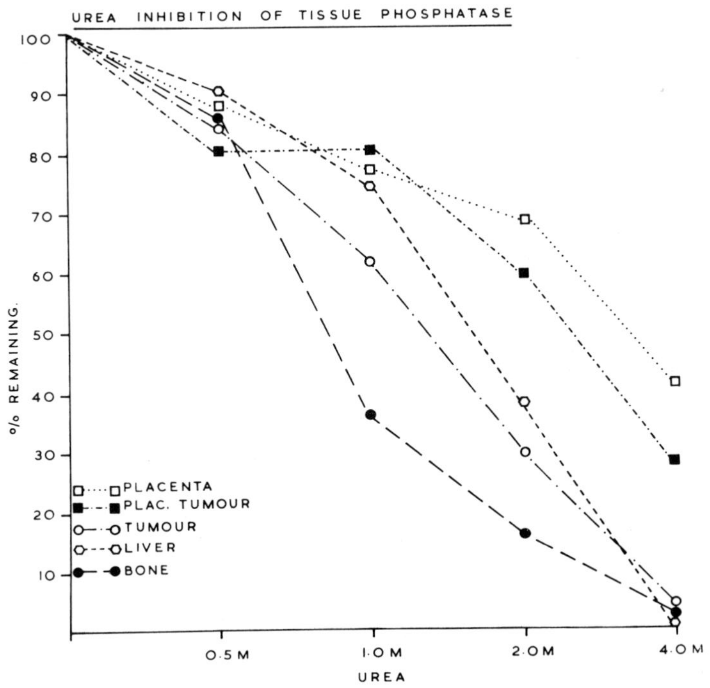

FIGURE 7. Percentage of enzyme remaining after treatment of various tissue enzymes with increasing concentrations of urea.

the type of inactivation in various tissues. At the lower concentrations, there is little difference between various tissues, but at 1 and 2 M concentration the patterns diverge, placental tissue and the placental tumor choriocarcinoma being most resistant, while liver tissue is less resistant and skeletal tissue most sensitive. The inactivation resulting in the serum of patients with liver and bone disease, respectively, is shown in FIGURE 8 and TABLE 5.

The phosphatase in patients with skeletal disease is most sensitive to urea; a mean of 21.6% ± 12.5 remains in those with Paget's disease and hyperparathyroidism, and a mean of 31.7% ± 8.7 remains in patients with metastatic bone disease. Phosphatase in hepatic disease is relatively resistant; 45% ± 4 remains in patients with nonmalignant liver disease, such as cirrhosis, hepatitis, and

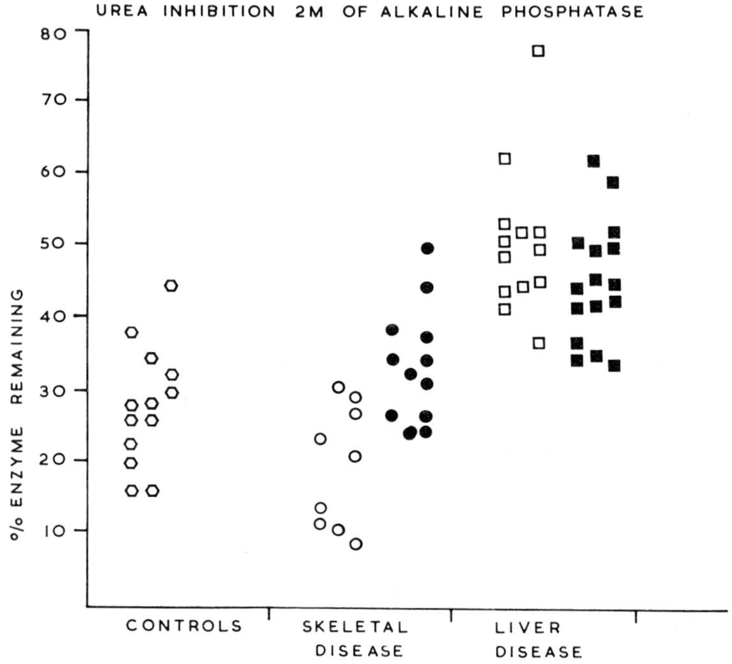

FIGURE 8. Inhibition of phosphatase by 2 M urea. Open symbols = nonmalignant conditions, closed symbols = malignant disease. (serum)

TABLE 5

ANALYSIS OF PHOSPHATASE REMAINING IN SERUM IN VARIOUS CONDITIONS AFTER TREATMENT WITH 2 M UREA

Conditions	No.	% Remaining Mean	St. E.
Control	19	32 ± 9	2.4
Bone Disease	8	21.6 ± 12.5	4.4
Bone Disease (Secondary)	12	31.75 ± 8.7	2.5
Liver Disease	13	45 ± 4	1.8
Liver Disease (Secondary)	16	44.8 ± 8.5	2.1
Bone and Liver Disease	4	34.5 ± 6.2	3.1

obstructive liver disease, and almost the same remains in metastatic liver disease, while serum of controls falls between 18 and 44% wtih a mean of 32% ± 9. Again, the difference between the groups is highly significant ($p < .001$) when comparing skeletal and hepatic disease.

In relation to control figures, it is important to remember that we are making calculations on very low levels, e.g., we may be talking of 20% of an enzyme level of 4 U%. At this level, minor variations in the estimation may cause large differences in ultimate results. The control group covers a wide age range from the teenage group to the sixties, the former showing a more skeletal pattern, while in the latter group the hepatic contribution becomes more evident, hence, the wide range of figures. Different types of liver disease did not show any variation in pattern, and the extrahepatic obstructive group showed the same patterns as intrahepatic disease.

Treatment of Enzyme Peaks by Heat and Urea

When heat inactivation was applied to the peaks obtained on gel filtration, we found that, whereas the enzyme in the peak B of skeletal disease showed marked sensitivity to heat, being reduced to 14.2%, the enzyme of both peak A and B in hepatic disease showed relative resistance, with 48.9% ± 6.1 and 48.7% ± 4 remaining in nonmalignant liver disease, and 43% ± 6.6 and 47.7% ± 5.9, respectively, in metastatic liver disease (TABLE 6). When the serum was heated before gel filtration, similar enzyme patterns resulted. When the separated peaks were treated with 2 M urea, the single peak B enzyme in skeletal disease showed marked sensitivity, while both peaks in hepatic disease were relatively resistant. Thus, the peak B enzymes present on gel filtration in both skeletal and liver disease were of different types as regards thermostability and urea inactivation. In sequential follow-up, changing patterns are clearly seen in some cases.

Patient E.F., on admission, had skeletal secondaries from breast carcinoma. The liver was not enlarged, though the BSP was abnormal, there being 20% retention at 45 minutes. Phosphatase was elevated, moved in one peak B on gel filtration, and was sensitive to heat (20% remaining). The pattern was followed over seven months, but then marked hepatomegaly developed. There was no change in total alkaline phosphatase, but the enzyme now moved in two peaks and was now much more resistant to heat.

Patient M.McG. FIGURE 9 illustrates the changing pattern in patient M.McG. who started on Stilboestrol treatment for skeletal secondaries from breast carcinoma. The total enzyme rose to 47 units, but retained the thermosensitivity of the skeletal enzyme, suggesting the phosphatase 'flare' of bone healing. This patient continues on treatment, but some months ago developed signs of chronic congestive heart failure with hepatic congestion, and associated with this, there was a moderate increase in BSP retention and a rise in the enzyme thermostability.

There is a good degree of correlation between thermostability and urea resist-

TABLE 6

DIFFERENTIAL THERMOSTABILITY OF PHOSPHATASE IN ELUTED GEL FILTRATION PEAKS

Conditions	% Remaining 10 Min at 56° C.		
	No.	A	B
Bone Disease	11		14.2 ± 8.7
Liver Disease	9	48.9 ± 6.1	48.7 ± 4
Metastatic Liver Disease	7	43.1 ± 6.6	47.7 ± 5.9

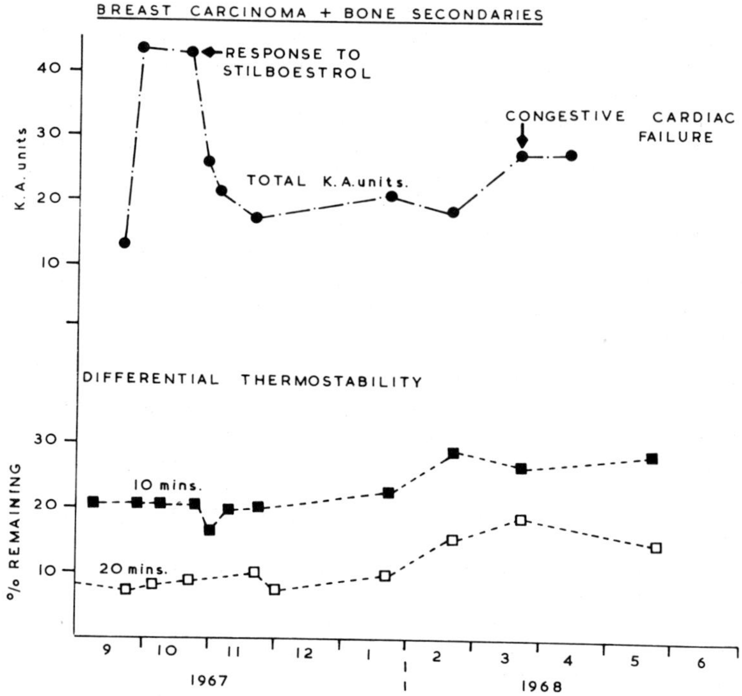

FIGURE 9. Effect of treatment and change in underlying conditions on phosphatase pattern.

ance, r = 0.83 (FIGURE 10). It has been noted that by raising the temperature of the reaction mixture, increased inactivation is produced by urea.[8] The correlation between urea resistance and the size of peak A enzyme, and between heat resistance and the size of the peak A enzyme, is not as clear.

Discussion

There is little doubt that with the methods now available, specific alkaline phosphatase patterns can be identified with increasing accuracy. When there is a simple method of differentiating the patterns of alkaline phosphatase, there appears little value in most clinical situations in relying on a more total level. The human being is such a variable subject, being prone to multiple system diseases, such as malignant disease, malabsorption and malnutrition, which may affect both the skeletal and hepatic systems, and he is affected by so many hepatotoxic drugs, that we must try to attach a little more meaning to our alkaline phosphatase assay. Who can say whether the rise in serum alkaline phosphatase in a patient with bony secondaries represent bone healing if there is a possibility that the drug being used is hepatotoxic? When we say we can identify the pattern of the circulating enzyme, we cannot guarantee that this pattern mirrors any underlying tissue pathology. Patients with combined bone and hepatic disease may show a pattern characteristic of one tissue or another. In our experience, the hepatic pattern tends to predominate in these situations.

Gel filtration of serum phosphatase gives clear separation of hepatic and

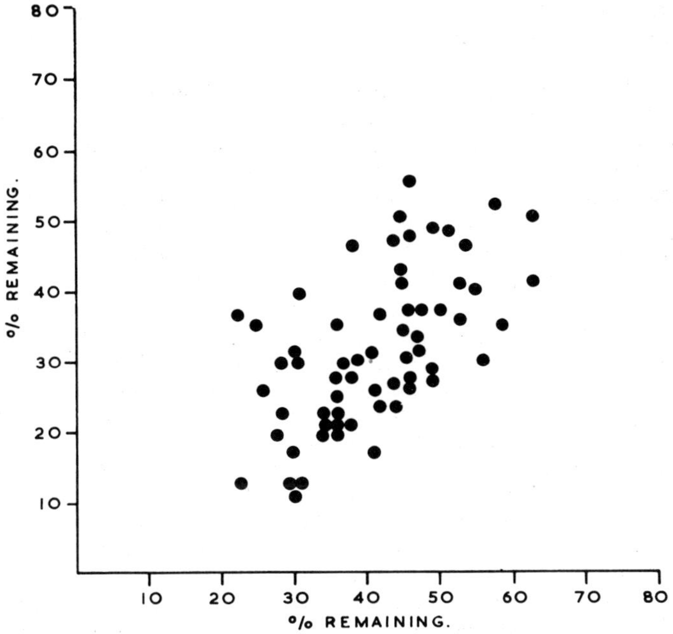

FIGURE 10. Correlation between phosphatase thermostability and urea resistance; r = .83. Ordinate represents heat inactivation and abscissa urea inhibition.

skeletal disease patterns in our experience. It must be emphasized that these patterns represent clear-cut, often advanced examples of the described disease. We feel it is difficult to correlate serum patterns with those obtained from tissue extracts, since the degree of purification may affect the patterns obtained. Estborn[18] noted that intestinal and liver enzyme eluted with both the excluded peak A and peak B, while bone enzyme eluted completely in peak A. In his experiments, as in ours, the serum phosphatase in Paget's disease eluted in peak B. Dymling[19] found that placental enzyme eluded completely with the excluded peak A.

The significance of the macromolecular circulating enzyme complex present in liver disease is not clear at present. Lipoprotein binding might be a factor, but precipitation of these with dextran sulphate has little effect on the size of the macromolecular enzyme peak. It is our opinion that the enzyme complex represents a polymer or an enzyme protein binding such as occurs when IgA protein is secreted through the epithelium.[20]

For practical clinical use, we have found heat inactivation and urea inhibition very satisfactory. The qualitative results from different diseases are quite similar, and there is a strong correlation between these properties. The sensitivity of phosphatase in skeletal disease to both heat and urea is in marked contrast to the relative thermostability of the enzyme in patients with liver disease. For differential thermostability, an accurate water bath is essential, since minor variations in temperature can cause great variation in results. Many incubators used in general laboratories are accurate only to 0.5 to 1.0° C. Our results using 10-minute inactivation figures are very similar to those obtained by Posen *et al.*,[5] who used a 15-minute sample. At times greater than 15 minutes, the amount of enzyme remaining is so low that minimal errors in the enzyme assay may become magnified.

Bahr and Wilkinson[6] have suggested that urea treatment brings about changes in the tertiary structure of the enzyme molecule. Urea is known to rupture hydrogen bands, and thereby to bring about unfolding of polypeptide chains. If change in molecular structure is a factor, we would expect to find a clear difference between the inactivation of the macromolecular moving enzyme (peak A) obtained on gel filtration, as compared with the smaller enzyme on peak B. There was little difference in the rate of inactivaiton in our experiments.

As regards the origin of control serum, it appears clear that control human serum phosphatase is derived mainly from skeletal and hepatic sources, the relative amounts of each being a function of the age of the individual, with skeletal phosphatase predominating in the early growing phase. A small intestinal component is contributed in subjects of blood groups O and B, who are secretors.[15] In our experience, the results from control subjects show gel filtration and thermostability resembling more the pattern of bony enzyme, but urea inhibition studies show a great overlap in figures between patients with liver disease and patients with bone disease, similar to the findings of Birkett *et al.*[7] Yong,[21] using agar gel electrophoresis, maintains that there is little or no skeletal enzyme in adult control serum. He supports his contentions with clear agar gel separation of the enzyme, but we feel his conclusion is too extreme

What of other enzyme studies in association with these? We are at present analyzing the sequential changes in our enzyme levels, such as glutamic pyruvate transaminase, glutamic oxaloascetic transaminase and lactic dehydrogenase in patients who have had attempted curative treatment for breast carcinoma. We do not have adequate studies yet to draw firm conclusions.

Gault and others[22] studied lactic dehydrogenase (LDH) phosphohexose isomerase (PHI) alkaline phosphatase and glutamic oxalactic acid tranaminase in patients with lung tumor. They found that changes in LDH and PHI preceded those of alkaline phosphatase. However, they did not study changes in phosphatase isoenzymes. It is our experience that changes in enzyme differential thermostability in many cases antedate those of total alkaline phosphatase by many months.

There is some evidence at present that phosphatase enzyme secreted by malignant tissues may have specific characteristics. Fishman and coworkers[17] have identified in a patient with carcinoma of the lung a phosphatase enzyme characteristic of placental enzyme on starch gel electrophoresis, heat inactivation and L-phenylalanine inhibition. Timperley[23] reported a similar patient who had a thermostable enzyme, but no inactivation resulted from L-phenylalanine treatments. Only one of our patients showed the kind of thermostability noted by Fishman. In that case of colon carcinoma, a markedly thermostable enzyme was found in serum and ascitic fluid. In our studies of Shay Chloroma tumor phosphatase, we have found an enzyme which, in the purified state is excluded from Sephadex G-200 and elutes in three peaks on DEAE cellulose. Two of these are changed in polyacrylamide gel mobility by neuraminidase treatment.[24]

In conclusion, we have studied the patterns of alkaline phosphatase in a large group of subjects using gel filtration, differential thermostability and differential urea inhibition. The patterns of patients with skeletal and hepatic disease can be identified with a high degree of confidence. The contribution of malignant phosphatase has yet to be clarified.

References

1. Dunne, J., J. J. Fennelly & K. F. McGeeney. 1967. Separation of alkaline phosphatase enzymes in human serum using gel filtration (Sephadex G-200) techniques. Cancer **20:** 1.
2. Fennelly, J. J., J. Dunne & K. McGeeney. 1966. Further studies of phosphatase in tissues and serum using gel filtration techniques. Irish J. Med. Sci. Series VI, No. 49.
3. Flodin, P. & F. Killander. 1962. Fractionation of human serum proteins by gel filtration. Biochim. Biophys. Acta **63:** 403.
4. Moss, D. W. & E. J. King. 1962. Properties of alkaline phosphatase fractions separated by starch gel electrophoresis. Biochem. J. **84:** 192.
5. Posen, S., F. C. Neale & J. S. Clubb. 1965. Heat inactivation in the study of human alkaline phosphatase. Ann. Intern. Med. **62:** 6.
6. Bahr, M. & J. H. Wilkinson. 1967. Urea as a selective inhibition of human tissue alkaline phosphatase. Clin. Chim. Acta **17:** 367.
7. Birkett, D. J., R. A. J. Conyers, F. C. Neale, S. Posen & J. Brudnell-Woods. 1966. Action of urea on human alkaline phosphatases with a description of some automated techniques for the study of enzyme kinetics. Arch. Biochem. **121:** 470.
8. Butterworth, P. J. & D. W. Moss. 1966. The effect of urea on human kidney alkaline phosphatase. Biochem. J. **99:** 9P.
9. Fishman, W. H., S. Green & N. I. Inglis. 1962. Organ specific behaviour exhibited by rat intestinal and liver alkaline phosphatase. Biochim. Biophys. Acta **62:** 363.
10. Bessey, O. A., O. H. Lory & M. S. Brock. 1946. Method for rapid determination of alkaline phosphatase with five cubic millimeters of serum. J. Biol. Chem. **164:** 321.
11. Walton, K. W. & P. J. Scott. 1964. Estimation of low-density (beta) lipoproteins of serum in health and disease using large molecular weight dextran sulphate. J. Clin. Path. **17:** 627.
12. FitzGerald, M., J. J. Fennelly & K. F. McGeeney. 1969. The value of differential alkaline phosphatase thermostability in differential diagnosis. Amer. J. Clin. Path. **51:** (No. 2) 194.
13. Kind, P. R. N. & E. J. King. 1964. Estimation of plasma phosphatase by determination of hydrolyses with antipyrene. J. Clin. Path. **7:** 322.
14. Davis, B. J. 1962. Disc electrophoresis II. Method of application to human serum proteins. Ann. N. Y. Acad. Sci. **121:** 404.
15. Langman, M. J. S., E. Leuthold, E. Robson, J. Harris, J. G. Luffman & H. Harris. 1966. Influence of diet on the intestinal component of serum alkaline phosphatase in people of different ABO blood groups and secretor status. Nature (London) **212:** 41–43.
16. Fennelly, J. J., M. X. FitzGerald & K. McGeeney. 1969. The value of differential thermostability, urea inhibition and gel filtration of alkaline phosphatase in the identification of disease states. Gut **10:** 45.
17. Fishman, W. A., N. I. Inglis, L. L. Stolbach & M. Krant. 1968. A serum alkaline phosphatase isoenzyme of human neoplastic cell origin. Cancer Res. **28:** 150.
18. Estborn, B. 1964. Separation of phosphatase enzymes by gel filtration. Klin. Chem. Heft. **2:** 53.
19. Dymling, J. F. 1966. Separation of serum and placental alkaline phosphatase by agarose gel electrophoresis and Sephadex chromatography. Scand. J. Clin. Lab. Invest. **129:** 18.
20. Holborow, E. J. 1967. Immunoglobulin physiology III. Lancet **i:** 942.
21. Yong, J. M. 1967. Origins of serum alkaline phosphatase. J. Clin. Path. **20:** 647.
22. Gault, M. H., M. W. Cohen, L. M. Kahanu, F. T. Lulin, J. F. Meakins & Aronovitch. 1967. Serum enzymes in patients with carcinoma of lung. Canad. Med. Ass. J. **96:** 87.
23. Timperley, W. R. 1968. Alkaline phosphatase secreting tumour of lung (C). Lancet **ii,** 7563:356.
24. Dunne, J., J. J. Fennelly & K. McGeeney. 1968. Purification and characterisation of Shay Chloroma phosphatase. Biochem. J. **110:** (No. 2) 12.

Discussion of the Paper

R. Keiding: I should like to refer to what I said two days ago—that this macromolecular phosphatase fraction in your first G-200 fraction is the main fraction is the main fraction of bile phosphatase. We find this fraction in 80% of hepatic disease; in 20%, we do not. We also observe this fraction in many situations where we can only find lung changes at autopsy; I mean that from pure lung diseases, we can also find this fraction.

May I also say that we have had several patients with breast cancer, with liver metastases, who have been hypophysectomized, and then this macromolecular fraction disappears.

DR. FENNELLY: We have studied the bile also, and find that it does seem to move in the macromolecular fraction as you suggest.

The lowest amount of enzyme we found in liver disease was 9% in one patient who actually had tuberculous granuloma liver disease. But this was a very stable enzyme. It was a hepatic-type of enzyme in this situation.

N. K. GHOSH: Just a comment on the very interesting observations made by Dr. Fennelly and his coworkers on the presence of 19 S fraction of alkaline phosphatase in serum of liver disease patients. I'd like to mention that in our recent studies on placental enzyme, when we separated the variant A and variant B, had a higher molecular weight. And variant B has been found to have greater antigenicity than variant A. So this finding that the 19 S form is present in all liver disease patients and that it disappears after the patient is cured, suggests that this high molecular weight of enzyme might have some role in fighting infection.

DR. FENNELLY: I would like to add to Dr. Keiding's comment that 20% of patients with liver disease don't have this macromolecular enzyme; I did make the comment in the discussion that the circulating enzyme does not always reflect the known underlying disease.

DR. FISHMAN: In relation to choriocarcinoma, there is the expectation, perhaps, that it would possess a residue of placental alkaline phosphatase, and this would be Regan isoenzyme. A comparison of the alkaline phosphatase pattern of two Regan isoenzyme preparations with that of choriocarcinoma and hydatidiform mole tissues (TABLE 1) indicates that the latter do not show the expected properties i.e., high L-phenylalanine inhibition and low heat inactivation. There is, likewise (FIGURE 1), failure of antisera at a dilution of (1:1000) to placental alkaline phosphatase (which effectively prevents the Regan isoenzyme and antibody complex to migrate) to alter the rate of migration of alkaline phosphatase

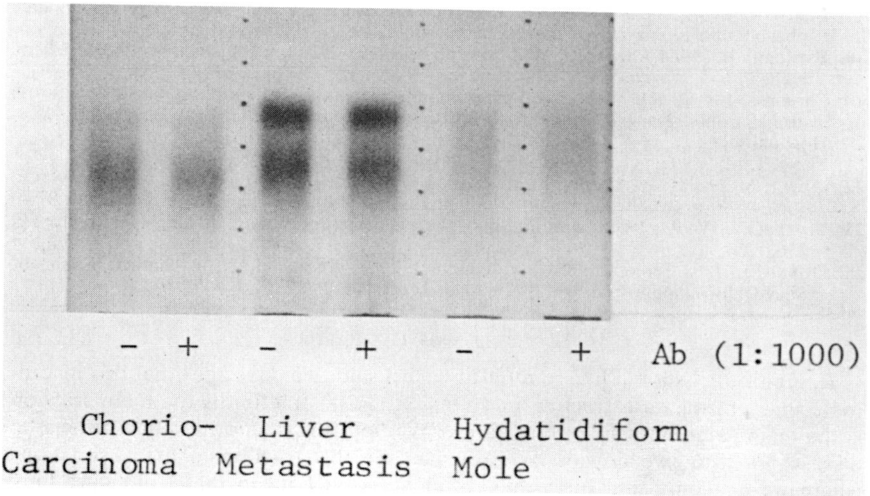

FIGURE 1.

TABLE 1

ALKALINE PHOSPHATASE ACTIVITY, pH 9.8, PHENYL PHOSPHATE, K.A. UNITS/GRAM

Tissue	Unheated Phenylalanine D	Unheated Phenylalanine L	LPSAP	% Inhibition by L-Phenylalanine	% Heat Inactivation Phenylalanine D	% Heat Inactivation Phenylalanine L	LPSAP
P.R. (Adrenal Metastasis)	1.22	0.36	0.86	70.0	14.5	14.5	0.0
A.N. (Lymph Node Metastasis)	17.5	4.07	13.4	76.0	17.0	17.0	17.0
J.P. (Choriocarcinoma)	3.12	2.67	0.45	14.5	89.5	90.4	84.1
M.S. (Hydatidiform Mole)	0.86	0.67	0.19	22.5	75.4	86.1	38.5

of choriocarcinoma and hydatidiform mole. It is of interest, however, that these phosphatases do migrate to the positions expected for placental alkaline phosphatase.

DR. FENNELLY: Thank you, Dr. Fishman. The only contrasting thing seems to be the urea inactivation and the heat resistance noted in our tumor, which resembles placental tissue. This is the one tissue we had.

DISCUSSION PAPER
STUDIES ON SERUM ALKALINE PHOSPHATASE ISOENZYMES

Hiroshi Suzuki, Masami Yamanaka and Toshitsugu Oda
The First Department of Internal Medicine,
Faculty of Medicine, University of Tokyo, Tokyo, Japan

Serum alkaline phosphatase (ALP) was separated into 7 bands on agar-gel plate by means of electrophoresis and diazo staining in its clinical surveys, and the clinical significances and tissue origins, as well as enzymatic characteristics against certain inhibitors were investigated.

Materials and Methods

Sera were obtained from 560 patients in our clinic. On these samples, ALP activity was determined by the modification of the Kind-King method or Bessey-Lowry's, and its isoenzymes were demonstrated by the method shown in TABLE 1.

Agar-gel electrophoresis was done according to the Wieme's method for one hour at 5° C with 15 volt/cm. Then, ALP was demonstrated by diazo dye staining.

Next, effects of urea and EDTA on serum containing each of ALP isoenzymes were investigated by the method as reported by Birkett *et al.*[1]

Results

1. *Clinical Significances of ALP Isoenzymes.*

Seven isoenzymes of ALP are shown in FIGURE 1. ALP I was found between α_1- and α_2-globulins, ALP II at the α_2-globulin fraction, ALP III between α_2- and β-globulins, ALP IV and IV′ as a narrow band between α_2- and β-globulins, ALP V at β-globulin fraction, ALP VI between β- and γ-globulins.

In normal adults, ALP II and sometimes ALP III, weaker than ALP II, were found.

ALP I was always associated with an increase of ALP II. ALP I accompanying ALP II was increased in obstructive jaundice, metastatic liver cancer, liver abscess, cholelithiasis, congestive liver and jaundice in leukemia. On the other hand, ALP II, not accompanying ALP I, was seen in hepatitis, liver cirrhosis, hepatoma and intrahepatic cholestasis (TABLE 2).

ALP III was found in umbilical cord blood, newborn, infant, hyperparathyroidism, metastatic bone cancer and hyperthyroidism, i.e., diseases with elevated osteoblastic activity.

ALP IV has been shown in nine cases so far (TABLE 3). All except the last patient died and were autopsied. In the surviving patient, ALP IV disappeared when his clinical condition was improved.

ALP IV′ was seen in the sera of the mother at delivery; that is, an elevation of ALP in the terminal stage of pregnancy.

ALP V appeared in liver cirrhosis with active change–positive in 20 cases (38.4%) out of 52. Chylous ascites induced by metastatic breast cancer and the sera of secretor of blood groups B and O received a high-fat diet and showed ALP V′ at the similar location of ALP V (TABLE 4).

In the case having ALP V, histological examination of the liver revealed ALP activity at the fibrous tissues, while such a finding was not seen in the cases without ALP V (FIGURES 2 and 3). And ALP activity at the fibrous tissues was

TABLE 1

METHOD FOR SERUM ALKALINE PHOSPHATASE ISOENZYME

Agar-Gel Electrophoresis:		
	Agar-Noble (Difco)	0.7 g
	0.05 M Veronal Buffer (pH 8.6)	100 ml
	100 Volt, 1 Hour	
Substrate:		
	Naphthyl Phosphate AS-MX	5 mg
	Fast Red Violet LB Salt	20 mg
	Dimethyl Formamide	0.5 ml
	0.1 M Tris Buffer (pH 8.8)	50 ml
Incubation:		
	37° C, 2 Hours.	

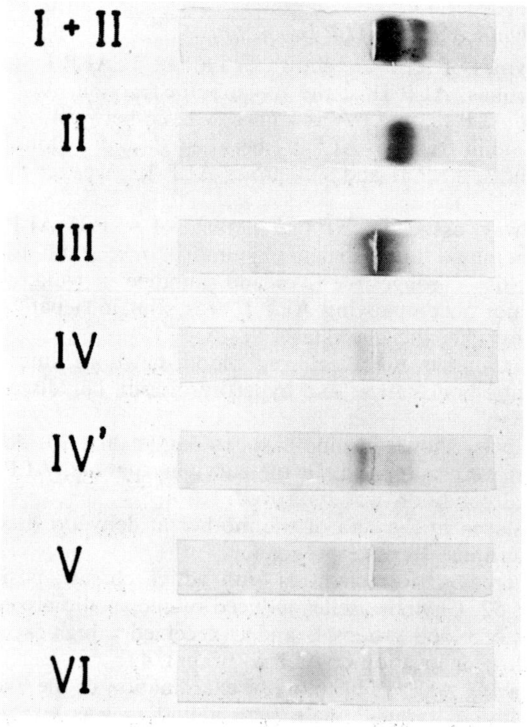

FIGURE 1. Seven isoenzymes of ALP.

TABLE 2

SERUM ALKALINE PHOSPHATASE ISOENZYMES IN DISEASES OF THE LIVER AND BILIARY TRACT

Jaundice	Diseases	No. of Cases			
		Total Cases	I + II	(I) + II	II
+	Jaundice in Leukemia	4	4	0	0
	Malignant Tumor of Biliary Tract	17	13	3	1
	Cholelithiasis and Cholangitis	12	7	3	2
	Toxic Liver Injury	4	1	2	1
	Cholangiohepatitis	7	1	2	4
	Acute Virus Hepatitis	16	0	1	15
−	Liver Abscess	5	5	0	0
	Metastatic Liver Cancer	29	25	2	2
	Congestive Liver	5	3	1	1
	Hepatoma	12	2	2	8
	Hepatitis	37	0	1	36
	Liver Cirrhosis	34	1	0	33

TABLE 3

DISEASES IN WHICH SERUM ALP IV APPEARED

Patient	Age	Sex	Diagnosis	S. ALP	S. LAP
H.H.	44	M	Cancer of Stomach With Liver Metastasis	9.6	28.1
M.T.	51	F	Cancer of Stomach	3.5	10.3
F.I.	53	F	Cancer of Stomach	4.9	10.3
K.N.	50	F	Cancer of Lung	5.8	16.2
K.S.	62	M	Cancer of Lung With Liver Metastasis	19.7	29.2
T.K.	40	F	Diabetic Nephropathy	5.6	12.1
S.E.	40	M	Acute Liver Atrophy	9.2	
S.I.	43	M	Liver Cirrhosis	8.1	23.2
S.Y.	65	M	Rheumatoid Arthritis	3.5	14.6

TABLE 4

CASES IN WHICH SERUM ALP V (V′) APPEARED

Diseases	No. of Cases	V (+)	V (−)
1. Liver Cirrhosis	52	20 (38.4%)	32
2. Chylous Ascites	1	1	0
High Fat Diet (Blood Group B and O)	6	6	0

inhibited by 5 mM L-phenylalanine. In contrast, ALP at the bile canaliculi and sinusoid was not inhibited (FIGURES 4 and 5).

ALP VI appeared in two cases out of six of ulcerative colitis, and ALP II was simultaneously decreased (TABLE 5).

2. *Effects of Inhibitors Against ALP Isoenzymes.*

(*a*) *L-phenylalanine*: 5 mM to 10 mM L-phenylalanine inhibited ALP II and III moderately. At 50 mM, L-phenylalanine inhibited all isoenzymes (FIGURE 6).

(*b*) *Urea*: ALP III and osseous ALP were markedly inhibited by 3 M urea; 5 M urea inhibited II, III, bone, liver and kidney ALP by more than 80%; ALP IV, IV^1, V, V^1 and intestinal and placental ALP were resistant to urea (FIGURE 7).

(*c*) EDTA: All ALP isoenzyme, except IV, IV′ and placental ALP were inhibited by 1 mM EDTA (FIGURE 8).

From these results, ALP isoenzymes can be differentiated by these inhibitors as shown in FIGURE 9.

DISCUSSIONS AND SUMMARY

Results obtained were summarized as shown in TABLE 6.

ALP I + II was seen mainly in obstructive jaundice and space-occupying lesion except hepatoma, and an increase of ALP II only in virus hepatitis and intrahepatic cholestasis and hepatoma. These findings are available for differential diagnosis of diseases of the liver and biliary tract.

Both ALP I and ALP II were demonstrated when the pressure of the bile canal

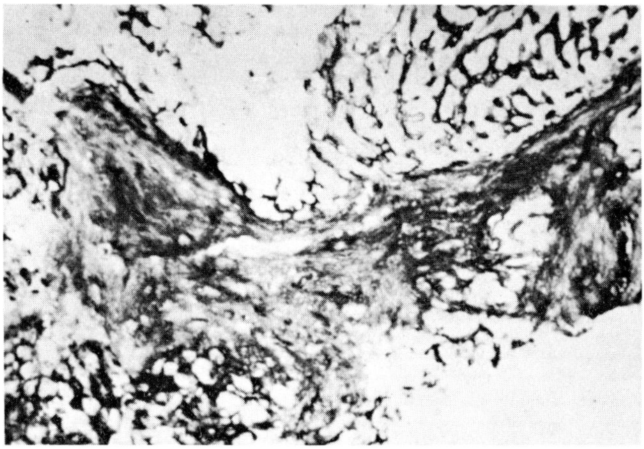

FIGURE 2. Liver cirrhosis with serum ALP V (Burstone's naphthyl AS phosphate method).

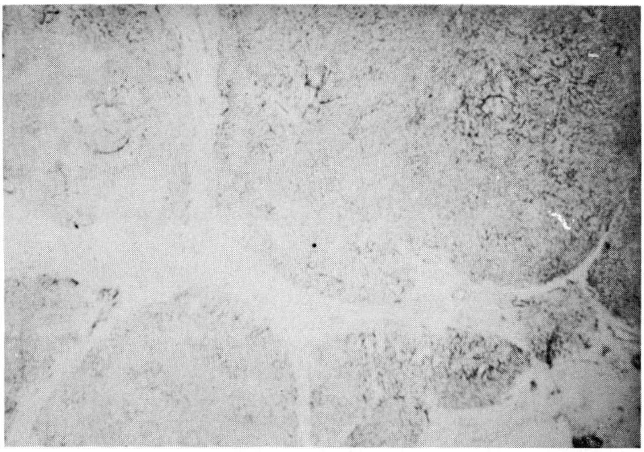

FIGURE 3. Liver cirrhosis without serum ALP V (Burstone's naphthyl AS phosphate method).

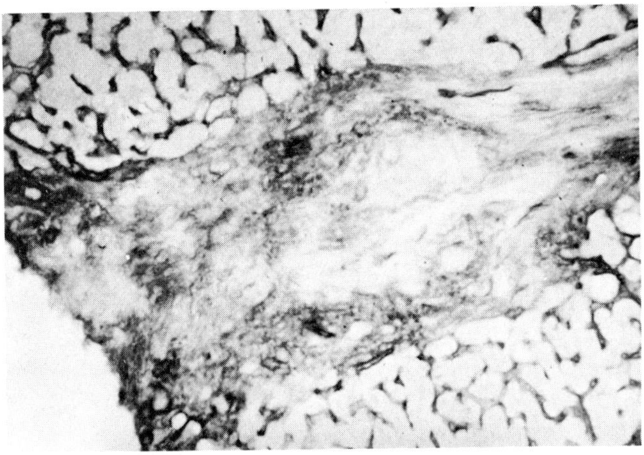

FIGURE 4. 5 mM D-phenylalanine (Gomoris' method).

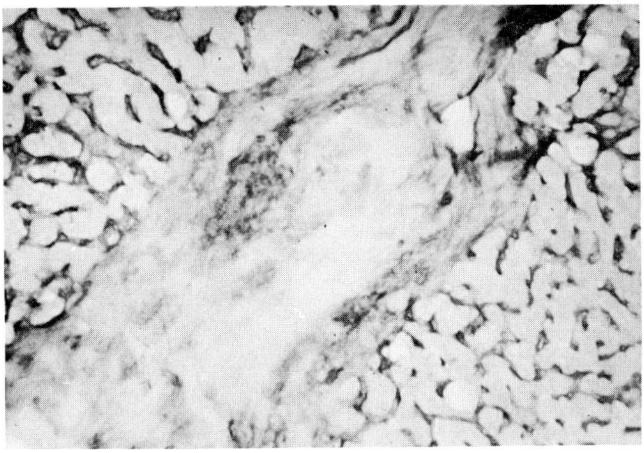

FIGURE 5. 5 mM L-phenylalanine (Gomoris' method).

TABLE 5

SERUM ALP ISOENZYMES IN ULCERATIVE COLITIS

Patient	Age	Sex	ALP*	II	VI	LAP
T.N.	28	F	9.8	±	Appeared	17.2
T.K.	27	F	9.4	±	Appeared	16.2
M.T.	19	F	6.7	+	—	16.4
A.M.	25	M	5.8	+	—	20.5
S.K.	24	F	7.3	+	—	16.2
T.V.	19	F	5.3	+	—	18.0

* King-Armstrong Units.

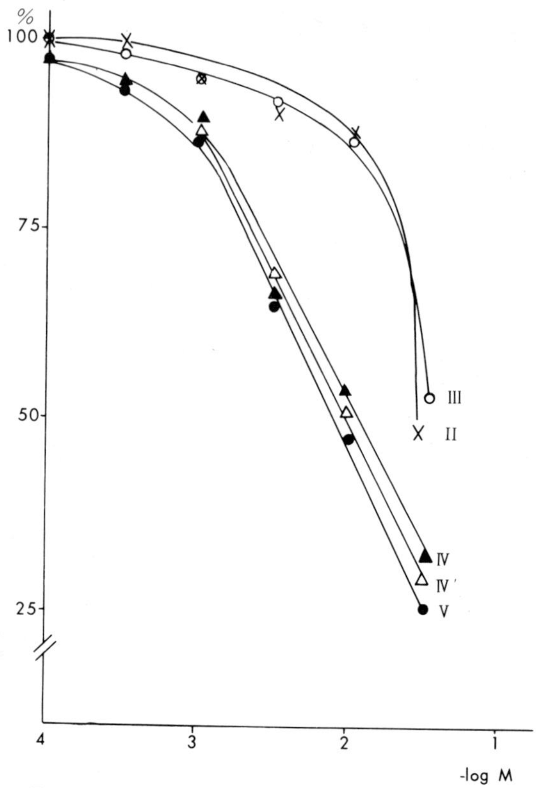

FIGURE 6. L-phenylalanine inhibition of serum ALP.

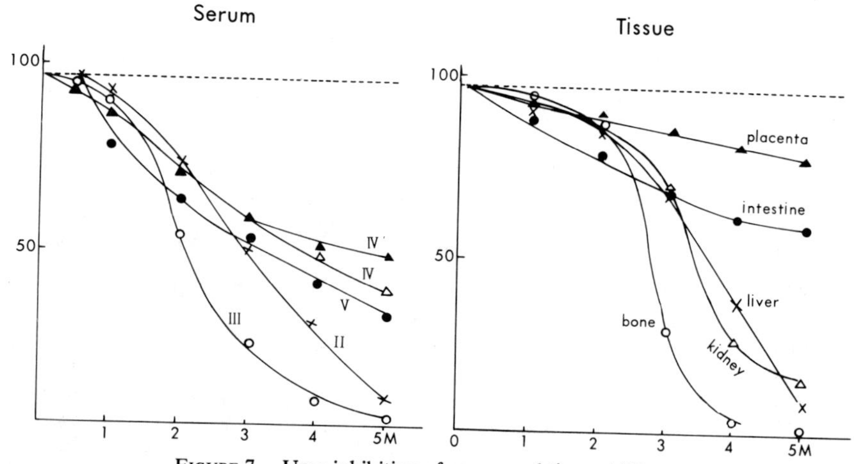

FIGURE 7. Urea inhibition of serum and tissue ALP.

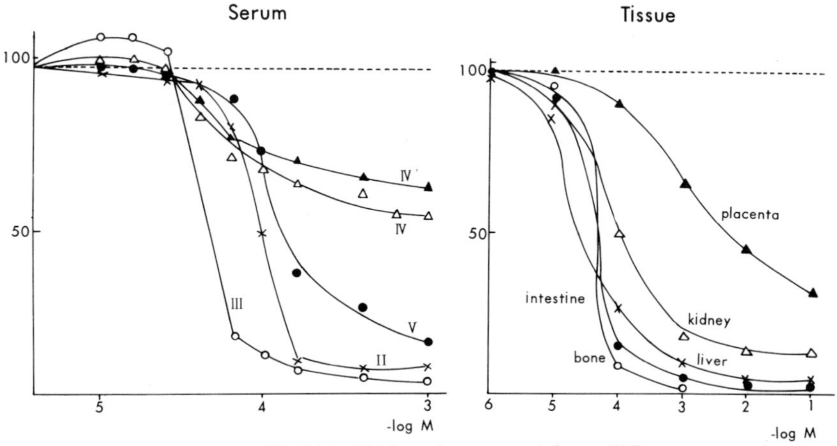

FIGURE 8. EDTA inhibition of serum and tissue ALP.

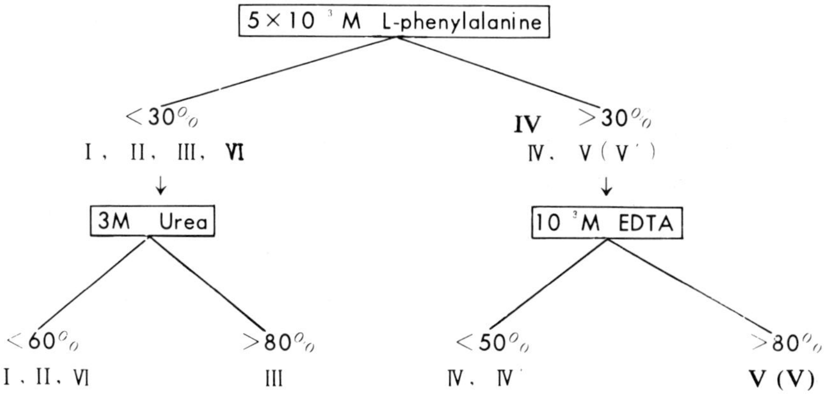

FIGURE 9. Differentiation of serum alkaline phosphatase isoenzymes by inhibitors.

was elevated. Therefore, Yamanaka *et al.*[2] suggested that the appearance of ALP I is caused by overproduction of ALP in the liver, possibly at the bile canaliculi, and disturbance of its excretion.

The origin of ALP II is still unknown, but it is not likely that ALP II originates from bone because of the difference in the electrophoretic migration and inhibitory effects by certain inhibitors, especially urea.

ALP III was increased in diseases with elevated osteoblastic activity, and is similar to osseous ALP in its pattern of inhibition by some agents. Therefore, it is suggested that ALP III originates from osseous ALP.

ALP IV′ coincides with placental ALP, as reported by Boyer.[3]

ALP IV is very similar to ALP IV′ and placental ALP. Fishman *et al.*[4] reported that ALP IV originated from ALP of cancer tissue (Regan isoenzyme). From our results, however, it comes from the other sources too, an aspect on which further investigation is needed.

It seems that ALP V′ originates from intestinal ALP as reported by Langman *et al.*[5]

TABLE 6

SUMMARY OF SERUM ALP ISOENZYMES

ALP:	I + II	II	VI	III	IV	IV′	V	V′
Diseases:	Obstructive Jaundice Metastatic Liver Cancer Liver Abscess Cholelithiasis Congestive Liver	Hepatitis Liver Cirrhosis Hepatoma Cholangio-hepatitis	Ulcerative Colitis	Newborn Infants Osteosarcoma Metastatic Bone Cancer Hyperparathy-roidism Hyperthyroid-ism	Various (terminal)	Pregnancy (terminal)	Liver Cirrhosis (40%)	Chylous Ascites, High-Fat Diet on Blood Groups B and O
Inhibitors: 5×10^{-3} M L-phenylalanine	(a)∼(b)	(a)∼(b)	(a)∼(b)	(a)∼(b)	(c)	(c)	(c)	(c)
3 M Urea	(c)	(c)	(d)	(d)∼(e)	(c)	(c)	(c)	(c)
10^{-3} M EDTA	(d)	(d)	(d)	(e)	(c)	(c)	(e)	(e)
Origin:	Liver (Bile Cana-liculi)	Liver ?	Unknown	Bone (Osteoblast)	Unknown	Placenta (Syntropho-blast)	Fibroblast in Liver or Intestine	Intestine

Inhibition Rate: (a) <10%
(b) 11∼30%
(c) 31∼60%
(d) 61∼80%
(e) >80%

Fishman *et al.*[6] suggest that ALP V coincides with intestinal ALP, because it is exactly similar to intestinal ALP regarding the location of electrophoretic migration and effects of inhibitors, as well as high incidence in blood groups B and O. But from this it cannot be explained why ALP V appears in liver cirrhosis only. On the basis of histochemical examination of ALP of the liver tissue, we suppose that ALP V originates from ALP of the fibroblasts in the liver.

ALP VI associated with the decrease of band II was seen in two cases out of six of ulcerative colitis. ALP VI is probably ALP II migrating to γ-globulin fraction for some reason.

References

1. Birkett, D. J., R. A. J. Conyers, F. C. Neale, S. Posen & J. Brudenell-Woods. 1967. Action of urea on human alkaline phosphatases: with a description of some automated techniques for the study of enzyme kinetics. Arch. Biochem. **121:** 470.
2. Yamanaka, M., H. Suzuki, T. Oda & Y. Yoshitoshi. 1966. On the mechanisms of marked elevation of serum alkaline phosphatase activity occurred by biliary obstruction, with special reference to its isoenzyme and histochemical demonstration. Proceedings of the 3rd World Congress of Gastroenterology : 415.
3. Boyer, S. H. 1961. Alkaline phosphatases in human sera and placenta, Science **134:** 1002.
4. Fishman, W. H., N. I. Inglis, L. L. Stolbach & M. J. Krant. 1968. A serum alkaline phosphatase isoenzyme of human neoplastic cell origin. Cancer Res. **28:** 150.
5. Langman, M. J. S., E. Leuthold, E. B. Robson, J. Harris, J. E. Luffman & H. Harris. 1966. Influence of diet on the intestinal component of serum alkaline phosphatase in people of different ABO groups and secretor status. Nature (London) **212:** 41.
6. Fishman, W. H., N. I. Inglis & M. J. Krant. 1965. Serum alkaline phosphatase of intestinal origin in patient with cancer and with cirrhosis of the liver. Clin. Chim. Acta **12:** 298.

Printed in the United States of America